## Praise for *The Alexander Technique: Twelve fundamentals of integrated movement*

There are many books in the marketplace about the Alexander technique, but this one is unique.

It provides a distillation of a lifetime of learning, practice, study, teaching and critical thinking. Penelope understands and explains the history and development of the Alexander technique and is not constrained by any one school or interpretation. Her original training in the technique was a standard "hands-on" training, and she has widened her horizons through her substantial subsequent study with remarkable teachers – Miss Goldie and Jeando Masoero come to mind.

In addition, she brings insights and knowledge from a wide range of scientific discoveries and mind/body disciplines which have developed since Alexander's time. And she weaves them into the intellectual and practical explorations which she offers to readers of this book. You might even call her book a contemporary update of the Alexander technique.

This is a book that you will keep coming back to, and working with. It provides rich experiential and intellectual sustenance and will certainly go onto the essential reading list for my Alexander trainees and on the highly recommended list for my yoga and Alexander students.

**David Moore**, Director of the School for F.M. Alexander Studies, Melbourne, Australia

Author of *Smart Yoga: Apply the Alexander technique to enhance your practice, prevent injury, and increase body awareness*
www.alexanderschool.edu.au/

Nowadays it is a well-known fact that musicians are particularly at risk from overuse injuries and anxiety or stress-related conditions. As a faculty member in a university music department, I have been delighted with the immediate positive impact the ideas presented in Penelope Easten's The Alexander Technique: Twelve fundamentals of integrated movement have had for the students in my Alexander technique class. No musician should be without a copy of this book. Read and study it, taking time to explore the various elements presented, and you will have the keys not only to wellness and reduced performance anxiety but also to enhanced musical technique and performance standard through an integrated and responsive body.

**Alison P. Deadman**, PhD, teacher of the Alexander technique, Professor of Music

This book is a treasure. In comprehensible language it helps us understand the multi-faceted science of the human body along with its functional anatomy, but at the same time it is very practically orientated. It provides a vast number of procedures for self-exploration which are also tools to teach students and groups. This book will become the modern encyclopaedia for Alexander technique teachers, bodywork practitioners of any kind, for the performing arts and for anyone interested in human nature.

In my practice as an Alexander technique teacher for actors, I find this profound work helps to free the actor's or singer's instrument. It unlocks natural breathing, free flow of emotions, and a more embodied way of speaking and thus enables the performer to come from a more truthful, authentic place.

**Annedore Kleist,** actor and Alexander technique teacher, Berlin
www.annedorekleist.com

Ms Easten offers us an e[...] ander's principles, rooted [...] of experience, and PLAY! [...] Alexander technique teac[...] sional who works virtually[...]

I'm an open-minded ske[...] classical Alexander train[...] Easten has upped both my in-person and online teaching game, deepened my anatomy understanding, as well as given me greater confidence. I am profoundly grateful for her gift to the future of the technique.

**Rebecca Poole**, cAmSAT, mACAT
www.NYalexandertechnique.com

Penelope is a humble genius with an incredible depth of knowledge and creative flair, making her innovating work exciting and irresistible! Working with Penelope has filled in the missing pieces of my Alexander technique jigsaw puzzle. I have now learned how to have appropriate tone without tension and stability without stiffness. As a classical dressage rider, this has hugely improved my back and seat, making me a much more effective rider, and I cannot thank Penelope enough for her wonderful pioneering work. I look forward to sharing these skills with other passionate riders.

**Chris English**, Alexander technique teacher and classical dressage rider and coach
www.riderselfcarriage.co.uk

The Alexander Technique: Twelve fundamentals of integrated movement *is a rich body of work in an accessible format that keeps delivering whenever you review. It is deep work and a great asset to self-understanding and self-care. So relevant for now!*

Penelope has brought Alexander's technique totally up to date. I have found the structure and format of the book has enabled me to teach AT remotely even more effectively than before. Her functional anatomy teachings offer us simple ways of improving our strength, vitality, poise. Our whole self is nourished with anatomical knowledge that aids better self-understanding.

My teenage pupils have appreciated the repeatable format enabling and empowering them to effectively apply this work to themselves during any activity. In particular, my Music Scholar pupils have benefitted greatly, introducing it as part of their Alexander practice and reaping the rewards of balanced, natural, and dynamic postural tone, essential knowledge to support a long term career as a musician in good health.

Medical imaging practitioners would be well-placed to follow Penelope's teaching; their detailed understanding of anatomy and all its different systems will enable them to build a self-care strategy themselves to help avoid the RSI and WRMSDs that are commonplace in this field.

**Angela Bradshaw**, MSTAT, DMU, DCR(R)

Author of *Be In Balance,* published by Balloon View, UK, 2014.

TEDxSWPS "Show Me How". DMU, Diploma in Medical Ultrasound; DCR(R), Diploma in Diagnostic Radiography; Alexander technique teacher
www.angelabradshaw.com

Finally, a comprehensive manual for Alexander technique teachers to work with clarity on biomechanics and neurological aspects of the discipline and to understand the roots of its different approaches.

*Penelope Easten also provides to professionals of the somatic field in general a complete guide on postural alignment and anatomy of movement: beautifully explained and precise on theory and practical explorations, it undoubtedly is a precious tool for training courses both for Alexander technique and Yoga teachers.*

**Sara Carissimo**, statistician and expert in sociology of health and non conventional medicines, Alexander technique and alignment-based yoga teacher
www.yogabodylab.com

*Penelope Easten's book has been an eye-opener for me and my training course students. So many new ideas – such as I've never encountered in 25 years of teaching – are inspiring me to look forward to the next 25 years! The new ways of understanding F.M. Alexander's work are contributing to a deeper understanding of how I teach my training course, group classes, and private students. The author takes Alexander's concepts of direction to a new level, bringing about an incredible coordinative strength in carrying out activities. No other course of study has influenced me more in how I approach teaching my trainees, groups, and private students.*

**Brian McCullough**, Director, Minnesota Center for the Alexander Technique (MinnCAT.org), Faculty Alexander technique teacher

*Penelope illuminates the Alexander technique with clear explanations of functional anatomy and neurological findings including polyvagal theory. This book teaches you to find more stability in your body and more calm in your self-regulative system. When I use Penelope's methods in the counseling and psychotherapeutic setting, people often say they feel more confident and with a quieter mind. I would recommend this book, not only for teachers and trainees of Alexander technique but also counselors and psychotherapists who are interested in adopting the psycho-somatic approach.*

**Kazuyuki Kajikawa**, clinical psychologist, public certified psychologist in Japan, Alexander technique teacher

*Engaging ideas and directed activities that create a conscious, constructive path toward rediscovering, and benefitting from, our intrinsic wholeness … the very essence of F.M. Alexander's work.*

**Aida McGugan**, RCST®, M.STAT, M.AmSAT, Michigan
Alexander technique teacher, biodynamic craniosacral therapist.

*This book has been a jewel to find, the best thing I could have come across after recently finishing my AT training course.*

*As I worked through each chapter, imbalances in my body were revealed. Penelope's The Alexander Technique: Twelve fundamentals of integrated movement has shown me how to work towards a potential for movement, freedom, and ease that has often seemed just out of reach.*

*As a yoga teacher, I have immediately been able to incorporate this revolutionary and fresh approach to my classes, seeing concrete and tangible transformation in my students. I am finally able to easily translate theory into practice as I teach. Penelope's deep understanding of functional anatomy and complex brain processes are explained candidly and many anecdotal stories enliven the book, making it easy and enjoyable to read.*

*In Penelope I feel I have found my own Miss Goldie, and I am forever thankful for this roadmap towards "a more balanced life."*

**Sara Robledo**, singer/dancer and teacher of AT, yoga and Pilates
www.namuyoga.com

*This new work by Penelope Easten is one of the most encouraging and exciting to emerge in the practice and theory of the Alexander technique. We are in an era where, if we want to really understand human nature, we can no longer retreat to the safety of what different individual disciplines offer us, whether that be neuroscience, psychotherapy, evolution, mindfulness or any host of others. This is an exciting time for thinking about what therapy is really about. With multitudes of old and new riches to choose from, whether established or unconventional therapies, this book is well placed to act as a guide to what we are learning about how to treat people in a really embodied way. As a psychotherapist who has benefitted enormously from many years of working with Penelope, I have seen the development of the insights and ideas presented here, and how they are transferable to my own work with clients in my everyday practice. This work is at the cutting edge of what it means to be an embodied therapist, and is applicable to many different therapeutic disciplines. Maybe the most important player in this new era of therapeutic work is neurobiology, and in particular our understanding of embodied intelligence. In this work, Penelope Easten gives us the theoretical background and development of this practice, and provides us with a practical guide to support the integration of the Alexander teaching with other bodily based therapies to bring about full integrated movement. I unreservedly recommend this work as an essential addition to every psychotherapist's toolkit.*

**Michael O'Toole**, Registered Counselling Psychologist and Psychotherapist in private practice. Co-author of *Transference and Countertransference from an Attachment Perspective,* with Dr Una McCluskey, 2020, Routledge, and author of numerous papers on clinical issues in psychotherapy in the Attachment Journal 'New Directions in Psychotherapy and Relational Psychoanalysis'. Group experiential facilitator with the Bowlby Centre, London

*Don't let the title of this book fool you. Yes, it is a deep and refreshing look at the Alexander technique – but it is much more than that. Easten has given us a bold inquiry into what it means to be embodied in this world, and to live from the ease, awareness and integrity of our most fully realized self. It is an inquiry that synthesizes an astonishing breadth of study, drawing from science, history, anatomy, psychology and personal experience. Better yet, it enables readers to experience its insights for themselves through a range of clearly presented practices. If you value a freer, richer way of meeting life, this book will be a cherished companion.*

**Philip Shepherd**, author of *Radical Wholeness and New Self, New World.* Facilitator of the Embodied Present Process
www.philipshepherd.com

# The ALEXANDER TECHNIQUE

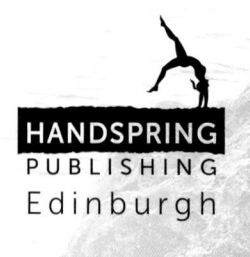

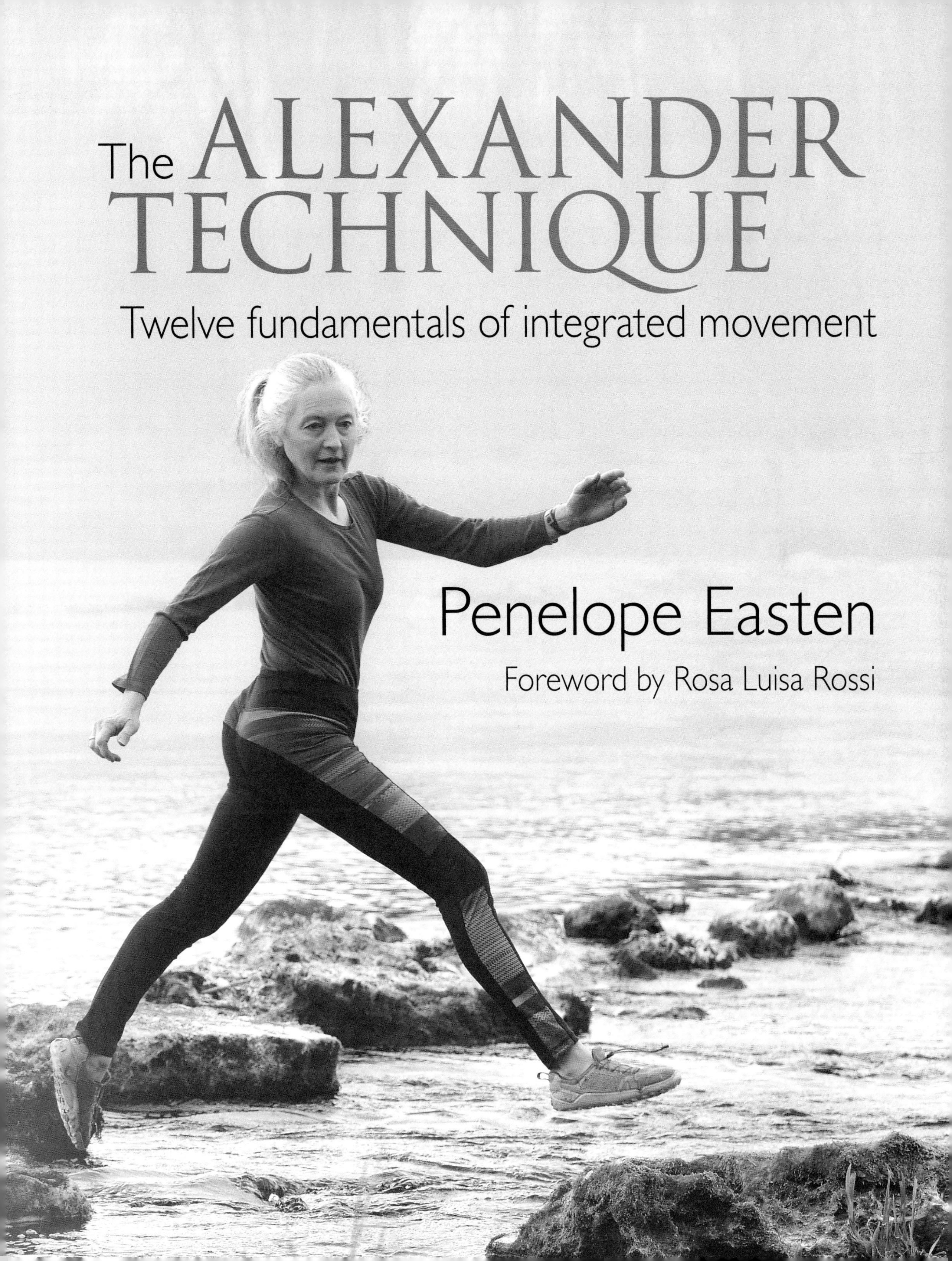

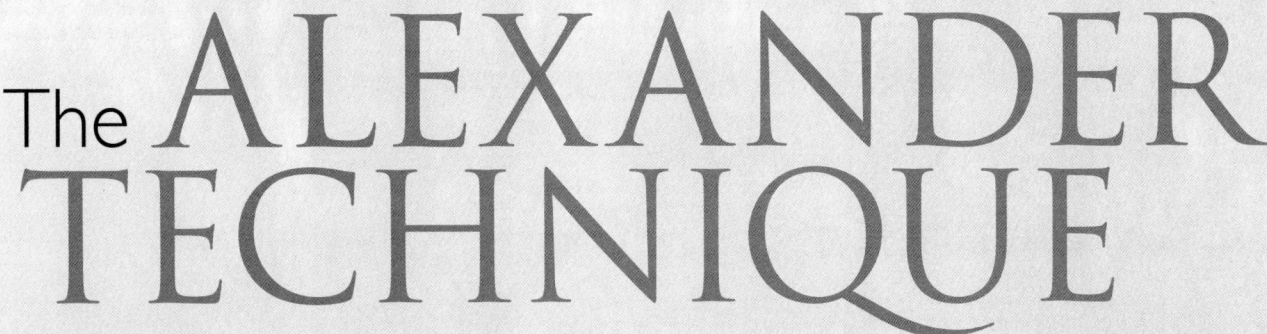

# The ALEXANDER TECHNIQUE

## Twelve fundamentals of integrated movement

### Penelope Easten

Foreword by Rosa Luisa Rossi

HANDSPRING PUBLISHING LIMITED
The Old Manse, Fountainhall,
Pencaitland, East Lothian
EH34 5EY, Scotland
Tel: +44 1875 341 859
Website: www.handspringpublishing.com

First published 2021 in the United Kingdom by Handspring Publishing Limited

Reprinted November 2021

Copyright © Handspring Publishing Limited 2021
All rights reserved. No parts of this publication may be reproduced or transmitted in any form or by any means, electronic or mechanical, including photocopying, recording, or any information storage and retrieval system, without either the prior written permission of the publisher or a licence permitting restricted copying in the United Kingdom issued by the Copyright Licensing Agency Ltd, Saffron House, 6–10 Kirby Street, London EC1N 8TS.

The rights of Penelope Easten to be identified as the Author of this text have been asserted in accordance with the Copyright, Designs and Patents Acts 1988.

ISBN 978-1-912085-85-9
ISBN (Kindle ebook) 978-1-912085-86-6

**British Library Cataloguing in Publication Data**
A catalogue record for this book is available from the British Library

**Library of Congress Cataloguing in Publication Data**
A catalog record for this book is available from the Library of Congress

**Notice**
Neither the Publisher nor the Author assume any responsibility for any loss or injury and/or damage to persons or property arising out of or relating to any use of the material contained in this book. It is the responsibility of the treating practitioner, relying on independent expertise and knowledge of the patient, to determine the best treatment and method of application for the patient.

All reasonable efforts have been made to obtain copyright clearance for illustrations in the book for which the authors or publishers do not own the rights. If you believe that one of your illustrations has been used without such clearance please contact the publishers and we will ensure that appropriate credit is given in the next reprint.

**Commissioning Editor** Sarena Wolfaard
**Project Manager** Morven Dean
**Copy editors** Stephanie Pickering and Fiona Conn
**Designer** Bruce Hogarth
**Cover photograph and all other photographs and videos of the author** Julian Easten
**Indexer** Aptara India
**Typesetter** DiTech, India
**Printer** Bell and Bain, UK

The
Publisher's
policy is to use
paper manufactured
from sustainable forests

# Contents

Foreword — xi
Preface — xii
Acknowledgments — xvi

## PART I The Basics of Fundamental Movement

**1 Introduction, aims, and a tropical tale** — 2
    Visions of free movement – a tropical tale — 3
    Aims of the book — 5
    How this book came about — 7
    Evolution of the Alexander technique, and finding the whole elephant — 8

**2 What has been lost, and the twelve fundamentals of movement** — 10
    Integrated movement – WHAT has gone wrong, and WHY? — 11
    Sitting is the new smoking — 11
    The five senses – one of the great myths — 15
    Changing our movement habits needs a change in thinking — 15
    Top-down vs bottom-up processing — 16
    Left hemisphere for the known, right hemisphere for the unknown — 16
    An evolutionary perspective puts the body first — 19
    Whole-body animal movement, the fulfilment of evolutionary potential — 21
    Introducing the twelve fundamentals of integrated movement — 23
    Time and space and rhythm — 29
    Seven new proposals for integrated movement — 29

**3 The fundamentals of structure** — 32
    Lesson 1  Waking up proprioception — 33
    Lesson 2  We are fighting gravity as we move — 35
    Lesson 3  Making your first changes towards a more mechanically advantageous structure — 41
    Lesson 4  Understanding the different models of body mechanics — 48
    Lesson 5  Control mechanisms of body balance and movement – the self-organization of the body — 61
    A summary of the engineering of the human body in nine layers — 62
    Appendix: Twelve teaching tips, and further reading — 64

**4 The fundamentals of awareness and thinking** — 68
    Lesson 1  Waking up external perception – tracking a visual line — 69
    Lesson 2  Clear brain choices and "inhibition" – the key to changing brain patterns of body use — 70
    Lesson 3  Interoception – the internal world of a hundred senses, and our reason to move — 73
    Lesson 4  Where we think from – mind in the brain, awareness versus feeling — 75
    Lesson 5  Whole-body awareness and embodiment – "liquid light" — 78
    Lesson 6  Finding our spatial awareness – of our surroundings and of ourselves — 84
    Lesson 7  Emergent integrated movement – discovering our fundamental bend led by focused vision — 87
    Lesson 8  Exploring semi-supine – a position of active rest — 89

# Contents *continued*

| | | |
|---|---|---:|
| **5** | **The autonomic nervous system – why we need to work from quiet presence and awareness** | 94 |
| | The three states of the autonomic nervous system | 95 |
| | The ladder from safety to danger to life threat | 96 |
| | Maintaining a balanced life with self-regulation | 98 |
| | Bringing the nervous system back to a place of safety | 99 |
| | Recovery by climbing down the ladder | 101 |
| **6** | **Finding the innate movements of breathing and walking** | 102 |
| | The evolution of our movement – finding the buried patterns | 103 |
| | Lesson 1  Natural breathing – finding the natural expansion of the torso | 104 |
| | Lesson 2  More breathing explorations | 114 |
| | Lesson 3  Finding our emergent rhythmic movement – walking and bouncing | 118 |

### PART 2 Linking brain and body with explorations of physical integration

| | | |
|---|---|---:|
| **7** | **The Initial Alexander technique, and a new model of postural alignment** | 124 |
| | Introduction to Part 2 – exploring Miss Goldie's model of the structural body | 125 |
| | The seven steps to a new body geometry | 127 |
| | The five stages to Alexander's path of discovery | 127 |
| | Lesson 1  How well is your body aligned with gravity? | 130 |
| | Lesson 2  Rebalancing the upper body | 136 |
| | Lesson 3  Making an integrated change | 141 |
| | Lesson 4  Rebalancing the lower body | 146 |
| | Lesson 5  Lengthening the back from top and bottom | 151 |
| | Lesson 6  Integrating directions within the expanded field of awareness | 156 |
| **8** | **Single leg balance** | 158 |
| | Lesson 1  Introduction to balance | 159 |
| | Lesson 2  The vestibular organs and the three directions of space | 161 |
| | Lesson 3  Finding our secure base – the ball of the foot and the sesamoid bones | 162 |
| | Lesson 4  Finding our secure base – the hip stabilizers | 165 |
| | Lesson 5  Finding our secure base – tilting the foot – the lower ankle joint | 170 |
| | Lesson 6  Placement of the feet – untwisting the leg spirals | 170 |
| | Lesson 7  Widening the hips with the breath – opening the femoral triangle | 175 |
| **9** | **Spatial relationships and use of the upper body and arms** | 178 |
| | Coming into relationship with our world | 179 |
| | Lesson 1  The supportive torso | 180 |
| | Lesson 2  The shoulders and upper arms – opening the deep back arm line | 181 |
| | Lesson 3  How safe do you feel? Opening up the chest and armpits | 183 |
| | Lesson 4  Opening the forearm flexors | 186 |
| | Lesson 5  Gripping without grabbing – balancing flexors and extensors as we grip | 188 |
| | Lesson 6  Delicate movements of the hand | 190 |
| | Lesson 7  Spatial relationships in the arms in everyday life | 192 |

| 10 | **Toned sitting – integrating the core muscles** | 196 |
|---|---|---|
| | Introduction – why work at sitting and standing? | 197 |
| | Lesson 1   Keeping the legs switched on while sitting, even at a desk | 198 |
| | Lesson 2   Sit to stand using the new alignment of the legs and feet | 201 |
| | Lesson 3   The anatomy of integration, finding our core muscles, and active hip folding | 203 |
| | Lesson 4   Finding the anatomy of integration by inclining back on a chair | 210 |
| 11 | **Walking as you've never walked before** | 216 |
| | The standard model of walking | 217 |
| | Lesson 1   Stability enables mobility | 218 |
| | Lesson 2   Stability enables coordination – finding fully active feet | 223 |
| | Lesson 3   Stability and mobility enable torque – finding the power in your walk | 225 |
| 12 | **Alexander's biomechanics for expansion of the upper body** | 236 |
| | Introduction | 237 |
| | Active, integrative stretching versus passive, single muscle stretching | 237 |
| | Lesson 1   Finding the supportive torso | 238 |
| | Lesson 2   Shoulders and clavicles | 244 |
| | Lesson 3   Opening, widening, and deepening the chest | 247 |
| | Lesson 4   Straightening the arms from both ends | 251 |
| | Lesson 5   Opening the top of the ribcage – the reverse whispered Ah | 254 |
| | Lesson 6   Classic Alexander technique procedures for arms | 256 |
| 13 | **Precise, springy alignment in sit to stand and "monkey"** | 260 |
| | Lesson 1   Anatomy and engineering play | 261 |
| | Lesson 2   Tilting the torso forwards into "monkey" | 263 |
| | Lesson 3   Balanced sitting – actively upright without bracing | 268 |
| | Lesson 4   Why the knees need to stay back as we tilt forwards to stand | 269 |
| | Lesson 5   Squatting and bouncing – testing our elastic resistance and mobility | 271 |
| | Lesson 6   Constructive conscious guidance and control – using Initial AT for yourself | 272 |
| 14 | **Freeing the neck, and Alexander's primary directions** | 276 |
| | Lesson 1   Why we need to free the neck | 277 |
| | Lesson 2   Finding length and adaptive tone in the neck extensors | 281 |
| | Lesson 3   Primary control and directions revisited | 284 |

## PART 3 Living in a flow of dynamic balance

| 15 | **Catching a ball – inhibition in action** | 290 |
|---|---|---|
| | Introduction – discovering the core of Miss Goldie's work | 291 |
| | Catching a ball in seven stages | 293 |
| | Fully responsive action for optimal coordination | 297 |
| | Discussion points | 300 |

# Contents *continued*

**16  New models of coordination and learning** — 304
   Lesson 1  Coordinating locomotion by using the whole-body intelligence network — 305
   Lesson 2  Coordination of reaching and grasping in everyday actions — 308
   Lesson 3  New models of learning a complex task — 316

**17  Embodied speaking** — 324
   Introduction — 325
   Lesson 1  Being present as you speak — 326
   Lesson 2  Embodying the voice — 327

**18  Relating and attuning to people for putting hands on others** — 332
   Introduction – we are not machines but self-integrating systems — 333
   How is non-verbal information transmitted? — 334
   Five key elements to bring about resonance with a pupil — 336
   Summary for hands-on work with a pupil or client — 344

References — 345
Index — 349

# Foreword

In 1988 I had lessons with Miss Goldie in London for one week: every day for thirty minutes. This happened two years after I had completed my Alexander technique training in Zurich, Switzerland. I remember Miss Goldie saying: "Much too much tension." Another sentence she repeatedly whispered into my ear was: "You just wish to be quiet throughout so that the right thing can happen to you." In other words, I needed to quieten my whole system in order for the entire system to reorganize itself. She explained to me that toward the end of his teaching career, this was what F. M. Alexander used to say to his students. I will always remember the extraordinary and powerful presence of Miss Goldie and these messages. Today I understand what she was "doing" or helping me to "un-do," but then I didn't understand, nor did I learn how I could continue on my own.

I always wanted to understand in depth the working and functioning of the Alexander technique. Thirty years after having worked with Miss Goldie and after uncountable continuous learning experiences in this technique, I met the author of this book, Penelope Easten. I listened and explored with great curiosity what she was teaching based on her study with Miss Goldie. I even went to Ireland for a week to take some lessons from her. At that time, she shared with me that she was writing a book about Miss Goldie's teaching. I told her about Jeando Masoero's work which had helped me to understand the mechanical advantages and the antagonistic pulls that F. M. Alexander mentions in his books. I was sure that a combination of the two approaches would offer what I had for many years been searching for: a practical guide to the Alexander technique which explains how to develop the quickening of the mental capacities, how to link those capacities to the mechanics of this work and how to relate it all to everyday activities.

With *The Alexander Technique: Twelve Fundamentals of Integrated Movement* Penelope has written a book of great value, including videos and a step-by-step plan, in which she explains and guides us through Miss Goldie's work. She presents current scientific ideas, particularly those associated with the autonomic nervous system and the right brain, hypothesizing their support for Miss Goldie's teaching methods – hypotheses that one hopes will soon be proven by scientific studies, but which readers of Penelope's book can explore right now.

This is not only a book to read, it is a book to study – a book for exploration. I am so pleased and inspired by it that I am going to invite people to discover these ideas together with me.

*The Alexander Technique: Twelve Fundamentals of Integrated Movement* confirms Penelope Easten as one of the most courageous, innovative, and effective teachers of the Alexander technique. Not only does her book advance the ideas and practice of Alexander technique teachers and students alike, it will be of great interest to anyone involved in related disciplines or with a curiosity about the mind–body connection.

Rosa Luisa Rossi
Rheinfelden, Switzerland
January 2021
*Member and former chair of SBAT (the Affiliated Society of Teachers of the Alexander Technique in Switzerland)*
*Member and current co-chair of the board of ATI (Alexander Technique International)*
*Co-director of the 8th International Alexander Technique Congress in Lugano, Switzerland, 2008*

# Preface

## Who is this book for?

This book is intended for everybody who is interested in improving their quality of life. Especially, it is for teachers and trainees of the Alexander technique (AT) as well as all movement educators and therapists, particularly those in the somatic field. It offers a broad, new theoretical framework of how integrated movement occurs, to be understood through theory, ideas from recent science, and practical explorations. The explorations are simple techniques aimed at enabling you to look after yourself in your practice and also for use with your clients or pupils to help them understand, integrate, and take advantage of what you offer them.

While most books for professionals are written in technical and complex language, I have opted to write this in more accessible language, so that the reader can flow easily between theory, explanation, and practical exploration and so facilitate their own discoveries, insights, and links. Technical and complex language speaks to the left hemisphere, which has no direct link to the body. Simple language communicates to our more playful, childlike essence and so more to the right hemisphere, which links directly to the body and to experiential learning. In this I draw on Iain McGilchrist's process-based model of the division of the hemispheres (2012). Theory that is not grounded in experience and discovery is less likely to be of practical use.

So, this is a springboard for your own process. The foundation of the Alexander work is self-exploration, and this is the core of the explorations presented here. These will be accessible to any therapist and to interested laypeople. But it is my wish that this material is *taught* much more widely – Alexander work has often been a well-kept secret. The Alexander principles can benefit everybody, in all spheres of activity, and deserve to be much better known, and there are simply not enough AT teachers for this task! So instruction is given on how to teach the material presented here, both for the Alexander world and also for other therapists or movement educators for whom some specific tools would be useful. Its applicability is then both for you, so you can look after yourself in your practice, and also for you to pass on to clients, either singly or in groups.

The basic tenet of Alexander technique is that physical problems are created over time when the body and mind are employed in an unbalanced manner, creating stress in the system. Alexander called this poor "use": it is held in habits programmed in our nervous system. By learning to move and live in a balanced fashion – by building better habits of use – we re-integrate the system and problems can then reverse. These changes can be held long-term because we are learning how to change the unhelpful "default" programs that have developed back to the "factory settings" for which we were evolved, and with which we moved easily as small children. Chapter 1 explores our untapped potential for movement, and how this book came about.

Our Western cultural bias is to treat (or teach) the structural body in isolation from other body systems, and Alexander work also is often thought of as "treatment" for posture, neck, and back problems and so on. This cultural mindset views the body mechanically and can be seen as a product of left hemisphere, linear thinking, which works from known experience and concepts. But as many therapists and movement educators know, the physical body cannot be considered alone in the quest for integrated movement – the nervous system is equally part of the process. What and how we think, where we think from, our degree of embodiment and of awareness – both internal and external, are all key players fundamental to integrated movement, allowing us to reawaken older, more balanced movement patterns. To access any of these keys requires a shift in how we think, to lead with experiential right hemisphere pathways. Then we link to the whole-body, to spatial awareness, to the present and the unfamiliar, allowing muscles and movement patterns that have gone out of play to be reawakened. This feels like a journey into the unknown, yet can bring us such ease of being and "homecoming." The theoretical basis for this approach is outlined in Chapter 2.

The main part of the book is a workbook, with many explorations to re-integrate the physical (and mental) body, through using the twelve fundamentals of integrated movement. This is not a book to read in a day! It is designed as a course to follow over several months, at your own pace. Part 1 gives you the foundations of thought and methodology, but one can do either Part 2 or Part 3 next, or bounce between them, as I do when teaching pupils.

The twelve fundamentals are introduced individually in Chapters 3 and 4 (these chapters will catch up anyone unfamiliar with Alexander technique); while Chapter 5 describes the crucial role of a calm nervous system. The fundamentals are used together to "re-set" our natural breathing in Chapter 6, and to discover how to let new movements come about for themselves.

The physical body is explored in Part 2, using Thomas W. Myers's Anatomy Trains® (referred to as anatomy trains hereafter), biomechanics, and spiral/curve/torque patterns. We will learn self-help tools for aligning the body more efficiently with gravity and taking pressure off joints; rebalancing and integrating different areas of the body by lengthening tight muscles for ourselves; finding our springiness again to feel younger, fitter, and stronger; moving as a flow of dynamic balance rather than imposing a movement, which brings ease, elegance and coordination (Chapters 3 and 7–14). These physical changes are integrated with what are thought to be Alexander's original protocol for brain programming.

But what integrates movement? Part 3 goes deeper into the roles of consciousness, perception, and embodiment in movement. While Alexander defined the head-neck-back relationship as the primary control that integrates the system, we can now take this further, discovering that the body and movement are self-organized around our awareness, focus, and goals. And while the brain has always been seen to be in charge, we can now be understood as brain/whole-body intelligence information networks. This is explored in Chapters 4, 15, and 16.

In addition, as we come into greater awareness and embodied thinking, it brings us into the parasympathetic – the "mindful" state of relaxed awareness. This can bring us into being more present, both in our lives and for our clients, deepening the physical connections we make, and developing our empathy and intuition. This is explored in detail in Chapter 5, then in Chapters 17 and 18, and I believe it can be of interest also for psychotherapists and indeed for anyone working with people.

After my Alexander technique training, I worked for four years with (Ellen Avery) Margaret Goldie (1905–97), known as Miss Goldie, one of Alexander's first teachers, who changed my whole understanding of the technique. In recent decades much has been discovered about the early history of his work that is very different to the story he left us in his third book, *Use of the Self*. In Chapter 7, I present a new interpretation of how Alexander developed the technique, some of which is well documented and some more conjectural. In addition to my work with Miss Goldie, this interpretation is based on the work of Jeando Masoero, the "Initial Alexander Technique." It is known that Alexander (1869–1955) evolved his technique over many decades, starting with his first teaching work in 1895 and only ending with his death, with radical changes around 1912, and then in the mid-1920s. In 1934, a schism arose on the first training course, in which several key students developed the "training course method." This became the modern AT, which some of the first teachers such as Miss Goldie perceived as very different. The further schism that occurred at Alexander's death then created several distinct training course lineages, and since then, others have developed new strands still, for the AT has many strands, and is always evolving and taking in new knowledge. Every one of these strands has positives to offer, and much healing work has been done to meld the

## Preface continued

different strands from the first-generation teachers and training courses, work that still goes on. I hope my book can add to that process by incorporating Miss Goldie's work and Alexander's initial work more explicitly into the mix – for this early work is, in many ways, implicit in all our work.

Other therapies might identify with this evolution of a method from the founder's discoveries (bottom-up experiential processes), from which his followers formalize the process (top-down methodology).

One of the hallmarks of the early work as I have experienced it is its precision of thought and action. This gave a clarity that enabled me to link the work to different structural models and neuroscience concerns such as the division between the brain hemispheres, interoception, polyvagal theory, and therapeutic attunement, the two visual streams theory, embodied cognition and others. Because of the wide range of science covered, I can only provide an overview of each area in the hope that this can stimulate further discussion and more detailed scholarly research. This is a starting point.

### For the Alexander technique community

In the Alexander sphere, different training courses have offered very different approaches to learning. My own training in the 1980s was completely technical-based. It was an apprenticeship – and a very good one – in how to improve a person's use by taking them in and out of a chair and working with them on a table. We came out very confident in what we were doing with our hands! But we had read no books, written no essays, studied no anatomy or science underlying the technique, delivered no talks. We learned very little about how to describe or communicate our acquired knowledge. When I started my practice, I realized I had no idea how to present the technique to the outside world. Other trainings addressed all this rather more than ours but were still largely technical, apprenticeship-based trainings.

In the last fifteen years particularly, our profession – at least in the UK and Ireland as I am aware – has moved toward much more professional training, but there is no textbook for this newer approach. Though Alexander considered that one could learn the technique from his own books, in practice they contain very little "how to" material; he even states that the directions given are of no use without the sensory experiences from a trained teacher to explain them (Alexander 1987: 108). Meanwhile the very recent science and theories, both of the nervous system and the new models of anatomy that underlie the technique and of integrated movement generally, is mostly not in any textbook. Most of the recent science that is helping to explain the therapeutic process is now to be found in psychotherapy books (see, e.g., Dana 2018; Siegel 2010) but generally not in those for somatic work. This book is offered to the AT profession as a contribution toward filling the gap for trainees and for teachers' continuing professional development (CPD).

Neither my initial lessons nor my training gave me sufficient tools to maintain the technique for myself in daily life. This was my personal experience; others probably had different experiences. (It never ceases to amaze me how people can go through the same training and come out with vastly different understandings.) It was the crisis that came out of this which first took me to Miss Goldie in 1990. Since then I have explored self-work as a core of the AT work, for myself and for teachers and trainees on workshops and courses.

In recent decades there has been increasing interest in the AT community in getting hands off pupils and teaching them to bring about their own change. The technique has always been promoted as a method that you learn to do for yourself, but trainings vary in how directly this is taught. While mainstream AT schools still focus primarily on how to put hands onto pupils to bring about change for them, there is growing emphasis on teaching the pupil directly to use different thinking and awareness to bring about change for themselves. This requires different teaching skills: in particular good observational skills, and better conscious understanding to direct the pupil's process. I observe that these skills build confidence in both teachers and pupils.

The material presented is ready to use with complete beginners (particularly much of Chapter 3) and the explanations given are those I use with my own pupils to help their understanding alongside their body learning. The hands-off format of the methods given makes it very suitable for groupwork, something that was not encouraged or even deemed possible in the early days of the technique. Likewise, it is suitable for online teaching. But as all AT teachers know, whichever way one works, one will always get the best results by thinking and directing oneself alongside thinking and directing the pupil. Therefore, the methods offered here are equally applicable for those who wish to continue with hands-on work, or – my own preferred approach – to use a mixture of hands-on and hands-off work.

Penelope Easten
Ogonnelloe, County Clare, Ireland
*January 2021*

# Acknowledgments

My journey has been a long one, taking many turns, with many supports and guides along the way. I'd like to thank my mother for passing me books on the Alexander technique originally and encouraging me to take lessons. In the last few years she has read everything I have written, tried out the explorations, commented in detail, and corrected my grammar, for which I am profoundly grateful. My understanding husband Julian has let me stay at my computer when we should have been holidaying or enjoying weekends, lovingly offering support and cooking great dinners. As a photographer, he has also used his personal experience of AT and Miss Goldie in doing the photos and videos with me. Our daughter Amelia has also patiently allowed me to write when I should have been fulfilling motherly roles! Thanks to her also for showing me weight-lifting approaches and physical training moves. Thanks to all my original teachers and trainers for setting me on the path and inspiring me that one can develop superb use, even without F. M.'s own hands. Thanks particularly to John Hunter for motivating me to go to Miss Goldie then to Erika Whittaker, and for his early workshops exploring their work.

To so many Alexander colleagues for their inspiring teachings and shares. Special thanks to Missy Vineyard for her book and workshops, Bob Britton for introducing me to functional anatomy, Ted Dimon for his books on anatomy for AT, Karen de Wig for explaining Dart's functional spirals.

My heartfelt gratitude to Jeando Masoero for his diligent research and patient teaching of his Initial Alexander technique methods; for answering my endless queries on the methods and history; and for his immense generosity in allowing me a free rein to use his work as I wished. I am indebted to Rosa Luisa Rossi for introducing me to his work.

Thanks to many other therapists and trainers I encountered on the way, who offered insights and experiences that changed my being and understandings. In particular, Peter Grunwald and his Eyebody method, and Philip Shepherd and Radical Wholeness training. Craniosacral therapist Stuart Walker has argued with me for hours, offering many insights on the nervous system, fascia and felt experience. To Camilla O'Callaghan, Viniyoga teacher, and Kate Bowes, Pilates teacher (sadly no longer with us), for introducing me to the core muscles in breathing and the role of the pelvic floor.

I am grateful to various friends and colleagues for helping me catch up three decades of missed reading. Missy Vineyard pointed me in the right direction. Everard Peters – osteopath, enthusiast for Alexander and Eyebody work and insatiable researcher of the scientific literature – has fed me many interesting papers of new ways of thinking within science and was a huge influence on Chapter 2. Thanks to Jean Fischer for answering historical queries patiently, and for the use of archive photographs. Thanks to Rajal Cohen and Patrick Johnson for their help and stimulating discussions on science versus speculation. Thanks to Tim Cacciatore also for patient emails and conversations, helping me integrate my experiential ideas with his scientific ones. Thanks to all friends and colleagues who have read and commented on chapters and encouraged me to keep writing: Sara Shepherd, Julia Woodman, Michaela Wohlgemuth, Rosa Luisa Rossi, Margaret O'Farrell, Malcolm Balk, Sarah McSwiney.

Thanks to all my wonderful pupils and groups with whom I explored and tested new ideas and methods; I could not have done this book without you all.

Thanks to all the Wwoofers – volunteers from around the world – who have stayed with us, cooked breakfast and lunch and looked after the garden, enabling me to write for more hours in the day and still relax in the evening. To the dogs for insisting I walk twice daily. Particular thanks to all at Handspring Publishing for believing in what I offered them and allowing me to bring my vision into being.

# Part 1
## The Basics of Fundamental Movement

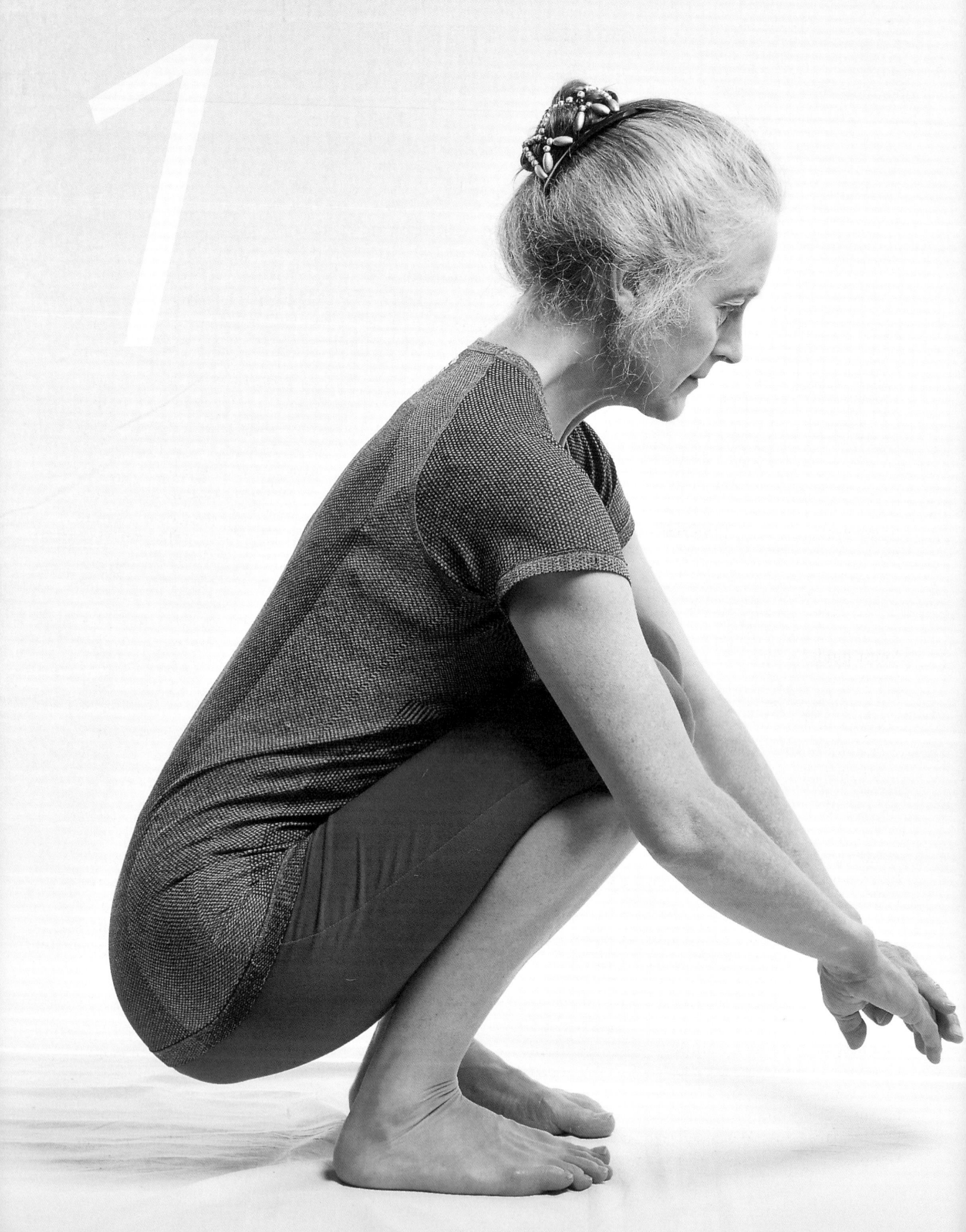

# Introduction, aims, and a tropical tale

## Visions of free movement – a tropical tale

On my twenty-first birthday I flew to the island of Borneo. The eight-hour time-shift meant that I only had sixteen hours of this precious day! I was a young scientist then, studying zoology at Cambridge University, and three of us were flying out to do an eight-week research project in the rainforest. I was ambitious and pushy, tense and stressy, very nervous about my first visit to the tropics. I need not have worried – Borneo was extremely safe and I loved it all. Alongside discovering cuisine I really enjoyed (more vegetables than meat, not boiled but stir-fried in flavorful new combinations), was the wonder of never being cold, the amazing insect life with saucer-sized butterflies among the ferns below skyscraper trees, the friendliness everywhere, and the size of the people, where my five feet three inches was considered normal while my six-foot five-inch boyfriend stood out like a freak.

But more than all this was how people *moved*. In every action they were so balanced, so free. Our forest guides simply shinned up the trees to collect the young leaves we needed. We had a go ourselves but couldn't get beyond our own head heights. In our last two weeks, we did an inland forest trek, staying in longhouses, off the tourist trail. We traveled by ferry up-river, passing women on the bank carrying pots on their heads. The ferry had no seating, everyone sat on the floor. I watched a group of wrinkled old women squat down with fluid ease, sit there comfortably, and stand just as fluidly at the end of the two hours. They had a whole-body movement that we would probably only see in three-year-olds.

For our trek we were allocated a group of six forest guides and bearers, all local men. They paddled us up-river in dugout canoes. We asked to have a go at paddling but they politely refused – we clearly hadn't the strength to force the boat against the fast river. The first day's route led through a part of the forest dissected by drainage ditches, bridged by fallen logs. They were slippery and sometimes rotten, but our barefoot companions went across them as if they were tarmac pavements. We in our leather boots stumbled, wobbled, and slipped. With my dance background I did better than my companions, but it still took a lot of concentration not to fall into the ditches. The men's movement seemed so effortless. We were exhausted after a full day's walking, while they just got on with making a fire in a safe place, preparing our meal, boiling water, and on one night, chopping down young saplings to make us all an open sleeping platform with leafy ceiling.

On day two, our guides squatted effortlessly for hours while they discussed our route. Hanging around waiting, I tried to imitate their action, and found I couldn't. I was astonished, for alongside science, dance was my passion, and I considered myself flexible. I couldn't take my eyes off these people, at ease in their bodies and their environment. In the evening they waded into the river and caught a fish to feed us all. Vegetables, including young fern fronds, and fruit were gathered as they went along; they knew their forest.

The entrance to the longhouse itself was up another wobbly notched slippery log; to them it was as stable as our front doorsteps. The longhouse consisted of a terrace of rooms fronting onto a long open corridor, each room a family home. There were chairs for us in the room we were housed in, evidently the "official visits room," but only we used them. The residents clearly preferred the floor.

*Everything* happened at floor level. The cooking fires were on veranda areas at the back and they squatted or sat around to cook, then we all sat on the floor to eat. For the toilet, you went down the wobbly log and into the wood, dug yourself a little hole and squatted over it. To wash, you went down to the river and squatted by the waterside. At night you unrolled your sleeping mat and lay on the floor. In short, everything involved getting on and off the floor, dozens of times a day.

They never wore shoes. They didn't have chairs or any other furniture for doing actions at a height. Although the children now went to school, the adults, I suspect, were mostly illiterate, so they were not bending over books. In 1981 there was no electricity, so no television and no electronic devices to bend over. There were no roads – you walked or

# CHAPTER one

paddled your dugout. Nearly everything came from the forest – hunted, gathered, or grown – or from the river, including water; the only shops were a long trek downstream. Everything involved physical movement. In retrospect, I also realize that they never sat back, never rested their backs against something. It seemed they didn't have the same urgency to stop and rest their bodies that we have, by collapsing onto sofas or comfy cushions.

Fluid, easy movement was required for life. There was not the "luxury" of being able to let their bodies degenerate that our "convenience" lifestyle gives us. I was young and didn't think to ask the questions I might ask now, such as what provision was made for disabled children or for those with disabling injuries. There must have been something, but I didn't really think at all, I just looked. And looked.

Yet the questions did come, each taking shape slowly until I could articulate it clearly. My initial question was simple: how were they so much more flexible than me, despite my dance training? Then when, two years later, I began taking Alexander technique lessons and my body began to change, I noticed, from pictures of other indigenous peoples, that their bodies were straighter, without the thrust-out chests and curving lumbar spines that ours have. Was there another model of alignment, different from our own cultural ideal? And what allowed these people in Borneo to *rest* as they squatted or sat upright? Did we need to "let go" to relax, or were we missing something?

Then questions flooded in about the senses: were there really only five? I kept coming across another and another sense, each introduced with the phrase: "and this must be the sixth sense" … only they were all different. Just how many extra "senses" did we have, and how did they all fit together?

It set me thinking: though we must have the same potential range of basic capabilities as those people I had met in Borneo, how have our extremely different cultural worlds and environments changed which capabilities we develop? Our own culture has given us such different ways of learning, working, and fulfilling our daily needs, with such different expectations and experiences. It must affect how we perceive and interpret our surroundings, and give us different priorities for our attention and awareness. I suspected that there was a whole pile of skills, perceptions, and goodness knows what else that I had missed out on.

I became aware that though many Western people are not moving well, the sense of movement is still in us all. We love watching fluid, natural movement: babies crawling, tiny children playing, and bigger children skipping or running. Or horses racing, cats rolling, natural history TV programs. People grieve that they can no longer move so easily, and wonder that such movement is even possible. What do we know of how movement really takes place? We think we need to be conscious of our movement, whereas animals and children clearly are not conscious of *how* they move – they just move.

Every so often, people can have a moment of free movement. It might be while walking, a moment when everything comes into balance and the walking seems to do itself. Or dancing with a partner when two people move like one being. Sports people call this being "in the zone," when movements look after themselves and coordination just happens. It brings a sense of inner peace. But how do we learn to be in this zone, not just occasionally, but whenever we want?

For all our technological advances, what have we lost? This book is an exploration of using the whole of our brain, and indeed all of our intelligence networks. With not five but perhaps thirty or more senses (look up senses on Wikipedia for some interesting lists) and all of our 700 or more muscles working together in a coordinated integrated network. Many of these processes are unconscious, but we can learn to access them, to live "in the zone" any time we choose.

> The number of muscles in humans depends on how you count them. Some sources count all the sub-muscles within a complex muscle, and then total up to 840 muscles. However you count them, it's a heckuva lot!

# Introduction, aims, and a tropical tale

By learning to use our unconscious processes consciously we can re-access brain plasticity in order to unlearn changes that have occurred. Then we can discover how to reprogramme our nervous system to redirect the musculoskeletal body and return to a more integrated state – closer to factory settings! Our culture has molded how we use our brains and how we learn, but not always for the better. We need now to balance our top-down learning – led by information from all we have read, seen, heard, or done – with bottom-up, sensory-led experiential learning.

In our own culture, is there a way a way to coexist comfortably with its technologies of shoes, desks and cars, computers and information streams, etc. to live our modern lives to the full? I suggest we can get there by finding a richer relationship with our bodies and the world around us.

## Aims of the book

Movement that is fully alive, fully optimal to our bodies, emerges out of a set of fundamental aspects, or "ingredients," just as cake comes from eggs, sugar, fat, and flour. But, unlike cake ingredients, the ingredients of optimal integrated movement are not just physical, but include consciousness, the way we think and make choices, the various nervous system networks, and the full panoply of our perceptions and senses, both external and internal.

Just as our movement has been limited and degraded by the constraints of our society, so too has our thinking, our perceiving, our consciousness. Many people will attempt to meditate or pray every day, as a separate practice apart from life. Likewise, they might exercise or practice Tai Chi or yoga as a separate activity. Here we will be exploring bringing consciousness, perception, and different thinking, along with full body exercise, to the daily activities of life, including sitting for hours at a computer!

The thinking and methods proposed here revolve around a re-evaluation of the Alexander technique according to what Alexander himself was originally doing. This older style of the work, which I stumbled upon in my late twenties, brought about profound and precise changes in me. These had such clarity that I have long felt they should be more readily understandable by science. And so it has proved to be, as I have delved into the broad spectrum of very recent research material and found scientific understanding which seems to back up my thinking. These new hypotheses challenge many deep-seated ideas that permeate our thinking about both our control of movement and how we orientate ourselves in time and space.

For instance, the purpose of vision is usually seen as being to create sharply focused images for object recognition, and to form an ongoing inner picture or perception of the world, from which we act. But early in evolution, before the ability to form and hold an image, vision was for coordinating the "eye" with the "arm" that stretched for food. This evolutionary development still underpins our dorsal visual stream, the unconscious and so mostly unknown aspect of the visual system that orients us for action.

Likewise, the idea is still around that the cortical brain controls movement, using mechanistic reflexes. In fact, the origins of the locomotion control system arose out of the early digestive systems in organisms like sponges, the nerve-nets which generate oscillating patterns to control peristalsis. Very few people have heard of central pattern generators, which by generating oscillating patterns, coordinate all rhythmical movements including locomotion. Along with other spinal microcircuits, they provide infinitely flexible movement programs, updated moment by moment with sensory information, that can act appropriately at immense speed. I hypothesize that these provide our innate patterns, and when unencumbered by overlaid patterns from higher up in the brain, they allow top sportspeople to find the predictive and responsive movement they need, mind-blowingly fast and deadly accurate! But often people work from predictive guesstimations based on the last experience, using information which will always be out of date. I suggest we can learn to sidestep this and discover more optimum use.

I present a new postural alignment model, which I believe is closer to our roots.

# CHAPTER one

Indeed each of our bodily systems has evolutionary roots. They are mostly disregarded, but they still play fundamental and essential roles, despite the huge overlay of increasingly specific processing and voluntary control that has occurred with their later developments. I suggest it is because we only focus on these new developments, and have lost touch with the underlying innate processes, that we have created such a gulf between those people I observed in Borneo and our modern selves.

The aim here is to weave these recent avenues of thought into a bold new framework of how movement happens, to give a very different perspective and a fresh approach to integrated movement. I offer this as an opening of a conversation.

This is an experiential book, because I consider that ideas are of no use unless they are grounded in practical experience. I will introduce each fundamental ingredient with explorations. Some might be familiar to you; others will be unfamiliar, or unfamiliar in the way they are approached. The problem with words is that our minds will assume we know what is being talked about, and will fit the idea or concept being offered to something already known and understood. But if one is willing to follow the instructions for the practical exploration, one can discover something quite different, which at first one might not understand, but only experience.

Experience provides opportunities for insights; real understanding comes later. This is a journey into the unknown which takes trust, and a willingness to return to "beginner's mind" (the Zen term for being open to all possibilities in a way we usually are not). But when we encounter experiences that do not fit our current paradigms, our belief systems lead us to reject them. We shall be learning to step out of such systems: our beliefs, habits, conditioning, and established learning patterns, which can imprison us within our known experience far more than we know. Understanding new ideas can enable our minds to get past these blocks, and risk something new.

Understanding is also *crucial* if we are to pass our new methodology on, especially when training the next generation of practitioners. (A lack of understanding has been a particular problem in the world of Alexander technique, for a variety of historical reasons, as we will find.)

We will explore these fundamentals of movement in the context of a series of everyday activities: standing and sitting upright, balancing on one leg, picking something up, catching a ball, walking, sitting at a desk, getting in and out of a chair and on and off the ground, breathing and speaking, touching therapeutically. Throughout each activity we will see how the fundamentals involved interact together and build on each other. We are a complex three-dimensional jigsaw of interconnecting and functionally interrelated parts and systems, and that jigsaw is maintained or changed continually by how it is used.

So this is a workbook to guide you on a journey into the unknown. To rediscover movement patterns, thought patterns, consciousness and embodiment innate in your body and nervous system that have been buried perhaps for many decades or even countless generations. As an undercurrent throughout the book (and explicitly in Part 3), we are exploring Miss Goldie's teaching on "stopping" as a state of quiet aliveness from which one discovers any action anew in the present, rather than replaying learned habits. This is how to live "in the zone," any time you choose, whether playing sport, sending a text or washing up. We also apply this to any therapy process, and to embodied speaking, to come fully present to those we are relating to.

To help with this quality of attention and thought, besides the "what" and "how" of directions for movement, many explorations have links to short videos. For this, I have selected the explorations where the material is most likely to be unfamiliar. Many of these will give a taste of using quiet spatial awareness to bring integrative change. However, these short videos cannot do justice to the richness of this work. See the inside front cover for details of how to access full tutorials that lead you step by step through each

# Introduction, aims, and a tropical tale

chapter, building your embodied understanding and experience.

## How this book came about

I did the Borneo trip because I was ambitious; I aimed to get a research paper out of our work there to further my career. The goal was achieved, and I was in the second year of my Ph.D. when I finished the paper and it was accepted. But by then my career in science was no longer important – I had discovered Alexander technique and was taking what seemed in 1984 a wild, even irresponsible, jump into the unknown.

On my twenty-first birthday I knew none of this. Although I could not yet name it, I was already ill with chronic fatigue syndrome (CFS), after having glandular fever at seventeen. I lived in a boom and bust energy cycle. I suffered from anxiety, panic attacks, depression, and strange sensations that nobody could explain. Our family doctor always assured me it was all in my head, and that I should just stop it, which was impossible. I put too much effort into everything, work or play. During my degree I would work too hard through term time, and then crash for a few weeks in the holidays. At Ph.D. level this was no longer possible. Once my research season started, with no breaks, I started to crack up, and was heading fast for a nervous breakdown. Fortunately for me my back gave out first – it seized completely – and that's what took me to my first Alexander lessons.

I was immediately hooked. At last, a method I could use to look after myself. I began to *observe* the scary processes that went on in my head or body without *reacting* to them, and to learn to let them go. Within a lesson or two I knew deeply that this is what I wanted to do with my life, although it was a while before I admitted it to myself. That was in 1983. I took lessons and explored my own process for three years, then trained in London between 1986 and 1989. After I qualified I quickly built a practice, and loved the work, where every new pupil brought a different challenge. With Alexander technique you have to look after yourself to work with the pupil. But after only a few months without the support of the training school, I couldn't do that; the pupil's energies would overwhelm me. I couldn't look after myself sufficiently, and knew I needed more help.

At that time there were still first-generation teachers around who had worked with Alexander himself. So in January 1990 I started lessons with Miss Margaret Goldie. Miss Goldie was then eighty-six, and she was a dragon, despite her mild, frail-old-lady appearance. She stripped away everything I knew and rebuilt it the way she understood the technique. It was a terrifying process, during which I continued to teach without any longer having a clue what I was doing, until the new understandings began to develop. Over and over again she told me that I knew nothing of the technique, and neither did anyone else in the profession – which seemed outrageous. I knew that all of those I had learned from until then were good people doing good work. But as she brought about something different, something deeper and more healing in me, slowly I began to understand her meaning: that Alexander had been doing something different. There were aspects of his work that had got sidelined, forgotten, misunderstood, or never articulated, and she urgently wanted to show them to me, and to others, before she was gone.

I talked to other people who had trained with her; I talked to other first-generation teachers or read their books, and the message stayed consistent. I have explored her work and her message for thirty years now, and it just gets clearer. As has happened with many disciplines, there is a level at which what is happening now is not what the founder intended. Alexander technique is a fantastic discipline. And yet there is much more to it. It had become a method in which you needed individual lessons for months or years, through which you slowly learned to do it for yourself. Even then, as I discovered, it's quite hard to hold on to it. But that is not where Alexander himself *started*; his technique started as a real self-help method. Thankfully, this is now changing again, as many teachers teach more of a self-help method from the start, needing far fewer lessons.

# CHAPTER one

Those first-generation teachers that I met were as phenomenal as the people of Borneo. They mostly lived incredibly healthily to a tremendous old age, with full practices still while in their late eighties and early nineties, as Alexander himself had done. They were active people. One of them was still riding her bike around Oxford until her death at ninety-eight. Another still gave "table turns" on the floor. There were no walking sticks, and they mostly died of old age, still with full mental faculties. I began to ask myself – what do I need to do to be as healthy, active and fully engaged with life as they were, when I reach my eighties or nineties? Several of them, I learned, had started with health just as poor as mine. And then, how do I make this knowledge accessible to anyone who needs it?

I cast a wider net than Alexander technique alone in my quest for such full health. Over the years I explored many different therapies and self-help systems. In particular, I used yoga and Tai Chi, craniosacral therapy, Bates's natural vision technique, then Peter Grunwald's EyeBody Method®, and Philip Shepherd's Radical Wholeness. They have important concepts and I will discuss them later. It was a therapy called Mickel (or Reverse) Therapy that finally freed me from the chronic fatigue syndrome, so that I could *enjoy* life rather than simply *minding* myself within it.

All these methods had something to add. But what intrigued me was that each had its own model of how the body worked. Several included a different model of the primary control of movement. This is one of the key elements of Alexander technique – in which the head leads the neck and back into movement. But here were at least four different explanations that evidently worked. In Tai Chi the dan tien (the belly center) leads movement; in EyeBody the eyes lead; in Radical Wholeness it's the pelvic bowl; and yoga – from everywhere. So that led to the question, how could they *all* be right?

I kept exploring it all experientially. One of the major problems I had experienced with the chronic fatigue syndrome was that it scrambled my brain and made me ill if I tried to read. For years I simply could not read. This became a tremendous gift as, alongside lessons, sessions and occasional workshops, I worked on my own, making my own discoveries. But there came a point where I needed more understanding to write. Fortunately, with the help of EyeBody, I have been able to read, write, and work on a computer again. Slowly, by reading science volumes and the accounts of first-generation teachers, and discussing it all with some wonderful people, this question has been answered, and a new model of how we move has emerged. It is a first attempt at a much more unified model of movement. Hopefully this will springboard a dialogue between Alexander teachers and other disciplines.

## AT info: Evolution of the Alexander technique and finding the whole elephant

I am attempting here to make explicit some of the core principles of the AT, many of which were not taught explicitly on any training course for many years, although this is now beginning to change. Alexander, like all original thinkers, was a true explorer. He was always observing, discovering fresh aspects of the work, characterizing what he found as best he could. Before he started the first training course in 1931, he changed his teaching several times – around 1912, again in the early 1920s, and then in 1925. He described each method in the first three of his books, and each new stage left key elements behind, unexplained. While these elements remained implicit in the work, they were mostly no longer addressed explicitly. Meanwhile he was still using them all himself. These included direct tuition of natural breathing; his initial focus on the torso and the movements within it, with his own biomechanics enabling pupils to produce profound structural changes for themselves; the early thought processes of his directions; how he used inhibition and the parasympathetic nervous system – coming to quiet attentiveness – to discover his innate movement patterns, from which he later formulated his theory of a primary control; and how he used vision as part of his process.

Even the first-generation teachers did not know all this explicitly, although it was imbued deeply in them

# Introduction, aims, and a tropical tale

through Alexander's hands and being. Goldie pre-dated the training course and so had seen the second stage. She was always close to him: she traveled with him to America, and after his stroke was housekeeper for him until he died, and saw where he was still attempting to take the work.

The first training course ran from 1931 to 1934, and during this period, several students worked together to formalize the teaching method that became the technique taught in AT schools from then on. Lulie Westfeldt tells the tale of this in her book (1985: 86); Erika Whittaker then named the little group as Patrick MacDonald, Marjory Barlow, Westfeldt, and Kitty Merrick (Hunter 2013) and Barlow confirmed it (2002: 81). This formalizing of a method is a necessary stage for any new discipline, if it is to be taught consistently and handed down to others. After Alexander's death, the inevitable schisms between the main trainers further split this knowledge pool, creating very different strands of work. Although much splendid work has now gone on to heal these rifts and share what was known, it has become apparent to many that it does not add up to a complete picture of what Alexander himself was doing.

We need to go back to what he was doing at these different stages, to reconnect with what was lost. But more fundamentally, we also need to return from formalized technique to re-access the discovery process itself. The path to this is largely through those who stayed outside these mainstream lines, holding to the original processes. Several of these teachers, of whom Miss Goldie was the most outspoken, expressed the idea that the mainstream technique as taught on the training schools had taken a different path from the discovery path intended by Alexander. Part 3 of this book explores this discovery work in detail, with a series of games that can quickly bring about the experiences that resulted from Goldie's lessons.

The book also draws on new material discovered by Jeando Masoero, of how as a young man Alexander was hugely influenced by the Delsarte system, of which he himself was a teacher. If Masoero is correct, the Alexander technique really did start as a self-help method, but quickly became a method of teachers working on pupils. This original material was perhaps even suppressed by Alexander, as it was gone by 1915 or earlier, once he discovered he could communicate the work through his hands. So even the first-generation teachers did not know of it, although it was intrinsic in their work. In Part 2, I will give a more detailed history, and the basic tools of Initial AT, to share their anatomical knowledge and precision. These have finally solved my puzzles of the anatomical model Miss Goldie was using in her "chairwork," and also answered the puzzle of giving directions "all together, one after another" (Alexander 1985: 64), in a new and more integrating way.

Everyone involved in the technique, including Alexander himself, has done the best they could to develop their natural abilities with the teaching they were given, and with the circumstances and understanding available to them at the time. Like the ancient parable of the three blind men introduced to an elephant, who all grasped different parts of its anatomy, believing that to be the whole animal, different schools have received and so given their trainees different pieces of the picture. We can scatter round forever gathering new and old bits, but what is needed now is a coherent structure on which to frame the understanding of Alexander's work. It is time for us all to grasp the entire elephant.

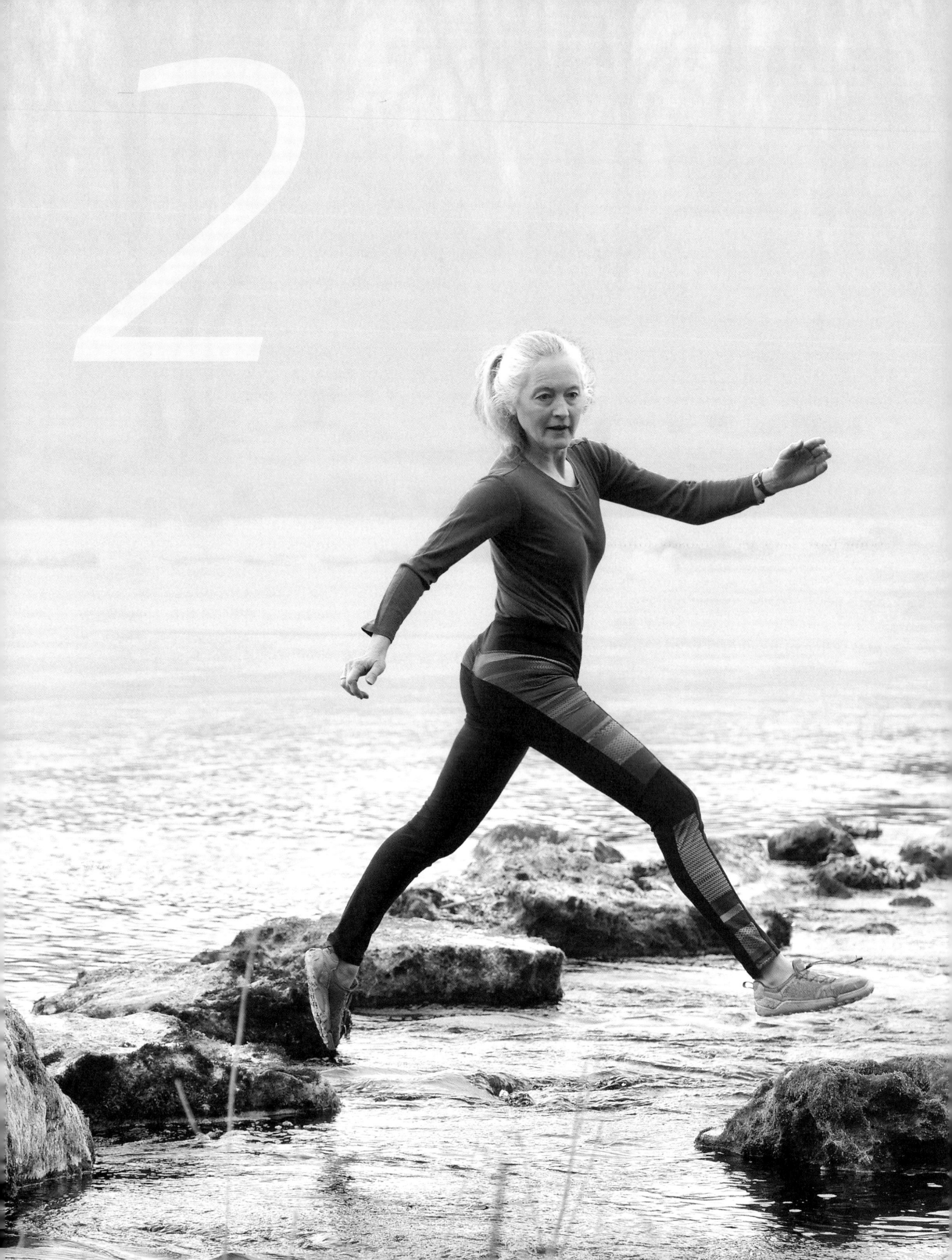

# What has been lost, and the twelve fundamentals of movement

## Integrated movement – WHAT has gone wrong, and WHY?

In Chapter 1, we saw that we have the human *potential* to be healthy in body and mind into extreme old age, to keep the full-body movement we had as children. I saw it in those people in Borneo, who had never lost it, and saw it later in those first Alexander teachers, who had reclaimed it. Yet in the West, generally our movement patterns degrade decade by decade, in slow decline through bent backs and stiff hips to walking sticks and Zimmer frames.

Estimates in the NICE guidelines (National Collaborating Centre for Primary Care (UK) 2009: introduction) suggest 84% of the population will at some point have back pain, mostly lumbar problems, no doubt along with a raft of neck and shoulder problems and tension headaches. Wrist pain, flat feet, and many other limb problems also abound. It is even common to think our bodies are not well-evolved for purpose. Most people think that a deterioration of structure is inevitable with aging, and consider hip and knee replacements inevitable.

From these worsening physical structures, our movement possibilities are degraded.

The natural squatting movement on and off the floor, with its simultaneous flexing of hips and knees and ankles, is long gone for many people in the West. Instead, people bend over from the waist or upper body with straight legs, and are then surprised when it hurts to come up again.

But surely sport helps keep us fit? My boyfriend at college avoided sports because he'd watched too many of his friends injure themselves, and had concluded it was dangerous to do other than walk. It's a view many older people are forced into, when they have to give up tennis, football, or running because their muscles and joints have been used in suboptimal alignments for too long. I believe that what is called old age can be misuse of the body catching up.

What has gone adrift? We will see that when muscles have unequal pulls, forces are applied across joints in the wrong planes, and harm will then result over time. But avoiding sport doesn't avoid the problem: the same also happens to musicians, computer users, factory workers, or anyone doing any repetitive movement. Even walking or swimming can cause harm when done with suboptimal alignment.

To see the patterns we are using, watch how old people painfully and slowly lower themselves into a chair and lever themselves out again. Watch them applying huge amounts of force in the wrong planes, such as pushing down hard onto legs that are trying to move them. These are the patterns that we are using, taken to their degenerative extreme. Most people move with these same patterns, but to a less visible extent.

With age, people lose the spring in their step, and with it their lightness of being. This stiffness is often what we define as "feeling old." Regaining springiness will be part of our explorations ahead, and with it comes a regained sense of youthfulness.

## Sitting is the new smoking

So why did this happen? Part of the answer is simply because our culture has lost its relationship with the floor. As a baby, you were probably allowed to roll and crawl around on the floor, tottering to stand, and then falling by folding onto your bottom. You flowed on and off the floor from sit to stand and back, and in and out of squat, with immense ease. But … the moment you sat up, you were given a high-chair, a buggy, and a potty. For activities with paper and paint, etc. you were seated at a table, which made life much easier for the adults. School intensified this. There you learned to sit still for many hours a day – it's our most practiced childhood skill! Then college, then perhaps a sedentary job, book-ended by car or train journeys (mostly) taken sitting … and evenings in front of the TV, with the remote control so you never have to leave the sofa.

This has worsened dramatically in recent years with all-day TV, streamed films, computer games, social

# CHAPTER two

media, or online shopping – all done sitting. Meanwhile the "strain" has been increasingly taken out of the physical tasks of the household: pre-prepared foods mean less active time in the kitchen, machines take the harder physical work out of most household tasks. We have become a sedentary culture.

Even those who take regular planned exercise at the prescribed target levels (an hour of brisk walking or its equivalent two to three times a week) are still largely sedentary the rest of the time. It is emerging that this sedentary habit is the real problem, causing serious health issues such as cardiovascular disease and obesity. Deborah Lou (2014) found that "On average, children and teens spend 6 to 8 hours per day watching TV, playing video games, and using computers. Relatively strong evidence links TV viewing with obesity ... and decreased academic achievement." While Lee et al. (2012) found: "Inactivity causes 9% (range 5·1–12·5) of premature mortality [worldwide]." Hence the new catchphrase: *Sitting is the new smoking.*

## What does all this sitting do to us, physically?

Our bodies are never fixed – the tissues are constantly being subtly re-molded to fit our circumstances. Areas that are receiving more tension or greater pressure are strengthened along the lines of force while areas working less are reduced. Bodies are economical – why maintain tissue you are not using? Women who have worn high heels all their lives may notice their heels no longer touch the floor when barefoot, as the muscles and tendons of the calves and thighs have shortened to the new length. The smallest units of muscles are sarcomeres (more about them in Chapter 3), and are like multiple groups of little chain links: if a muscle stays shortened, after a while the body takes links out of the system, while a muscle continually stretched may be lengthened (Bowman 2017: 70).

Sitting is our greatest cause of this inequality of muscle use. The quads, psoas, iliacus, and erector spinae are all tightened and shortened, working overtime to hold the torso, arching the lumbar spine and tilting the pelvis (Fig. 2.1A). But with little support from passive, overly relaxed legs, switched-off feet and with a tilted, and therefore unstable, pelvic base, this is hard work. So the torso collapses into a "comfortable" reverse curve slump (Fig. 2.2). The legs rest passively. The gluteal muscles and hamstrings will relax and spread, the pelvis tilts back. In this, the torso is compressed and shortened down the front. Over the years it all adjusts to the new position.

Whether arched or slumped, the overall shortening caused by these muscle imbalances means that when we stand, a fully upright stance is no longer possible (Fig. 2.1B). To balance upright we have to be either curved back or curved forward, or some awful mix of the two. There are many variations of poor sitting and standing, but overall the picture is of imbalance, with some muscle groups tightening and other groups slackened and weakened. Consequently, every single one of our actions is colored by these underlying imbalances in muscle length and action; our walking patterns will be less graceful, running will be harder, and so on. We will have to work harder all the time to overcome the underlying lack of balance in the system.

To this physical picture we can add the effects of stress and trauma, which can cause deep physical tension that will embed into the body if not resolved quickly. The tension patterns created are often the same: the pelvic floor and psoas tighten, the body slumps, and the neck constricts.

In contrast, there is only one balanced, upright posture, in which everything is lengthening but not rigid (Fig. 2.3).

## Why did we get caught in this trap?

There must be principles we can use that work with us, not against us? You might expect me to launch straight in with physical explanations of how we can change all this. Instead, I am going to ask some more fundamental questions, such as "Why do we have to go to school all day?" Most children would rather be running around and playing. Schooling was

# What has been lost, and the twelve fundamentals of movement

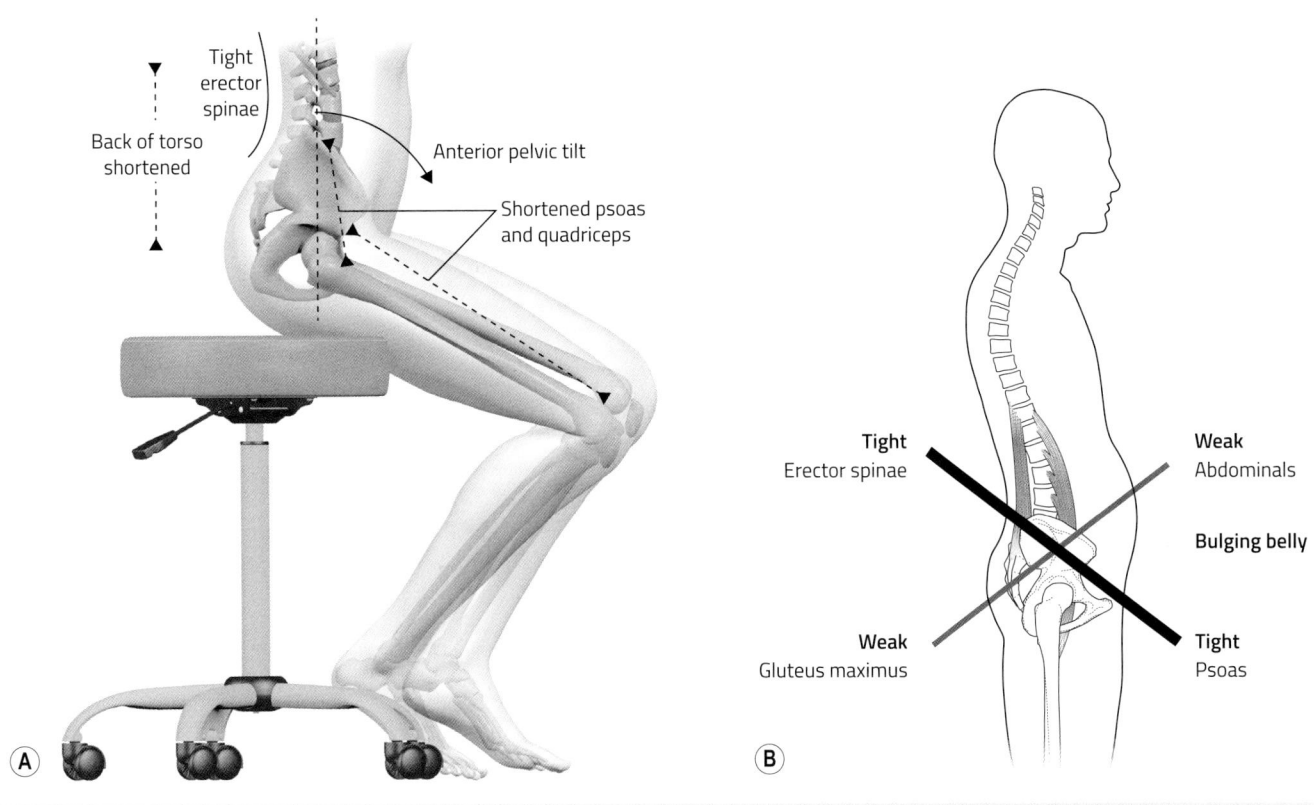

Figure 2.1A, B
How we sit affects how we stand

instituted to learn through reason rather than through experience. Initially, it was for the elite only, and now it is for everyone. It is vital we all learn essential knowledge and skills, but also *to learn how to learn*, and how to think clearly about ourselves and our situations. The whole process of what is taught, and how, needs a radical rethink.

There is now a lot of evidence that we learn much faster and remember it better when all our senses and movement are also involved. Maria Montessori was a pioneer in multisensory learning for children, which is especially used where children have disabilities. But the more this is researched and proven, the more mainstream education often goes in exactly the opposite direction, so that even practical and creative subjects, such as woodwork or art, now demand written commentary.

The origin of this imbalance between experiential and intellectual learning is often traced back to French philosopher René Descartes (1596–1650), who declared that the mind and body are separate. In his vision, "mind" is intelligence and reason – the interesting bit – while the body is a machine, worked by nerve reflexes from the brain. These ideas are a lot older than Descartes, however: in around 450 BC the ancient Greek philosopher Parmenides stated that the body is unreliable. Its emotions and drives will lead you astray, and only pure reason can be trusted

# CHAPTER two

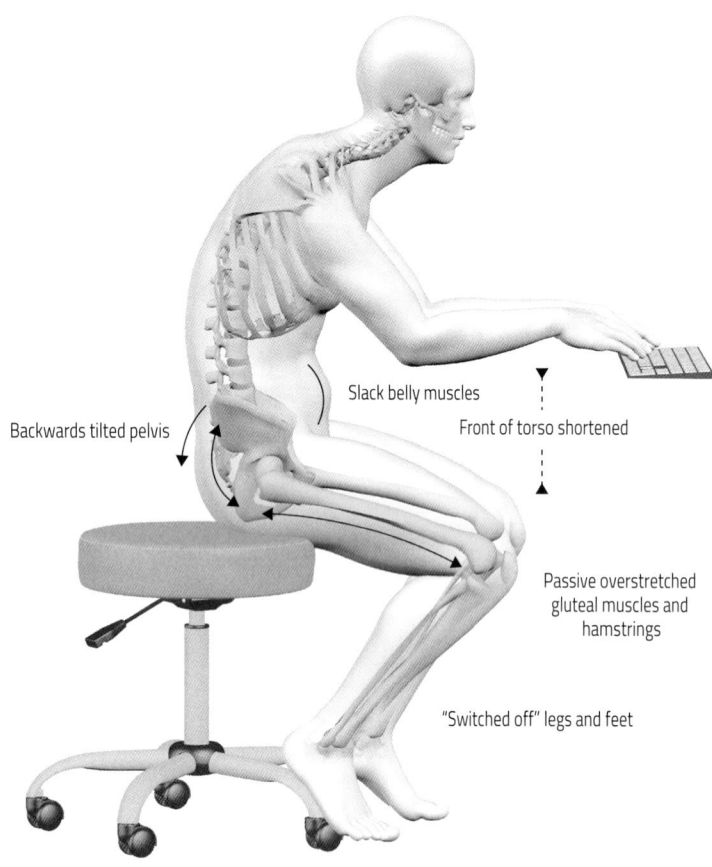

**Figure 2.2**
Slumping compresses the torso

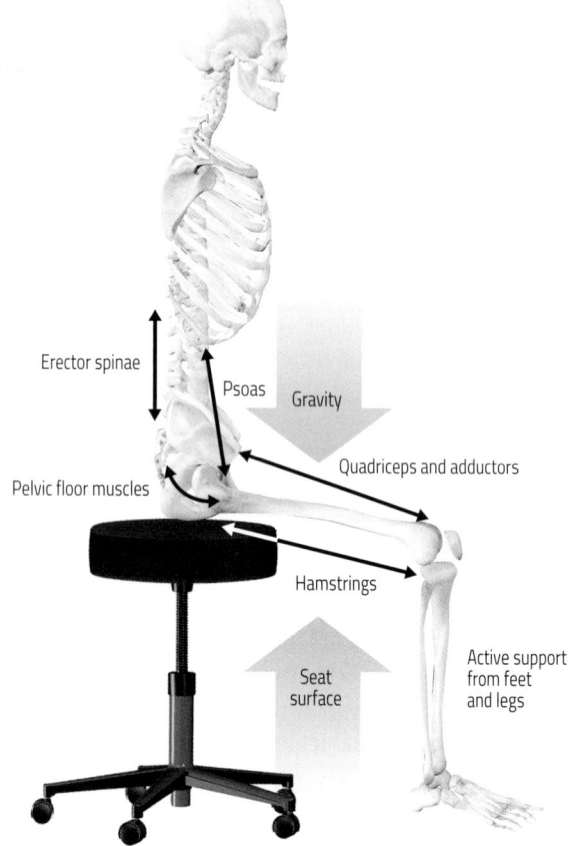

**Figure 2.3**
Balanced sitting

(Shepherd 2010: 51). Slightly later, it was Aristotle who first proposed the body as machine.

This set the stage for later Western thought and civilization. The head and cold reasoning (mind) were idealized and were to be trained, while the physical, feelings, and instincts (body) were mistrusted and suppressed. This is top-down thinking, where the reasoning brain is seen as more important than the experiencing body, and consciousness is seen as emerging from the brain. Even within neurological research, the cortex – the newest region – has been seen as the most important one to study. This is why, beyond these first two chapters, all the ideas presented will be backed up by opportunities for experiences and discoveries. Without this bottom-up experiential process, knowledge is not integrated and is of no practical use.

# What has been lost, and the twelve fundamentals of movement

## The five senses – one of the great myths

Once you have a top-down model of reality, where thinking is prized above being and experiencing, you can put what you like in it and leave other stuff out (Philip Shepherd, Boghill Retreat Centre, November 6, 2019). It was Aristotle who defined the five senses, and conventional Western thought still teaches this – it's what we learned at school. Notice that these senses – sight, hearing, taste, smell, touch – are all communications from the outside world of "other" into the inside world of "me." Each inputs through its own sense organ, its information being fed directly to the brain's processors. This is *exteroception*.

The various "sixth" senses I encountered included proprioception – our internal sense of position and movement. The vestibular system, often called the balance organs, contributes to our spatial sense and sense of boundary. There is our sense of time. Then there are all those less tangible senses that are often distrusted in our rational society, such as gut instinct, intuition, knowing what another is thinking or feeling, or inner guidance through dreams or signs. People perceptive to these often find themselves labelled "weird."

These last all probably fit into *interoception* – sensing the internal environment. Interoception includes survival drives, emotions, and pain signals, and also awareness of others' states. It is here that the legacy of Parmenides is clearest: if the body is unreliable, you should not pay attention to its information. Hunger, a need to pee, pain, feeling tired or ill, grief, frustration, etc., even feeling loved – we have all been taught, to a greater or lesser degree, to deal with these by putting them on hold till later. Many schools and most working environments can be impatient, even ruthless, with people who insist on listening to their body's internal messages. It is inconvenient for getting the work done.

Many illnesses today can be traced to this denial of internal body messages. When our heads overrule our bodies, how tightly do we have to hold our bellies and muscles to ignore their input? All movement suffers from this approach to life. Our eyes learn to spend hours tracking horizontally across flat and mostly black and white surfaces. Exercise mostly consists of repetitive movements. We learn to concentrate – to use a narrow band of focus, restricting other input. In this top-down approach to life, so many movements, visual patterns, sensory possibilities and awarenesses have simply been thrown away. Worst of all, we think it is normal.

All this restricts our flow of breathing, leaving it shallow and tight – restrictions in our life force itself. How can we fulfill our real potential when we are bound and hampered by these invisible bonds? Our amazing culture brings us many benefits, but it has also let us down.

## Changing our movement habits needs a change in thinking

Fitness and movement gurus all tell us we need to be more active, for more of the day, using different movement patterns that use our joints properly. But this advice alone cannot lead to fully integrated movement.

Firstly, we tend to use repetitive movements, whether in life or exercise. Not only were indigenous peoples active for longer, but they had a greater range of movements through the day, often on uneven surfaces and with crude tools, calling up multiple differing balance patterns. For us, with already a more limited movement range, flat surfaces and well-engineered equipment mean that repetition really is that (Bowman 2017: 35). This functionally employs only a limited number of our 700 or more muscles.

But more fundamental than this is that movement patterns are held in the brain. To change a habit we must make a real change at brain level. This requires not learning, but unlearning, which involves a different way of using our brains. To experience how ingrained we are in our habits, try crossing your arms. Now cross them with the other hand on top. Is it comfortable, or does it feel all wrong? Known habit patterns feel not only familiar, but also correct. This is still so even when they are creating considerable harm, such as bending from the waist to pick up

# CHAPTER two

something heavy. This is called **faulty sensory perception**, a crucial concept that has been very little articulated other than by Alexander.

> To experience how ingrained we are in our habits, try crossing your arms. Now cross them with the other hand on top. Is it comfortable, or does it feel all wrong?

To make a change, we have to allow unfamiliar movement, and our whole systems seem to rebel against this. If you continue to sit with your arms crossed in the unfamiliar way, once your attention is elsewhere you will probably unconsciously return to the familiar position. Why are we so attached to the familiar?

## Top-down vs bottom-up processing

There are (at least) two ways of nervous system processing by which we represent reality. One is based in language, story, thinking, and is conceptualized, while the other is experiential, sensory, perhaps more image-based. We can call the first top-down processing, and it happens in the conscious brain alone. It is based on prior experience from which we create an interpretation of what is happening. In making this re-presentation, we take ourselves away from direct experience of the moment. When we come present to the sensory information, we are in bottom-up processing and involving information from our entire body and being. We need both top-down and bottom-up processing, but our culture pushes us towards the former.

This division has been long associated with the division between left and right hemispheres of the brain, which is in all vertebrates. The old approach of asking what the two hemispheres did (left for language and reason, right for emotion and creativity, etc.) was abandoned by neuroscientists when further research showed that every aspect of brain work – language, emotions, creativity, etc. – is represented on both sides. Then, in *The Master and his Emissary* (2012), Iain McGilchrist asked "*how* do the hemispheres *process information*?" And a whole new picture emerged.

## Left hemisphere for the known, right hemisphere for the unknown

There are two ways of being in the world, whatever your species, which require completely different forms of attention. Consider a bird pecking seeds on your gravel path. It needs close focused attention and sharp sight to spot the little seeds between the stones – now here, now there – and aim the beak accurately to peck them. Yet simultaneously, the bird needs to be continuously scanning the entire scene for the unpredictable – for cats or sparrowhawks – and for what other birds in its social group are doing. These are *two competing needs*, requiring two different nervous system processes to function simultaneously. The solution is a piece of biological genius: keep them separate! Close focus, requiring a narrow attention beam, is organized by the left hemisphere. Watching for social interactions, predators and the unfamiliar in the environment, which all need a broad attention beam, is organized by the right hemisphere (McGilchrist 2012: 25–8).

Many other aspects of being and processing follow from this division of labor. Key to it all is that the right hemisphere is open to the unknown; it is curious and exploratory (McGilchrist 2012: 40). It looks at the whole picture for new subtleties and new patterns. New information is passed to the left hemisphere, which classifies it according to known information. The left hemisphere deconstructs the new information, names it and files it in fragments, to be used for the focused tasks of life. This is essential for predicting the world, needed for, say, tool use: for example, knowing that if you turn your car key the engine will start. The left hemisphere loves machines because it sees the world – and the body – in a mechanistic way (McGilchrist 2012: 55).

*Left hemisphere processing is top-down*. It utilizes previous experience of the familiar, to predict what will happen next to control and manipulate its world.

# What has been lost, and the twelve fundamentals of movement

It is an interpreter, hard at work seeking the meaning of events and creating stories to explain them (Gazzaniga 1998). But because it doesn't have access to the full facts, but only the facts it already knows, its interpretations are often wrong. Faulty sensory perception comes from this. *Right hemisphere processing is bottom-up*, utilizing new information streaming in from all the senses, both external and internal, to explore and relate to its world. So it can experience the unfamiliar crossing of the arms (for example) without judging it wrong.

A red apple on the table is processed by the right hemisphere in the context of the whole scene – the pretty dish with other fruit and the room behind it, and the fact that I could give it to my upset friend. The features that make us truly human, such as artistic appreciation or empathy, have their roots in the right hemisphere. The left hemisphere sees a pre-formed concept of apple that I can grasp and eat. It asks, "what can this give me?" This has given us tools, innovation, and business, equally crucial human capabilities (McGilchrist 2012: 55).

*Space and time are processed differently.* The right hemisphere's world is the present, seen in three dimensions, with depth and color. We are in relationship to it, inseparable from it. It is the right hemisphere that holds sustained attention, perceiving the flow between actions, giving a sense of the fullness of time. It sees the relationships between jobs to be done, and that I can flow from one to another (McGilchrist 2012: 75).

The left hemisphere works out of past and future. It draws from a memory bank of all that it has known, so it needs only brief attention to identify something as useful to it or not. Its attention is fragmentary and two-dimensional. Because it experiences life as fragments, the left hemisphere has no real sense of time, no flow, just of "jobs to be done" now (McGilchrist 2012: 76).

### The right hemisphere links to the body, the left hemisphere predominantly links within itself

Although both hemispheres have sensory and motor links, each to the contralateral side, they experience the body differently. It is through the right hemisphere that we experience the body's positions, balance, feelings and drives, in real time and real space. The left hemisphere lives in the realm of ideas. It seems to see the body as an assemblage of parts that do not touch it at any deeper level (McGilchrist 2012: 67). We need both hemispheres.

I always enjoy asking people "where are your hip joints?" Doctors or chiropractors, with their vast memory bank of anatomical knowledge, are often taken by surprise, "*my* hips?" They are used to finding other people's hips, but not their own. Then I watch them work it out, logically, until they can point to the correct place. In contrast, if I ask, say, a farmer or musician, they will bend around and explore until they feel the hips working, and can then point to them. A top-down exploration of known facts in the memory bank, versus a bottom-up exploration led by the senses.

In the right hemisphere we connect the internal perceptions with all the external senses to create a richly complex, dynamic, three-dimensional and coherent world. This is deeply calming to the whole system. Our trap, when the left hemisphere dominates, is to live in our heads, in a realm of ideas and interpretations, in past and future. To envision realities outside the present is an amazing capacity of humans, but this can come with problems, as we may not cope well with the present or may experience a sense of alienation from a loss of real relationship with the world (McGilchrist 2012: 407).

### Which should lead the show?

We have been taught that the left hemisphere, with its facts and logic, should lead our lives. McGilchrist holds that this is where we have gone wrong. Because the left hemisphere is self-referring and can be ignorant of right hemisphere's insights and contributions, it can see them as unimportant. When the left leads, the right hemisphere is dumbed down and belittled – we become dominated by the left's logical approach to life (McGilchrist 2012: 209). The reverse is not the case, however: when the right hemisphere leads, the left works in context, under the guidance of the right.

# CHAPTER two

Only the right hemisphere can see the overall picture. It needs to lead in any task, overseeing the actions and watching for the unexpected arising while the left hemisphere takes charge of the detail. This allows us to keep the task in context (2012: ch. 5).

For example, a parent envisages an activity in the context of their day (RH), then oversees the child's play: engaging in the detail (LH), peripherally watching for danger (RH) and staying attentive to the child's needs (RH), then is able to choose the moment for ending and moving on (RH). The parent's calm authority makes the child feel safe and relaxed to focus on their play. In the same way, when the right hemisphere determines, from the overall context, what we need to do, the left hemisphere can relax and get on with the detail, knowing the bigger picture is being dealt with. The nervous system can relax into the parasympathetic, muscles can relax and engage as they need, and all aspects of the body can function optimally. And it all happens simultaneously, subconsciously, without our active knowledge.

The way we pay attention to ourselves, and to the world, changes what we perceive, and in the process, also changes us and the way we inhabit our bodies (McGilchrist 2012: 28). This, in many ways, is the focus of this book. For, as McGilchrist concludes, our Western society has increasingly prioritized the left hemisphere at the expense of the right to a level that is now creating serious harm.

## Updating McGilchrist's theory

I am told that McGilchrist's book speculated beyond the level of the data in its conclusions. The brain is increasingly understood to work in networks, only some of which are highly lateralized, with language (particularly speech) and the default mode network (from where we mind wander) to the left and spatial attention to the right (Corballis and Haberling 2017). Other networks, such as the two visual streams (see Chapter 14), may be behind other processing divisions mentioned. Siegel (2010: 104) suggests that interpretation vs experience may be mediated in the vertical columns lining the neocortex. Bottom-up data from subcortical areas and body moves from layer 6 to 5 to 4 while top-down prior learning information flows from layer 1 to 2 to 3. Layers 3 and 4 where these meet give us awareness in the present, but only if we have not allowed the top-down flow to predominate. Along with top-down interpretive processing/bottom-up experiential processing, I will continue to use left/right hemisphere, though it may be partly metaphor.

## Real change of muscular habits requires right hemisphere/experiential processing

Much bodywork in the West has become left hemisphere/top-down led, dictating instructions to specific body parts, seeking to strengthen or flex the body one bit at a time. Moves are done with little internal awareness, and maybe to pounding music. This is "treating" the body as an objective thing that must be minded. For integrated movement, we certainly need new learning of muscles, joints and methods, etc. But more than this, *we need a perceptual shift in the way we think and how we pay attention.*

Top-down processing is self-referring and can only recruit known muscles, the ones in play. It can fire these in different patterns to create an overlay that looks like a change, but can never do anything fundamentally different. The underlying pattern will still be there; meanwhile we have increased the tensions in the system. For real change, you need experiential processing, with access to the full body, to all muscles with their innate programs and integrating networks. Then overworking muscles, seen as essential by the left hemisphere because familiar, can let go and muscles that are currently not being recruited can swing into play, involving new nerve pathways. This is stepping into the unknown. We need to let something come about that the left hemisphere will think is wrong. We need to return to child learning – right hemisphere learning, exploratory, curious, unafraid; this is what we will be exploring.

When we allow the unknown to guide us, we are bringing consciousness to unconscious processes. This

# What has been lost, and the twelve fundamentals of movement

also is a theme of this book, and we will explore different aspects of it. The old estimate that we only used 5% of our brain capacity was of conscious thinking. This was changed by the advent of MRIs, CAT scans etc., providing images of brains in action, showing that the whole brain is involved. Neuroscience can now map and explore the 95% that is unconscious, which has created an explosion of new research. By tapping into this, I consider we can unleash our real potential – both of physical movement and of many other aspects of self.

### Whole-body being: left and right, top and bottom, front and back

As we have seen, our culture values the left hemisphere over the right and the brain over the body – the head over lower areas. It also values the front more than the back. We need to step into our whole beings. The right hemisphere doesn't just provide another way of *being in* the body, but of *whole-body being*. Another author who wrote a very similar book to McGilchrist's at the same time, in the strange way these things happen, is Philip Shepherd (2010). He points out that when we say things like "I'm looking after my body" or "I'm listening to my body" this still indicates that I am seeing *myself* as separate from *my body*. He coined the phrase "radical wholeness" for the state in which we experience ourselves as one being, not as brain and body.

Where McGilchrist defines left hemisphere and right hemisphere, Shepherd defines head brain and belly brain, and his experiential work teaches one to utilize other intelligences within the nervous system that have long been forgotten by our mechanized view of the body. Shepherd sees head brain as isolated within its own structures and thinking, while belly brain is in touch with the whole. To him, thinking happens in an axis of communication between the two. He writes: "Our primary wound … [is] an underlying schism in our culture: the separation of your thinking from your being" (Shepherd 2010: 24). Science is now beginning to unravel the connections between right hemisphere and belly brain to what has been called our primary consciousness (Schore 2003). We will explore these ideas further in the book.

The third plane is front/back, and this has particularly been the focus of Alexander work. Our thinking culture emphasizes the frontal lobes from where it is thought we plan. Rodin's sculpture *The Thinker* shows how this emphasis draws us into the front of the body. We try too hard to control and do everything, overusing our front flexor muscles. We have often lost touch with the back – with its real strength to hold us up and with the calm that comes when we "step back for a moment" or become more "laid-back" about life. When we come back in the head, we reawaken insight that comes from the visual cortex above the occiput, and also the cerebellum, right at the back of the brain, which recent research suggests may be a crucial part of all planning, smoothing both movement and complex thought (Williams 2018).

McGilchrist, Shepherd and Alexander all observe that when you step out of the over-emphasized left hemisphere/head-brain/front, and balance it with the right hemisphere/belly-brain/back, you "unlearn" your habits by stepping out of them and instead, step into the unknown. Then something is unlocked in you. You allow a new way of being to emerge, new movement patterns to happen that somehow you knew were there all along.

So what are we unlocking? I consider that all our body systems have underlying innate aspects that are fundamental to our optimal functioning with which we have lost touch, and which science until recently has disregarded.

### An evolutionary perspective puts the body first

When we look from an evolutionary perspective, it is obvious that the body must precede the brain. When Descartes proposed that mind and body are separate, he did so nearly two centuries before Darwin was born, and Adam and Eve were still viewed as fact. All scientists then believed the Bible creation story (Genesis 1) that God had created man fully formed, with his resplendent

# CHAPTER two

intellect and language, morality and culture, superior to and separate from the animal kingdom.

*On the Origin of Species* was published in 1859, with Darwin's shocking concept that we are descended from apes. Subsequent science (anatomical studies of fossils particularly, and now genetics, alongside geological studies, etc.) has confirmed repeatedly that evolution, not creation, was the path to modern man. But other areas of human biology were slow to catch on. Descartes's thinking quietly pervaded each field, with the intellect and brain as king, and the body a mechanical second. However much they espoused evolution intellectually, most scientists and thinkers were still living out Descartes, so that in effect, creationism still unconsciously underpinned much scientific thinking.

The revolutionary new science that has emerged in the last twenty to thirty years is changing this, often with evolutionary hypotheses. These recognize that the body is always in intimate association with the brain, in close partnership. Many of these are not yet widely known, or well linked together. The following are the main new theories I will explore in the book:

Biomechanics (Bernstein and others, Chapter 3) and biotensegrity theory have described new models of body structure, showing we are not constructed like machines (though I describe problems with the biotensegrity model). Posture itself has been surprisingly unstudied until recently. Tim Cacciatore explores the postural regulation of tone as a dynamic modulation in response to gravity (Chapters 3 and 10).

Goodale and Milner have given us the two visual streams theory, showing how vision's primary evolutionary function is to coordinate movement (Chapter 15).

Sten Grillner's work on central pattern generators shows how movement emerges from bottom-up processes, built up from innate patterns in the spinal cord and brainstem (Chapter 6), with patterns conserved through evolution.

Neuroscience increasingly sees the brain as a predictive machine. However, the brain is not a composite of specialized areas as was long thought, but a set of informational networks that link not only within lower and higher areas, but also between brain, body and environment, giving a much more embodied vision to this (Chapter 4, Miller and Clark and others).

Stephen Porges (the polyvagal theory) identified the evolution of the autonomic nervous system, and has explained our awareness of safety in relating to self and others (Chapter 5). This has implications for all therapeutic work, especially with trauma.

In psychotherapy, polyvagal theory has been linked with the field of attachment theory to change the model of child development: the right hemisphere, linked to visceral awareness and an intuitive relationship with the mother is our primary consciousness and underpins a healthy mental and social life (Allan Schore, Chapter 5). How this all applies to any therapy process, and adult human relationships generally, is also being defined (Deb Dana, Chapter 5).

Even thinking and language, the bastions of the "created" intellect, are coming under new scrutiny. Antonio Damasio argues that reasoning must be underpinned by the body's emotion and feeling, without which coherent reasoning is lost (2006). David McNeill describes the evolution of language, and how gesture and language evolved inseparably together (Chapter 9), with gesture as primary.

These new developments in science and thought are not only seeing the primary importance of the body but also of our interconnectedness with each other and our surroundings. "Mirror neurons," first discovered in 1991 by Giacomo Rizzolatti (in Blakeslee and Blakeslee 2008: 163), are what allow us to watch someone else perform an action and reproduce the action ourselves. They are probably involved in empathy as we model someone else's emotion internally to understand it (Dan Siegel, Chapter 18). Science has shown how the brain links with the space around the body (Chapter 18).

The brain, once thought to be fixed beyond age ten, is now known to be plastic and changeable (Norman Doidge, Chapter 16). When we focus on the task of

# What has been lost, and the twelve fundamentals of movement

movement instead of on instructions to control our bodies we learn experientially and much faster (Gaby Wulf, Chapter 16), very different from traditional, top-down learning approaches.

Bernstein recognized that movement does not emerge from mechanistic, predetermined patterns that we switch on and off but is always in adaptive response to the environment. From this, Michael Turvey and others see the nervous system as always switched on and responsive, coordinating with information experientially, rather than existing to gather and process information from which to respond (Chapter 16).

All these and more are describing how bottom-up processes evolved us into the complex beings we are today. They each show how the brain needs the body's underpinning to function. I observe neuroscience moving towards the idea that there is no primary control of the body by the brain; instead there are multiple networks and feedback loops. It seems that the body runs the brain just as much as the brain runs the body.

Recent research on fascia and its connectivity suggests it to be an integral part of movement, sensing, and communication through mechanotransduction, though little is proven as yet (Chapters 3, 4, 18). Kinetic muscle chains and functional anatomy (Chapter 3) are linking the physical body into one cohesive unit, rather than being a series of separately operated parts that somehow were supposed to add up to make a whole. This more unifying approach may bring our biological structures more in line with the findings of quantum physics, that everything is connected to everything else, something biology has been very slow to espouse. The old top-down, dualistic model is slowly being toppled. We will look at how this affects Alexander's concept of primary control in Chapter 14.

> This book draws on well-researched science but also on theories from established researchers, some of which are quite speculative as yet. While I have attempted to cover relevant neurological, physiological, and psychological research, I have not explored the biomechanical research as it was too big a field to tackle for this book. Therefore, my new biomechanical models are presented experientially, drawing also on other practical work that runs ahead of the research.

## Whole-body animal movement, the fulfilment of evolutionary potential

So what are the fundamental components and dynamic processes that interplay for integrated movement?

Structure has to be a prime factor since in nature, structure and function go together. A giraffe will move differently from a whale or a rabbit – you cannot separate movement from structure. It is less obvious that neither can you separate movement from orientation, perception, choices and consciousness.

Think of a cat hunting a mouse, and marvel at all that evolution has brought about over the 350 billion years since life first appeared on the planet:

The integrated *structure* of the cat's body facilitates the *movements possible* – the flexible spine enabling slinky stalking on silent paws, powerful muscles to spring, retracting claws to grasp.

But before hunting begins, a *series of perceptions* are needed, *to orient* the hunter within the environment: firstly, to gravity – the cat needs to be the right way up! Other *orientation and proprioception mechanisms maintain postural stability*, enabling the cat to balance as it stalks, crouches, and springs. The cat also needs to be aware of its *internal drives* – that its need is hunger (or the drive to hunt), rather than sleep, or mate finding. Then, *perception* of the mouse – the sight, sound, and smell of it – *orients the action itself*.

Simultaneously, it must perceive and respond to more peripheral elements in the environment – stones to step over or plants to weave around. It must try to *predict* what the mouse might do and what actions

# CHAPTER two

will be needed. It needs a *good spatial sense* to gauge the pounce accurately. The cat needs *clear brain choices* throughout the process, and for this it needs a *calm nervous system*. It needs to "inhibit" – to hold back on pouncing too soon and choose to proceed only when the moment is right. It also needs to be fully present – conscious – to carry out the hunt successfully. Distractions usually result in losing the mouse. When all these factors are employed well (our cat is presumably always *embodied*) the resulting *responsive movements* – stalking, pouncing, catching and eating – have a good chance of being successful.

In hunting and other similar activities, cats have several advantages over the average Westernized human. The cat's body is probably organized efficiently, with free joints, lengthened muscles with dynamically modulating tone, the bones well aligned. They breathe easily and freely, and appropriately for their activity (did you ever see a cat puffing?). Cats don't go in for overthinking the procedure, so they can let their natural abilities work for them without anything getting in the way. Neither, probably, do they have negative beliefs such as that hunting always fails for them. Being present, they receive all the information of their environment – the plants and scents, wind direction, etc. in spatial relationship, updating yesterday's maps of the garden moment by moment, rather than taking yesterday's remembered environment as most of the story. In the moments of stalking and leaping their whole being is organized in relationship to the mouse, in the context of the environment. The more that this is so, the higher the chance of success.

### The gains and losses of human evolution

But as human evolution dovetailed into human history we moved in a very different direction. Our evolution from primates has been an amazing process, where body and brain have evolved together. It is theorized that brachiation – swinging through the treetops –required much greater acrobatic skill, with attention, spatial perception, and an ability to do fast complex calculations of trajectories that required a vastly bigger brain which could plan ahead (Barton and Venditti 2017). Brachiation also built different arm muscles for hurling ourselves forwards. These developments meant that when we returned to the ground, we could be bipedal, with arm muscles that could hurl a spear, and with the visual, spatial and planning abilities to do so.

Bipedalism opened the way for tool use, and a different use of the mind, which now could move around – into the body, into the tool, or into the world. Our brain maps acquired the plasticity to extend to include the tools in our sense of ourselves – as when you use a fork, you have the sensitivity you would have in your fingertips (Blakeslee and Blakeslee 2008: 139).

When language began to emerge (50,000–70,000 years ago,) it hugely developed the left hemisphere with its sequential thinking. A whole new neural architecture was developed that allowed us the necessary cognitive fluidity to invent, store, and retrieve thousands of symbols, all with grammatical constructions and associations. Language liberated thought and communication from the experienced present and from the constraints of time and space, allowing our minds to soar in creative freedom. But the right hemisphere was still hugely involved – giving language its tone, emotion, and rhythm, bringing depth, color, context, and social connection to our communications.

Literacy (only a few thousand years old) has hugely increased this liberation of thought from the present reality, and with increasingly sophisticated symbolizing of our world. This has now speeded up exponentially into the computer age, where we can live our days in virtual reality, switching consciousness modes as easily as switching TV channels. But at a cost. Our modern challenge is to maintain any awareness of our embodied selves, in the face of this enormously powerful and immersive left hemisphere-based symbolic thinking. This is demanded increasingly by our society and is insidiously displacing the primary knowledge of ourselves.

The cost is not just to our movement patterns, but also to our sense of ourselves, our connection to each other and to our world. A sense of nihilism, alienation,

# What has been lost, and the twelve fundamentals of movement

and increasing despair is the legacy of neglecting our right hemispheres. This huge social and emotional cost is to ourselves individually and to society as a whole (McGilchrist 2012: 407).

Living in the head, in abstract thought, is not fully living. The journey back to integrated movement not only reclaims the whole-body and its full range of fluid action, but also reclaims the embodied self, the calm content self, the nicer, more socially comfortable self, and the more open and exploratory self. They are indivisible. We need to learn to bring our primary neural architecture, such as the cat or monkey possesses, back into play alongside our new neural architecture as we raise and educate children, learn new skills, work on computers and live fulfilling lives. We are currently only accessing a fraction of our neurology. What potential might we possess if we learn to use all our brain and body networks together?

## Introducing the twelve fundamentals of integrated movement

The twelve fundamentals defined here encompass the principles that lie behind the cat's unconscious and elegant movement (Fig. 2.4). They are our keys for

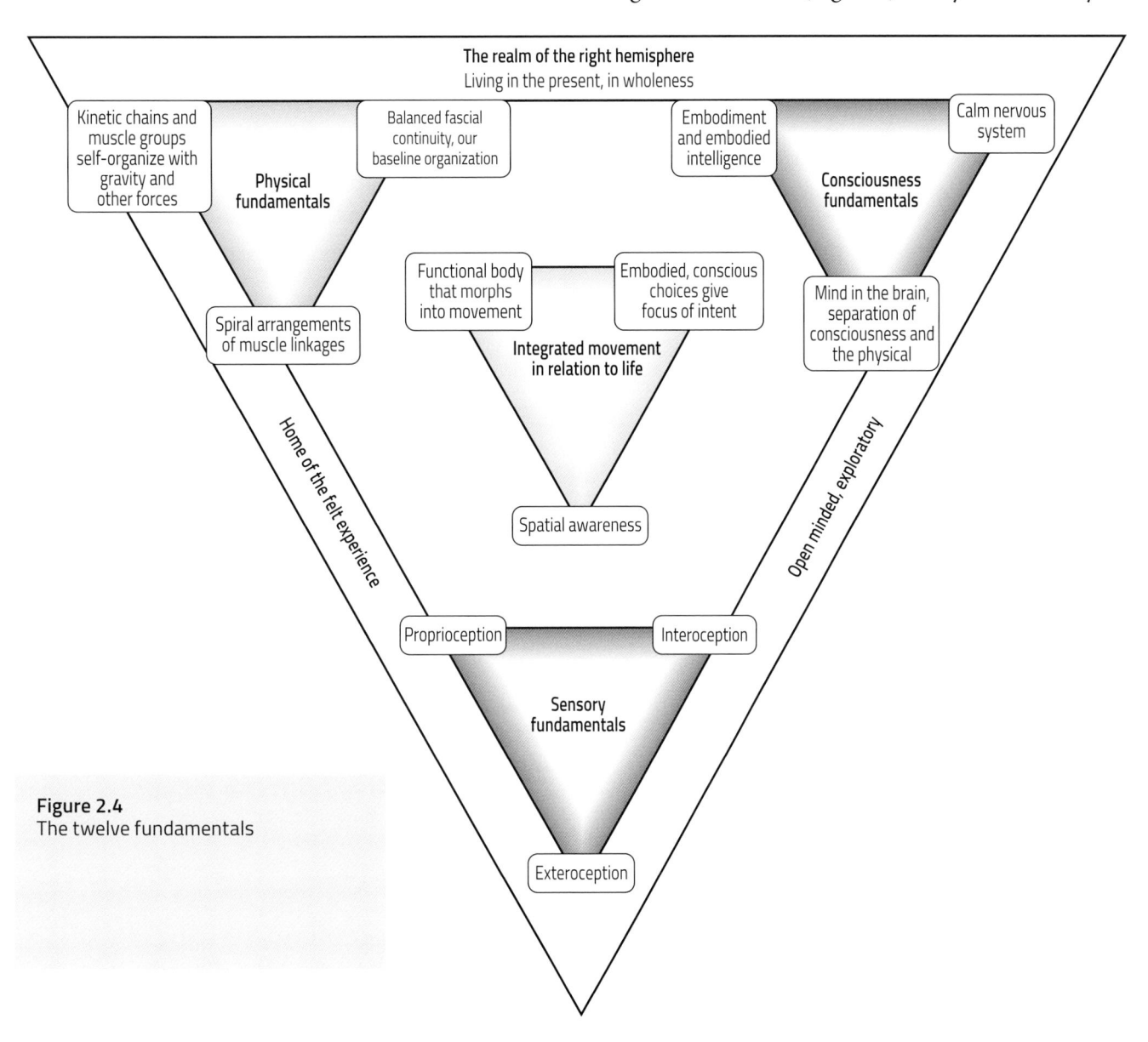

Figure 2.4
The twelve fundamentals

# CHAPTER two

returning our structure and functioning to its birthright, and in doing so, to reclaim our whole-brain whole-body networks. But unlike the cat, we need to learn to work consciously with the unconscious processes.

Integrated movement is a cake that could be cut in many ways, but to find a doorway into new experiences I have picked out twelve fundamentals that are usable as tools for our process. These can be divided into four groups of three or three groups of four. To the body, though, they are all one, and as we get deeper into the book, distinctions will become less meaningful as we work with the whole. If it suits you to redraw the lines for yourself, then go ahead!

Be aware as you read through them that they may not resonate with you as true if they are currently outside your experience. As you proceed through the explorations, my hope is that they will explain themselves. The next three chapters introduce each of these fundamentals (though not in the order given below).

### Summary of the twelve fundamentals

Four structural fundamentals

1. **A balanced fascial continuity**, our baseline organization.
2. A self-organizing structure of muscles, ligaments, tendons, and bones, in lengthening antagonistic relationships, **aligning with gravity** and other forces.
3. **Spiral arrangement** of muscle linkages, enabling movement.

4. These together give:
   - a **fully functional body, balanced with dynamic modulation of postural tone, poised for action**. This, along with all the other fundamentals, enables *emergent integrated movement*.

Four sensory fundamentals

5. External perception of the world around us.
6. Proprioception.
7. Internal perception of drives, emotions, moods, intuitions.
8. Together, these give:
   - **spatial awareness:** of the body and environment, and orientation to gravity.

Four consciousness fundamentals

9. A calm, balanced nervous system.
10. Where you think from: mind in the brain.
11. Embodiment, leading to embodied thinking throughout the brain/whole-body intelligence system.
12. Together, these enable:
    - **clear choices from the brain/embodied intelligence.** "Inhibition" of old patterns (verbally, or as a quiet, tonic state) allows new choices to be made, *giving a clear focus of intent*.

This allows new movements to emerge.

# What has been lost, and the twelve fundamentals of movement

## Alexander's fundamentals

While I believe Alexander was using all the fundamentals I have listed, he only defined seven of them:

1. The need for a balanced physical structure, lengthening and widening with free joints.
2. Self-observation – i.e. of proprioception.
3. Calming reactivity.
4. Clear thinking with inhibition (stopping), from which a new reasoned choice can be made.
5. Thinking directions – the lines along which the body expands and moves.
6. A goal of movement – to be carried out with "means whereby" (with conscious reasoned directing of the body), rather than with "end-gaining" (only task-focused, with no thought or awareness of how it is carried out).
7. By employing these six factors, the resultant movement then brings about a new level of integration.

Alexander did not define where we think from, or the need for embodiment, although Goldie, from whom I learned these, indicated she got them from him. Neither did he define the need to be in relationship to the task, or to the external environment and spatial perception – aspects that were clearly understood by Irene Tasker, Miss Goldie, Erika Whittaker and Marjory Barlow, the teachers involved in the small school– though there was a sense that he knew all about this.

Interoception was not defined by any of them, though they would have included it in self-awareness.

"Direction" is not a clear-cut concept, and is a source of endless debate, because it is not a fundamental at all. With directions, we use deliberate conscious thought (Alexander's "constructive conscious control") to bring the physical structure of the body back into an expanded, balanced, embodied state, and into integrated movement. As such, it a reparative process which animals do not have. I see it as a composite process involving varying brain and nervous system fundamentals (see Chapter 4).

Likewise, inhibition has been greatly misunderstood. On its own, it is a recipe for shutting down the life force. "Non-doing" can become "not-doing." The deeper inhibitory process, which Alexander used to develop the technique and which I learned from Goldie, was rarely made explicit. One inhibits fully to quieten all reactivity, from which one can review and make a fresh choice, saying "yes!" to the next move. This brings us more fully alive (see Chapter 15).

# CHAPTER two

### *The twelve fundamentals in more detail*

The three primary physical fundamentals

1  A balanced fascial continuity (fascintegrity), our baseline organization (Chapter 3, lesson 4).

2  A self-organizing structure aligning with gravity and other forces: finding physical balance. Every part is in lengthening, tensioned relationship to every other part (Chapter 3, lesson 4).

3  Spiraling arrangement of muscle linkages: these bend, flex, and twist the structure in all planes (Chapter 3, lesson 4).

Our physical bodies are immensely complex, with 700 or more muscles in dynamic interplay with 206 bones. These need to be aligned precisely for an optimal relationship with gravity and to have every part in both opposition and harmony with every other part – a balance of lengthening antagonistic relationships. The spiraling arrangements create not only movement within the structure itself but also the torque that powers movement. We need to understand and learn how to use these forces together, to give stable, strong, and versatile bodies. In such a structure, every joint is free to move with every muscle working with adaptive muscle tone to be available for use in every moment, so that the structure can flow into dynamic movement with appropriate force.

The three primary sensory fundamentals

4  External perception (Chapter 4, lesson 1). The five external senses. Mostly we live in our heads, without truly seeing, hearing, or touching what is around us as an artist or musician might, not tasting our food as a chef might. We need to be *receptive* to what we see, hear, taste, smell, and touch, present to what is really happening around us, rather than assuming we know. This is a prerequisite for spatial perception. When we allow what we see and perceive to "touch" us, then we link with our interoception; this is a prerequisite for fully embodied, focused movement.

5  Proprioceptive awareness (Chapter 3, lesson 1). We need to bring our proprioception – our sense of what our muscles and joints are doing – more into conscious awareness, so we can improve our brain "maps" and redirect our physical functioning.

6  Internal perception – interoception (Chapter 4, lesson 3). Movement evolved to meet our internal needs: our hunger or thirst, need for shelter or a mate, need to escape danger or boredom. Having perception of our drives, emotions, moods, joys, and urges allows us to link our internal states with our external actions, giving them more clarity and integration.

The three primary consciousness fundamentals

7  A calm and balanced nervous system. We need the parasympathetic nervous system to be in charge, even in the face of strong stimuli. Without this, we lose awareness of self, our sense of the whole environment, and our capacity to think clearly – we are stressed (Chapter 5).

8  Where we think from: *mind in the brain* (Chapter 4, lesson 4). This immense physical complexity cannot be controlled directly from the individual body parts: when one part is prioritized over another, imbalances and tensions will be created. If you want to drive your car, you don't push the wheels and swipe the windscreen wipers, you get into the driving seat where you have access to all the controls. The control panels of posture and movement are in maps in the brain and spinal cord. We need to bring the mind to the brain, where it can interface easily with these maps, and to stop it interfering directly with the body. Later, we can move to whole-brain/embodied thinking (see Chapter 4, lesson 6). So your brain is the physical control system (i.e. the switches and controls of the car) but the mind is the conscious driver that works the controls.

# What has been lost, and the twelve fundamentals of movement

> The definition of "mind" is a controversial topic, with countless books and theories having been written about it. I follow Miss Goldie's practical explanation of "mind": the element of consciousness which can move around.
>
> Consciousness is another huge subject of debate. My practical definition is: *consciousness* is the awareness of some phenomenon, in the world or within the self, which allows us the option to choose our response.

9  Embodiment and embodied thinking (Chapter 4, lesson 5). There is a paradox in that we need to get our conscious processes – our mind – out of the way of the body, not *feeling* into it, and yet with full *awareness* of the body so the brain maps are always updated and there is a fully flowing connection between brain and body. The resolution of this paradox gives us embodied thinking: when we are consciously present in our fronts and backs, left and right, up and down, we can utilize and integrate all our neural networks. Embodiment is like having your TV on stand-by, always ready to go into action when needed.

   Are we back at the age-old split between mind and body? Or is this different? Previously, the mind (spirit/consciousness, or later the brain) was seen as in charge of, and superior to, the physical body. But where science seems to be heading, and what I trust you will experience for yourself, is that the brain is just one part of the body's systems, connected to them all in a vast, cooperative, and highly communicative network, separate and yet inseparable from it. Mind in the brain is one part of embodied consciousness and embodied thinking, again separate yet inseparable. And the embodied consciousness (or as some scientists are calling it, the "experienced body"), together with the networking physical body, are in an interweaving dance together – separate yet inseparable.

## The three emergent fundamentals

10  Spatial awareness: *3D perception of body and the environment* (Chapter 4, lesson 6). To navigate us through the world, the nervous system must give us an internal three-dimensional representation of ourselves – our own avatar – as well as a three-dimensional representation of the external world, along with a sense of how the first fits inside the second. Spatial awareness is the key to both, and some systems, such as the vestibular system, are involved in both. Spatial awareness is such a crucial factor for all aspects of life and health, and is so rarely discussed. Our visual spatial awareness of the environment is handled through the dorsal visual stream (Chapter 15). Spatial awareness is processed mostly unconsciously, in the right hemisphere, in the present, and when working well it brings us into the flow. But when we are working more from the left hemisphere, we are working more from a conscious, remembered state which is less efficient (Chapter 16). Our three primary coordinates of space, perceived by the vestibular system (Chapter 8, lesson 2), are also part of this. The primary of these is gravity, with which we need to be in precise alignment. When our sensory inputs are in play together in the embodied self, we have a unified field of attention in the present.

11  Embodied conscious thinking: clear brain choices (Chapter 4, lesson 2; Chapter 15). Clear brain choices allow us to stop and take stock of a situation rather than to react; the process of stopping is "inhibition." From there we can make new choices, form plans with a clear focus of intent, and then give the go ahead. (Inhibition and excitation are originally neurological terms; they are yes/no gates. An inhibitory process stops a nerve or neuron from firing, an excitatory process stimulates it. This is synaptic inhibition.) Inhibition is the key to neurological change. Our nervous systems are now primed for many habitual patterns of action that are unhelpful. We can only bring about change by inhibiting the old pattern.

# CHAPTER two

But inhibition is not an end in itself and if used this way it stops life flowing. Unfortunately this was part of many of our childhoods – "stop this," "stop that …" – so that the word "no" often has negative connotations. Alexander work often uses phrases to access inhibitory processes, such as "I can do less"; however, we need to remember to use these. There is also a deeper level of inhibition which is very different. Miss Goldie taught that inhibition is a moment of quiet attention, of waiting, so that previously unknown movements can emerge. We say "no" to say "yes." This is a positive, right hemisphere process where we can pause a moment to observe – finding the bigger picture – and then modulate our responses.

This process of quiet inhibition facilitates dynamic modulation of postural tone. Then it feels as if the action does itself. Any action or process – breathing and swallowing, seeing and touching, running and grasping, rational thinking or intense grieving – can be modulated by inhibition to reawaken the natural balance that has been lost, and allow an easier flow in the present.

12 Emergent movement (Chapter 4, lesson 7). When we are in relationship with our world there is always a focus of movement: maybe a cup to be grasped; a friend we are walking towards; a purpose to scan a website. This contrasts with the state of being lost in thought, or aimlessly net-surfing, in which there is little clear perception or relationship. When the whole-body system perceives the goal of movement, then it is in relationship to it with real metrics, attuned to it. The focused goal then draws the appropriate movement from the whole-body system in an explosion of changing spatial relationships. The whole-body moves as a coherent unit, not as a collection of body parts where one leads and the others are pulled along.

When the first eleven fundamentals are in dynamic dance together, with the fully functional physical structure informed by the fully operative sensory systems, along with embodied conscious presence and choices, then the quality of movement changes. We do not move as a deliberate willed act, forcing the movement. Instead we morph into movement with dynamic modulation of tone, feeling as if the body moves us, drawn and directed by the attunement to the goal. Emergent movement then has clarity, strength, purpose, coordination, and fluidity.

In this, the body with its senses, nervous systems, and consciousness is "self-organizing." This phrase comes from dynamic systems theory, and was taken up by the movement sciences in the 1990s.

"Behaviour emerges from the interaction of multiple sub-systems, including experience. Behaviors are assembled in the moment and context of the current movement task. While it is efficient to develop stable behaviors for recurring task categories, these behaviors need not be encoded in detail in the system. Flexibility and adaptability can coexist with stability when solutions to movement problems are softly assembled and remain plastic" (Buchanan and Ulrich 2001).

This could be called Alexander's key discovery: that behavior is not dependent on learned habits, but can self-organize to the requirement of the moment.

### A new approach to voluntary activities

Innate movement patterns such as breathing, swallowing, even walking, are organized in the central pattern generators CPGs – oscillating mini-circuits in spinal cord and brainstem. They provide a whole network of little modules that can interact in different combinations for flexibility of movement. But mostly I consider we have overlaid these with inefficient movement habits held higher in the brain. By inhibiting these overlaid habitual tensions, we can return to our natural movements. But what about voluntary actions, like turning a tap? Much is written in modern neuroscience about movement pathways being predictive, so that the brain does not have to work from scratch each time, and has pre-formed responses ready to roll out at speed as the moment requires. The hand approaching the tap is already shaped to the grasp required, the muscles tensed for the strain needed.

# What has been lost, and the twelve fundamentals of movement

Prediction is necessary, but it also needs to be accompanied by conscious awareness. Modern life encourages us to be reliant on prediction, taking us into autopilot. We can make a predictive response to, say, opening our kitchen cupboard, because the spatial details are unchanging. For people picking berries, every aspect of the movement varies for every berry, needing responsive touch, not predictive. The environments we evolved in were always changing; modern life is more invariant. We then "satisfice" – making "good enough" predictions from a limited range of sensory data.

Miss Goldie wanted me to become conscious in the present of my actions. Surely that is what the great sportspeople or musicians are doing, with their phenomenal coordination and energy? I believe we can all have this ability. By bringing the nervous system to quiet calm, with full attention in the present, our predictive mechanisms have fully updated sensorimotor information and there is internal time to process it fully. We can respond intelligently in any given moment to the situation; we can be in the driving seat of our lives. This also opens the way for accelerated learning, rather than the laborious left hemisphere, trial and error methods we expect to use. We can learn to use our brains more intelligently (see Chapter 16).

## Time and space and rhythm

The following story illustrates how many Westernized people, stressed at work, experience time and space, and how for my pupil Terri this was redressed. Terri is a pharmacist. Every month she must sort and double-check all the prescriptions for a nursing home, a huge piece of work; even the thought felt overwhelming. Terri would often over-check (the left hemisphere can get stuck on tasks and cannot move on). Her whole-body would tense, making the work slow and exhausting (left hemisphere has no sense of body or movement), despite wanting to jump quickly from one to another to get it done (left hemisphere has no sense of time and snatches at tasks).

We worked to find her spatial relationship to the task. Before doing each prescription, she found she could step back, finding her own space and body (right hemisphere perceives and connects to the body), and her spatial relationship to the task (right hemisphere has depth perception and spatial relationships). Next, she looked at the photo of the person, finding relationship to that individual (right hemisphere recognizes faces and has empathy). Then she could step forward and allow the movements required to happen with much more flow and integration, that freed off the tensions and kept her relaxed through the task (spatial perception brought in whole-body coordination). She then found she could check her work once and let it go. As each prescription was completed, she took another moment to step back and repeat this process (right hemisphere has a sense of time and flow). Soon, the task felt like it was doing itself, and became an integral part of the flow of the month, rather than a mountain to be climbed. Her anxiety and tension around the task, along with the sense of not enough time, all melted away. Terri became a much happier person!

The differences between the old and new approaches outlined here can be summarized as shown in Table 2.1.

## Seven new proposals for integrated movement

Emerging from the twelve fundamentals, I offer seven bold new proposals. They all are based on my experiences and observations and all need research. Some of these spring-board from the work of others, as will be described later. I believe Alexander and Miss Goldie were using these, whether consciously or not:

1. A new model of postural alignment, that optimally facilitates stability and mobility together (Chapter 7: torso and Chapter 8: legs and feet). All muscles are toned in lengthening antagonistic relationship.

2. A proposed model of embodied perception and whole-body intelligence (Chapter 4, lesson 5). All senses are awake and we are present.

# CHAPTER two

| Table 2.1 Old and new science models | |
|---|---|
| **Old science models** | **New science models** |
| Our parts add up to our whole | You cannot separate the parts from the whole |
| Our structure is purely gravity stacked | Our structure is self-organized by lengthening antagonistic relationships, many in curve / spiral patterns, aligned with gravity |
| Muscles work in antagonistic pairs | Muscles work in groups, in relation to the whole |
| Movement happens independently | Movement emerges out of relationship to ourselves and our environment |
| The head makes us human, the body is animal | The body is a key part of being human |
| Reason is superior to emotion and intuition | Reason is underpinned by emotion and intuition |
| Body envisaged as machine | Body envisaged as process |
| Organization is top-down, brain-led | Organization is in networks, whole-body, sensory-led |
| Left hemisphere leads | Right hemisphere leads |
| Time is uniform | There are multilayered flows of time |
| Thinking is two-dimensional | Thinking is three-dimensional |
| Science underpinned by Newton's physics | Science may be underpinned by quantum physics |

3  That there are two distinct types of inhibition: the processes of executive inhibition (whether reactive or proactive/selective) and the state of tonic inhibition, which for many years I have called the state of quiet, or deeper inhibition (Chapter 4, lesson 2).

4  When these three work together in the quiet, tonic, right hemisphere-led state, all our fundamentals network together, self-organizing, to give us integrated movement (Chapter 4, lesson 7).

5  I suggest that not only posture, but also movement can happen through evolutionarily older, self-organizing hindbrain pathways using dynamic modulation. I call this morphing into action, as our plastic, self-organizing systems sort the optimal body geometry required in the moment. With greater stability from this, only the phasic muscles needed for a precision task are recruited, increasing dexterity (Chapters 6 and 15).

6  Through bringing the nervous system to an alive place of non-reaction and open possibilities, we can then act responsively to coordinate with tasks, solving the challenge of coordinated movement anew each time. Learning becomes an experiential process of connection rather than top-down orders and repetition drilling a new pathway (Chapters 15 and 16).

7  That movement is led both from the senses – for us mostly the vision, which organizes the head and then spine to follow (Chapter 4, lesson 7) – and simultaneously from the lower torso, organized and stabilized through the lumbar and sacral spine and thoracolumbar fascia (Chapters 6, 10, and 11), with its links to the whole-body and limbs. I suggest that finding this is the real purpose of chairwork.

3

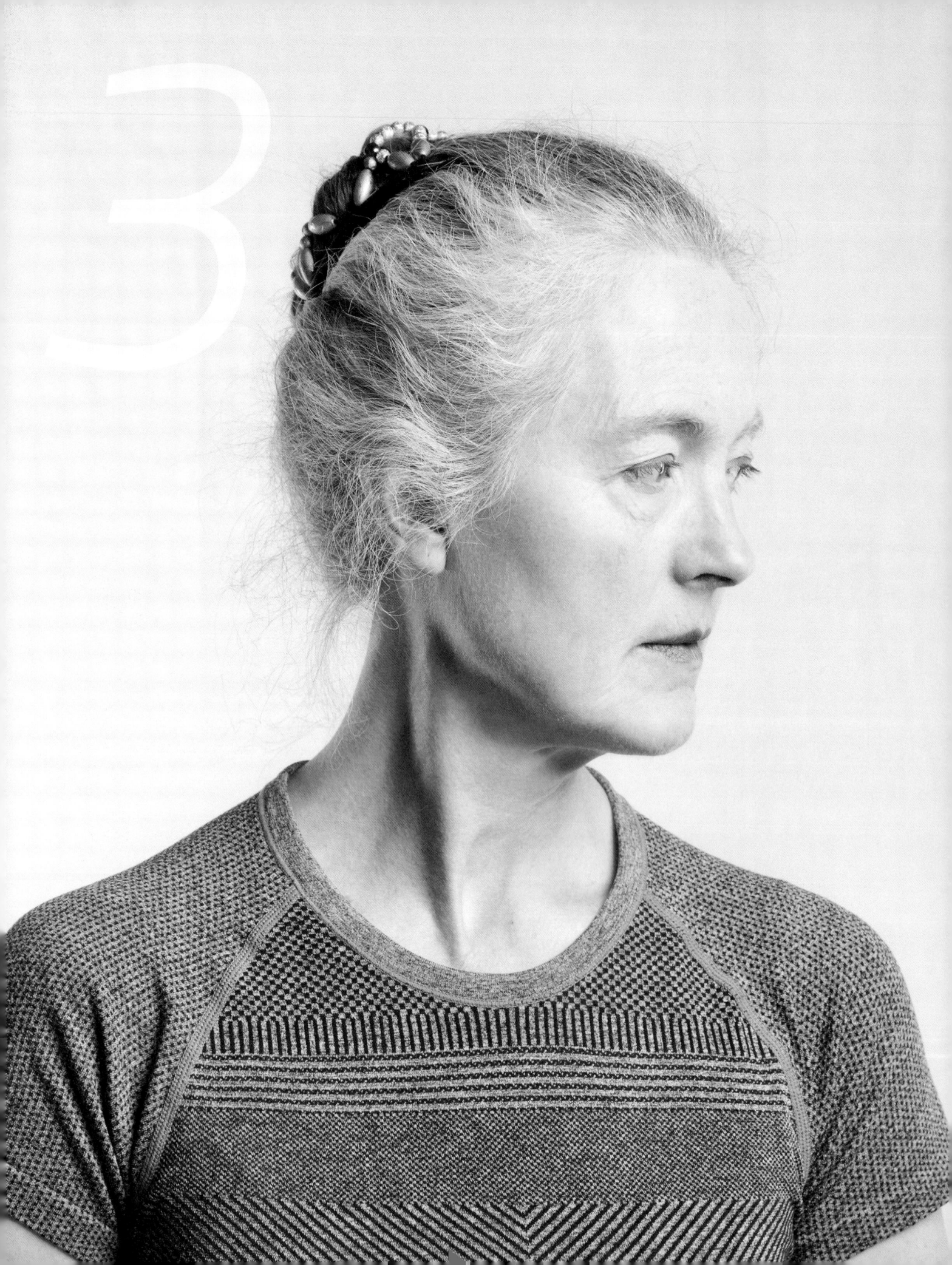

# The fundamentals of structure 3

## Lesson 1  Waking up proprioception

### Becoming aware of how you stand, sit and move, and discovering our tensions from the inside

If we are to reawaken what we've lost – that is, our evolutionary legacy – changes are needed to both structure and nervous system. But first we need to know what we are doing right now: we need to reawaken awareness of the body.

### Exploration 3.1  Getting in and out of a chair

- *Start by sitting down in a chair and then standing up, and ask yourself, how did I do that?*

If you are unfamiliar with the Alexander process, you probably have no idea. You may be aware of an area hurting, but this does not tell you what the body is doing. For instance, your shoulder may be hurting, but that does not inform you if it is higher than the other one, or lifts and crunches up to your ears as you sit and stand, etc. You will need a friend to observe or a selfie video to discover this, or, if you think you do know, to confirm that your self-observation is correct. *Actions that we perform repeatedly are mostly subconscious, and we need to bring them to consciousness by waking up the proprioceptive sense.*

Notice whether you are in the top-down approach of left hemisphere thinking, referenced as it is to right or wrong, where we are more likely to feel criticized or "caught out" by noticing something, and so less likely to explore. Instead, come to the right hemisphere place of curiosity – observe yourself as a scientist would observe animal behavior, free of judgment. I invite you to come to beginner's mind and have a go, whatever your thinking tells you. At birth we were given these amazing bodies and minds, but nobody gave us the instruction manual! This book (with its accompanying video tutorials) is such a manual, and we start from where we start from. If you do still have a critical voice (I'll never be good enough/I'm a mess, etc.) then say hello to it, thank it for its help in your life so far, and tell it that now you will travel a different path. Let it be there and learn to ignore it.

- *Sit and stand again. What do my hands do? Do they go to my legs? If so, do they push, lightly or hard? Or slide? Do they go for the chair? Or do they swing forwards?*

Watching ourselves intently can change our use. Instead, observe yourself lightly, without getting involved – just sit down, then just stand up again.

Try videoing yourself side on, for an objective look. Is this what you perceived internally? Have another go without the video. Can you now pick up the sense of what you saw on the video?

### Video link  for exploration 3.1

### The proprioceptive sense and faulty sensory perception

We are tuning into *proprioception*, the internal sense of our body's position and motion in space. There are several sense organs for this. *Muscle spindles* are stretch receptors. Sited in fascia and muscle, they are little coiled springs registering how stretched or contracted the muscle is. The *Golgi tendon organs* tell us how much force of contraction is being generated by the muscle. *Joint receptors* tell us the joint angle, how much pressure there is across the joint surface, and, when moving, how fast it is bending.

All this data is fed back to your brain, brainstem, and spinal cord, and processed there. In particular, the brain asks "is this data different from the usual data?" If not, it is deemed unimportant and stays subconscious, unless we choose otherwise. It is like walking into a room with a bowl of hyacinths on the table. Initially the heavenly scent of the flowers hits us, but after five minutes our brain has screened this out and we don't smell them anymore – until we choose to

# CHAPTER three

do so. We are choosing to bring information to consciousness that the brain thinks is okay and safe to ignore.

But it may not be okay! When change happens slowly, the brain adjusts to the new patterns and now considers them the correct ones. The held information against which actions are compared is now incorrect. To use a computer analogy, we are using the wrong default settings. We call this **faulty sensory perception,** and it particularly seems to apply to the muscle spindle data. Because of it, "wrong" use feels right, and when we do start to make changes, we might notice that "right" use feels wrong. So wrong and right cease to be useful concepts.

We need simply to observe what is happening, with no judgment. "Body use that is more or less efficient" is a more useful way of viewing it. Your hands may swing wildly forward to hoist you out of the chair – but they achieve the goal. Without them you'd be stuck on your backside till someone pulled you out. Whatever our bodies are currently doing *does* work, even if it is giving us pain.

If we want fully efficient, fully integrated movement patterns we need to change these default patterns. Chronic pain or tension mostly comes out of how we are performing everyday movements, yet their discomfort often prompts people to rush into fixing the "problem" with no regard for their own part in it.

### The importance of proprioception

It used to be thought that proprioceptive sensors were only in muscles. It has been suggested that the fascia has about six times as many sensory nerves as red muscle (Schleip 2012). Fascia is the connective tissue that weaves around and through all tissues, and provides the gliding interfaces between shifting layers of muscles and the more immobile skin. Therapists working with fascia notice that when muscles are chronically shortened or lengthened, the fascia around them becomes disorganized or thickened and cannot glide.

With no stretch on the muscle or fascia, it seems that the stretch receptors are disabled, and proprioception diminishes, reducing body awareness. This may increase potential for injury (Scheirling 2017).

### Exploration 3.2   Noticing every part of your body

Now ask questions for each part of the body. Keep standing up and sitting down, using feedback from video, mirror, or helper, so the answers are from experience, not assumption – you'll probably want to guess the answers. If you do the action differently each time, you are noticing all the movements in your current "movement bank."

Some people tune in to this more easily than others. If you are one of those people that cannot feel anything, don't worry! Just use video or a partner's help. With time the internal awareness will come. If you think you imagine it, that's ok. Imagining is a pathway that sensitizes us to a to new awareness.

- *What is happening in your hands, arms, elbows, shoulders?*
- *Does your back curve forwards, curve back, or stay straight? Does your pelvis rock forward or back?*
- *What gets you out of the chair? Is there some propelling thrust or weight shift? What gets you into the chair?*
- *Do your legs work hard, or your feet? What do your knees do?*
- *What do your neck, head, and chin do?*
- *Do you stay straight on to the chair, or do you twist to one side? Overall, does your body use feel light and easy, or heavy and labored?*

Stay present with what you see.

- *When you notice something, can you stop, be present with it, rather than immediately changing it?*

# The fundamentals of structure

- *If, for instance your head is pulled back on your neck, notice if it feels comfortable to you. The brain may tell you this, because it is your normal use. But stay with it, and you may become aware of the pressure on the neck joints, or tension in the muscles, which are uncomfortable. This lets your brain register what is really happening and updates the brain maps.*

Video link for exploration 3.2

Our culture tends to weigh everything as wrong or right, and when something is wrong, it must immediately put it right. This is left hemisphere, top-down thinking, where everything we do comes with an interpretation and a story, and it makes us reactive. The right hemisphere, led by bottom-up sensory awareness, simply notices and explores what it finds.

### Patterns of contraction and the problems they cause

You are probably noticing patterns of contraction. Figures 3.1–3.3 show three common patterns in their more extreme archetypal forms, often seen in older people. But if you observe closely, you can see the same patterns at work in younger people – and maybe in yourself.

## Lesson 2   We are fighting gravity as we move

All these tensions are serving to hold us up and to stop us falling as we stand, sit, or move. We are fighting gravity. Movement into the chair is often done carefully, particularly as people get older.

### Exploration 3.3   Fighting gravity

- *Look again at the pattern of your movement and ask: where am I tensing in order not to fall as I sit down? In my back? Arm or shoulders? Neck? Legs or hips?*

People will often use hands on their knees when moving on and off a chair to take pressure off a weak or painful back. But I feel that there is often a subtler pattern at work. I notice that we put our hands onto our knees, even with the lightest touch, because the upper body is misaligned and could fall forwards; hands on knees are preventing or guarding against this. People who let their hands hang by their sides as they move often put extra tension into their spines. Or we might instead brace the knees, or across our shoulders or upper back. When misaligned people don't tense, they drop into the chair. To stand again they have to push or pull the weight of the body against gravity.

### The reasons for physical problems

If you have physical problems, you may now have clues as to why they are occurring. For instance, neck/headache problems are associated with forward-held head and lifted chin (protraction), while shoulder problems usually occur when we tense, lift, or pull them as we sit or stand. You may be letting one part of the body weigh down heavily on a lower part. If you lean back with your upper back while standing, the upper torso collapses down onto the lower lumbar spine, compressing it and causing problems. Knee and foot problems often occur when people bear down heavily on their knees or legs. People with hip problems likewise may be moving heavily and/or standing misaligned. Since most people do some version of one or more of these patterns, it is little wonder that so many people have problems or pain.

### Layers of muscles work together to hold the skeleton in alignment

Standing upright is a precarious business. The human skeleton is the opposite of any classically engineered stable structure with a wide base: 206 bones, six major leg joints to hinge or rotate, twenty-six vertebrae supporting a prominent ribcage topped by a heavy, nodding head, all balanced on slim, multi-jointed feet.

# CHAPTER three

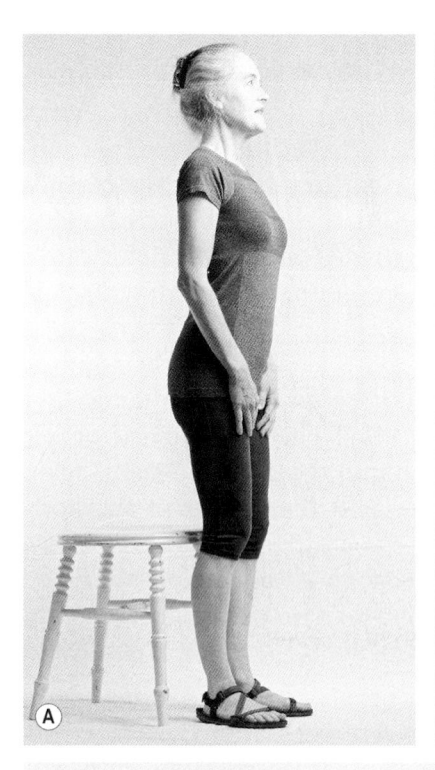

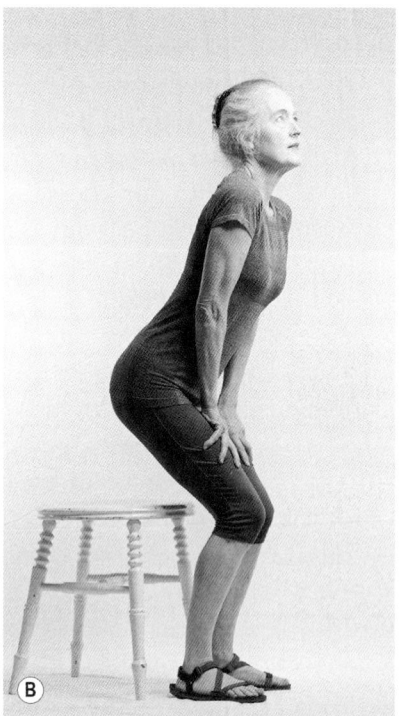

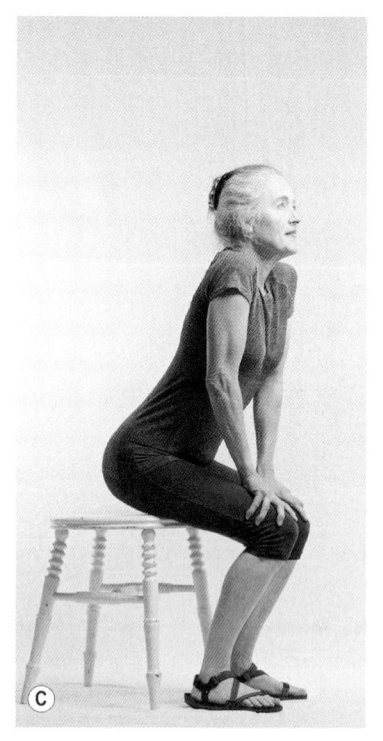

**Figure 3.1A–C**
"Tight secretary" sitting. Often starts with a stance in which chest and chin are lifted. Constricted neck, arched lumbar, weight supported by hands on thighs, which raises and compresses the shoulders, knees falling together

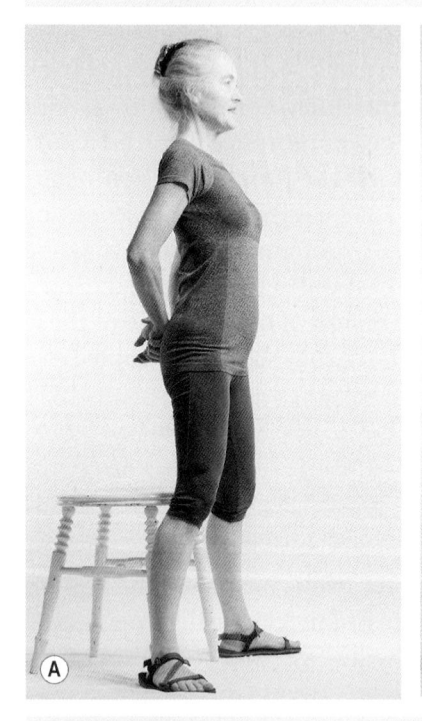

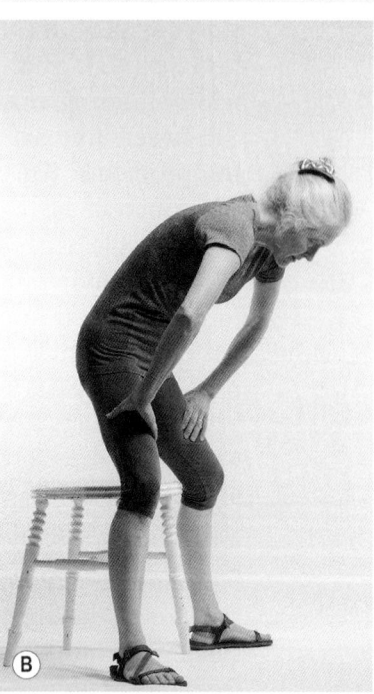

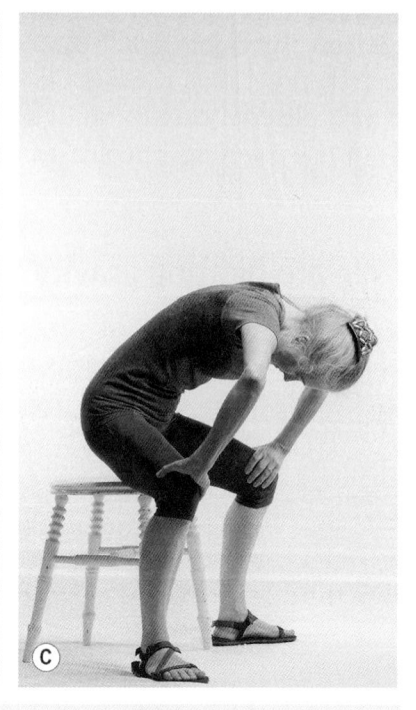

**Figures 3.2A–C**
"Big man" sitting. Often starts with a pushed forward stance in hips and ribs. The head and upper body drop, supported with hands on knees, the shoulders raise, and the hips round. On sitting, the legs are often wide apart and the lower back and pelvis are completely rounded, giving no support to the upper body, which then must round also

# The fundamentals of structure

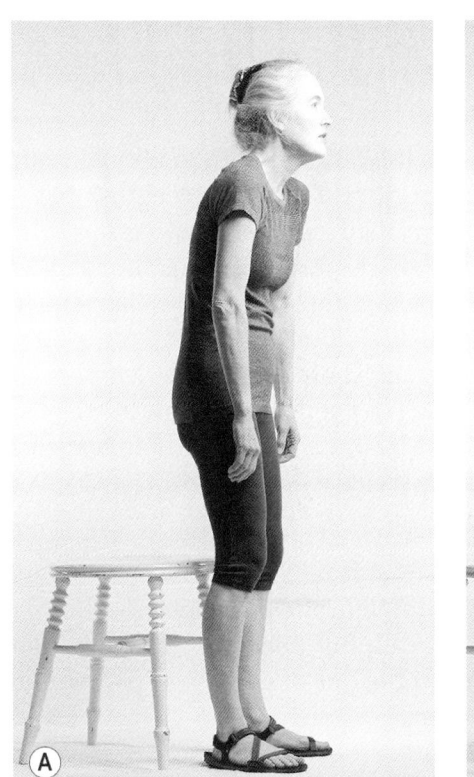

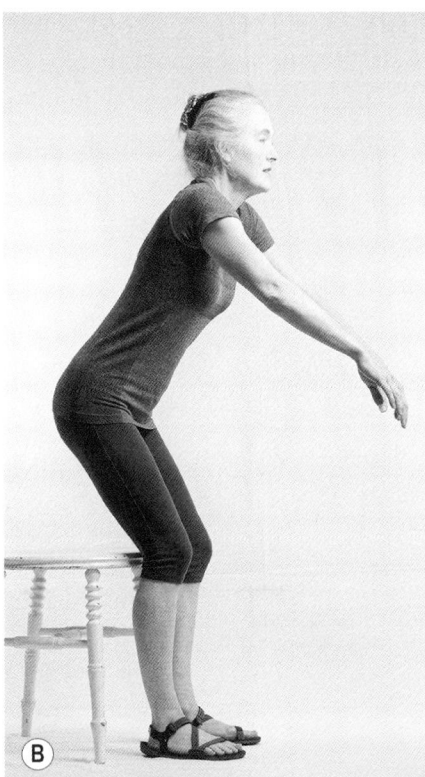

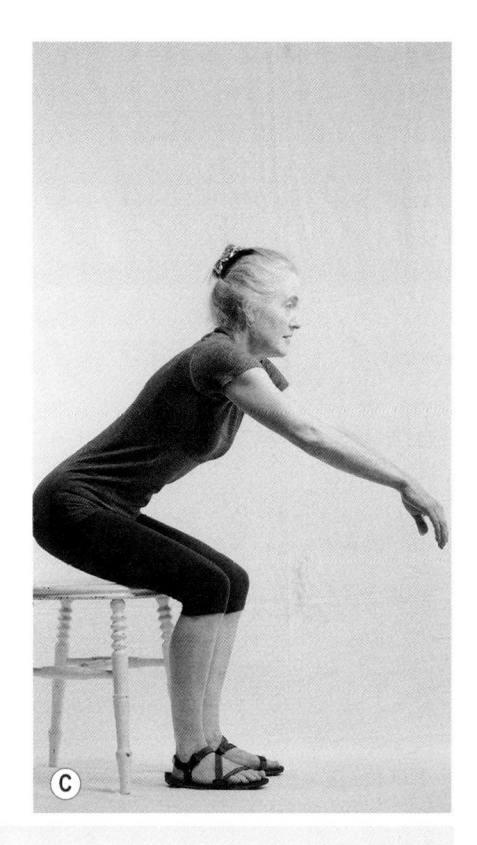

**Figures 3.3A–C**
"Fat old lady" sitting, where the backside goes too far back towards the chair, the arms hold forward in a struggle to maintain balance, and then lose it at the last moment, so the person drops heavily into the chair. Getting out is even more of a strain, requiring substantial lifting of the shoulders. The next stage, when this no longer works, is to need one of those chairs that catapult you out!

Even the torso base, the pelvis, has three bones. How do we keep it all together?

The musculature is arranged in several layers, with *postural muscles* deeper in, and action muscles overlaid. The slender postural muscles have slow twitch fibers that can sustain contractions continually. They are controlled by oscillating "programs," like Christmas tree lights where different groups of lights fade in and out continually making a slow dance. At any given time only a third of the nerves are firing so that one third of the muscles are contracting, then the next third in sequence. This needs high oxygen levels so postural muscle is richly vascularized and is red in color (like chicken leg meat).

Our big *"action" muscles* are superficial, and are sometimes called phasic muscles, because they often work in oscillating patterns of contraction and release, such as in walking or throwing actions. They have solely or mostly fast twitch fibers, designed for fast, strong movement and then release rather than for sustained contraction to hold us upright. They have much less vascular supply as they work more anaerobically, so are pale in color (like chicken breast meat).

### There are three main layers to the back

The deepest layer, the tiny muscles that run between the vertebral spines, are true postural muscles

# CHAPTER three

(Fig. 3.4) that between them twist, tilt, and bend the vertebrae on the tiny facet joints. A healthy spine is fully mobile.

The next muscle layer is the *erector spinae* muscles. They run the length of the spine from the base of the skull down to the tail bones (Fig. 3.5). These are the postural muscles that extend the spine, bringing it erect.

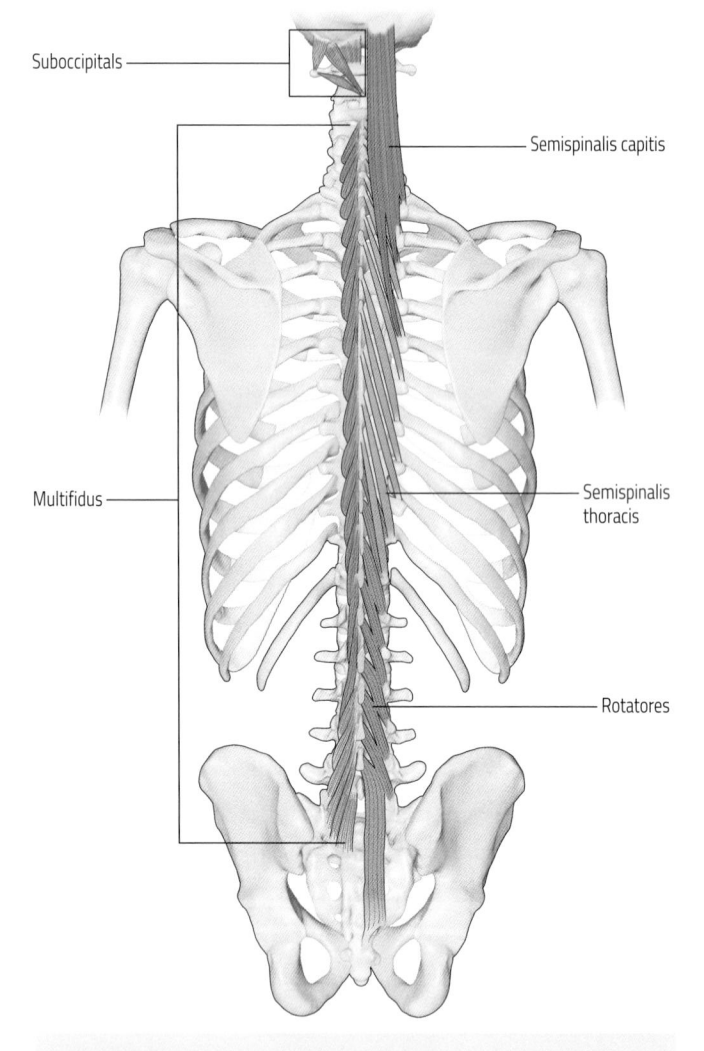

**Figure 3.4**
The deepest layer of spinal muscles

The outer muscles of the trunk and limbs (Fig. 3.6) are those that gym bunnies can name: trapezius, latissimus dorsi, rhomboids, gluteus maximus, and deltoids.

With good body use (aligned with gravity) all our muscles are operating over the correct lengths, maintaining the bones in their rightful relationships. The different layers of the back are then in dynamic balance, each taking their share of the muscle tone appropriate to their size and function. But where body use is poor (fighting gravity) some muscles are over-lengthened (resulting in straining or floppy tone), while the opposing muscles are over-shortened (giving tightness and tension), pulling the skeleton out of alignment.

Load and weight are not the same thing. When we are aligned, the weight of the body is held evenly by the musculoskeletal system and transmitted smoothly through to the ground. But poor posture, by taking weight further from the line of gravity, is loading the body at many points.

> During computer tablet use, when users sit with forward bent neck and head, the mechanical demand on the neck muscles has been estimated to increase 3–5 times compared to seated neutral posture (Vasavada et al. 2015).

Now the muscles must work harder to hold the structure up – tensing together instead of in phase, a process called *co-contraction*, which stiffens us. My understanding is that the small postural muscles tense together to help stabilize the spine. As the spinal curves become accentuated, such as a lumbar arch, the tight erector spinae muscles can often be felt like ropes either side of the spine, effectively locking the imbalanced vertebrae together to hold the torso. The further the weight is held from the line of gravity, the bigger the leverage required to hold it. Then the outer "action" muscles must also work to hold us up, in complex pairings across the layers of the torso, work for which they are not designed. These over-working muscles are then holding chronic tension, and become locked long or locked short (Fig. 3.7).

# The fundamentals of structure

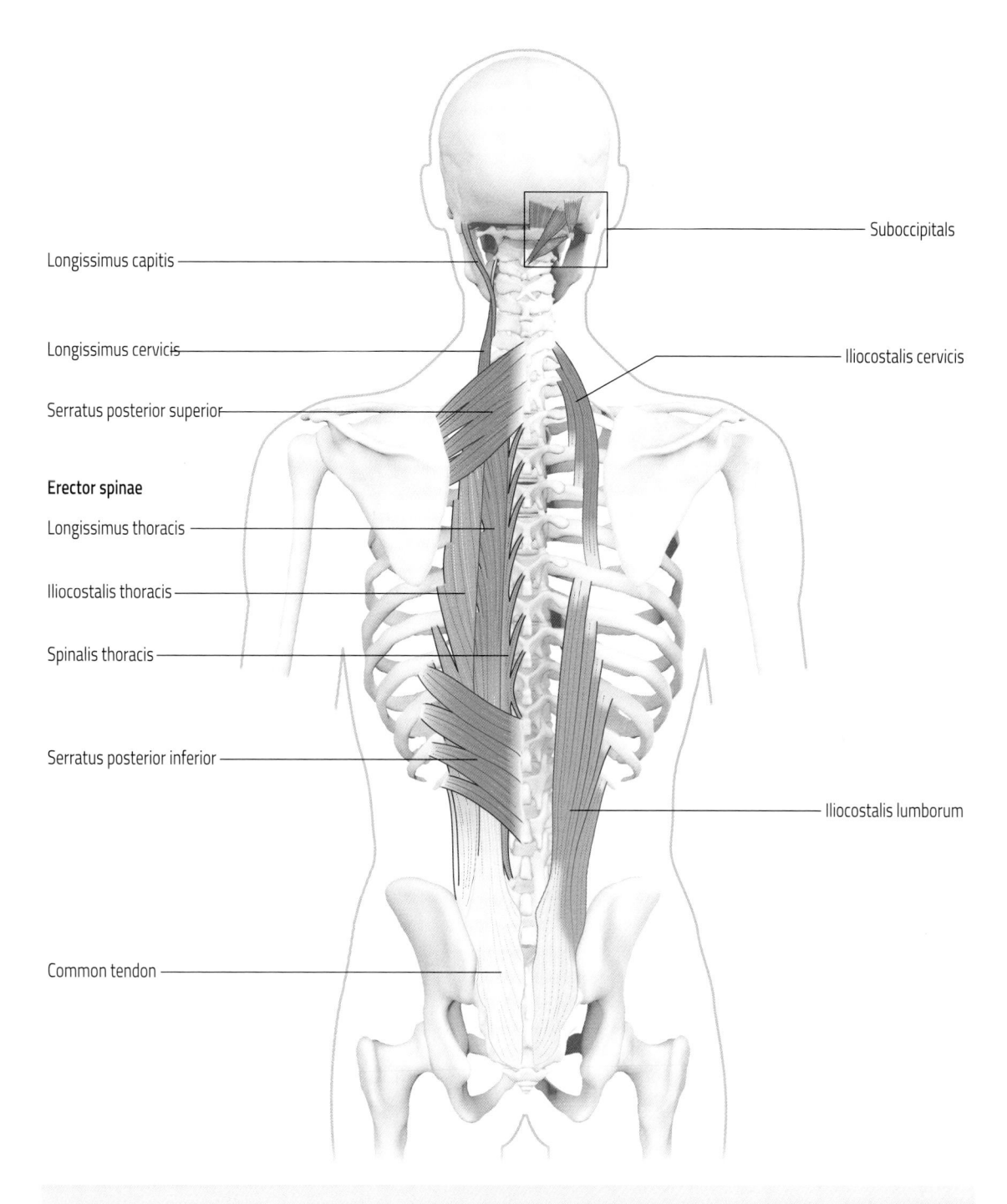

- Suboccipitals
- Longissimus capitis
- Longissimus cervicis
- Iliocostalis cervicis
- Serratus posterior superior

**Erector spinae**
- Longissimus thoracis
- Iliocostalis thoracis
- Spinalis thoracis
- Serratus posterior inferior
- Iliocostalis lumborum
- Common tendon

**Figure 3.5**
The erector spinae, the middle layer of the back muscles

# CHAPTER three

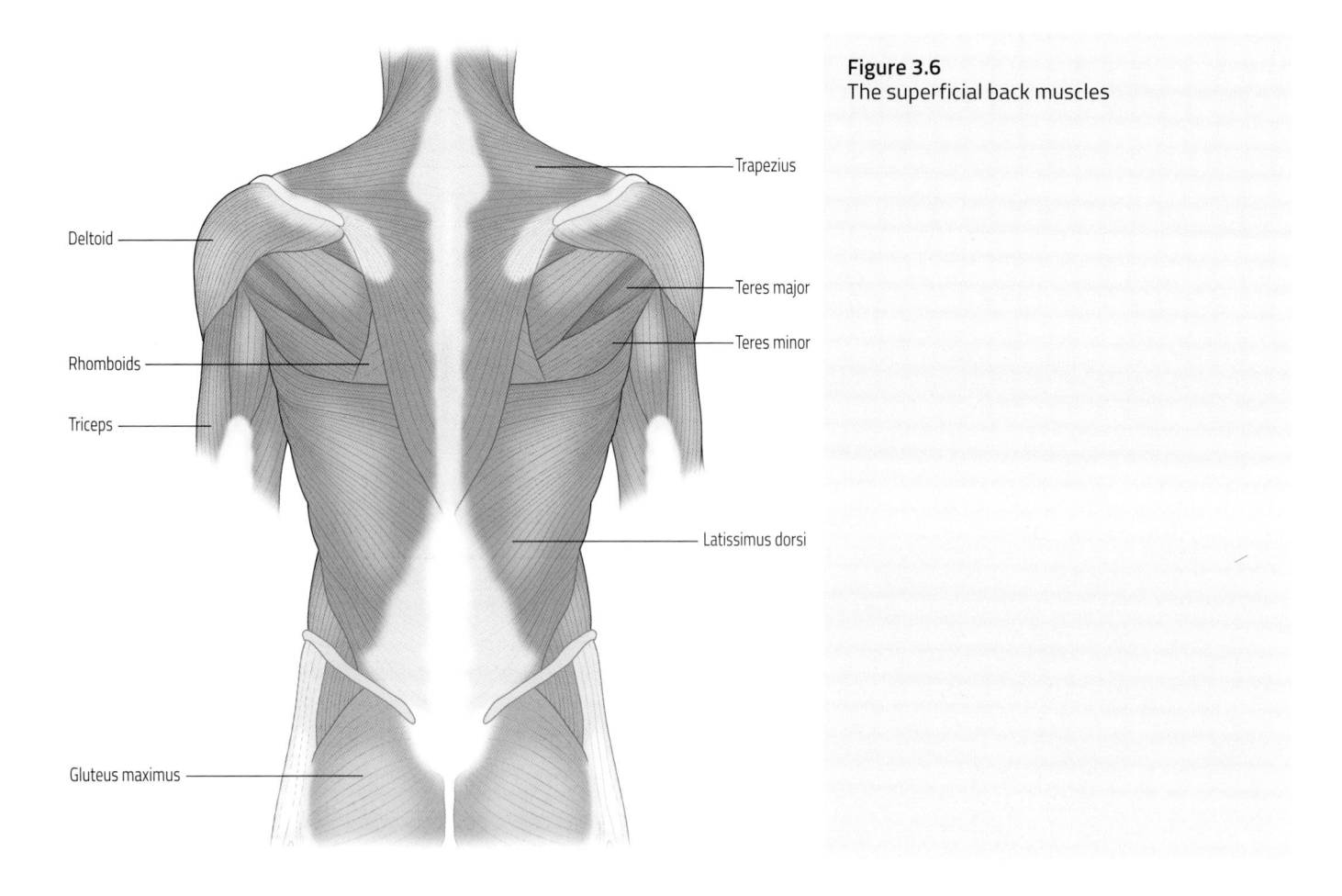

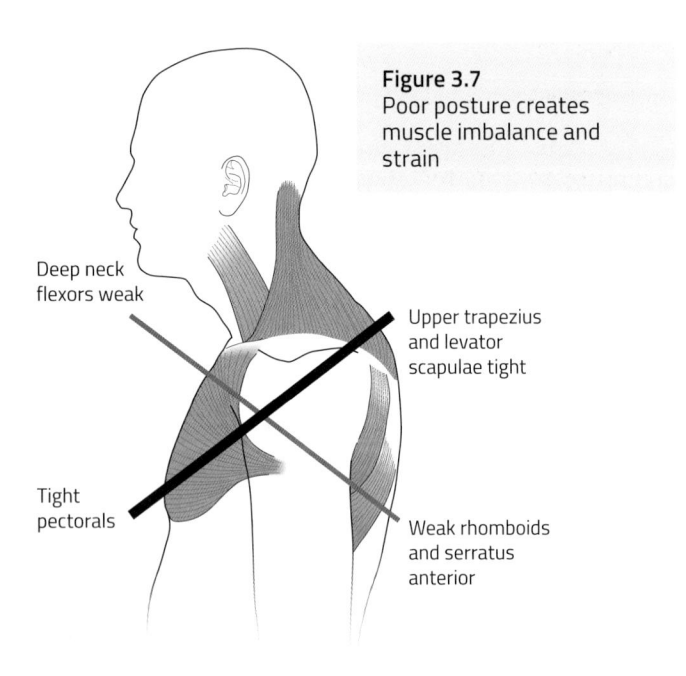

**Figure 3.6**
The superficial back muscles

- Trapezius
- Deltoid
- Teres major
- Teres minor
- Rhomboids
- Triceps
- Latissimus dorsi
- Gluteus maximus

**Figure 3.7**
Poor posture creates muscle imbalance and strain

- Deep neck flexors weak
- Upper trapezius and levator scapulae tight
- Tight pectorals
- Weak rhomboids and serratus anterior

The first hard evidence that we overuse superficial muscles and under-use postural muscles for posture comes from Jull et al. (2009, cited in Cohen 2019). People with high neck pain were using sternocleidomastoids to tilt their heads forwards from supine; when trained to use these less, they used deep cervical flexors instead, which reduced pain levels.

Normally, by contracting and releasing in phase, there is circulation within muscles that oxygenates, cleanses, and renews them. But when the outer muscles are conscripted into postural support, they are permanently contracted. There is then reduced efficiency of the blood and lymph circulation and less natural dynamic movement in the muscle, so they are neither oxygenated nor nourished efficiently, nor are toxins being cleared. This is exhausting, and leads to pain, stiffness, etc.

# The fundamentals of structure

### Exploration 3.4  Wakening this awareness in our lives

- *Notice how you get on and off kitchen chairs, office chairs, sofas, toilets, in and out of cars. Notice how you sit at a desk. Notice shape or tension, such as all the tensions and collapses we employ to sit with crossed legs and arms, which we feel is comfortable. Anything you observe, whether a little or a lot, is good (Fig. 3.8).*

Faulty sensory perception is, in my opinion, one of the most useful concepts for any teacher of movement, exercise, or music, and yet mostly it is not addressed or even recognized. It explains two common problems that frustrate teachers and pupils: that the pupil either cannot follow the instruction, however hard they try, or cannot even see there is an issue to be addressed.

## Lesson 3  Making your first changes towards a more mechanically advantageous structure

In Westernized societies, I suggest we are fighting gravity as we move. We contract and tense to some degree in everything we do, getting heavier and less springy year by year. But small children don't fight gravity. Instead they fold and unfold, their bodies springing and bouncing in and out of different positions with adaptive muscle tone. It makes them a joy to watch. In Borneo, the entire native population moved as fluidly as small children.

To move, we need stability and mobility together. There are two ways of solving this movement problem. We have described how a misaligned body is held upright by co-contraction. In order to move, then, we must use compensatory patterns, which are often hard work. But when the body is aligned, the musculature can adapt moment by moment to every changing circumstance – this is adaptive (or responsive) muscle tone.

So let's explore our way back to our birthright. In the following explorations, we are returning our structure to a better alignment with gravity, which reduces the gravitational load on us and makes us feel lighter. But also, we are learning to reduce co-contraction – recognizing consciously when this tension is no longer necessary, and saying "no" to it.

### Exploration 3.5  Finding your stable base

- *Look at how far apart your feet are. Are your heels under your hips, closer together than this, or further apart? Explore each state, and how it affects your lower back.*

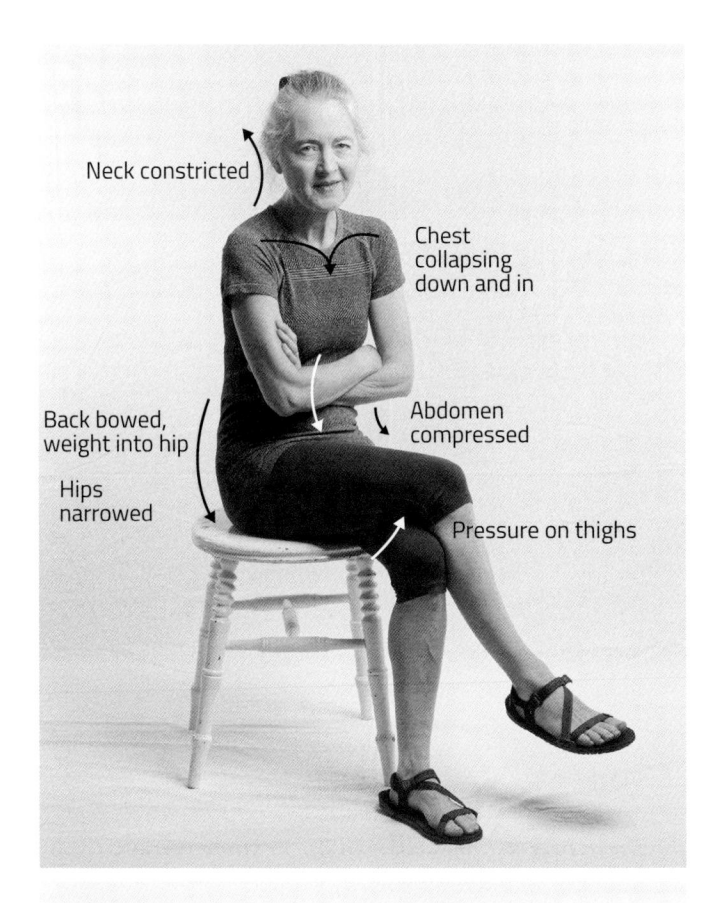

**Figure 3.8**
Sitting with legs crossed compresses the body

# CHAPTER three

- *If you were building a porch to your house, would you put the columns in any other position than vertical? To give the body a secure, stable base, your heels need to be underneath your hip joints. This allows the legs to be vertical and the pelvis to be horizontal, like a porch. The torso then has a secure foundation (Fig. 3.9).*

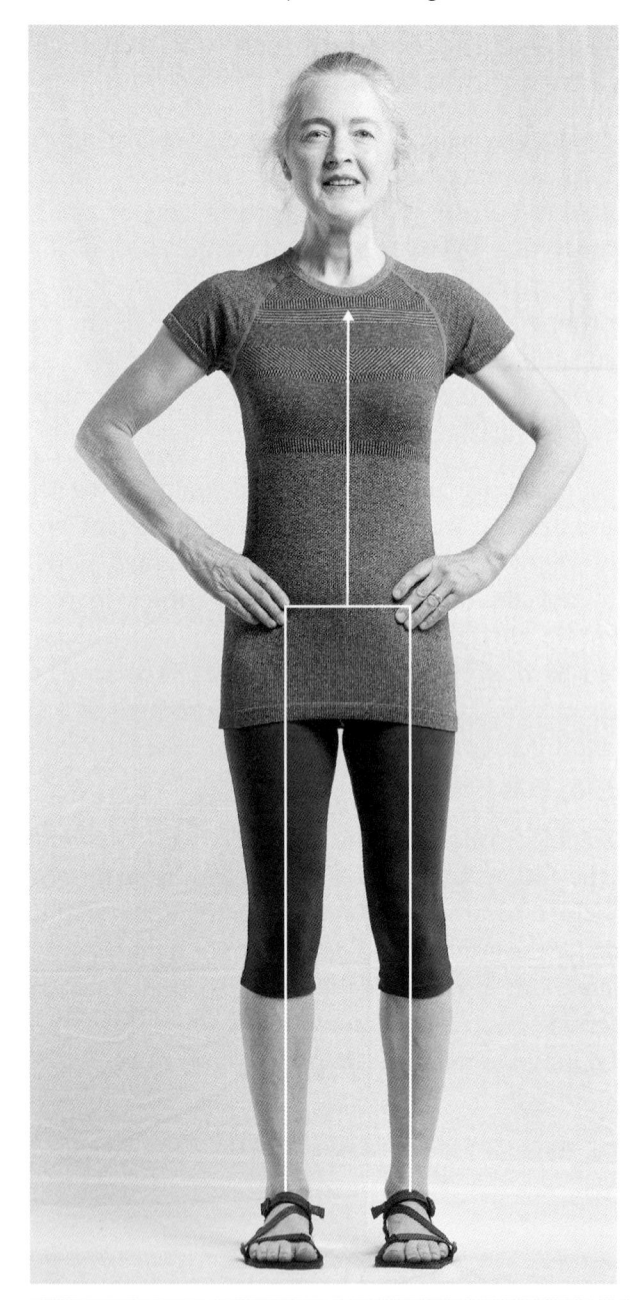

**Figure 3.9**
Optimal support for the torso is when heels are directly under hips

## Two voices of positional "right" and "wrong"

To change the distance between your feet is such an apparently simple change, yet it can be profound. For some, it may feel strange, or wrong, even unsafe, while others may experience it as a welcome relief.

There are two sensory "voices" competing for attention, telling us what is right and what is wrong. Faulty sensory perception, when present, tends to shout loudest. It derives from the stretch receptors' data of muscle lengths and is based, as we have seen, on the premise that our usual body positioning is the right one. But there is another, often quieter sense that was never named by Alexander and that seems to be more truthful. This is the sense of relief that we get when we find balance and can include a sense of lightness, ease, freedom, poise, stability, or body harmony. It derives from the joint receptors, when pressure is lessened and equalized across all the joint surfaces. So often pupils ask me "Am I in the right position?" But we cannot feel the right position because of faulty sensory perception. If instead, we look for a quality of freedom, we will do better.

### Exploration 3.6    Freeing the knees

- *Observe your knees. Are they pushed right back? Do you stand with them slightly bent? Do you hold the muscles tight around the knee joint?*

- *The knees always need to be free to move, with the leg bones simply balanced one on top of another.*

- *Wobble your knees to free them from habitual tension around the joint, and bring them straight, inviting yourself not to tighten them up again.*

- *If they want to tighten again, try thinking "I can do less with my knees." Notice any faulty sensory perception, such as feeling you will fall over. The brain is not used to standing with this little tension and may think it wrong. We have hugely protective mechanisms built in to stop us falling over, but they can be over-zealous!*

# The fundamentals of structure

### Exploration 3.7 Freeing the ankles

Most people are totally unaware of their ankles; they are simply too far from the control tower of the head. To find them:

- *Stand 30 cm from a wall, facing away from it. Allow yourself to fall gently back, catching yourself on your hands. The aim is to let your whole-body pivot on your ankles, so that the front of the ankle opens.*

- *Play around until you can lower yourself back safely to the wall in a straight line from your feet, the toes staying down. Your hips and back of the knees are also falling back. This brings the hip joints back, as they are often pushed forward.*

- *To come up again off the wall, notice if you push forward with your hips. Invite this not to happen; push with elbows and hands to pivot yourself back up.*

- *Stand and notice if your habit is to push your hips forward. Explore bringing your hips back a little bit, to open the ankles and hip joints (Fig. 3.10).*

### Exploration 3.8 Rebalancing the head on the neck (atlanto-occipital joint)

Your head weighs 8–12 pounds (4–6 kg) or even more. This heavy weight is the keystone of the body. The skull pivots on the top of the neck at the atlanto-occipital joint, which is level with the hollow under the ears. However, the center of gravity of the head is both in front of and up from this point. So the head wants to nod forward on the top of the neck, delicately balanced by tiny muscles. If the balance is off, these tiny muscles cannot hold such a heavy weight, and the big muscles of the neck, such as the trapezius, come into play to hold the head on the neck. This creates tension and the neck feels stiff. Freeing the atlanto-occipital joint is a major concern for many therapies, yet we rarely then observe how the head is balanced in daily life.

- *Place your forefingers in the hollows under the ears. Imagine a "raindrop" rolling slowly down your nose and*

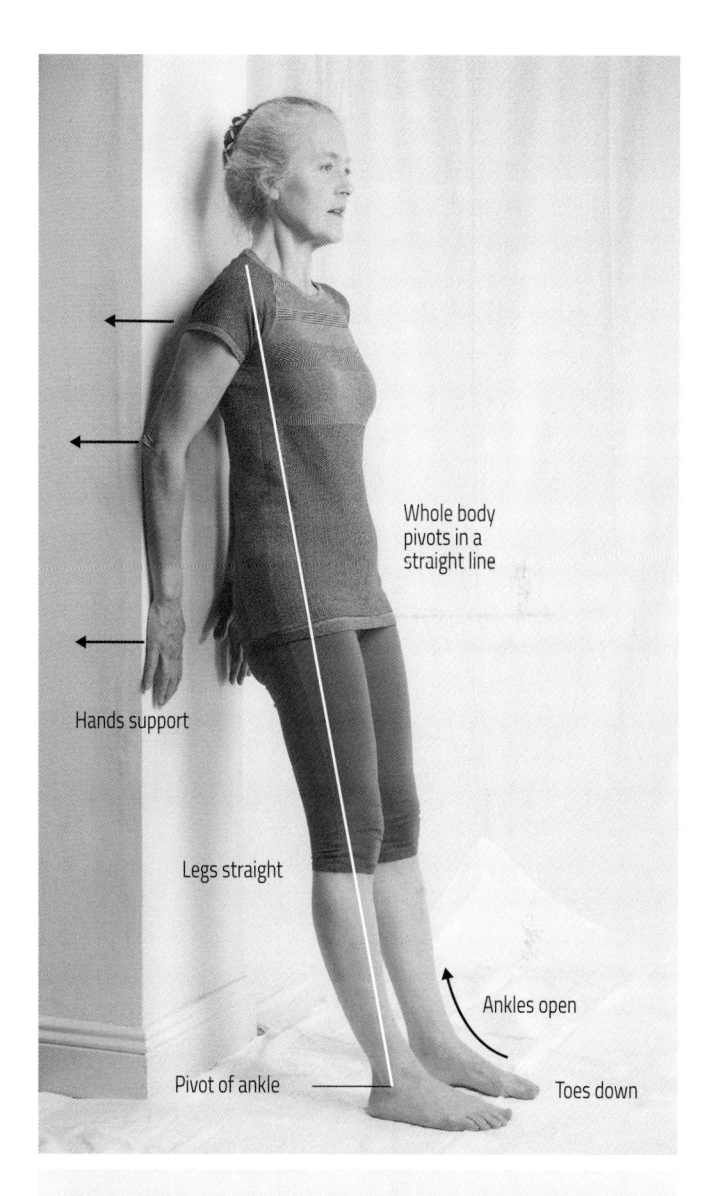

**Figure 3.10**
Opening the ankles by leaning back on a wall

*LET the head very gently roll forwards following this imaginary "raindrop". Be aware of how the head rotates forwards somewhere between your fingers, and there is a gentle stretch just under your skull (Figs 3.11 and 3.12).*

The top of your neck might now feel higher up than usual, as the big outer muscles are able to let go and the top joints and tiny muscles come back into play. Maybe you are aware of the whole spine lengthening upwards after it, and the body subtly rebalancing.

# CHAPTER three

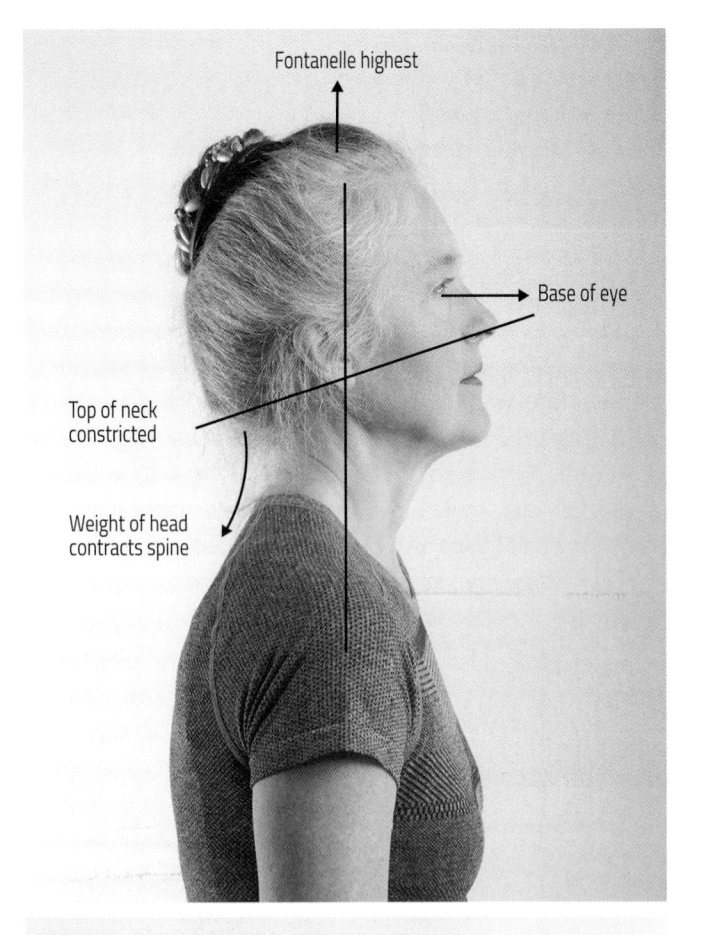

**Figure 3.11**
Head tightened back on forward neck constricts top of neck

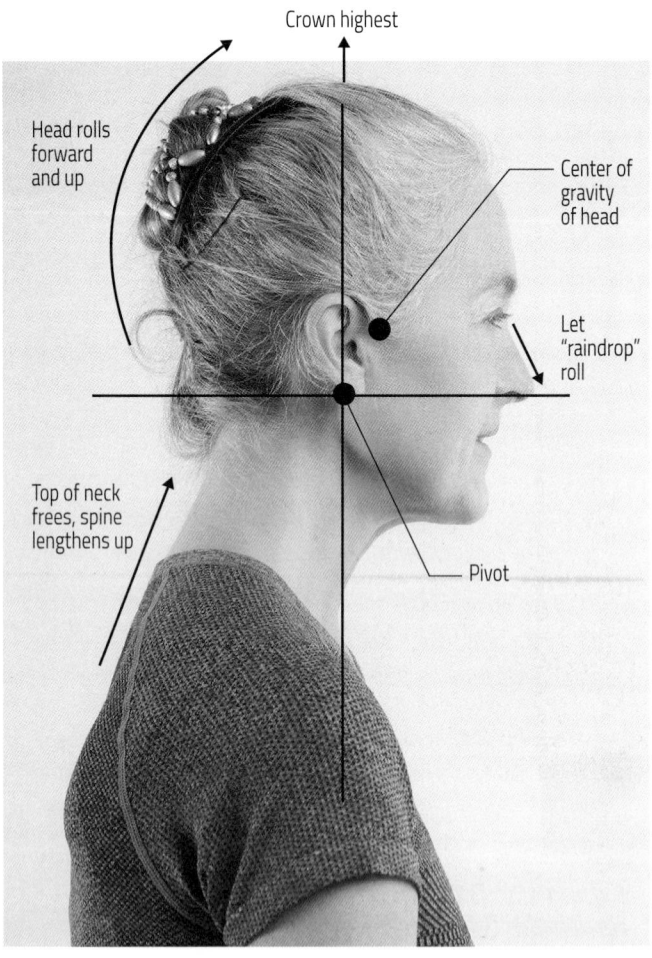

**Figure 3.12**
Head rolling forward to balance

- *Bring the head gently up again by lifting your eyeline, letting the head follow it. Then let the "raindrop" roll down your nose again to nod the head forwards, while letting the eyeline slide down again. Do this a few times, but keep it subtle.*

Notice the difference between only letting movement happen from the atlanto-occipital joint – the very top joint of the neck – and allowing all the other joints to be involved, especially the bottom one (Fig. 3.13). Whenever possible, we do not want to bend from these other vertebrae, as the head is now off-balance on the neck, as in text-neck, and is a recipe for problems.

**Video link for exploration 3.8, part 1**

Your eyes may now feel wrong. You may be looking down, or seeing from under your lids. The eyeball muscles have their habits too: if you habitually pull your

# The fundamentals of structure

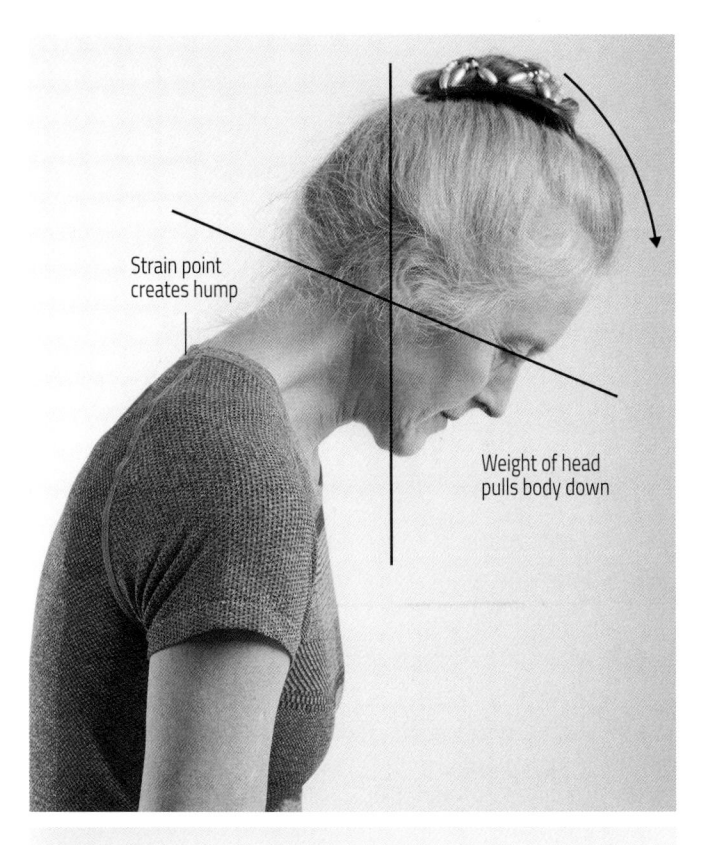

**Figure 3.13**
Head and neck forward from base of neck

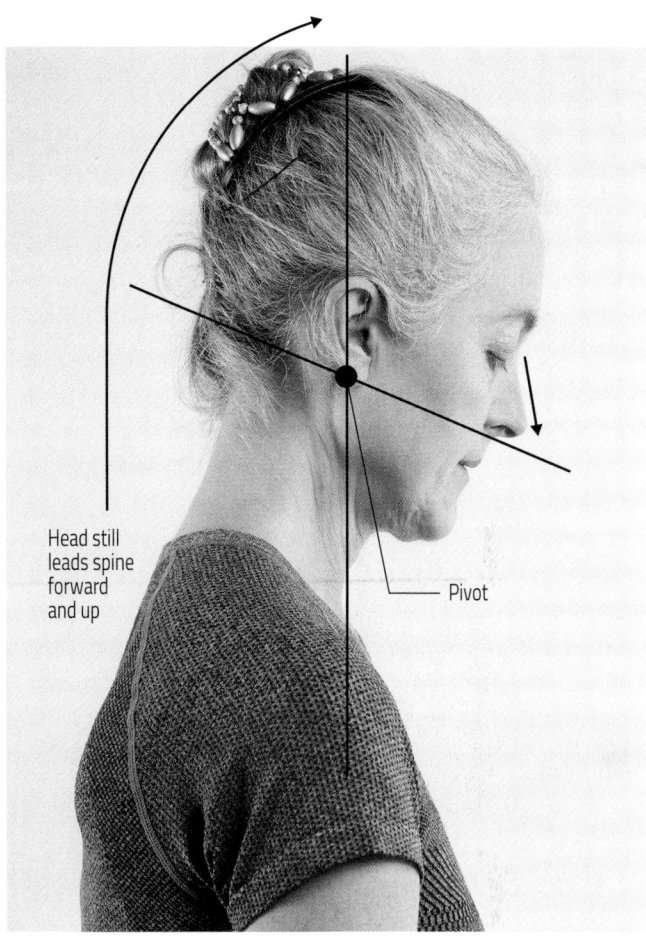

**Figure 3.14**
Looking down led by the eyes

head back, your habit is to look out of the bottom of your eyes (Fig. 3.11).

- *To rebalance the eyes and sight line: look forwards and track your eyes up and then down, letting the head gently follow the sight line, until the eyes rebalance with the new head alignment.*

When the head is level you can look forwards comfortably, out of the middle of the eyes, while seeing the ground nearly to your feet with your peripheral vision. I call this *the lower visual quadrant*. If your head is tilted back, you will see more sky than ground peripherally – *the upper visual quadrant*. This cannot be right! If your head rolls too far down you will see too much ground, including your feet and body. You can use this as a check

that your head is level. When you need to look down – maybe to lay the table, lead with your eyes and "raindrop" from the atlanto-occipital joint only (Fig. 3.14).

## Exploration 3.9    The turning joint (axis joint)

The turning joint is just below the nodding joint.

- *After nodding your head forwards, let your eyes go around to the right, allowing your head to follow without lifting your chin. The head should turn easily until your eyes are looking over your shoulder (Fig. 3.15).*

# CHAPTER three

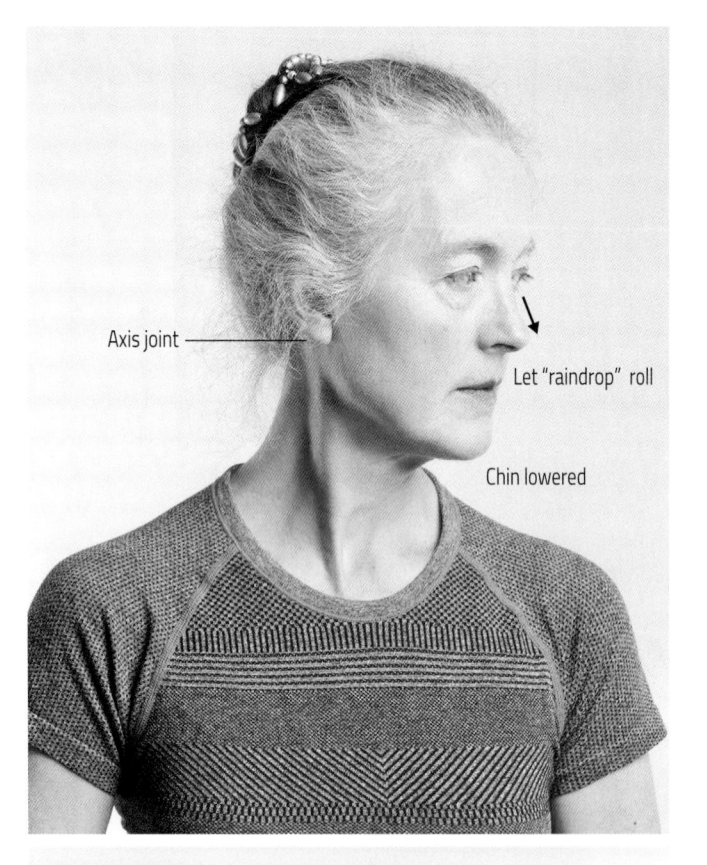

**Figure 3.15**
Balanced head/neck turns from axis joint

*Axis joint*
*Let "raindrop" roll*
*Chin lowered*

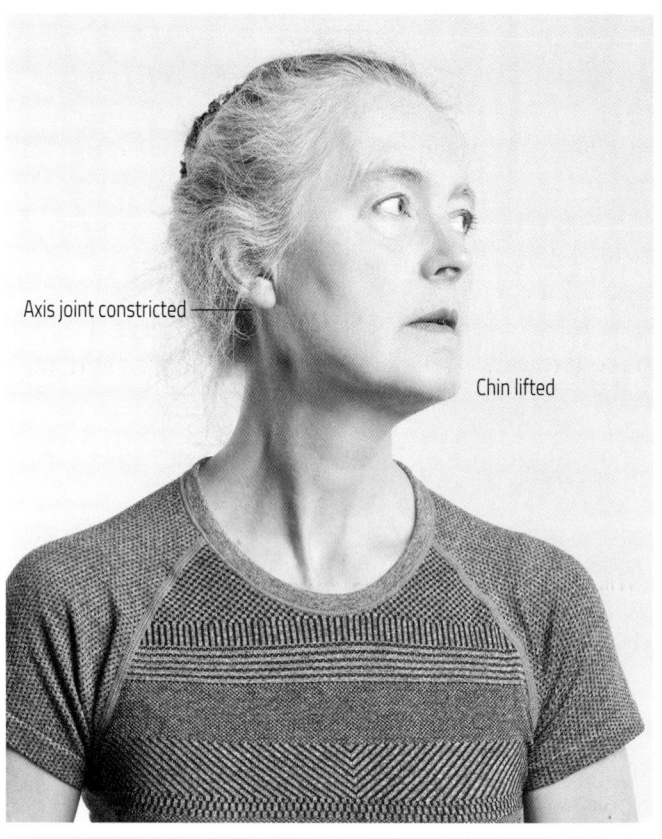

**Figure 3.16**
Constricted head/neck turns from other neck joints

*Axis joint constricted*
*Chin lifted*

- *Bring your eyes back to center and let your head swing back again, then take your eyes left to go the other way. Do this a few times and be aware of your neck loosening up.*

- *Notice that if you attempt this with the chin slightly in the air, the head will not turn very far before it sticks, and if you do this too fast you will crick your neck (Fig. 3.16).*

This is because with the chin raised, the top two joints go out of play, and the other joints do not have the same range of motion in that plane of movement.

I love to play with the mobility of these two joints for a few minutes each day, to wake them up. The atlanto-occipital and axis joints are the only joints of the spine with full independent movement.

### Exploration 3.10   Freeing up your jaw using "directions"

(Thanks to AT teacher Carolyn Nicholls for this one)

Many people hold a lot of tension in the powerful muscles of the jaw, and may grind their teeth at night. Since the jaw joint is above and slightly in front of the atlanto-occipital joint, freeing this will also help the head/neck balance.

- *Invite your jaw back into a more balanced tone by thinking "I let my lower back teeth drop away from my upper back teeth, and I let my upper back teeth lift up and off my lower back teeth."*

# The fundamentals of structure

- *Think this thought clearly a few times, to invite a successional rebalancing of tone, and allow anything or nothing to happen. You are opening to the possibility of change.*

In the Alexander technique such intentional sentences are called *directions*. They work best when they are clearly articulated thoughts, and you are aware of their link to the body. Mushy thoughts and meaningless recitations don't work. Alexander called such directions "orders" or "commands." This is a bit dictatorial to modern ears – I prefer "possibilities" or "invitations."

### Exploration 3.11  *Going up to your crown*

Think of a tree. Its crown is carried by the trunk up to the sky, while the weight of the crown is carried down by the trunk into the roots. There are equal and opposite forces going up and down the tree trunk, but the tree does not move. For us, having flexible bodies, "down" is usually winning, causing us to slump, or if "up" is winning, we pull up too tightly, like a soldier on parade. We want an equal force of up and down through from our heels to our crown.

- *As you stand normally, where is the highest point of the head? Is it the crown (where the hair line spirals) or the forehead (the fontanelle)? Notice that if the forehead is higher, the head is tipped back. Notice that when you roll the "raindrop" to rebalance your head on your neck, the crown becomes the highest point, and the whole spine lengthens to follow (see Figs 3.11, 3.12, 3.17, and 3.18).*

- *Stand with your weight all on one hip. What has happened now to your up-force? Notice how the downforce puts pressure in all sorts of incorrect places.*

- *Bring your awareness back up to your crown (keep seeing out). Wait a moment and see if your body wants to follow upwards, and move with this impulse till you are balanced evenly again on two feet. Think "up" through your crown every time you notice yourself slumping down on one hip, until it stops being something you want to do.*

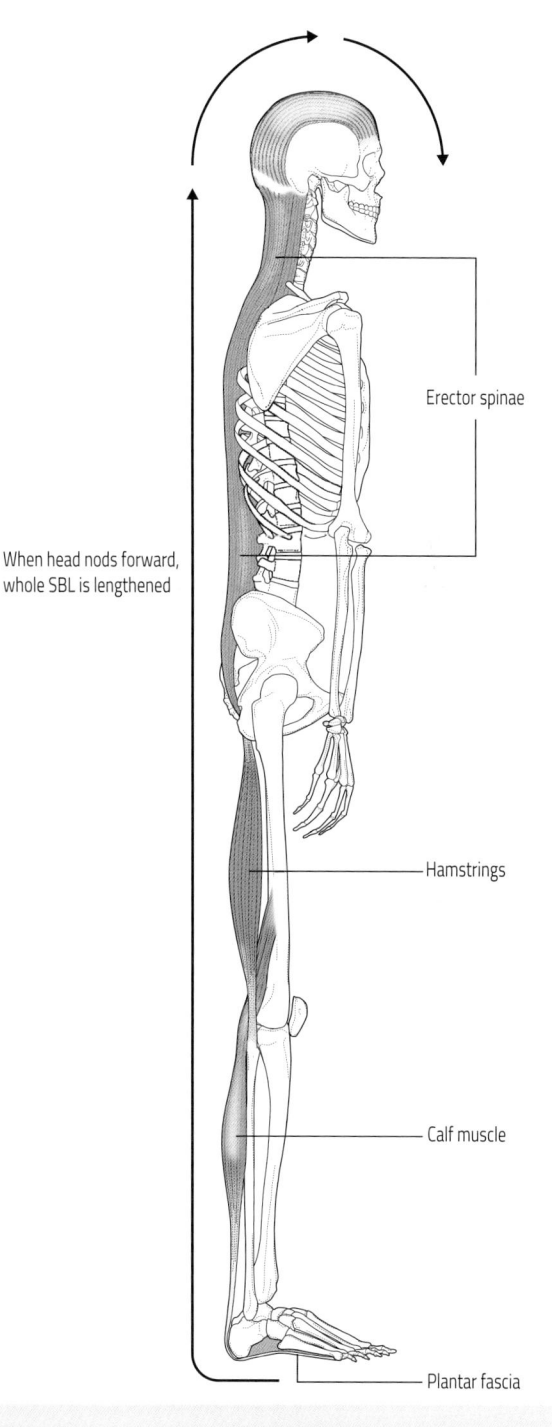

**Figure 3.17**
Superficial back line of body (SBL), side view. When the head nods forward, the whole SBL of muscles is lengthened

# CHAPTER three

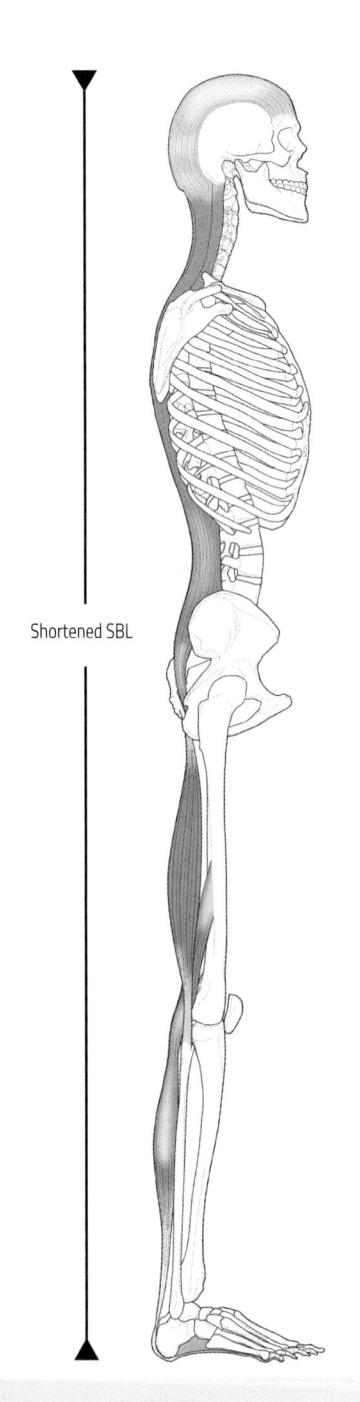

**Figure 3.18**
Head pulled back on constricted neck causes compression and shortening of the SBL of muscles

(Shortened SBL)

*Gravity and "anti-gravity"*

The primary axis of the body is the vertical axis: down to the feet – the gravitational force – and up to the crown, that feels like an "anti-gravity" force.

Why is it that when we free the head on the neck, the whole spine and body lengthen up away from gravity? The answer can be found in the linkages between muscles and the fascia. To know more, we need to look at our assumptions about anatomy.

## Lesson 4    Understanding the different models of body mechanics

*The old paradigm of descriptive anatomy*

Meticulous dissections of corpses over many centuries allowed anatomists to understand the body as an assemblage of parts, to be described in detail and named. Anatomy courses for therapists teach the origin and insertion points of muscles, and what each muscle does to move the bones around: for example, the biceps runs between points on the scapula and radius and its contraction lifts the forearm. This has been called *descriptive anatomy* and I will refer to it as the old paradigm.

From this, modern medicine has come to see the body in parts – to be mended, cut out, or replaced if they malfunction. Forces in this model are seen as localized: so, for instance, if you have a blow to the knee, most doctors will only examine and treat the knee. This reductionist paradigm is the logical conclusion of investigating bodies only when dead, with a knife. It fits with most people's conception and experience of their bodies as a set of parts to like or dislike, own or disown: head (with brain – myself), back (often achy), shoulders (tense), belly (fat), legs (to move us around), etc.

From this came the first biomechanics, which only understood the body as a gravity-stacked structure. The head weighs down on vertebra C7, the torso

# The fundamentals of structure

holistic bodywork methods. In the Western world, this paradigm is still embedded into how we think, pre-dating any new understanding. Unless we can clarify the differences, we will not be able to explain our discipline clearly to others. The confused thinking that results from two paradigms at war with each other can result in saying one thing and doing another.

The new paradigm is one of connectivity, and it is being explored not only in anatomy but also in many areas of science. At last, we can begin to understand our work as Alexander teachers or other holistic somatic therapists. More specifically, it has helped me understand Miss Goldie's work: why she maintained there can be no switching off, not even of one muscle, without collapsing. Her work was about integration and the natural strength that comes from that, rather than release.

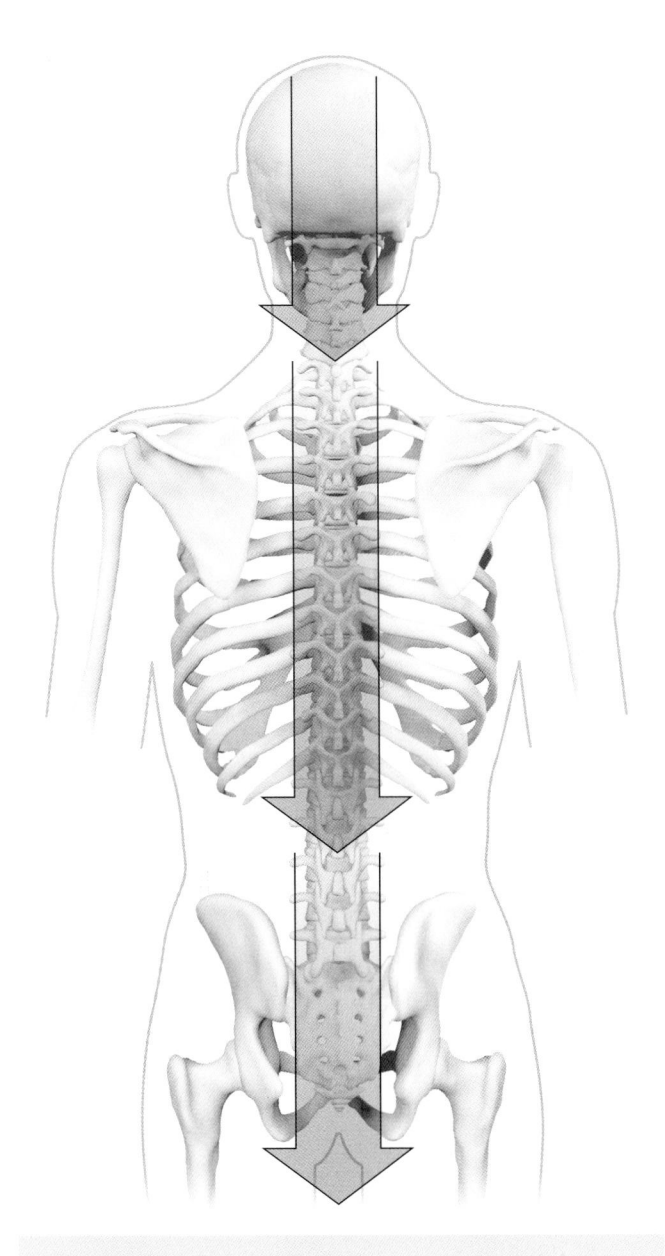

**Figure 3.19**
The continuous compression model (gravity-stacked) of human structure

on L5, and the whole weight rests like a stack of bricks on the feet (Myers 2014: 48) (see Figs 3.19 and 3.20).

When in the 1930s Alexander attempted to explain his technique he struggled because this culturally accepted paradigm did not fit with his experiences, as was true also for those attempting to explain other

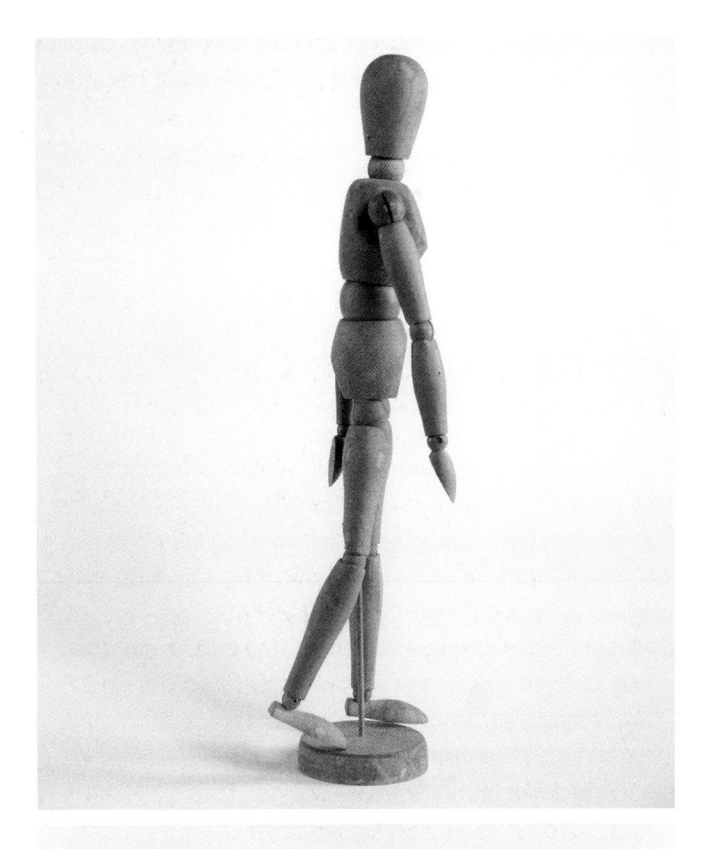

**Figure 3.20**
Animal forms are top-heavy. With gravity-fed forces alone this figure could never balance or walk on its small feet

# CHAPTER three

## Anatomy trains – linking up the body

*Functional anatomy* looks at the relationships between anatomical elements; muscles and bones always work in groups for stability and movement. Groupings of multi-joint muscles that work together – for example, to extend a limb – are known as kinetic chains. But personally, like many holistic practitioners, I am drawn to the work of Rolfer Thomas Myers and his Anatomy Trains® (2014). Myers wondered how muscles might operate together after coming across Raymond Dart's muscle spirals. Anatomists for centuries have sought to do clean dissections of individual muscles, by stripping away all the fascia that connects them to everything else. Instead, Myers did dissections looking for the fascial links between muscles at the same level (deep, medial, or superficial), and found clear linking lines that he calls myofascial trains (Myers 2014: 6–7). The "stations" where these trains pause are the muscle attachment points on the bones. The major myofascial trains provide the main body tension cables of the body, catching and holding the bones in place.

> Fascia is the white filmy stretchy stuff you see between the flesh if you cut up meat. For centuries viewed simply as the padding between tissues, fascia is now recognized as a complex and chaotic web that connects everything to everything (Myers 2014: ch. 2). While the myofascial trains are the large-scale connectors, the fascia wraps around and through every muscle, organ, or tissue, from skin through to bone. The fascial web *forms* the total body structure, and all the elements of the body – organs, nerves, vessels, muscles, and bones – are nestled within it. "Muscle never attaches to bone. Muscle cells are caught within the fascial web like fish within a net. Their movement pulls on the fascia, the fascia is attached to the periosteum, which is the membrane that wraps around the bone like clingfilm, and the periosteum pulls on the bone" (Myers 2014: 41).

The superficial back line of the body (SBL) (see Fig. 3.21) is a key line we are working with as

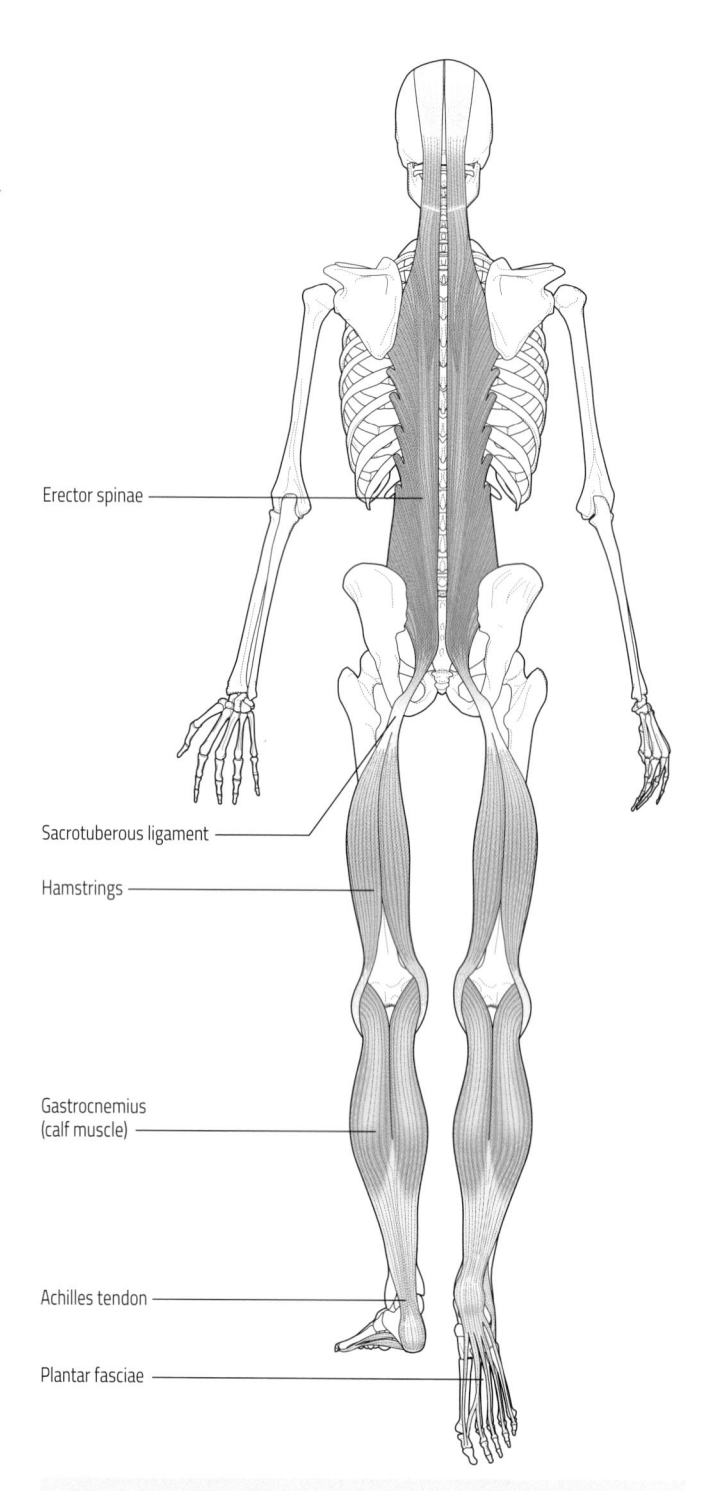

**Figure 3.21**
Superficial back line of body (SBL)

# The fundamentals of structure

Alexander teachers: it lengthens the head, neck, and back up, right from the heels. This continuity of muscle and fascia starts with the thin layer of muscle over the scalp, runs down all the erector spinae, along the sacrotuberous ligament across the pelvic girdle, down the length of the hamstrings, the calf muscles and Achilles tendons, and then runs as the plantar fasciae along the soles of the feet to the tips of the toes.

I see any constriction within this line as disturbing the relationships between the parts of the body – legs, torso masses, or head/neck balance – taking them further from the line of gravity, putting a compressive loading on the spine. Then the whole line of muscles will contract in response, tightening around the joints of the spine and limbs, and the body will become heavier and stiffer (Fig. 3.18). Conversely when the parts of the body are returned to optimal relationships, muscles can relax and this whole superficial back line will lengthen upward again, from the sole of the foot to the crown. This allows all the joints to expand and free up, and the body will lighten upwards (Fig. 3.17).

Though we play here with doing this from the balance of the head, we will see in Chapter 7 that the real culprits of imbalance are constrictions and imbalances further down the torso. When the torso provides coordinated support, one can tip the head around with little disturbance to the rest of the system.

The SBL is then balanced by the superficial front line (SFL): muscles running up the front of the feet, the legs, the torso, and then up the sternocleidomastoids (SCMs), that finish on the mastoid bone under the ears. These all act to lift the front of the body, which anatomically hangs down from the skull and neck, and so can tend to drag us down (see Fig. 3.22).

> Myofascial trains are used effectively by many somatic practitioners and movement instructors. But Myers (2014: 1) stresses that his model is not established science; it has leapt ahead of the research. While there is some evidence that the fascial elements of the trains can transmit the necessary force-load, others are disputing it (Zügel et al. 2018). More research is needed here. Kinetic chains – the linkages of overlapping multi-joint muscles (muscles that cross two joints such as the biceps femoris which cross knee and hip) and their underlying single joint muscles are more proven, and these comprise a large part of anatomy trains. I invite you to play around with the anatomy trains and come to your own conclusions.

### Exploration 3.12    Think up the legs

- *Most of us stand very heavily on our legs, viewing them almost as props under us. Explore this while standing, by lifting one heel forward and then dropping it back down again. Do you notice the weight settling back into that leg and foot? Play with the other leg likewise.*

- *Lift the heel again, but this time lower it slowly, as you think a line running up your leg from heel to Achilles tendon, up your calf muscle, up the back of the knee, up the lower, middle and upper thigh, across your backside and to your sacrum (the solid bony area of four fused vertebrae at the base of the spine, and above your tailbone).*

- *Repeat on the other foot, and then again on both feet. Does the whole-body feel lighter?*

### Balancing with gravity

The compressive forces of gravity are carried down the spine through the sacroiliac joints, which is why the lumbar vertebrae are bulkier than the neck vertebrae – they are transmitting more weight. They are also coping with ground reaction forces, pushing up with every footstep into knees and hips. When the superficial back line (the extensor chain) is in balance with the superficial front line (the flexor chain), then the forces will be equalized across the discs, and the structure will be optimally aligned with gravity. But when the neck pulls back, as in Figure 3.18 above, this will create an imbalance, loading one side of the intervertebral discs more than the other side.

# CHAPTER three

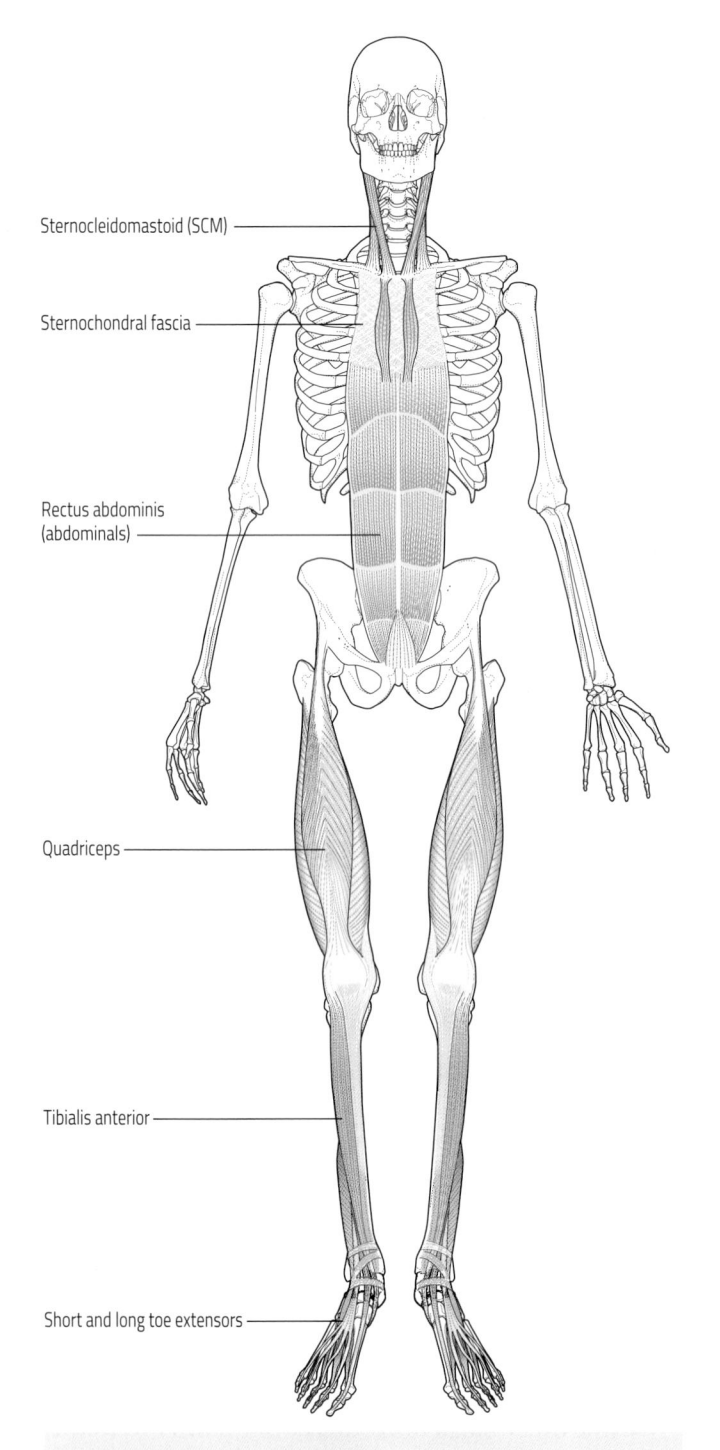

**Figure 3.22**
Superficial front line of body

Labels: Sternocleidomastoid (SCM); Sternochondral fascia; Rectus abdominis (abdominals); Quadriceps; Tibialis anterior; Short and long toe extensors

This creates more force load at this point, and will feel heavier. This sets up compensatory patterns throughout the body and one can speculate that over time, this is what compresses the vertebral discs (or joint capsules for limb joints) and can eventually lead to arthritis as cartilage and then bone is worn away. In this work we are always looking to align the structure with gravity in any position, allowing muscles to lengthen and inappropriate pressure across the joints to be removed.

### *The new paradigms – three models of connected body structure*

Myers places his anatomy trains hypothesis within the larger theory of biotensegrity. Proponents of biotensegrity often describe the shortcomings of biomechanics, while proponents of modern Bernstein-derived biomechanics can be dismissive of tensegrity. Additionally there are other theories of structure, including Dart's muscle spirals and torque chains (discussed later in this chapter).

Our standard response in Western thinking, when offered several models, is to ask which is right, and then to set about proving that the others are wrong. In contrast, East Asians see their world as "complex, containing inherently conflicting elements. Where Chinese students try to retain elements of opposing perspectives by seeking to synthesise them, American students try to determine which is correct so that they can reject the other" (McGilchrist 2012: 455).

I consider that these models are not competing but rather are describing different aspects of structure and movement. So I will describe them all (along with the shortcomings of the tensegrity model), and attempt to weave them into a whole that can better explain integrated movement.

The biotensegrity model – everything connects to everything

The concept of tensegrity was developed in the 1930s by the architect R. Buckminster Fuller, with structures such as geodesic domes. He looked to the forms

# The fundamentals of structure

of nature for solutions "because it is structurally and functionally efficient, lightweight and dynamic, and adjusts itself to its surroundings" (Scarr 2018: 4). The theory was first applied to whole animals in the mid 1970s, when Stephen Levin MD questioned how dinosaurs held up their necks.

The word tensegrity is made from combining the words "tension" and "integrity." In tensegrity structures, compression and tension forces are always in balance. The basic model is the icosahedron, which can be modeled with a set of rods and elastics (see Fig. 3.23). The rods – the compression structures – are held in relationship in a continuous sea of balanced tensioned elastic, so that at no point do the rods touch. The structure is a closed system of continuous tension transmissions and so can work any way up. If the forces of compression and tension are balanced, the structure is stable. Think of putting up a tent: one struggles with poles, until the covering fabric sheet and the guy ropes are in place and tightened, and then magically the structure self-supports, withstanding considerable wind and rain. You can lean on a well-constructed tent and it will take your weight, distorting slightly, returning to its full shape once the stress is removed.

This biotensegrity model demonstrates several paradoxes of living structures:

Lightness, springiness, and poise come out of an antagonistic balance of lengthening forces.

- *The compression rods do not touch*. Our bones do not sit on one another – there are severe problems if they ever do. There is always a space between them, visible on X-rays.

- *The tensioned integration of forces makes structures light and strong – highly mechanically efficient from minimum materials.* Think of a wagon wheel, whose sturdy struts must take the whole quarter-weight of the cart when directly below it, yet carry nothing at other angles. In a bicycle wheel, the many metal spokes are tensioned into the rim, continually distributing the load of the rider. The result is light, springy, strong, and speedy.

- *The antagonistic balance of lengthening forces means the system always has stored energy.* Like the stretched guy ropes and sheets of a tent, the resting structure is a balance of opposing forces. When that tension is lost, the system loses efficiency. Think of one guy rope slackening on a tent; the structure will sag a little and lose some resiliency, but will still stand. Then slacken another rope, then another, until the structure collapses.

- Forces through our bodies are evolved to be carried equally by the bones and the tension of the muscles and tendons, etc. Poor posture has progressive slackening of some parts of the structure, while other parts must then work harder to maintain uprightness (think of slumping on one hip). The whole structure then holds more compressive tension, with imbalanced loading across joints. The more some areas slacken, the worse this gets, and the result is heavy, tension-laden movement.

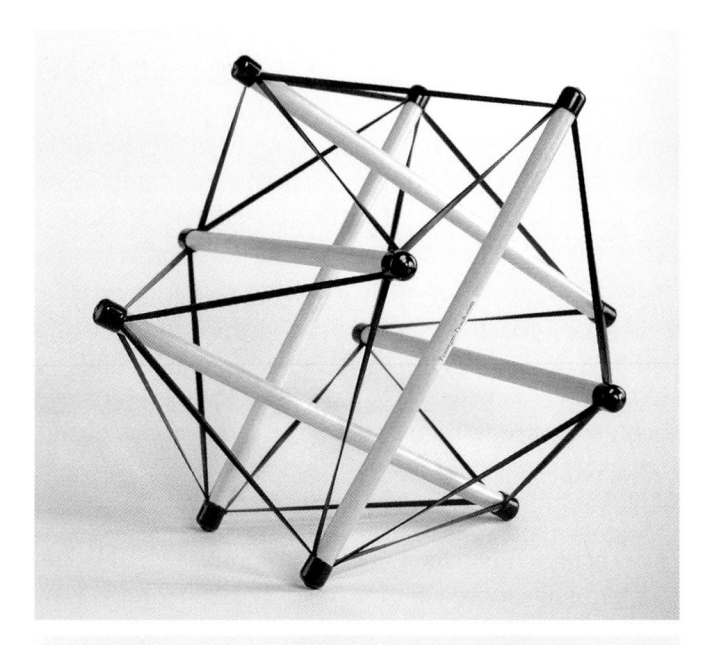

**Figure 3.23**
Icosahedron – tensegrity model of rods and elastics

# CHAPTER three

- *Non-locality of effects.* Put force on a tension–compression structure and something will eventually break – but not necessarily where the force is applied. This happens in the body, as when a knee problem has its cause in the back.
- *Biotensegrity structures are hierarchically nested.* The whole-body is a dynamic balance of opposing forces, and so is every part within it, down to organs, cells, organelles, enzymes, and DNA, all connected through the fascial network. Every part of the system takes its share of the total load, appropriate to its size (Scarr 2018: 30). This means that every part of the body is self-supporting rather than collapsing onto the area below; for example, the shoulder girdle is self-supporting on the ribcage.

## Problems with the tensegrity model

While the tensegrity model is hugely useful as a teaching tool to demonstrate these principles, it does not relate directly to our gross anatomical structure – we have no crossing struts. Physicist and AT teacher Patrick Johnson (2019a) also considers that the force-reduction claims and other calculations made by tensegrity theorists are inaccurate. Modern biomechanics has models that also work as a balance of compressive and tensional forces, using kinetic chains, and cover this same ground. Johnson points out that biomechanical robots look human, while biotensegrity robots look alien.

Clinical anatomist John Sharkey now refers to "living Biotensegrity." He says that the icosohedronal model (Fig. 3.23) is both friend and enemy to biotensegrity, as it gives no sense of living materials. The tensioned element of the body is the endless web of fascia that gives our bodies structure. In this, muscles, tendons, ligaments, muscle sheaths, and septa are all part of a continuum. This structure is always in dynamic flow with breath, heartbeat, and other body rhythms. It is fluid, soft, and alive, a pulsing living structure. Like a Mobius strip, inside and outside are all part of a continuum that connects every part to every other part (Sharkey 2016).

So the skilled somatic practitioner can put hands on a client and receive information about the whole structure through the fascia. From this conscious awareness, maybe also communicated through the fascia, they can effect changes in the client's body.

Tensegrity is more widely recognized as working at the level of the cell, where the cytoskeleton transmits externally applied stresses throughout the cell and into the nucleus. Linkage also connects with adjacent cells, giving a body-wide connectivity for mechanotransduction (Myers 2014: 56–8; Turvey and Fonseca 2009). I think of this as a *balanced fascial continuity*. Bordoni et al. (2019) call this living, connected, ground of the body "fascintegrity."

## Bernstein's biomechanical model – mastering complexity

Another problem with tensegrity theory is its claim that living structures are independent of gravity: they work any way up. But all land-based life is precisely oriented with gravity; it is the primary force on us.

Biomechanics is the study of *how mechanical forces affect biological systems, both externally and internally.* The old biomechanical model set precise roles for each muscle, working as agonists and antagonists around a hinge joint. The brain's role was then to order them to move, like pressing keys on a piano, one instruction per muscle. Repetition of movements, such as walking or tying shoelaces, created learned patterns in the brain, which, once acquired, could be switched on as needed. Different external conditions, such as walking on cobbles, were seen only as obstacles to be overcome. It was also assumed that when movement feels good, it is right.

Bernstein identified many problems with this mechanistic approach. He saw that the number of joints and muscles, each with a set of movement possibilities, created a vast number of potential positions and movements (the problem of degrees of freedom).

# The fundamentals of structure

He asked how does the nervous system control this complexity? He also saw that context changes which muscles come into play. For instance, if you pull your arm slowly down against a resistance, the latissimus dorsi is engaged, but if you simply lower it, you use the deltoid. With either movement, the forces on all the other joints (and tissues) will also be continually changing, and in different ways (Turvey et al. 1982). Environmental forces acting on us are also drawing different muscles into play, such as walking in mud, on hard ground, or on ice; uphill, or on the flat.

A more integrated approach was needed. Parts of the body are interdependent: "The co-ordination of a movement is the process of mastering redundant degrees of freedom of the moving organ, in other words its conversion to a controllable system. More briefly, co-ordination is the organisation of the control of the motor apparatus" (Bernstein 1967: 127).

In kinetic chains linked muscles are all directionally related so that when they are activated they will move the limb or part of the limb in a well-defined direction, reducing unnecessary movement possibilities. (When these are not limited, legs can kick sideways as we run, knees wobble as we sit, etc.) Optimal coordination of movements leads to economy of nervous system control. For this we need conscious guidance so that we step out of using feeling and coordinate the parts together. As we learn a new movement the kinematics of the body (body geometry), the forces involved, the nervous system input, and the homeostatic state of the body (energy levels, health, etc.) are all in relationship together.

With the repetition involved in learning we are not reinforcing new nerve pathways (the standard theory), because movements can never be identical. We are solving a movement problem, and the repetition of learning is about repeating the process of solving the problem, building knowledge in the system that can be applied to any such situation (Reed and Brill 1996) – for example, a proficient cyclist can tackle any new road surface.

> Nikolai Bernstein (1896–1966), was a brilliant mathematician turned neurophysiologist. He worked in Soviet Russia in 1930s, analyzing poor and excellent use of movement in factory workers. Like Alexander, he developed a new vision of possibilities of coordinated movement, though his work was not known in the West until 1967, when his first book, *The Co-ordination and Regulation of Movements*, was published in English. Biomechanics is mathematical and precise, using engineering principles to analyze the complexities of movement generation, and how the nervous system controls this complexity.

Spirals, curves, and torques take us into movement

*Spirals build from the micro to the macro level to facilitate structure and movement together.*

In the body, larger molecular structures are often formed of smaller molecules strung together, such as proteins made from strings of amino acids. These often form spirals which can be directionally left- or right-handed. Such helixes can then coil around each other to produce complex hierarchical structures with specialized functions. By altering bonds between the coils, the molecule will flip between precise shapes. This is the essential geometry behind protein chains such as enzymes, or actin and myosin – the active proteins of muscle.

Collagen, the main component of fascia which binds the body together, is our most widespread structural molecule. There are many types, which can be more elastic (by combining more helixes with the same twist) or more resistant (by combining helixes of opposite twist). These then pack together to make microfibrils, fibrils, and fascicles within bone, tendons, ligaments, and fascia (Scarr 2018: ch. 6).

Flexible tubes in the body, such as arteries and gut, are reinforced by concentric layers of collagen fibers, in alternating left- and right-handed helixes. This provides reinforcement to the tube, allowing bending without kinking and safe expansion and contraction

# CHAPTER three

in response to volume changes. Similar arrangements of muscle and collagen in the heart walls allow for left- and right-handed twisting motions as the heart chambers contract, resulting in a staggeringly efficient organ (Scarr 2018: 66).

The double spiral of muscle, our primary and secondary curves

At the whole-body level, our torso is wrapped around with a similar double-helix of muscles that encloses the abdomen and chest cavities, strengthening the tube of the torso, while allowing expansion and contraction (Figs 3.24 and 3.25). In this, "the single superficial sheet [of muscle], formed by two opposed, diagonally-running flexor muscles in front, is continued through a deeper-lying extensor sheet on each side of the spine behind" (Dart 1996, first published 1950: 69). Anatomist Raymond Dart identified this pattern following Alexander lessons, and then used it, along with Alexander principles, to help undo his own and his child's scoliosis patterns. From Dart's work, two overarching movement patterns were defined, our primary and secondary curves. The primary curve comes out of spinal flexion, the fetal curve. Birth then begins the long road of expansion – extension of the spine – the secondary curve, culminating in standing fully upright. The primary curve takes us in on ourselves, the secondary takes us outward into the world.

### Exploration 3.13  *Primary and secondary curves*

- *Play with these by crouching over, in a squat if you can, arms wrapped around your trunk, head down, knees and feet turned slightly in. This is the primary curve.*
- *Then expand out with head, back, arms, legs, and feet altogether, coming fully upright and into a star pose, expanding up, out and arching back – the secondary curve. Go between the two a few times.*
- *Notice that between the two there is a place of neutrality, where outer and inner, primary and secondary curves, balance.*

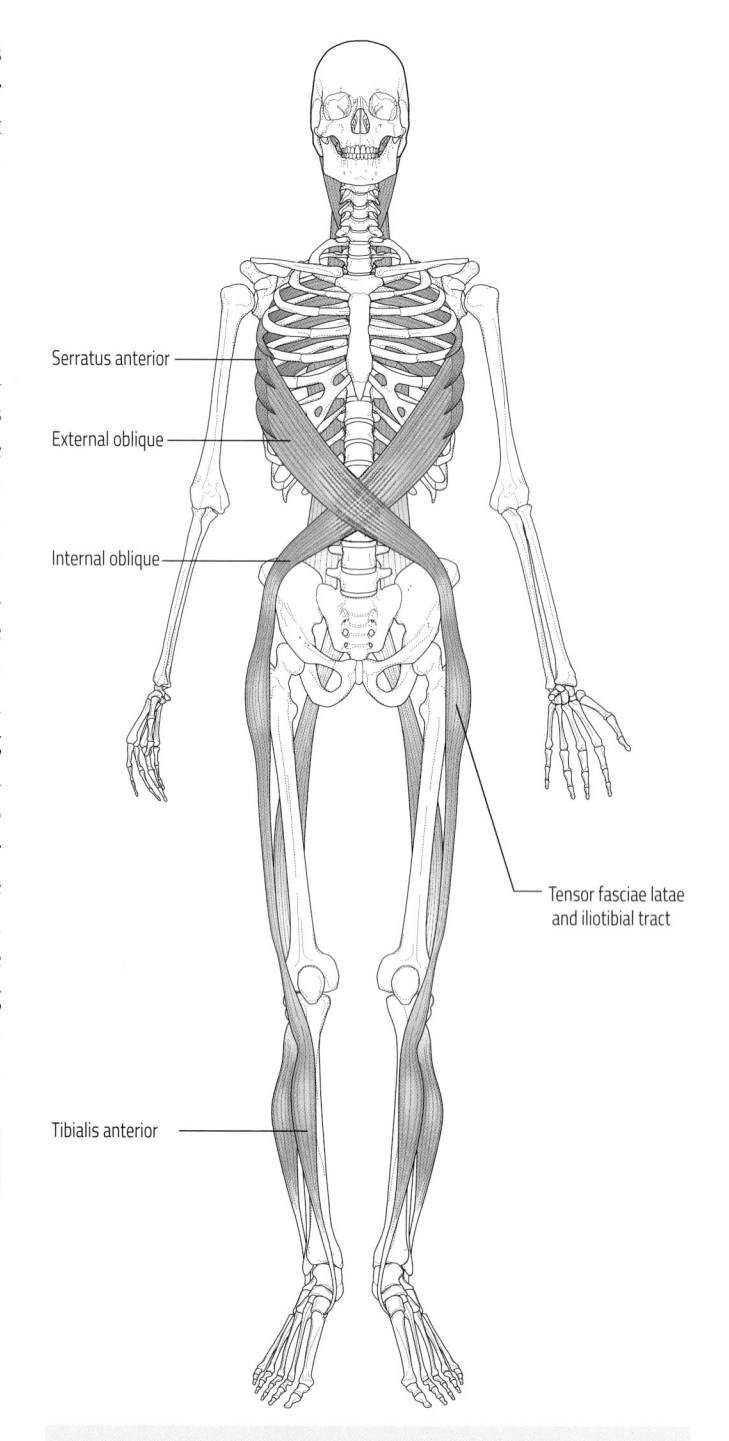

**Figure 3.24**
The spiral line, front view

# The fundamentals of structure

In daily life, we are going between these two curves all the time as we move between our inner and outer worlds. They are also happening within us continually as the curves of the spine: the sacral and thoracic curves being primary, and the cervical and lumbar being secondary; there are similar curves in the legs and arms (Nettl-Fiol and Vanier 2011). When we twist, we have diagonals between hips and shoulders, one of which is in primary, supporting us, and the other in secondary, extending us. When these curves work in dynamic cooperation, flowing easily throughout the body between primary to secondary and re-setting back to neutral, there is fluidity in our movement; when that process is interfered with, there is rigidity. Think of throwing a frisbee backhand: ideally the hand holding the frisbee leads the arm and whole-body into a downward and inward spiral, building the energy required, then propelling it out along an outward and upward spiral in which the whole-body unwinds, then returns easily to neutral. Then think of the awkward thrower who blocks this flow through the body, using only the throwing arm while holding the body rigid to avoid being destabilized by the propulsive force (see Figs 11.9 and 11.10).

## Torque – the power that drives movement

Julien Pineau, originator of the StrongFit system, observes that functionally, all muscles produce either internal or external torque, and that this is consistent however the muscle is deployed (Pineau 2018). In descriptive muscle theory, muscles are described by how they rotate or move a joint – for instance the pectoralis major (the pecs) is described as an internal rotator of the humerus. But if you take a plastic pipe, hold it in front of you and bend it by engaging your pecs, they externally rotate the humerus. Many muscles show this sort of confusion of classification.

Rotation only gives positional information. But torque – the twisting power generated by a muscle across the joint – gives a muscle's function – to create tension towards or away from the body.

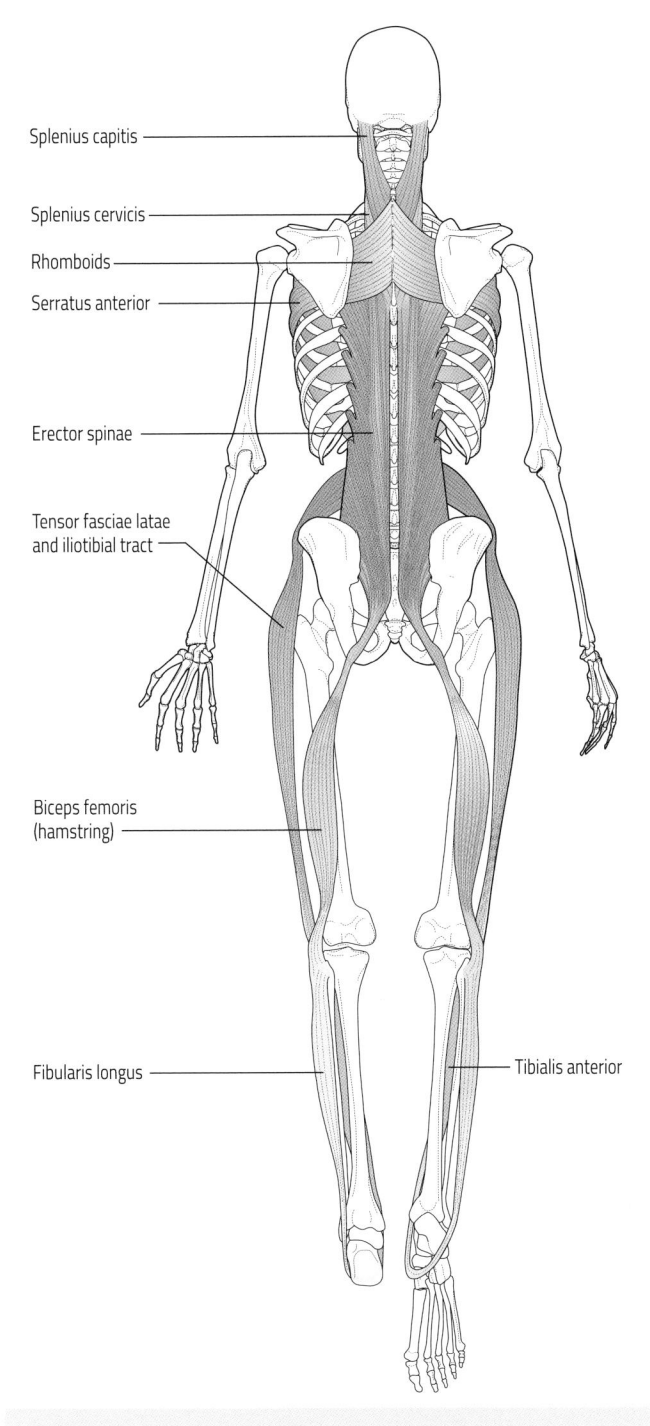

**Figure 3.25**
The spiral line, back view

# CHAPTER three

Torque is created because almost all our muscles are offset to the bone, causing a twist as the muscle contracts, that puts the power into movement.

Chains of muscles work together to create torque, and Pineau finds that these groupings are constant (Fig. 3.26). While internal torque chains draw the body in on itself, for example clasping something heavy, external torque chains expand it, for example drawing the arm back to throw something. While pectoralis major creates internal torque, the latissimus dorsi create external torque. External and internal torque chains need to be in balance together as we stand and move, with one chain moving and the other stabilizing us in any moment.

> How do primary and secondary curves relate to external and internal torque chains? Are they different ways of describing the same groupings? I am not sufficiently versed in the anatomy of both systems to answer this. Both these spiral models need more research verification; again, I invite you to play with them and make your own judgment.

### Western postural ideals emphasize secondary curves and external torque patterns

Most Westerners are out of balance, with either primary or secondary curves dominating. Many are only too aware of their primary curve patterns – round-shouldered, rounded spine, slumping in a chair – but are unaware of secondary curve patterns. In fact, much of what we think of as good posture – shoulders back, chest up, chin up, feet turned out – are an overshoot of the neutral balanced position and are secondary curve patterns. This can equally be reframed as an imbalance in our internal and external torque chains. Pineau points out that most training overemphasizes the external torque chains (see Chapter 5). Part 2 of this book looks in detail at our patterns, and will often seem wrong to our eyes because we will be rediscovering the true balance between the spiral patterns that will return us to full biomechanical balance.

### The flow of dynamic balance

The models presented above are overlapping: they all involve kinetic chains of muscles or myofascia in oppositional tone along tensile lines and sheets balanced with compressive forces. So why define three structural fundamentals? I see them as building on each other to give a fully functional body.

*Fascintegrity*: the living structural ground of the body facilitates body-wide connectivity through mechanotransduction, giving our baseline organization.

On this, mechanical forces (including gravity and movement) act and can be analyzed through modern biomechanics.

The curve patterns and torque chains act in combination for a wide range of fluid, integrated, and powerful movements.

> I notice that these models draw different groups. Somatics practitioners, communicating with the body through touch, are drawn to fascial continuity ideas. Biomechanics is highly theoretical and mathematical, designed for movement analysis, and attracts researchers and analytical-based practitioners. The curve models provide elegant simplicity for movement analysis for dance, body building, fitness, etc.

Bringing the kinetic chains into balance gives the body a geometric framework poised to morph or thrust into action that can perform well in any situation. This makes a fully functional body, in a *flow of dynamic balance*.

# The fundamentals of structure

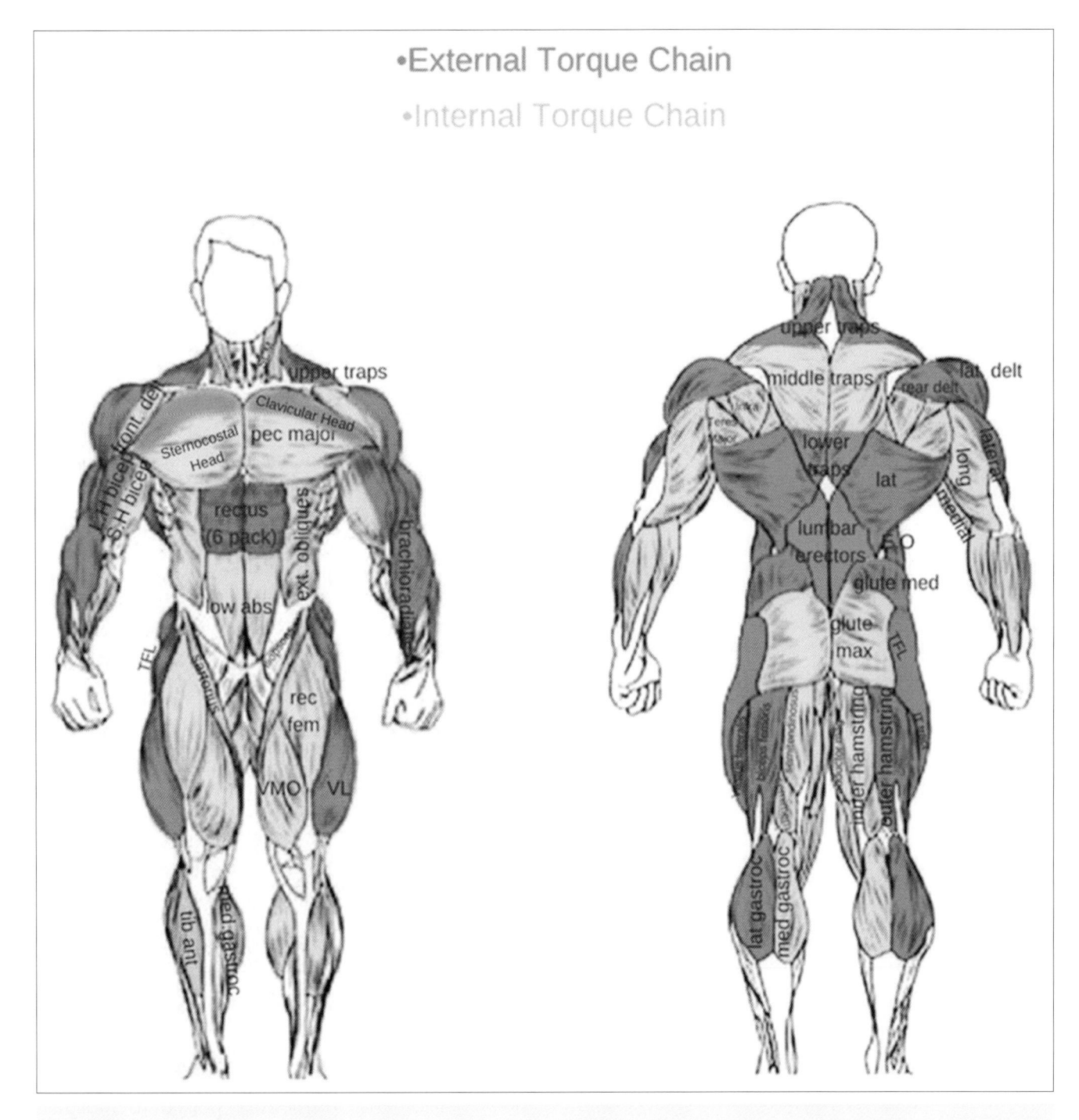

**Figure 3.26**
External and internal torque chains. Reproduced with kind permission from Julien Pineau, wwwStrongFit.com.

# CHAPTER three

> Picture two people playing tennis. The first is stable, with their myofascial trains and curve patterns in balance together, aligned with gravity. With no co-contraction, all joints will be fully mobile and fully available for fluid whole-body movement patterns. This dynamic balance is maintained moment by moment by the nervous system, using sensory feedback, requiring minimum work to maintain it. Any thrust to move will be aligned with the movement, giving optimal power for the energy used.
>
> The other person is not well aligned, with maybe upper chest collapsed, protruding neck and other areas tensed and co-contracted for support. Each imbalanced part loads the part below and it requires more overall work to maintain stability. Sensory feedback from muscles is reduced, consciousness of the body is dulled. The co-contractions stiffen and shorten the whole system, reducing adaptive responsiveness of muscles, mobility of joints, and tying areas together that should move separately. Myofascial or kinetic chains now cannot operate as a whole, but are divided into partial patterns. Because springiness is lost, areas of the body – for example, legs – must be pushed into movement, while other areas that are not joined up get carried along, or involved inappropriately in compensatory movement patterns such as hip twists, upper body tilting, etc.
>
> It is not hard to imagine who will win the game!

### Exploration 3.14  Linking up the body, coming into a flow of dynamic balance

(a)  *Stand balanced on two legs, and perform some simple movements such as lifting an arm up, or out to the side; turning your head or looking up. Let your eyes lead the movement.*

(b)  *Now repeat this, but before each movement, soften your knees so that they are free to join in the movement as needed. Go between (a) and (b) until you can notice differences. What are they?*

You may be aware that (b) is freer.

- *Notice that if the movement is done with unresponsive legs, then the unmoving parts of the body must resist the movement happening to maintain stability.*
- *If the knees soften first, then the whole-body is free to move in a dynamic balance, moving and stabilizing together. You may notice spirals and curves coming into play as part of this, and that the muscle trains can all join up.*

Tai Chi, with its flow of movement along a continuity of balanced moments, can be seen as a study of the flow of dynamic balance.

> **AT info:**  Alexander referred to this flow of dynamic balance as a position of mechanical advantage (PMA). The modern AT only defines "monkey" (Fig. 13.8) as a PMA, whereas Alexander himself defined many different ones, such as leaning back in a chair (Alexander 2011: 158). When using this term, he is not referring to static positions but freeze-frames in a flow of balanced movement, so that the torso stays in expansion whatever the limbs are doing, for instance between leaning back in the chair, sitting, and standing.

### We are relaxed in activity when in a flow of dynamic balance

Many people think of relaxation as letting everything go, such as lying back on a bed or sofa. This relaxing is really collapsing. Lying flat and letting the body tone go is needed at night when we sleep, but is not much use for getting the shopping done. Others relax by reading a book or other activities to distract the mind so that the body can let go. I prefer it when people tell me they relax by walking, easy running, or swimming, as balanced, rhythmic movements can gently realign the body.

With the flow of dynamic balance, I suggest we have a new definition of relaxing, *in which every part of the body is working!* With the muscles in active, lengthening relationships, the separate parts are brought into alignment, and the whole system will operate with

# The fundamentals of structure

least strain. This can go against everything we believe about relaxation. In particular, we need a well-functioning internal torque chain, which includes our core muscles that stabilize the structure (deep front line, Chapter 10, lesson 3). These also link to a calm nervous system. Then big outward movements can occur fluidly and easily, with easy coordination, and with full mobility across joints.

## Lesson 5  Control mechanisms of body balance and movement – the self-organization of the body

What we are seeing in all the explorations is the self-organization of the body: if we find the right cues for the nervous system, the body will self-correct.

How is this balanced network of lengthening muscles maintained?

There are several control mechanisms for organizing posture and movement. Alexander knew two of these (1 and 3 below):

1. The stretching of muscles produces an elastic recoil response which is greater when muscles are toned (i.e. stiffer rather than floppy) and actively lengthening in eccentric contraction. I suggest that we are springy when we have elastic resistance along with responsive muscle tone, so that the body can utilize the elastic recoil.

2. Central pattern generators (CPGs) that run rhythmical movement patterns were discovered in 1930s but did not receive recognition for many decades. See Chapter 6.

3. Reflex arcs, discovered in the 1930s, were thought to control movement, but are now understood to be only one of several sensory inputs to movement.

4. Spinal microcircuits and the dynamic modulation of postural tone.

These elements have been studied separately for decades. Recent studies have begun to integrate them into one model (Prochazka and Yakovenko 2007).

### *Reflexes and the maintenance of lengthening tone – old and new understandings*

The balanced network of lengthening muscles is maintained by both feedback and feed forward systems. Feedback systems include reflex arcs, such as the simple knee jerk reflex. When your knee gives under you, the quad muscle suddenly lengthens, and this is detected by the stretch receptor in the muscle, which relays a signal along the sensory nerve to the spinal cord. This is then processed in the gray matter of the spinal cord, initiating the firing of a motor nerve, which causes the quad to contract, and stops you falling.

Alongside these are the Golgi tendon organs – sensors in the tendon of each muscle. These detect the force of a contraction and relay this information to the brainstem, from which the brain can adjust the contractile force of the muscle. Between these two sensory systems, we have detailed feedback of what our muscles are doing, from which postural tone or movement can be adjusted according to our needs. Other receptors in joints give information of pressure and shear across the joint, while pressure receptors in the skin, particularly in the soles of the feet, also contribute with their information.

But if all our postural tone was maintained by one-on-one reflex feedback in this way, it would absorb all the nervous system. Modern cell recording techniques have shown multi-synaptic connectivity and large-scale integrative circuits: that information mostly does not come piecemeal into the spinal cord, but comes in from several types of receptors (skin, touch, joint, tendon, and stretch receptors) and groups of receptors, onto each receiving cell body. From this, it is suggested that whole limb kinematic information is available not just to the brainstem and cerebellum (the brain areas responsible for background control and smooth movement) but even at spinal cord level (Bosco and Poppele 2001).

The old model of reflex action was of feedback pathways, continually responding to postural instability after the event. Modern neuroscience talks a

# CHAPTER three

lot about feed forward pathways, which are detecting current use and predicting what is needed next, refining it with incoming sensory input, including those of stretch receptors. "The nervous system uses sensory information to develop and recalibrate internal models of the musculoskeletal system itself" (Bosco and Poppele 2001: 541).

### The dynamic modulation of postural tone

Researcher Tim Cacciatore and his colleagues are the first to study postural tone directly using the "Twister," an incredible contraption they have developed that isolates postural tone. The first study with this showed that on twisting, stiff people tended to have fixed muscle activity while less stiff people's muscles changed length dynamically in response – one set of muscles freeing off as another set took up the slack (Gurfinkel et al. 2011). He then demonstrated that AT training makes one much better at such dynamic modulation of postural tone than healthy untrained adults (Cacciatore et al. 2011).

In the white matter of the spinal cord, there are *two pathways of muscle action*, transmitted by motor neurons down the spinal cord. The *pyramidal pathways* (also called the corticospinal tracts) conduct signals from the cerebral cortex and some brainstem nuclei. They are involved in the generation of skilled movements. The *extrapyramidal pathways* conduct signals from subcortical regions – nuclei in the medulla oblongata and pons, and from the cerebellum and brainstem – and are involved in the complex patterning of postural control and locomotion. So, for instance, when you pick up your full mug of tea and bring it to your lips, the pyramidal pathways organize the precise holding and moving of the cup so you do not spill a drop, while the extrapyramidal pathways organize the background tone of the body, so that the weight of the cup and of the moving arm is accommodated, and balance maintained. The cortical output is almost all phasic, while the extrapyramidal output is tonic.

In the gray matter of the spinal cord, interneurons interface simply or in complex formations of spinal microcircuits. It is hypothesized that these form a pattern formation layer that recruits appropriate patterns of muscles to coordinate all the other muscles in dynamic and appropriate play (Guertin 2012).

But what happens when we are fighting gravity to stand and move, with some muscles working overtime to hold us up while others are switched off? My understanding is that when muscles become over-contracted, we lose this dynamic instinctive relationship with our muscles. Instead, we have to hold the body contracted to stand, and then further contract them to move.

While it can feel satisfying to sense muscles working, I speculate that what we are feeling is muscle imbalance; in contrast, fluid, integrated movement gives very little sensation.

## A summary of the engineering of the human body in nine layers

We will explore each of these in more detail in other chapters except 2, which is the study of craniosacral therapy. Deep AT work touches this system, and is worth exploring by any serious AT teacher.

1. The deepest layer of muscles of the spine and its link to the occiput are a fascial unity.

2. Inside this is the craniosacral system of spinal cord and brain, surrounded by strong membranes; and a balance of fascia within the spine and skull that can also pull the body out of shape when imbalanced.

3. Erector spinae, with their myofascial links to the balance of the head, give us the primary extensor system maintaining the upright spine.

4. Several structures hang down from above: the jaw hangs down from the skull by the masseter muscle; the windpipe and larynx hang from the styloid processes of the skull; while the throat and the start of the digestive tract is slung from the front of the occiput at the base of the skull. While the ribs are supported by sternum and spine, they are also suspended from above: from the skull by

# The fundamentals of structure

the SCMs, from the neck by the scalene muscles, and from the spine by posterior serratus muscles. Each structure has its relationship to gravity and is also hugely supported by continuous muscular tone and a complex fascial web providing support in all planes. These are the evolutionarily oldest structures, present in all vertebrates before limbs were added, but now operating vertically in humans.

5  The organs also hang from above and are encased and supported by the spiral lines and the superficial front lines along with the transversus abdominis, which all enclose the torso and particularly the abdomen. (This is obvious in quadrupeds where the organs hang below the spine.) The weight of the organs wants to take the body into a fetal curve, opposed by the erector spinae and latissimus dorsi extending us up, and the obliques, transverse abdominals and latissimus dorsi widening. Upright stance is a counterbalance of these curves.

6  Limbs were added for terrestrial locomotion, connected to these central structures by pelvic and shoulder girdles. The double spiral of curves that runs through the torso continues into the limbs, facilitating and powering complex movements. Because of our bipedal stance, humans have the strongest, most connected and least flexible pelvis, along with the least connected shoulder girdle allowing the greatest possible movements of the arms. The pelvis is commonly understood as an arch structure, sitting on the legs and supporting the torso, supported by many muscles that balance and spread the load at that point. While the arms hang down at rest, their tone is as vital to whole-body dynamic balance as any other part.

7  Our overall structure is supported by the upright stance of head, torso, and legs, on which the shoulder girdle and arms float. This central structure is stabilized by superficial front line, superficial back line, lateral line, and spiral lines all working together.

8  Within all this are the deep front lines that link and support from within and provide support for the internal organs. The adductors and deep muscles of legs, pelvic floor and psoas, belly muscles, diaphragm, the throat, larynx and floor of mouth are all part of this continuity.

9  The surface layer of the body, with gluteus maximus, hamstrings, latissimus dorsi, trapezius and deltoids – comprising the functional lines – propels kinetic force from the feet and legs through the back and to the arms and hands.

In summary, the head–neck–trunk–legs makes a functional unit that is led from the head, but driven and supported from the pelvis and back, legs, and feet. The ribs hang down from this for independent movement, although their width gives the lateral expansion of the torso and is also key to postural support. The shoulder girdle and arms float on top of the expanding ribcage and are then free for a wide range of independent movement. This is key to human structure, but it is usually not working fully.

We will see again and again in subsequent chapters that when the central structures are not offering sufficient support and the ribs are not moving freely, the shoulder girdle, arms, and outer back muscles have to take over. This is to their detriment, and to the neck which is tightened and pulled down. The reverse is also true: when the outer layers are imbalanced, the inner layers are compromised. Because the throat and voice-box are slung within all this balance of opposing forces, their optimal functioning is completely dependent on balanced relationships being maintained throughout the system. Any torsion or collapse will be reflected in forces on them, making voice a very accurate indicator of alignment. No wonder that Alexander, Delsarte, and others began their discoveries with an analysis of voice production.

The chapter Appendix that follows gives some teaching tips for this book.

# CHAPTER three

## Appendix: Twelve teaching tips

**Staying on-script, going off-script.** Most healing methods have undergone a shift in focus: from the discovery process of the founder, a right brain-led exploratory process of moving into the unknown, to a left brain protocol, a "this is how you do it to get this result" process. This is always necessary to establish the process and define the method, but is not the end of the road. If a technique just becomes protocols it risks becoming "cast in stone," drawing only from the experiences and ideas of past "experts," and not a living process in the present.

We need both. When teaching only happens from remembered actions, there is no inner life for the pupil to resonate with, and little true learning can occur. But we need to start with the method, to learn its rhythms and purposes, its usefulness and its limits, from where we can then begin to play. These procedures work, they are tested, and the words are all carefully chosen. Use the steps and even the language given to master them and get the feel of them. But they are only a starting point for you. Then if you pay attention with your whole being to yourself and the pupil, you can follow your own guidance and inspiration of how to proceed with them and begin to make your own discoveries.

"Mr Alexander would make more discoveries making a cup of tea than most teachers make in their entire lives!" said Miss Goldie to me in 1990. I think we have moved on from here, yet there is always more to learn as we become conscious that every action can be a journey of discovery.

However, I suggest not going off-script too quickly. I notice that when I follow a new cookery recipe, my inclination is immediately to add "my own touches"; this feels creative and self-determining, but leads inevitably to food that is no different to my usual creations. To discover something radically different, I must follow the new recipe exactly a few times, and then a new flavor can be discovered with which I can experiment.

**Go through it twice yourself.** The first (and obvious) step in teaching anything is to have a good-enough grasp of a procedure yourself – both of the process and what it is trying to achieve. This usually requires going through each exploration at least twice – depending on your own learning rhythm. My own strategy for learning is to go fully through a chapter or lesson once, and then go back and have another go at each section in more detail. Rather than bashing away to try to understand something, leave a few hours, or preferably a day or two between these readings, so that the brain has a chance to process what was read. Be patient with your own learning rhythm – these are three-dimensional concepts rather than linear facts and they need to be felt within the body, which takes time.

**Get in there and have a go!** The best way to learn something and deepen understanding is to teach it! Play with each little technique with someone you know well – a friend, colleague, or longer-term client/pupil – and have a go, in a very simple way. It need only take a few minutes.

**Hands off or hands on?** There are four options: (1) the old way was to do it for the pupil and not explain, but I feel these days are past – for any therapy; (2) you can use your hands to do it for them, and then explain after what has happened; (3) you can talk them through doing it for themselves, but with your hands on to monitor what is happening; or (4) you can work through verbal direction alone. I think these four options are stages on the path many Alexander teachers are now exploring – it certainly charts my own path as I have found my confidence in taking hands off. Many teachers, including myself, are now also working online, in which this is the only option. If you do put hands on, then light touch is needed both for your receptivity and for effective somatic communication. This is discussed in Chapter 18.

**Finding the words.** Most manual therapists and many AT teachers are so used to "talking" with their hands only that it can be very unfamiliar to use words alone. Words enable us to refine understanding – for us and the pupil – and make us develop our observation skills. The first time you work primarily or

# The fundamentals of structure

solely with verbal directions you will be searching for the right words, remembering sequences, etc., but this fumbling start gets the process of understanding underway. You can talk it through with yourself first to help this along. Reread the instructions in between attempts until you can find your own words to put the concepts across. *Always watch for the effect of different words or phrases – they can change the outcome for better or worse.*

With time, you can explore the directions fully for yourself alongside the client (see below); this makes it a much more internal process. Then you will be envisaging it and embodying it as you describe it, and your own three-dimensional understanding will communicate (see Chapter 17 on whole-body speaking).

**Use pictures and toys.** Show your pupils the pictures, get charts, get a tensegrity toy, find videos. A picture is worth a thousand words, and a three-dimensional model is worth more still.

**How do I begin?** If you are shy of trying a new approach, you could preface it with "Can we try something different to help your neck (or back, or balance etc.)?" or "I read about this yesterday and it makes sense to me, can we give it a go?" If it works, you both learn something. If it doesn't, then quietly steer them into something more familiar, and try again another day with someone else. Or you could say: "I'm not sure we're getting this working yet, we'll come back to it some other time."

**Look confident!** Remember the pupil does not know what you are trying to do, so will usually not know if it has worked or not.

**Start simple.** See if you can talk them through "rolling their raindrop" or getting their feet hip-width apart with free knees. It takes a couple of minutes only and begins to give you a sense of how directing their action with words alone works in practice. It is my fervent wish that, if nothing else, these two simple skills are taught by every therapist and movement educator to every client and pupil who is ready to hear, as they can make such a difference!

**Thinking alongside the pupil.** Once you have a grasp of the method, it is crucial that, whatever you are asking the pupil to do and whether your hands are on or off, you are also going through the procedure yourself. Firstly, it means you are engaged with the process. If you are only remembering and communicating steps by rote, this is left hemisphere learning and will be much less fun for the pupil (and you), and will not hold as well. By making it an exploration for yourself, this awakens your own interest in it which brings you into your right hemisphere/whole-body consciousness. You are then teaching at an *embodied* level in the present, which engages the pupil's nervous system with the right hemisphere to right hemisphere communication (Chapter 18).

**Observe your pupil.** Your pupil might not be "getting it" because they have their own blocks. Watch continually whether they are responding as you intend, enjoying the process or becoming frustrated or bored. Is their voice/face/body relaxing or tightening, engaging or withdrawing? Watch for the moments to press on, or the moments to back off or change direction; sometimes people are not yet ready for this stage. Use your eyes, your ears, your intuitive senses. These skills will build with time.

**Attuning to yourself and the pupil together.** For deep change, your whole nervous system is communicating what is happening for you to the pupil, and you are also attuned to what is happening for them. Then you are alive to what their systems need and can modify the process accordingly – you can feel into what is needed. This is what we are aiming for.

All this is discussed in more detail in Chapter 18, where we look at how to put hands on a pupil, and how to maintain spatial relationship to them.

### Professional protocol when sharing this material

Training to teach the Alexander technique requires several years of intense study with a certified AT teacher. I am inviting any somatic or movement practitioner to share this material as appropriate for their

# CHAPTER three

practice and clients. However, please do not claim to be a teacher of the Alexander technique without the full AT training. Instead, I suggest saying that you are sharing methods/procedures/explorations that come from Alexander technique and this book.

## Further reading

Blakeslee, S. and Blakeslee, M., 2008. *The body has a mind of its own*. New York: Random House.

Bowman, K., 2017. *Move your DNA. Restore your health through natural movement*. USA: Propriometrics Press.

Dimon, T., 2001. *Anatomy of the moving body. A basic course in bones, muscles, and joints*. Berkeley, CA: North Atlantic Books.

Dimon, T., 2011. *The body in motion: Its evolution and design*. Berkeley, CA: North Atlantic Books.

Grunwald, P., 2010. *Eyebody. The art of integrating eye, brain and body*. 2nd edn. Auckland, NZ: Condevis Publishing.

Jones, F.P., 2016. *Freedom to change. The development and science of the Alexander technique*. 3rd edn. London: Mouritz.

McGilchrist, I., 2012. *The master and his emissary. The divided brain and the making of the Western world*. New Haven, CT: Yale University Press.

Myers, T., 2014. *Anatomy trains. Myofascial meridians for manual and movement therapists*. 3rd edn. Edinburgh: Elsevier.

Pert, C., 1998. *Molecules of emotion. Why you feel the way you feel*. London: Simon and Schuster.

Porges, S.W., 2017. *The pocket guide to the polyvagal theory: the transformative power of feeling safe*. New York: Norton.

Shepherd, P., 2010. *New self, new world*. Berkeley, CA: North Atlantic Books.

Shepherd, P., 2017. *Radical wholeness*. Berkeley, CA: North Atlantic Books.

Siegel, D., 2010. *The mindful therapist*. New York: Norton Books.

Vineyard, M., 2007. *How you stand, how you move, how you live*. MA: Da Capo Press.

Wolf, J., 2014. *Art of breathing* [video download]. Available at: <http://www.jessicawolfartofbreathing.com/> (last accessed 31 July 2020).

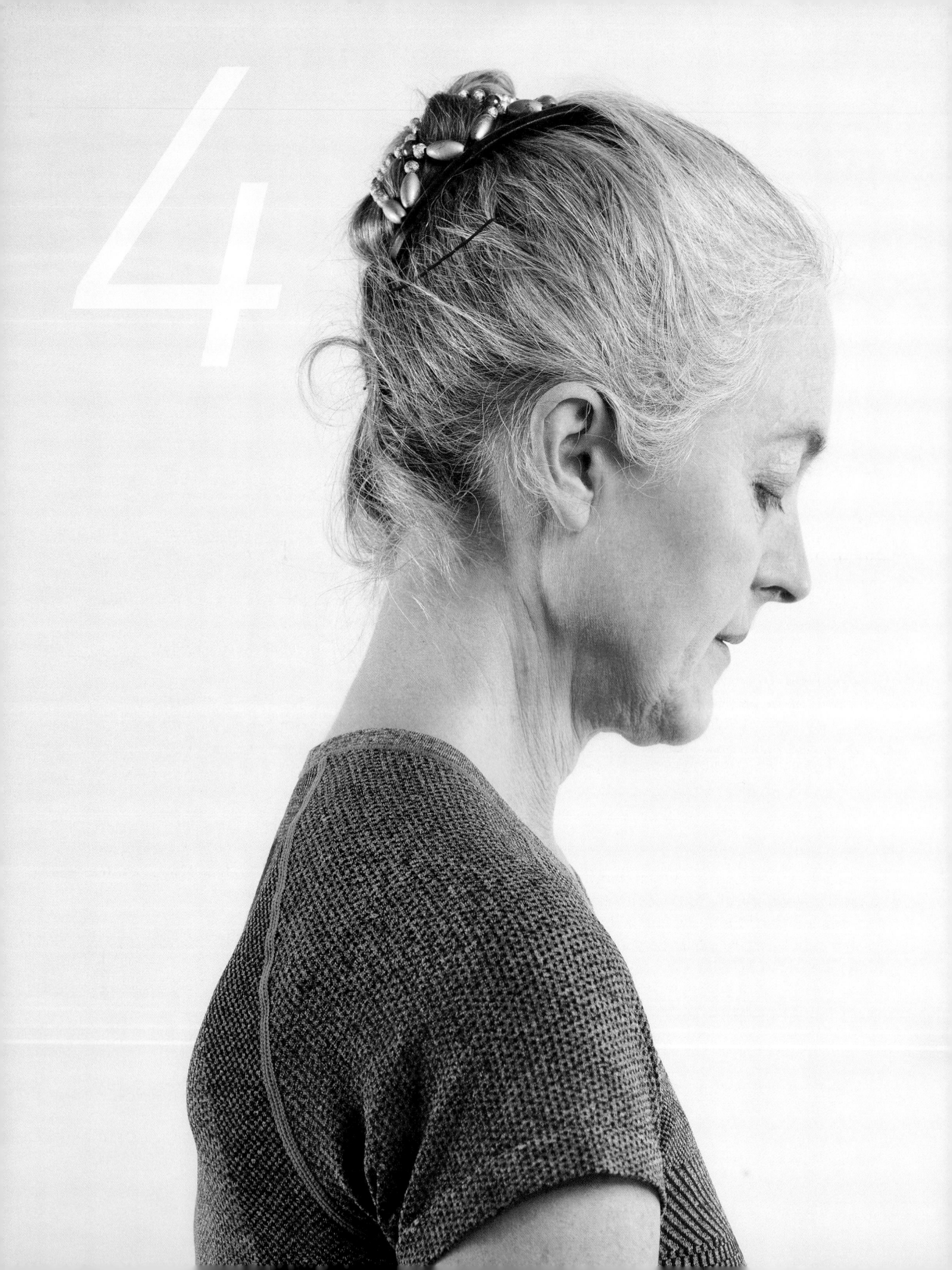

4

# The fundamentals of awareness and thinking 4

Our thoughts, our tension levels, and our sense of embodiment and energy go together, along with the awareness of our surroundings (Shepherd 2017). For instance, if one is anxious, the body will tense up slightly, as if something has risen up the body. At the same time, one may feel less grounded, less in contact with the world around or with the sense of one's own body – embodiment. In another scenario, when feeling depressed one may feel "down" and heavy on the ground, the body slumps with loss of tone, the energy becomes sluggish, one will probably withdraw into oneself. It is tempting to add causality, to choose one of these and say it caused the others, but in practice they all occur together. When these imbalances happen, our spatial sense becomes skewed, reduced to focusing on what concerns us most – whether one gets stuck in thoughts or emotions, or lethargy, in watching for danger, or on physical discomfort. Since imbalance of the physical body is part and parcel of this, we lose optimal movement patterns. Our sense of the whole self is also diminished.

Science might define these phenomena with the general word "stress" and relate it to the autonomic nervous system, which we will look at in the next chapter. But here I want to highlight and explore these more subjective phenomena, discovering how to work with them. The methods are those I developed to bring about the quality of Miss Goldie's lessons, in workshops often titled "Come to quiet." From the scientific viewpoint, much of this chapter is highly speculative. Where there is research, it is often outside standard paradigms of thought, or is only beginning to be accepted, and I have sometimes pushed the speculations that come from it further still. So as ever, I invite you to play with the explorations and be your own research subject. One can discover that working with any one of these aspects can swing us back into a felt sense of coherence, and so into balance and integrated movement.

## Lesson 1  Waking up external perception – tracking a visual line

Do we really see what is in front of us? Or do we in fact see what we expect to see?

### Exploration 4.1    Tracking side to side

- *Stand balanced (as Chapter 3, lesson 3).*

- *Look straight forward at an interesting view and focus on something a comfortable distance away. See the colors that are really there – they may not be as you expect. Are the leaves really green? Is the cloud white?*

- *Now take your eyes for a little walk to the left, over the objects they encounter, and over the surfaces between objects too, as if your vision is a little dog sniffing its way over the ground. Your head will follow easily on the axis joint, as the eyes lead the head.*

- *It can help to envisage a long feather (or alternatively a paintbrush) from your nose to the items viewed, brushing each as the vision explores it. Involving your nose will help balance the head and help both eyes to converge on the point of your attention.*

- *Then track attentively back to center and to the right, and so on.*

- *Do your eyes willingly track a smooth path? Do they hop from object to object? Do they stop and glaze over, go to sleep? Invite them to track smoothly, open to seeing all the unexpected detail, color, shape, shading of each object and area in turn, without analysis.*

Initially this can be difficult. I find my eyes usually begin in jumping mode but then settle to tracking, and on each arc I see more than the time before, which is deeply calming to the whole system.

Video link for explorations 4.1 and 4.2

### Exploration 4.2    Tracking a line

- *Now track away from yourself, from below your feet out as far as you can to the horizon (or in a limited space:*

# CHAPTER four

*across the floor and up the wall) and back again. Trace a path: follow any lines available, such as floorboards, fences, etc. or follow an imaginary line. Track it gently along, inviting the eyes not to glaze out or jump. Use your nose feather to help both eyes and your attention engage at the same point.*

- *Track out and back again a few times. You may notice that as you go up to the upper limits, your head gently follows your eyes up. Then when your eyes get back to the floor below you, your head nods forwards a little on the top of your neck. Discover that the eyes can lead the head on the nodding joint.*

### Tracking in real time

As my eyes and I become calmer as I track, I feel that time expands. One is seeing so much more, yet there is a wealth of time to use. In this, I propose we are transitioning from left to right hemisphere dominance (McGilchrist 2012: 75–6). Left hemisphere vision is fragmentary: notice that when the eyes jump between objects, they see nothing in between. There is no flow of time, only an urgency to "get there," "get the job done," even though in this moment there is nothing to do. In this way of seeing all objects are disconnected, nothing is linked to anything else, or to me, while in the flow of vision it all hangs together and everything has its place, including me.

One can play with this while out walking, especially while "getting the shopping done." What would it be like to see the pavements, the walls, the people you pass, rather than rushing from shop to shop? (I notice that displays of goods are designed to grab our attention which fragments our vision again.) If you feel that sustained attention takes too long, remember that this is a left hemisphere illusion. Invite yourself to trust time, and notice what happens.

### Lesson 2  Clear brain choices and "inhibition" – the key to changing brain patterns of body use

We are discovering habits of use that are unhelpful, and setting an intent to change them. But we cannot make changes from the physical body itself, as most physical work assumes. This is because these habit patterns are held in the central nervous system of brain and spinal cord, and when habits change, the brain resets to our current habit patterns leaving us unaware. Alexander called this faulty sensory perception. In exploration 3.2 we learned to observe our habits by choosing to become conscious of them.

### Exploration 4.3  Observing without reacting

- *Become aware now of a habit – maybe your head is tipped back or your feet are too close together. Can you simply observe this without reacting? Or, when you notice something "wrong," do you instantly move to correct it?*

*Inhibition is the moment of not reacting to a stimulus.* (Its opposite is excitation.)

### Saying "stop"

Having a choice of how to act is at the heart of the technique.

- If we react to a tipped back head by pulling it forward again, we simply exchange one tight muscle group for another. Instead we could think: "stop" or "don't react" or "let it alone." By stopping the desire to act, we gain a moment of reflection in which we can choose to do something else.

- From this reflective moment we can remember some different possibilities: such as that the natural balance of the head is forward, and that the direction for enabling this is "rolling a raindrop down the nose" (exploration 3.8).

- Then we can action that change: to let the new movement happen by itself. We are usually over-involved with every action we do. *There are simpler, older pathways in the nervous system that will work beautifully for us, if only we would let them work without interference. These have no sensation in them, and so it feels like we are not-doing the action, that it somehow "does itself."*

# The fundamentals of awareness and thinking

This requires moment by moment inhibition, continued presence, to stop the usual pathways swinging back into action.

Psychological research on inhibition focuses on inhibitory control as part of our "executive functioning," along with working memory and cognitive flexibility. The ability to choose our actions and to say no to unwanted actions is a crucial part of living, for ourselves and for society to function. "Reactive inhibition" is mediated by simple pathways in the frontal and subcortical brain, and it stops the firing of motor nerves that would carry out the action, which allows for a new action to be chosen and initiated. This is a stop/go, whole-body response process, such as stopping at traffic lights, or a sportsperson changing direction to dodge a tackle. We all make such decisions daily and they do not usually, in themselves, change our tension levels.

In general in AT we are doing something more subtle than this that changes the body state. Psychologists now talk more of proactive and selective inhibition, for where there is time to choose a response and prior knowledge of what to do in working memory. The description given above of remembering how to rebalance the head fits this model. These are also executive inhibition processes. Both Rajal Cohen (2019) and Patrick Johnson (2019b) explore the degree to which the processes of executive inhibition are relevant to the AT.

But this cannot be the whole story. Johnson points out that the executive function model is of short-term processes, changing from one action to another. He cites Cacciatore et al. (2014), who noted that while AT teachers could perform a *very* slow, smooth, and sustained sit to stand movement, control subjects attempting this *always* lurched to lift themselves off the chair, however much they understood cognitively that they should not. In that moment, they could have performed any other executive task, so why not this one? There is something different going on. Cacciatore (personal communication, February 11, 2020) and Johnson both think that this inhibition is not a short-term process but a *state* we can inhabit, of quiet, tonic functioning, which enables the system to self-organize and modulate responsively. It is probably not a simple pathway, but a more complex state of networks involving many aspects of being.

This could also relate to left and right hemisphere. According to McGilchrist (2012: 91), left hemisphere inhibition is stop or go, while right hemisphere inhibition is more about finding space, a moment of quiet waiting from which something new can emerge, a place of *modulating* an action rather than *stopping* and then resuming. This may involve whole-body decisions rather than the hierarchical top-down/brain-in-charge approach.

Johnson and Cacciatore's scientific perspective fits with my experiences in Miss Goldie's lessons. She taught me to find inhibition as a state of quiet aliveness from which clear choices could be made and the body could flow responsively into movement. This deeper level of inhibition often does not need thoughts or words and could be part of how animals or small children stay free, for they are clearly not saying "let my neck be free," or imagining raindrops rolling. We will return to this in lesson 7, activating this positive state from quiet presence using the fundamentals of perception, orientation and embodiment.

### Exploration 4.4    Using inhibition to reduce whole-body tension

To come out of patterns of co-contraction and into better physical balance, we need to maintain a background awareness of current tensions and imbalances, and *not* to change what we observe. Then we can use phrases to cue the nervous system response. The simplest inhibitory phrase is "I can do less."

- *Say: "I can do less with my shoulders/knees/wrists" when you notice individual body areas are tight or working too hard. Notice whether the tension reduces.*

But individual tensions are always part of a bigger picture of tension.

# CHAPTER four

- *Use "I can do less" any time when you are aware of using too much tension and effort overall. Perhaps rushing to catch a shop before it closes, or using too much force to open a door, or holding the steering wheel too tightly.*

For either of these:

1  *Observe the tension.*

2  *Do not react to it.*

3  *Think of the phrase needed.*

4  *Say/think the phrase clearly.*

5  *Notice what happens, and trust the brain to sort it without your help.*

This does not necessarily mean that the body does less overall. Movements may become smaller, or they may become more expansive, freer, bigger, as the freedom allows the natural movement to surface. The "doing" we are reducing is our interference, not the action in itself.

### The "muscle tension control board" of the brain

These self-organizing centers are probably in the hindbrain. I picture them as having control boards like those of sound engineers at a rock concert, with levers for guitar, singer, and drums. By adjusting each lever up or down they can keep the balance of the music. Just so, when we bring the brain's attention to the overall imbalance, it adjusts the control for each muscle or muscle group to restore the tensional balance. This is the *dynamic modulation of postural tone* (see Chapter 3, lesson 5).

### We are not "releasing" our tension

Releasing muscle tension has become a modern obsession, with such instructions as "release your neck," "give me the weight of your leg, let it be heavy," and so on. While this is sometimes necessary initially with very tense pupils, it is not useful beyond that point. "Release" invites "let go," which can result in collapse of tone in the dynamic balance of the system, like letting the guy ropes slacken on a tent. To stay with "release" work, usually also done on the table which itself encourages passivity, will never strengthen someone's body. To bring the body back into a balance of lengthening relationships which will then *maintain* ease between all areas, we need to be developing tone, not reducing it.

> The word "release" was despised by Miss Goldie, and also by Marjorie Barstow. I heard both these senior teachers observe that it was a common pattern to over-release the shoulders, and so partially collapse the upper back.

Equally, we are not "relaxing." I see true relaxation as a state of toned balance throughout the whole-body, where nothing is either over- or under-working. When we think to "relax" an area of the body, we are usually inviting release there. Inhibition must always be done at brain level just as to reduce a lightbulb's intensity you must use the dimmer switch.

### Exploration 4.5  "Negative directions" given to the activity itself

This form of inhibition was discovered by Missy Vineyard (2007: 169).

- *Verbally deny the activity you are doing, such as "I am not walking," "I am not opening the door," or "I am not vacuuming," and notice what happens.*

I suspect this works because we let go of cortical interference patterns. Alexander thought these stemmed from our preconceived ideas of walking, opening doors, or vacuuming, which may also be part of the picture. This leaves the deeper, tonic pathways freedom to work, and the action becomes freer. It also addresses the activity rather than the body directly, which can be more successful (see Chapter 16, lesson 3).

# The fundamentals of awareness and thinking

*Five tips for making long-term change in our patterns*

1  *Change default patterns in muscle use and consciousness by thinking these thoughts regularly.*

   It is easy to make a change using inhibition, but the brain usually resets quickly to the old pattern, its current "default." We need to repeat and repeat until the new patterns are taken into sub-cortical layers and become the new default. I notice that some defaults reset easily; others fight you all the way.

   In the early days of my lessons, my throat area was very tense. One night I woke and noticed that my tongue was held tightly against the roof of my mouth. I thought "let the tongue be free" and it relaxed into the floor of the mouth. A few minutes later I noticed it had tensed up again. I repeated the phrase, and again it freed then tightened. I decided to stay present, rather than "switch off" once change occurred. I watched it free, and saw that within a microsecond it was tensing again. Immediately I repeated the phrase and the same thing happened. I continued this, seeing no change in the pattern, until I fell back to sleep.

   The next night I woke again to a tense tongue, and repeated my procedure. It still tightened again but not quite as fast, maybe staying free for one tenth of a second. Again I repeated the process until I fell asleep. The next night the tongue stayed free for maybe a quarter of a second. This went on for perhaps two weeks, until one night only one instruction was needed, and it stayed free. This has held over the years: any time my tongue tightens, it only takes one thought.

2  *"If only I could hold onto the change!"* Holding on always involves tension. When a nerve fires, it happens in a microsecond, and then has to reset before it can fire again. The only way to repeat is to re-send the message.

3  *"I know what I'm doing now."* Once we have experienced, say, a free head/neck joint, we latch onto the feeling, and when it tightens again try to recreate the freedom using muscles instead of using the unfamiliar thinking work. Goldie talked to me about "always returning to first principles." This is "beginner's mind," a place of no expectation. In other words, *every* time we want to make a change, we need to inhibit the desire just to get in there and reproduce the feeling, and instead do all the thinking again *as if we have never done it before.*

4  *"I can't be aware all the time."* That's ok. While autopilot changes nothing, it won't worsen it either. It is those small but powerful moments of quiet, sustained attention that change brain plasticity (Doidge 2007: 53).

5  *"How long do I need to think these conscious thoughts for?"* The left hemisphere wants us to fix the problem and move on. But life keeps changing and we need to be awake! Alongside changing our movement patterns, think of building new habits of staying conscious and present, of being in right hemisphere thinking.

## Lesson 3   Interoception – the internal world of a hundred senses, and our reason to move

You move to service your internal needs: to fetch food, meet friends, go to bed, or to escape something you dislike. Life is movement. But how much attention do we pay to our internal promptings? We can become so involved in what we are doing that we forget to eat or sleep.

Emotional awareness is another matter. Do you know when you are angry, sad, or frightened? Bored or lonely? Frustrated or irritated? Like many chronic fatigue sufferers I had little awareness of my emotions. I used to get very tense in social situations before I realized that my tolerance for people was much lower than the social norm, and my legs were tense because they needed to walk away. Like many people I could spend an evening net surfing or watching TV, feeling increasingly dissatisfied because I was not stopping to ask my real feelings – a need for people, to move, or to sleep.

# CHAPTER four

Emotional awareness is a huge topic in its own right. For this book it is important because when our actions are in complete harmony with our feelings, intuitions, and drives, our movements will be more purposeful, clearer, stronger, and we will be healthier.

When I listened to my feelings, I found myself moving much more.

All internal sensing is interoception. It includes all senses from our internal organs, brought to us up the sensory fibers of the vagus nerve: whether the stomach is hungry or nauseous; the bladder is full; the sex organs are excited, or the womb aching premenstrually; whether the immune system feels well or under the weather, or ill; the pulse of the heart ... a mass of continual information.

Emotional feelings have physical sensations also carried in the vagus nerve: feeling heavy hearted, butterflies in the tummy, lump in the throat, gut clenching at the horror movie. Internal pain is carried in the same pathways and processed in the same part of the brain, the right frontal insula, which is why emotional pain and physical pain often are profoundly interlinked. The map that forms here links the body state and brain state, to give us emotional awareness (Craig 2003).

When we engage in activity, the impulse – or motivational drive – to move comes from a decision-making process that involves body and brain, exteroception, interoception, and conscious choices. Hunger may impel us from within to seek food – from which perhaps an idea emerges to go to the fridge, or desire may prompt us to reach for a biscuit in view. These often have many more unconscious layers than we are aware of, including responsiveness to other people and to our surroundings that we might call intuitive or instinctual responses.

Benjamin Libet's famous experiment asked subjects to move their finger spontaneously. He showed that they were conscious of their urge to move a finger 0.2 seconds *after* the readiness potential that would initiate the contraction (Libet 1985, cited in McGilchrist 2012: 188). It showed that the decision to move had already been taken. This prompted discussion of whether we have free will. Libet did more experiments showing that people could veto the muscle contraction before it went ahead. He concluded that what we have is "free won't" –the free will to *stop* an action. But McGilchrist comments: "Libet's experiment does not tell us that we do not choose to initiate an action: it just tells us that we have to widen our concept of who 'we' are to include our unconscious selves" (2012: 188).

Humans have more access to their internal sensations than any other animal. "Your primary visceral map [of all your organs] ... is uniquely super-developed in the human species, and it gives you a level of access to the ebb and flow of the internal sensations unequalled anywhere else in the animal kingdom. You feel lust, disgust, sadness, joy, shame, and humiliation as a result of this body mapping. These visceral inputs to the psyche are the wellspring of the rich and vivid emotional awareness that few other creatures even come close to enjoying. The activity in this map is the voice of your conscience, the thrill of music, the foundation of the emotionally nuanced and morally sensitive self" (Blakeslee and Blakeslee 2008: 11).

Research shows that the more aware we are viscerally, the more emotionally attuned we are (Blakeslee and Blakeslee 2008: 181), giving us emotional intelligence. The reverse happens when emotions or pain become overwhelming, and we cope by dissociating from the body and from our feelings. Interoception is also part of our rational intelligence: both Damasio (2006: 190) and Philip Shepherd (2017: 19) give evidence that reasoning is underpinned by gut feelings. Our cognitive functions only work well when they are working in alignment with the belly and heart brains. Stock market traders who were more in touch with the inner life of their bodies made more money (Shepherd 2017: 21)!

### Exploration 4.6   Interoceptive awareness

- *Practice interoceptive awareness by paying attention regularly to those disregarded internal messages, asking: "What*

# The fundamentals of awareness and thinking

*am I feeling right now?" Then having felt it, allow yourself to move to carry it out. You can come back to what you were doing after your need is met, if it feels right.*

- *Thirsty? Get up and have a drink.*
- *Bored body and legs? Stretch or dance around the room a bit.*
- *Lonely? Phone a friend, cuddle the cat. Feeling unsafe? Acknowledge it, then make a change to help yourself.*
- *Watching a film? Acknowledge the fears, longings, or sadnesses that stir in us from what we are witnessing, and which require processing afterwards.*
- *Really hear and feel what someone is telling you – empathy requires interoception too.*

  Discover your "free won't."

- *You may also become more aware of actions that previously would have gone "under the radar" such as reaching for another biscuit or cigarette. Then you have a choice to say "no."*

## Lesson 4 Where we think from – mind in the brain, awareness versus feeling

### *Mind in the brain, one of Alexander's lost instructions*

When I first started Alexander work, it was a joy to find my body. To discover my hips, my lower back, to feel into it and be able to send instructions directly to it. I thought I knew my body as a dancer, but it turned out I only knew it from the outside, not from the inside. This involvement with my body was encouraged by my first teachers and my training school. Then when I went to Miss Goldie, she wanted something completely different, that I should bring my mind out of this over-involvement with the body.

"Your mind is in the brain, and your brain is in the head," Miss Goldie would often tell me, sometimes adding "and your head is at the top of you!" In the technique we talk a lot about thinking, but rarely about from where we think. *"Mind in the brain" gives us the key how to become conscious of the body without interfering*: if my mind is not in my brain, then it is wandering round my body checking on myself. (This may be conscious or unconscious.)

Mind in the brain is a key concept in the technique that was never explicitly articulated by Alexander, though he did say: "There must be a clear differentiation in [the pupil's] mind between the giving of the order and the performance of the act ordered and carried out through the medium of the muscles" (Alexander 2011: 167).

This story, which Goldie told me and I think originated with Alexander is a clear metaphor for mind in the brain.

A boss in charge of a typing pool worked in his office all day with the door shut; the typists sent the wrong letters to the wrong people and chaos reigned. One day the boss realized there was a problem and went out into the typing pool to sort it out. But in his effort to help he found he was getting in the way, making them self-conscious and creating more errors. He was in despair. If mistakes happened while he was in his office not watching, and mistakes happened because he was in the typing pool trying to help, then what was he to do? Suddenly he got it. He had to go back into his office, but leave the door open. Then they could ask for help through the open door if needed, and he could give help from the office.

Goldie seemed to define "mind" as the place from where one is thinking, which can move around the body (or be outside it). She contrasted it with the brain, which is a fixed organ, in the head. Some people feel resistance to bringing the mind to the head, but it is a starting point that most people need, to come out of the mind being in the body. We will go on to embody mind shortly. Even if you do not personally need this step, many of your pupils/clients certainly will.

> Mind in the brain can seem like a return to dualism. Delsarte's work was underpinned by dualism, that spirit and mind (the immortal soul) are enveloped in a corporeal body, and they are totally separate entities. Alex-

# CHAPTER four

ander (1985: 21) made a huge shift in thinking when he realized "that it is *impossible* to separate 'mental' and 'physical' processes in any form of human activity." He named this "psychophysical unity." However, Goldie was implying that he understood that there were still two linked entities, "psycho" and "physical." How do we understand this? This has been debated by philosophy for centuries and continues to be so. Some modern philosophers continue to see them as separate, while neuroscience tends to see "mind" as by-product of "brain" and slave to it. Daniel Siegel (2010: 4–12), who writes on the synthesis of psychotherapy and neuroscience, also sees two linked elements, which he describes as two sides of the same coin. Mind gives us the experiential side of reality; brain gives us the physical side. The first is subjective, the second objective, but they occur simultaneously and indivisibly.

### Exploration 4.7  Discovering mind in the brain

- *Stand, or sit in a chair.*
- *Put your mind into your toes of one foot, bring all your attention to your foot.*
- *Wiggle your toes, and be aware of the sensation.*
- *Then bring the mind right up to the brain, above your eyebrows, are you aware of something moving up?*
- *Look out at the room, and see what you are looking at.*
- *Stay looking out, and give consent from the mind in the brain for your toes to wiggle. To prevent yourself zooming back down at the thought of toes, think of it as sending an email, rather than delivering a letter by hand. Be aware of the sensation.*
- *Observe the difference. Was one lighter? Freer? Less defined? Was one more definite? More involved? More contracted?*
- *Put your mind into your other foot. Do you notice something moving down?*
- *Notice whether you are still really seeing the room? Or has it faded out a bit?*
- *Likewise notice whether you are aware of the rest of your body, or only of your foot?*
- *Now give consent to wiggle the toes of the foot. Notice the sensation.*
- *Bring your mind right back up to your brain. Do you notice something moving up?*
- *Look out at the room, notice that you can pay full attention to what you see, with detail, color and shape, relationships and spaces.*
- *Now staying looking out with this clarity, give consent from the mind in the brain to wiggle the toes. Send an email, don't dive down to deliver the letter. Notice the sensation.*
- *What is the relationship now between your foot and the rest of your body? Is it isolated or integrated?*

### Video link for exploration 4.7

I find that most people can clearly perceive something – the mind – moving downwards and up again.

With the mind in the foot, people notice that the toe-wiggling sensation is definite, that they feel in *control*, but it feels tight. They are only aware of the foot, excluding the rest of the body. Their vision (and hearing too) dims, there is pulling down and in, the world is lost to them. I define this sensation as *feeling into* the body.

In contrast, with the mind in the brain and eyes seeing the surroundings, they need to *trust* that the message will reach the toes. Many find it hard initially to think of giving consent to wiggling the toes without going down there. When they succeed though, there are clear differences: the physical sensation is much less, but there is a sense of the foot integrated with the rest of the body; of greater freedom and lightness in the movement. I define this different sensation as *awareness*

# The fundamentals of awareness and thinking

of the body. The vision and connection with the world stays clear. Miss Goldie often emphasized that you need to trust that the brain messages will get through (just as we need to trust that emails will arrive).

The paradox is, that by bringing my mind out of my body, Miss Goldie brought me into the body as nobody before had ever done. I discovered from her that the *mind* needs to come out of the body, it is the *awareness* that needs to come into it. Mind and awareness are not the same thing.

The differences are summarized in Table 4.1.

Our Western culture teaches us that we can be aware of only one thing at a time – because the left hemisphere works sequentially, and it cannot conceive of a different experience. With mind in the brain, and the following embodiment and spatial awareness games, we are working towards finding an expanded consciousness, in a unified field of awareness. In this, we become aware of all parts of ourselves at once while still being aware of the task we are engaged in, and our surroundings also. We are bringing our right hemisphere dominant again.

### *Allowing an unfamiliar experience*

We have learned to process through mental understanding, but such understanding can only happen after the event. It is from embodied understanding, after years of experience, that I am writing this book and articulating left hemisphere concepts to explain it. What matters for you right now are the experiences. But a dominant left hemisphere will try to screen out anything different. Keep a constant watch for anything that is different, anything that tells you something has changed.

> My mother, who has lived her adult life among academic, "left brain" thinkers, struggled with the unfamiliarity of "mind in the brain." She attempted to rationalize it according to her current reference frames, which initially stopped her perceiving changes that were happening. She played with it while walking, and noticed the trees against the sky were clearer, somehow more present. Her right hemisphere was coming more online, but her left hemisphere tried to discount this "strange" perception, which I encouraged her to accept as real. Then she discovered that by keeping her mind in the brain, she was no longer over-involved with her feet, and could trust them to walk safely on the uneven path, improving her stability.

Don't be too worried about defining the words such as "mind," "feeling," etc. If you are not sure about a word (particularly if your first language is not English, as these concepts rarely translate directly), then come back to the *experiences*, and from there choose the word that best fits your experience. Our hardwiring was there before we put ideas and constructs on it, and this is what we are looking to get back to.

| Table 4.1 Mind in the brain versus mind in the body (e.g. foot) ||
|---|---|
| **Mind in foot** | **Mind in brain** |
| Sensation is a definite FEELING | Sensation is less distinct, a peripheral AWARENESS |
| Only aware of the foot | Aware of the foot in relation to the rest of the body |
| Sense of being in CONTROL, involved | Need to TRUST that the message will reach the toes |
| "Delivering a letter yourself" | "Send an e-mail" (or post the letter) |
| Pulling down and in | Expansion |
| Vision and hearing dimmed | Vision and hearing stays clear |
| Loss of connection to the world | Continued connection with the world |

# CHAPTER four

## Lesson 5  Whole-body awareness and embodiment – "liquid light"

Having insisted I keep my mind in my brain, Miss Goldie would then talk of keeping the whole-body alive, not switching off in the legs. She also told me that on the first training course Alexander would talk of "intelligent knees," which puzzled his trainees. Throughout this work we are solving the paradox that we need to keep the mind in the brain to stop interference in the body, yet without shutting off from the body. This paradox is rarely articulated but is key to finding integrated movement. We need to be conscious of the body, but in a different way to "feeling." This is particularly crucial for the many people who are dissociated from their bodies.

To solve this paradox, here is another exploration. We will pour "liquid light" through the whole-body, to waken awareness of all areas: top to bottom, front and back, outside and inside. Do this first with eyes closed, so that the sensations are definite. Then repeat with the eyes open to find the awareness without having to go there directly. Using the imagery of "liquid light" is not an "Alexander style" procedure (the basis of it came from a healing workshop) but it works. It tracks the same path as "the boss in the office": first going down into the body, and then finding awareness of the whole-body through an open channel from the brain.

### Exploration 4.8   "Liquid light" with eyes closed, to find the body

- *Sit upright, with feet firmly planted, and eyes closed.*
- *Let your head fill with warm "liquid light". (Don't worry if you're not very good at visualizing, the sense of it is sufficient!) Let that "liquid light" fill your whole skull, brain, and sense organs. There is an infinite source of this light.*
- *With your mind, find the "trapdoor" at the base of the skull, where the brainstem becomes the spinal cord. The connection here may be flowing well or it may feel closed, like a trapdoor. Open the trapdoor and let the "liquid light" flow down into the neck.*
- *Now all your neck is filling with warm "liquid light": bones, muscles, and throat, right to the base of the neck. This is the next trapdoor, where there can again be a constriction of flow.*
- *Continue in this way, opening trapdoors at the base of the neck into the chest – flowing front to back, into lungs, heart, upper spine and ribs, back muscles and breasts:*

    *at the solar plexus and diaphragm, the "liquid light" flowing into the belly with its abdominal organs, the lower spine, the abdominal and back muscles, to the pelvic floor*

    *at the hips opening into the thighs filling them from top to bottom*

    *at the knees opening into the lower legs*

    *at the ankles opening into the feet and toes.*

- *Then at the shoulders opening into the upper arms:*

    *at the elbows and wrists and into the hands and fingertips.*

- *Take your time till the whole-body is flowing with "liquid light", of which there is an infinite source.*
- *Open your eyes and observe how you feel, in yourself? And in relationship to your surroundings?*

### Exploration 4.9   "Liquid light" with eyes open, to bring about an integrated flow between head and body

Having connected to every part of the body, repeat this whole procedure, this time keeping the mind in the brain and with the eyes open, alive to your surroundings.

We will give a simple brain thought of what is required, without "going there" with the mind. You may be less aware of "liquid light," more a sense of each part switching on with awareness and presence, becoming included in "you."

Your brain has many three-dimensional body maps within it, particularly in the parietal region of the cortex

# The fundamentals of awareness and thinking

(the band arching over between the ears) and so knows the location of every part of you (see lesson 6). Trust it!

- *Sit upright with planted feet. Looking out at your surroundings, let your eyes move around gently, seeing what is there, engaging with the world.*

- *With mind in the brain, give consent for your head to fill with "liquid light", and keep seeing, you are just allowing the light, or sense of presence, to fill your head, all through the skull, brain, and sense organs.*

- *Now, give consent for the trapdoor to open and the light to flow into your neck. Keep the mind in the brain and keep seeing out. Trust that you can be aware that the neck has filled, and from front to back, top and bottom of the neck: filling the spine, muscles and throat. Your whole neck is now included in your perception of you.*

- *Continue in this way, opening trapdoors at the base of the neck, solar plexus, hips, knees, and ankles and into the feet and toes; at the shoulders, elbows, and wrists and into the hands and fingers; allowing the light to flow into all the body spaces, the muscles, tendons, bones and organs.*

- *Keep reminding yourself to keep the mind in the brain, to keep looking out and engaging with the world, so that the mind does not go down; we are including the awareness of these areas in our perception of ourselves, the awareness of these areas lighting up with presence and life.*

- *Now you are aware of your whole-body pulsing with "liquid light", your whole-body is present as you continue to look out with mind in the brain.*

- *Check how you feel? Are you physically lighter or heavier, more or less present? How is your relationship to your surroundings compared to where we started? And how does this compare with the first time?*

- *When the procedure is complete, notice again how you are, in body, mind, and relationship to your surroundings. When you move, is it different? Be open to all discoveries!*

After doing this people often observe a sense of lightness, wholeness.

*Thinking from spatial awareness and whole-body intelligence.* The awareness of the whole-body now becomes a peripheral awareness akin to visual peripheral awareness, and similarly spatial in nature. One can experience this as a "consciousness cloud" which is both around and permeating throughout the body. I define embodiment as coming present not just *to* the body but *within* the aliveness of the body (which *includes* the brain), coming present within its sensitivities, and awakening its whole-body intelligence and consciousness. In many subsequent explorations we will begin by finding spatial awareness and whole-body intelligence in order to encompass mind in brain, embodied intelligence, and our surroundings together.

### The experienced body and the physical body are separate

*Embodiment is not a direct physical sensation (as proprioception is), but an experience of the spatially expanded, present, conscious self.* After years of viewing the body completely mechanically, neuroscience has now found a path to defining the experienced self as separate from the physical self. While this fits with our experiences here, neuroscience sees this experienced self as rooted in the brain.

"Your body schema is a physiological construct. Your brain creates it from the interaction of touch, vision, proprioception, balance, and hearing. It even extends it out into the space around your body ... Your schema is updated constantly by the flow of sensation from your skin, joints, muscles, and viscera. Your continuous sense of inhabiting a body embedded within a larger world stems in large part from this mental construct" (Blakeslee and Blakeslee 2008: 32). "When you work with instructors of dance, yoga, Tai Chi, Pilates, Alexander technique, Feldenkrais, or dozens of other kinds of movement training, you are basically working on body schema awareness. These methods teach you to purposefully attend to the many core elements of your schema as a means of self-exploration" (Blakeslee and Blakeslee 2008: 37).

This stance seems rooted in the implicit belief of most neurologists, that the senses of embodiment and consciousness are purely a creation of the brain. This

# CHAPTER four

is because, following Descartes, they mostly believe that the brain is the only site of intelligence. But *there are systems of connection and communication within the body that predate the nervous system*, going back to single-celled organisms: the chemical network of hormones and neurotransmitters and the fascial network, along with the evolutionarily later glial cells. There are speculative schools of thought that all of these are involved in embodiment and consciousness.

## Embodiment, consciousness, and the whole-body intelligence network

### 1   Fascia and mechanotransduction

Fascial research is a burgeoning new field. For centuries only viewed as the padding between tissues, fascia is now recognized as a complex and chaotic web that connects everything to everything. While the myofascial trains are seen by Thomas Myers (2014) as the large-scale connectors, the fascia wraps around and through every muscle, organ, or tissue, from skin through to bone, and from whole-body structures through to the internal cytoskeletons of cells, right through to the DNA. It is sometimes strong (like tendon and muscle sheath) and often delicate as spiderweb. These connections are fluid, fractal and ever-changing, so that tissues are elastic in any plane, and layers of tissues can slide over one another. Dr. Jean Claude Guimberteau (2014) has made beautiful videos of living webs of fascia.

This provides a communication network of mechanotransduction – older than the nerve networks, and over three times faster than the fastest nerves (Myers 2014: 33). When we are touched, the mechanical "vibrations" ripple through the body and are felt throughout; we are very aware of this when we receive a severe blow. The same is happening with the lightest touch also, but much more subtly. Mechanotransduction through fascia, muscles, and bones is happening all the time within our bodies, whether from our weight bearing down on the ground giving a counter-pressure relayed back up through the body, or the touch of air on the skin. Every breath we take and every movement we make sends ripples throughout the body.

A healthy body allows a smooth transmission throughout this continuous interconnected web, so that the pressures, pulls, pushes, and shearing forces of movement and touch are easily transmitted. But an imbalanced body has areas of tension that block this smooth flow, not just mechanically, but also at this communication level.

### 2   Consciousness in the fascia

How are we conscious of this communication network? "The fascial network is one of our richest sensory organs" (Schleip 2012: 77), with a greater density of receptors even than the retina; with a multitude of different receptors for proprioception, pain, touch, and more. But as we saw with stretch receptors (Chapter 3, lesson 1), it is thought that only when the fascia is free to move, stretch, and lengthen do its myriad receptors hum fully into being; stuck tissue ceases to be so receptive or sentient.

Fascial tissue also links to the nervous system through the glial cells. These are specialist fascial cells that support and nourish the nerves. Now they are understood to have intelligence of their own that interacts with nerve tissue (Field 2009). The relationship between fascia and nerve tissue is a whole new field of current research (Oschman 2012). This linkage between the nervous system and fascia could link our consciousness to every cell in a new understanding of intelligence networks. It gives some substance to the speculation that consciousness travels in the fascia and is present in every cell in the body.

Fascial tissue is organized by movement, aligning along the force lines, but also changing with the quality of that movement. It resists forced stretching, but complies with the gentle invitation to expand, such as from natural breathing and flowing movement. This could explain why, where muscles are habitually tight and fascia is correspondingly resistant, there is often little sense of embodiment – the mechanotransduction messages cannot be transmitted easily through the tissue. By lengthening and softening shortened and compacted tissues, we may not only be working on this mechanically, but at the consciousness level

# The fundamentals of awareness and thinking

too. This process seems to work both ways, so that bringing embodied consciousness into an area by methods such as "liquid light" encourages the area to wake up and reorganize.

3  Emotions, moods, messenger molecules, and embodiment

You may have found "liquid light" easy, and could flow it through all parts of your system. Or you may have found that some areas seemed blocked or absent. You may have found that as you came into an area it released emotional feelings, or you may have felt strange or weird sensations, maybe spacy, dizzy, or overwhelmed. These are all signs of unprocessed emotions.

All our emotions, moods, feelings, and "drives" such as hunger and thirst are mediated by chemical messengers: hormones and neurotransmitters. This system also predates the nervous system, going back to single-celled animals, and its vast scope and complexity has only been explored for a few decades. Science assumed that molecules of emotion would be only in the brain, but work by Candace Pert (1998) and others has found them in every cell in the body, deeply affecting cell processes.

These molecules produce emotional states or moods and activate neuronal circuits which generate behaviors involving the whole creature (Pert 1998: 145). For instance, one does not just have a *feeling* of anger: with it comes a rising of energy through the body, with a flush of red to the face and neck and rising blood pressure, tensing of the big muscles – particularly fists and across the chest – angry facial expressions with narrowed eyes, tense lips, etc. The emotion and its physical and physiological expressions cannot be separated. Watch a child's moods: a happy child is upright, his whole being lights up. A sad child collapses throughout his being: in energy, posture, and mood.

While all cells produce these information molecules, "nodal points" are particularly rich in them. Pert (1998: 142) believes they act as decision makers in the choices we unconsciously make. There are many nodal points in the brain, in all the organs, and all the way through the gut, giving a location for gut feelings. The molecular basis of memory is created by biochemical change at this receptor level, not just in the brain but in a psychosomatic network extending into the body. The decision about what becomes a thought rising to consciousness and what remains an undigested thought pattern buried at a deeper level in the body is mediated by the receptors.

*The interplay of posture and feelings*

Emotions and bodily sensations are intricately intertwined through nodal points in the spinal cord, in a bidirectional network in which each can alter the other. This could explain how mood and posture are so intertwined. You can "Sit up and you'll feel better," or share your feelings, which will "lift a weight from you" and lets you stand straight again. I observe that for the best results one usually needs to work with both processes. Another of Descartes's ridiculous legacies has been the separation of body therapies from talking therapies; we need to know about both.

*We only see what we want to see*

The external senses are entry points for information into the nervous system. The nerve pathways from these entry points all have nodal points in series to provide a filtering system. This enables us to pay attention to what our body-mind deems important and to ignore the rest, so that what we perceive as real has been filtered along a gradient of past emotions and learning. In other words, we only see what we want to see, both visually and emotionally.

So faulty sensory perception is not just internal, such as being unaware that a shoulder is up, but also external, when we "choose" not to see what is in front of us. This is why someone with a raised shoulder, who *internally perceives* their shoulders as level, then *sees* them as level when they look in the mirror. This gives us what I call our "autopilot" mode. When we pay attention, and "wake up" to what is in front of us, then reality can be perceived, internally and externally.

# CHAPTER four

*Conscious embodiment shifts deep emotional blocks*

This is why just becoming conscious of our muscles is not enough. Many therapists have observed that when we take the time and patience to focus our consciousness deeper into all the tissues of the body, we come to that quiet place from which the body can make clearer choices deep in our systems, with far-reaching changes to our physical and emotional well-being. We come deeper into the fascial network and encourage it to reorganize, opening up access to physically and/or emotionally stuck areas. We come into the nodal points and enable them to make fresh decisions. Then any movement work is likely to flow more easily for us.

*Keeping our body's network of communication flowing*

Science now sees that there is a multidimensional *network* of communication linking all the systems and tissues of the body, always bidirectionally. There is constant exchange of processing and storage of information, with multiple feedback loops continually adjusting "settings" throughout the organism to maintain homeostasis – the physiological balance required at any moment. When these feedback loops are rapid and unimpeded, the system is healthy and will move easily. Stress of any type reduces this free flow of information, and with time will impact our health at all levels (Pert 1998: 184, 243).

> If I put a biscuit on the floor for our little dog, she hears it drop, sees and smells it, all her senses come alert. The sensory messages are associated in the memory with past experiences and imagination of what is to come. Messages start to be fired out all around the body. Her interconnected body starts walking her towards the biscuit, led by her head with all its sensory organs and urged on by her whole-body intent for the food. Her tongue is already licking her lips – her salivary juices already flowing and messages already received further down the gut to prepare digestive enzymes. Pleasure signals are flowing throughout her body. We see a whole coordination of behavior, physiology, and psyche.

"We see that there is an intelligence running things. It's not a matter of energy acting on matter to create behavior, but of intelligence in the form of information running all the systems and creating behavior" (Pert 1998: 185).

Goldie told pupils that her work brought the gift of life. When we learn to bring our consciousness *into* the body, *through* the body, the cells and tissues are enabled to wake up to the decisions they have made, and to change for fresh decisions by the touch of our own consciousness. (Methods such as craniosacral therapy's somato-emotional release, or somatic experiencing, work in this way.) By keeping the expanded field of consciousness, we also help this integrate with the whole system.

4   The brain/body intelligence network

Most Western thought has taken for granted that the cranial brain controls the body. The concept that other parts of the nervous system could have autonomous control of an area was first put forward by Byron Robinson in 1907, with *The Abdominal and Pelvic Brain*. He showed that the day to day running of nutrition, gestation, elimination, and general health of the viscera and other abdominal organs is controlled entirely by these nerve plexuses; the cranial brain only influences its speed of action. "The abdominal brain is not a mere agent of the brain and cord … It is the automatic, vegetative, subconscious brain of physical existence. It is the centre of life itself" (Robinson 1907: 123–4). However, the Western world was not ready to hear this, nor was it ready when John Langley, who first defined the autonomic nervous system in 1921, initially defined its *three* divisions as sympathetic, parasympathetic, and enteric. The abdominal brain was finally accepted as a serious study in the 1980s with Michael Gershon's work and popularized with his book *The Second Brain* (2003). It is now a burgeoning field of study, not just of autonomic function, but also of its role in mental health and personality through the gut biome.

The heart brain has been studied extensively by the Heartmath Institute, showing its role in intuition and reducing stress. Eighty percent of the vagus nerve is

# The fundamentals of awareness and thinking

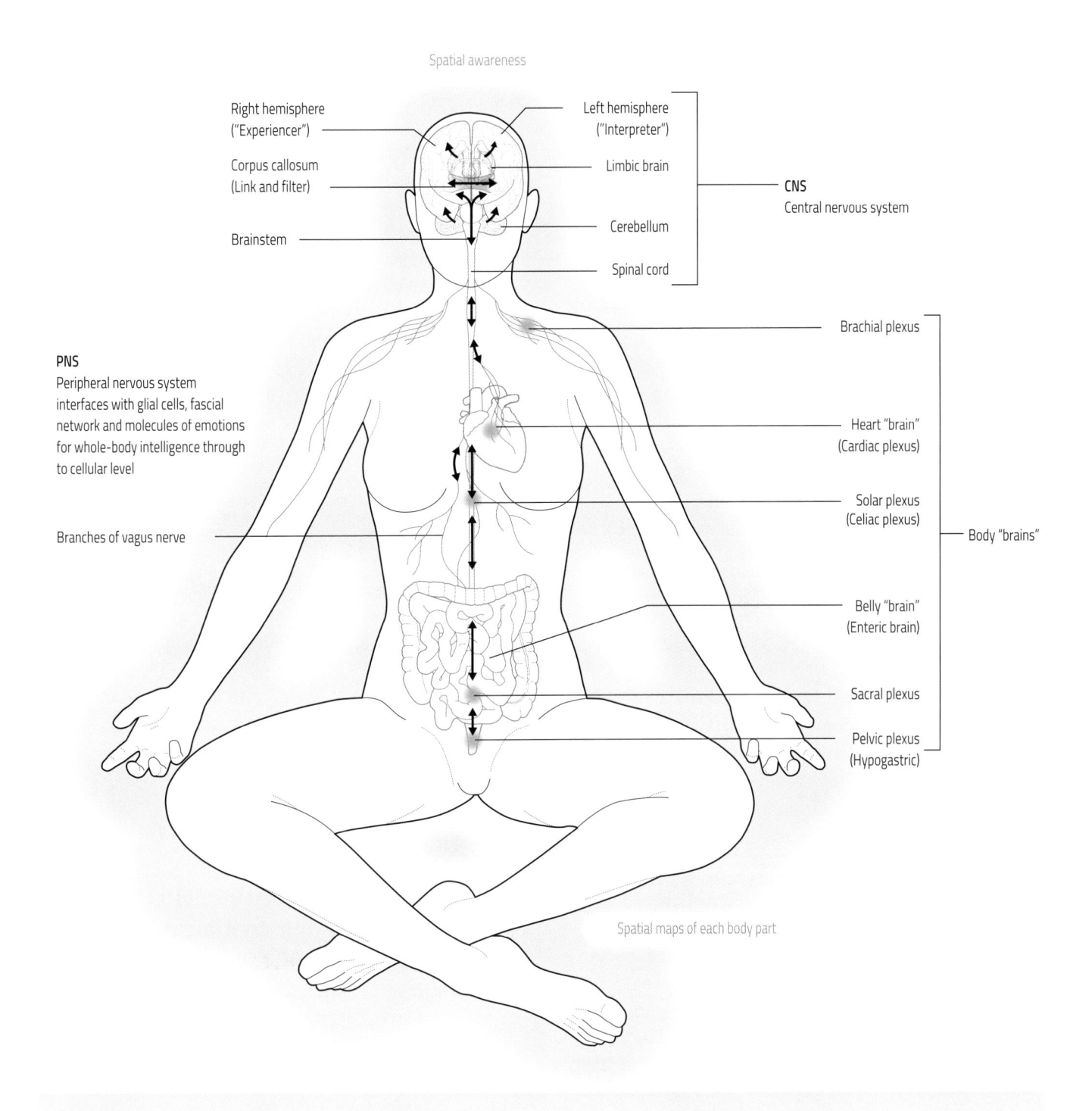

Spatial awareness

Right hemisphere ("Experiencer")
Left hemisphere ("Interpreter")
Corpus callosum (Link and filter)
Limbic brain
Brainstem
Cerebellum
Spinal cord

CNS
Central nervous system

PNS
Peripheral nervous system interfaces with glial cells, fascial network and molecules of emotions for whole-body intelligence through to cellular level

Branches of vagus nerve

Brachial plexus
Heart "brain" (Cardiac plexus)
Solar plexus (Celiac plexus)
Belly "brain" (Enteric brain)
Sacral plexus
Pelvic plexus (Hypogastric)

Body "brains"

Spatial maps of each body part

**Figure 4.1**
The brain/body intelligence network. Information flows between all parts of the network and the environment

# CHAPTER four

sensory, carrying information from body to brain. For both enteric and heart brains, there are many more signals going from guts and heart to cranial brain than vice versa.

Even skin can make intelligent decisions. Neuroscientist David Linden says: "Our entire skin is a sensing, guessing, logic-seeking organ of perception, a blanket with a brain in every micro-inch" (Gopnik 2016).

A new way of thinking is emerging, as I understand it. Instead of the tyranny of the cranial brain there is a democracy in which each part has its own expertise and the whole system is in constant dialogue before decisions are taken – just as you see in a business corporation. This operates at every level – even neurons and cells are being understood as individuals that often work together to make decisions.

The modern view sees the nervous system as a set of networks, summarized beautifully by Olaf Sporns in the following three passages (2010: 2):

"The collective actions of individual nerve cells linked by a dense web of intricate connectivity guide behaviour, shape thoughts, form and retrieve memories and create consciousness. No single nerve cell can carry out any of these functions, but when large numbers are linked together in networks and organised into a nervous system, behaviour, thought, memory and consciousness become possible."

"Brain networks span multiple spatial scales, from the micro scale of individual cells and synapses to the macro scale of cognitive systems and embodied organisms."

"We cannot fully understand brain function unless we approach the brain on multiple scales, by identifying the networks that bind cells into coherent populations, organise cell groups into functional brain regions, integrate regions into systems, and link brain and body in a complete organism. In this hierarchy no single level is privileged over others."

This view is echoed by Miller and Clark (2018). In their vision, online cognitive function emerges from the tight coordination of looping networks between cortical and subcortical layers that weave bodily and emotional information with top-down predictions, to give an embodied process of decision making.

Figure 4.1 is my simple portrayal of the whole-body intelligence network. In this, each plexus or area is potentially a site of information exchange and decision making at a level appropriate to that area, and there will be many more smaller ganglia and plexuses where this occurs. While conscious processes are 5% of cranial brain processes, the total amount of information we process without being aware of it is at least a trillion times greater than the information we process consciously (Herbert 1994: 185). Apparently, the conscious cranial brain is a *very* small part of total intelligence.

> **Teaching tip: Maintaining conscious attention quickens the process of change**
>
> It can often feel easier to let our pupils'/clients' attention wander off, getting them out of our way while we work. But by engaging with them, inviting them to pay attention to what's going on, the process of change is quickened because there is more intelligence at work in their systems. One needs to play around to discover how to help each person think, in this moment. Our aim is to help clients *observe* their own process, to *be present to it without reaction,* to help them *understand* it, to have *clear intentions* for the process, to make *clear choices* to inhibit reaction or send directions.

## Lesson 6    Finding our spatial awareness – of our surroundings and of ourselves

Finding full three-dimensional vision and spatial awareness will be easy for some, while for others, particularly anyone who wears spectacles, it may take time and may bring up strange sensations – so take it gently. You may be entering into very new territory, so keep observing what happens, and invite yourself to use less effort ("I can do less") – straining will not help! You may notice the world getting more three dimensional, or it might get fuzzier first. It may also get brighter, with clearer color or other changes.

# The fundamentals of awareness and thinking

### Exploration 4.10    Finding depth perception

- *Stand or sit where you have an interesting view. Let your eye gently track around what you see, without jumping, stalling, or glazing. See the colors as they really are, the textures, movement, shapes, patterns. Keep renewing your interest in what you see.*
- *Use your nose feather (exploration 4.1); you are at one end and the object is at the other end. Imagine all the little wisps of your feather in between, bringing you aware of the fullness of the space between you. You may see a glimpse of your nose, hair, clothing, etc. You are receiving the view across the space, not pushing out onto it.*
- *Notice the spaces between the objects in view. There are spaces either side, in front, and behind.*
- *Where do you see the world from: your eyes, in front of yourself, or from inside your head?*

Just as we can shift the mind – the place from where we pay attention – up and down the body, we can shift it within the brain itself, so that the whole brain is involved in receiving the visual input and in seeing. This may gradually activate the optic pathways.

(This is the work of Peter Grunwald and his Eyebody method, which I highly recommend to anyone interested in exploring their eyesight and vision capabilities.)

*Invite yourself to receive the light that carries the visual information successively:*

*from the front of the eyes*

*from the retina, the light sensitive layer at the back of the eye*

*from the middle of your head*

*from the visual cortex at the back of the head.*

Video link for explorations 4.10 to 4.12

You are like a photographer behind his camera, seeing through it and out to the world. The light reflected from objects is received through the cornea, iris, and lens, deep into the eye to the retina and then along the optical pathways to the visual cortex. You see from the visual cortex at the back of the skull, through the retina and eye, and out to the world. Play with this in both directions.

How is your depth perception now? Is the world more three dimensional than before?

### Exploration 4.11    Finding full peripheral vision

- *While still looking straight forward, and seeing from the back of the head, bring your hand up to the side of your head and some way away, and wiggle your fingers. Take your hand back gently until your fingers are out of sight then bring them back to the limit of your peripheral vision to stimulate it. Repeat on the other side.*

*How is your depth perception and three-dimensional awareness now?*

- *Become aware of how gently you can move the eye in the eyeball socket, giving you an awareness of where the eyes are in relation to the world. Explore the thought that the lens inside the eye turns before the eye moves, to invite the ciliary bodies that hold the lens to move freely.*

*When you find this, you will come into three dimensions.*

### Exploration 4.12    Adding spatial awareness of the body

Now you are in spatial awareness to your environment. Notice whether you are seeing from mind in the brain, or perhaps from a more fully embodied place of mind in the brain/body intelligence network that includes awareness of the full height and volume of the head.

Add in awareness of your own body, while still focusing on the chosen item.

# CHAPTER four

- *Notice the huge distance from your crown and upper brain (parietal and upper visual cortex areas) to your feet on the floor.*
- *Be aware of your hips, and their distance from your brain. Is your torso longer than you expect?*
- *Now work through the whole-body in this way, finding the vertical space to your knees, hands, ribs, elbows, shoulders as you continue to see forward. Are the distances bigger than you expect?*
- *With mind in the brain, become aware of how wide your body is – how far apart are your shoulders, ribs, elbows, your hips, knees and feet, your ears? Do they seem further out than you expect?*
- *Observe any changes in your body, e.g. grounding, lengthening, breathing, lightening.]*

What did you notice about your spatial awareness? Do you normally contract space, either in the world, or in your own perception of yourself?

### Spatial awareness is not only perceived by the brain, but by the whole-body

If you were able to explore the above from an embodied state you may now be aware of seeing objects and their background spatially from the whole-body. We were taught that the sense organs are localized, and only feed to their relevant cortical sensory region, from which motor regions make responses; for example, the eyes, in the head, link to the visual cortex then link to the motor regions for grasp. Current research is seeing that ordinary perception involves multiple senses. Each part of the body has its own spatial map, tracked by multisensory cells. Blind people can track sounds around their bodies using such cells (Blakeslee and Blakeslee 2008: 115–19).

### Waking up our brain maps

It is thought that by coming into our spatial awareness we are waking up our brain maps and so are improving our body schemas – our felt experience of ourselves that we use to plan movement.

Our brains are full of maps. The simplest maps of the body were discovered by Penfield in the 1930s while probing the parietal cortex of an epileptic; his needle elicited either a *sensation* in a particular part of the body or a simple *involuntary action* as muscles fired. He put these together to make the first brain maps. Though every part of the body is represented, the sensory map is weighted for the areas with most sensations (such as the hands, key areas of the face and the feet), while the motor map is weighted for the areas requiring most dexterity. Search the web for images of Penfield's "homunculus" to see that every part of the body is there – your brain knows where your body parts are.

From these basic maps, other maps become increasingly complex, building up from simple involuntary actions into complex movement patterns, and the lines between sensory and motor become a lot less distinct. While the parietal cortex has been most extensively mapped, maps are now turning up in many other areas of the brain and brainstem, and we will discuss several of these in later chapters.

This all looks nicely consistent and reliable. But in practice our body maps get corrupted by how we use ourselves – neuronal pathways are disconnected where areas are little used. For many people, the experienced body is compressed, along with their sense of space around them – so that they feel small or insignificant in the world. For others, the opposite may be true.

By finding our spatial awareness, as we have just done, we are probably inviting the various body maps to reactivate and/or rebuild connections and perceive the physical layout of the body in the optimal fully expanded state in which our muscles come into balance. By working with these programming layers within the brain we can already begin to change our tension patterns. I consider that we can only work with body maps directly in this way if we work from embodied awareness while staying out of *interfering* with the body. The body can then be experienced in its depth and fullness as a peripheral awareness, in the same way as peripheral vision, as we go about our day.

# The fundamentals of awareness and thinking

## Spatial awareness for sounds and smells

Why on earth should we come receptive to sounds and feelings in a big city, with its sirens, arguing neighbors, and cars with blaring radios? Noise pollution is one of the huge and often unspoken stressors on us today. I had my own journey with this when we lived just off a main city road in the UK. Most Friday evenings a nearby shop's burglar alarm would set itself off, and ring incessantly until the owner returned on Monday morning – or on a public holiday, Tuesday morning. He was oblivious to complaints, so we endured this for several years until he sold to someone more considerate. At first, the awful sound seemed to ring inside my head, which made the weekend agony. After a while, I learned to block it out. This was preferable, but it took energy and tension to maintain. At last I thought to apply spatial perception to it, noticing that the offending bell was a street away while the air around me was silent. It worked. I could then let it ring over at the shop and notice that our bedroom was quiet. This took no energy, involved no fight, and it no longer bothered me.

One can apply this to any noise, and even to smells.

### Exploration 4.13   Depth perception for sounds and smells

- Find and maintain focus and interest on a chosen item, with depth perception and peripheral vision that includes yourself, then add your awareness of sounds. Notice how far the sounds are from you; and that the area around you is silent. Do the sounds impose on you as they might normally?
- Add awareness of smells, temperature etc. Can you allow these more freely than usual? Let there be an exchange between you and the environment, visually, olfactorally, any other way.

The full spatial awareness available to us is an interplay between our whole-body and the whole environment around us. A full sense of embodiment – proprioception, balance, touch – brings a spatial sense of the body, its metrics and volumes, along with our sense of personal space. The full visual field is in play, with background and foreground seen together, and other senses – hearing, smell – also active and spatially aware.

## Pain control through mind in the brain and spatial awareness

I have found that one can use these new ways of thinking and being for pain control. How might this work?

Most alternative therapies hypothesize that problem areas are separated to a greater or lesser degree from the flow of the body by some variety of tension and imbalance. I notice that when we have pain, the mind goes to it, feeling it. But as we saw in lesson 4, mind in the body is a point focus, creating tension, losing the whole picture of self and the world. This would isolate the painful area further from the body, potentially worsening its chance of healing. It also loses our sense of perspective so that the pain becomes our whole world. By bringing the mind to the brain/whole-body intelligence network, we come out of over-involvement with the painful area and let it take its place as one part of the body. The world comes back into focus also. This non-involvement through spatial awareness seems to open up the tissues, and I observe it can speed the healing processes.

## Lesson 7    Emergent integrated movement – discovering our fundamental bend led by focused vision

Attention organizes our response. If we are only in our heads, our response will be an idea, unintegrated with the body's current reality. If we are embodied, our attention organizes us. Think of a child who has found some feathers – the child's delight, her vision, thinking and chatter, her hands clasping the feathers and whole-body following this movement, are all organized around her attention on the feathers.

# CHAPTER four

Here we will discover the fundamental folding bend of the human being – of the small child, or the Bornean people. They bend for a purpose – say, to reach for something on the floor. Led by the attention, the head/neck/spine alignment stays in one piece, while the hips, knees and ankles fold around the line of alignment with gravity. It is a whole-body experience.

### When our kinetic chains are working in dynamic balance we can morph between shapes

From an imbalanced state, with only partial patterns operating, we must pull and push ourselves against gravity to move. When we move with balanced use, we are allowing our structure to reorganize its shape in space, using dynamic modulation of postural tone. Whether stationary or moving, we are in a *flow of dynamic balance*.

My hypothesis is when we are in the quiet, tonic, right hemisphere-led state, all our fundamentals network together. Then the *fundamental bend* is led by perception and focus – our attentiveness. For us, this is primarily visual, but also includes kinesthetic input (especially in the visually impaired). The head orients and takes decisions (in communication with gut feelings and desires) and the body follows responsively, engaging our kinetic chains. Eyes and movement centers may be linked through the dorsal visual stream (see Chapter 15) and superior colliculus in the brainstem (see Chapter 16, lesson 1).

### Exploration 4.14. Organizing a bend consciously

- So maybe now you are standing comfortably – balanced equally on two legs, with feet hip-width apart and knees that are not locked back, muscle-bound or bent but instead balanced across the joints. With head balanced on the neck, articulating on the nodding joint, looking forwards, and free to move into a nod or turn. With your crown going up, and an up-force flowing up from your heels to your sacrum. Not over-involved in your standing.

- To move, you could carefully organize this balanced structure into a bend. Have a go at sitting down from this position. Where does your mind go? Are you still seeing forwards or, in the moment of moving, does your attention get pulled into your body? When that happens, do you still see the world in front of you? Sit and stand several times, and notice whether, as you move, you stop seeing the world with any detail. We assume we are still seeing, but often we are not.

### Exploration 4.15    Discovering the fundamental bend, led by perception and orientation

1    Perception leads movement.

- Track your visual line out to the horizon and back again. As you come into spatial awareness of your surroundings, it will bring calm and awareness of the body. (Use your nose feather and "liquid light".)

- If you let the vision arc outward (keeping your spatial sense), the head will tilt a little upward on the nodding joint, and when the vision arcs back to your feet, the head will follow. Perception leads the head.

2    One can think of two "up-forces" orienting and integrating the body. The "anti-gravity" force, the body's extensor response to the gravity down-force, that springs vertically up from the heels to the crown, uses the extensors of the superficial back line. A second "up-force" that runs along the head/neck/spine orients the body to follow the head.

- If you take your eyes a little lower, using the nodding joint but not allowing any bend in the rest of the neck or spine, the next joint available for tilting is the hips. Allow your eyes to lead the torso into a forward tilt on your hips. It can help to imagine a ladybird crawling down the wall and across the floor towards your feet. To come up, use the "anti-gravity" line – thinking the top of the back of the neck away from the heels. The eyes track the visual arc/ladybird, but do not lead, or the chin would lift and the back would arch.

- Repeat the tilt, keeping your attention out on the visual arc/ladybird, letting your knees bend responsively too. Go only

# The fundamentals of awareness and thinking

as far as is comfortable, then again use the anti-gravity line to unfold back to standing, tracking with your eyes.

3   Muscle tone requires consciousness and presence, so that if the perception "switches off," the movement is less free, and also less controlled.

- *Notice that once the body begins to fold, your attention may be drawn away from what is in front of you and back into looking after your body, feeling into it. Do you notice tensions creeping back in? Instead, stay in spatial awareness to it.*

4   We might be aware of our reactivity, habits, and beliefs about what movement is possible. To let a new way of moving happen, we need to "inhibit," to stay out of our own way. Then we will move into the unknown. We are discovering what can happen next, allowing the body to surprise us.

- *Keep paying attention to your visual line. What is different? It may feel very unfamiliar, even unsafe or out of control, as you do this – but this is faulty sensory perception. Without being drawn in again, are you aware of the freedom of the bending action?*

- *You may be aware of the spatial relationships of your whole-body folding and unfolding responsively, and perhaps the world around you also flowing by as you move. Can you go into a squat and out again in this way?*

Video link for exploration 4.15

### Exploration 4.16   *Using vision to sit down into a chair*

- *To sit down into a chair, there are two arcs to follow: the first takes your visual arc/ladybird down and towards your feet, until your backside touches the chair.*

- *STOP without moving, and find the "anti-gravity" line, leading with the back of the neck away from the heels, rotating the torso on the hips until you are sitting upright. The eyes track the visual arc/ladybird, upwards away from ourselves.*

- *Reverse these to stand. Can you allow the adaptive muscle tone to sort the challenges of moving so that you can flow onto your legs and up to standing? (See Figs 4.2 and 4.3.)*

## Lesson 8   Exploring semi-supine – a position of active rest

Modern Alexander technique incorporates one activity that pupils are always encouraged to do daily: to lie down for 10–20 minutes on your back, with knees bent and head resting on some books. Known as semi-supine or active rest (and in lessons as tablework), it is a position that invites the lengthening and widening of the whole-body structure, and so facilitates returning to our flow of dynamic balance. It is a simple way of taking time out, and keeping the principles going.

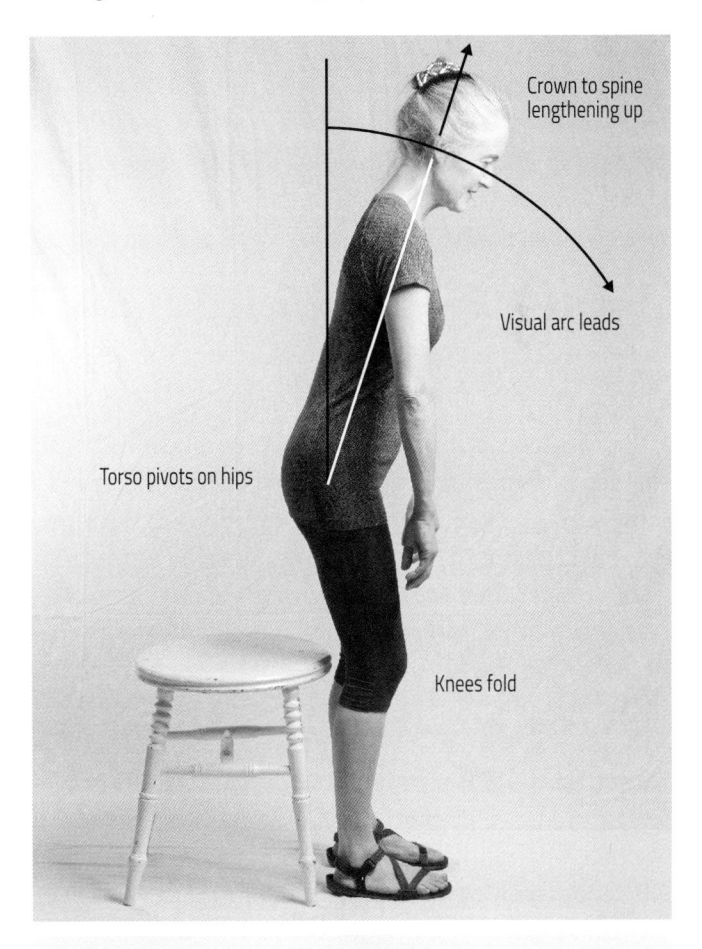

**Figure 4.2**
The visual arc leads the body into folding

89

# CHAPTER four

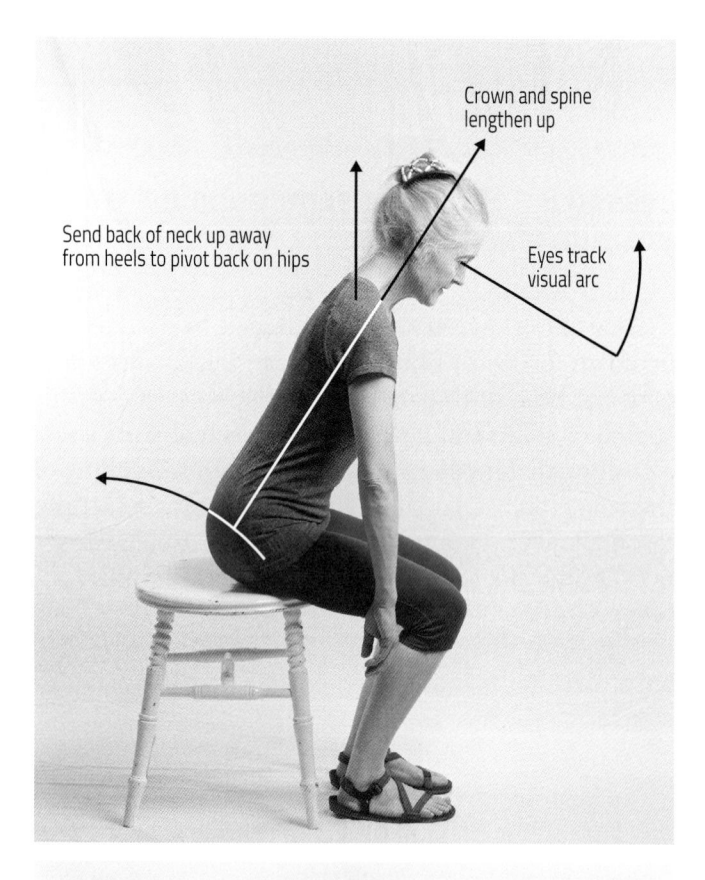

**Figure 4.3**
Tracking the visual arc while tilting back to upright

*Labels: Crown and spine lengthen up; Send back of neck up away from heels to pivot back on hips; Eyes track visual arc*

This was why Goldie hardly ever used tablework in her later years. The real nature of the Alexander technique is not about releasing muscle tension, it is about getting the whole-body *working*. I want to shout this as loudly as possible. Tablework was little used by Alexander himself, probably for this reason.

### Exploration 4.17 Semi-supine – a position of active rest

1  To find your number of books:

- *Stand against a wall, with your heels, backside and shoulder blades against it. Let your head find its natural position from the wall then use your hand as a measure – this is your number of books. Lie down on your back, on a carpeted floor (not a bed), with your head on your books, and your knees up (Fig. 4.4).*

2  Observations on lengthening and widening:

- *Notice that without the books, the back of your neck would curve back and shorten, and your head would fall back. The books are there to lengthen your neck spine.*

- *The bent knees, with feet flat on the floor, open the lumbar spine. If the feet are too far from the hips, notice*

I introduce mind in the brain, embodiment and spatial awareness together to pupils while they are in semi-supine, usually on their second lesson with me. After which I mostly never do tablework with them again, unless they are too tired or ill for anything else. I do ask them to do semi-supine most days at home, as it forms a useful basis of self-practice. In modern Alexander practice, tablework usually forms at least half of every lesson: it is increasingly dominating our work. But there is a problem with this. Firstly, pupils tend to remember the lying down part of a lesson – the nice bit – and forget the bits that were hard work. Alexander's niece, Marjory Barlow, told me she never did tablework in the first lesson for this reason.

Secondly, one cannot strengthen anybody's back or teach them better movement by lying them down.

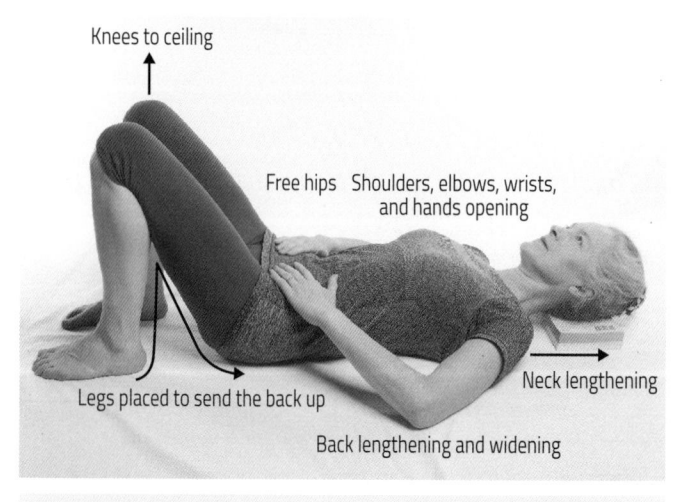

**Figure 4.4**
Lying in semi-supine

*Labels: Knees to ceiling; Free hips; Shoulders, elbows, wrists, and hands opening; Legs placed to send the back up; Neck lengthening; Back lengthening and widening*

# The fundamentals of awareness and thinking

that it pulls on the back. The feet need to be parallel, and comfortably close to the hips, so the feet and legs support the back.

- *When the feet are hip-distance apart, it widens the body at the hips.*
- *With the hands on the lower belly, and not touching, the upper back and shoulders widen.*

3   Staying present in semi-supine:

- *Stay in semi-supine for 10–20 minutes, coming to calm, seeing the ceiling and gently tracking round what you see, using your nose feather. This will bring calm, and awareness of the body.*
- *Find your spatial awareness to the ceiling, and to each part of your body, from mind in the brain and the consciousness cloud.*
- *Inhibit – say no to – any desire to wriggle or help with sensations that may occur as the body expands.*

4   Find a regular time slot: before or after a meal, on coming in from work, or just before bed. A regular slot will become part of a daily routine, and provide a starting point for more active thinking or movement work. Also use active rest as a restorative at other times, if you are exhausted, aching after strong activity, or in pain (use the pain control technique from lesson 6). You may find it more effective than resting in bed or on the sofa.

### Exploration 4.18   Rolling off the floor with adaptive movement

For each stage of this, maintain gently tracking eyes, with the mind in the brain. Use spatial awareness to find each body part needed and allow it to move without interfering. This will feel different – allow the unexpected!

- **Stage 1** *Let your eyes slide across the ceiling, to one side, and let your head follow. Let vision lead the head. See the direction in which the head is now pointing.*
- **Stage 2** *Waggle the fingers of the hand on the opposite side, so that they come alive. From mind in the brain, imagine light coming out of the fingertips of this hand, and let the fingers follow this imaginary light so that they come off the body. Now let the fingers lead the arm across you, as if they are pulling the elbow, so that the arm follows. Take your time about this, leaving the shoulder behind so that you get quite a different movement of the arm. Stop before you distort your shoulder (Fig. 4.5).*
- **Stage 3** *From mind in the brain, know where your knees are, and let the legs roll you onto your side.*
- **Stage 4** *Let the leading hand come onto the floor right by your shoulder, palm flat. Keep rolling until the weight of your body comes right onto that hand. With body weight on it, the arm may naturally want to push, and the lower elbow will join in, to push you up. up (Fig. 4.6).*

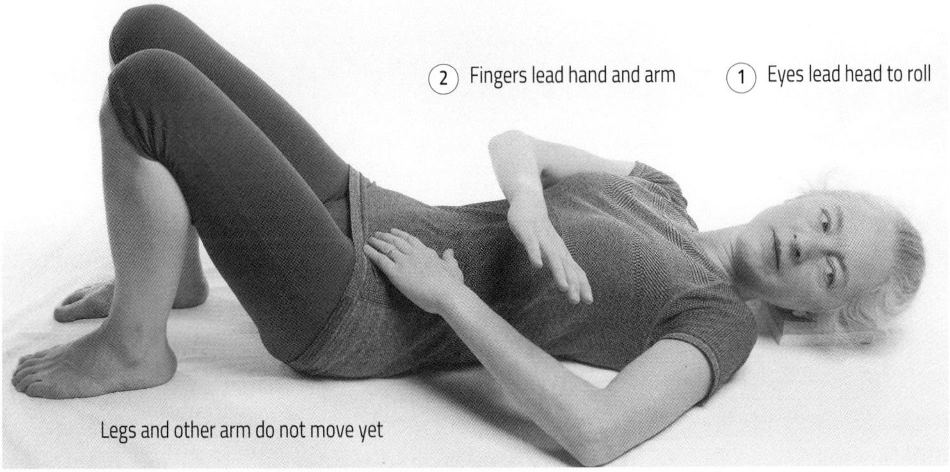

**Figure 4.5**
Rolling out of semi-supine, stages 1 and 2

(2) Fingers lead hand and arm    (1) Eyes lead head to roll

Legs and other arm do not move yet

# CHAPTER four

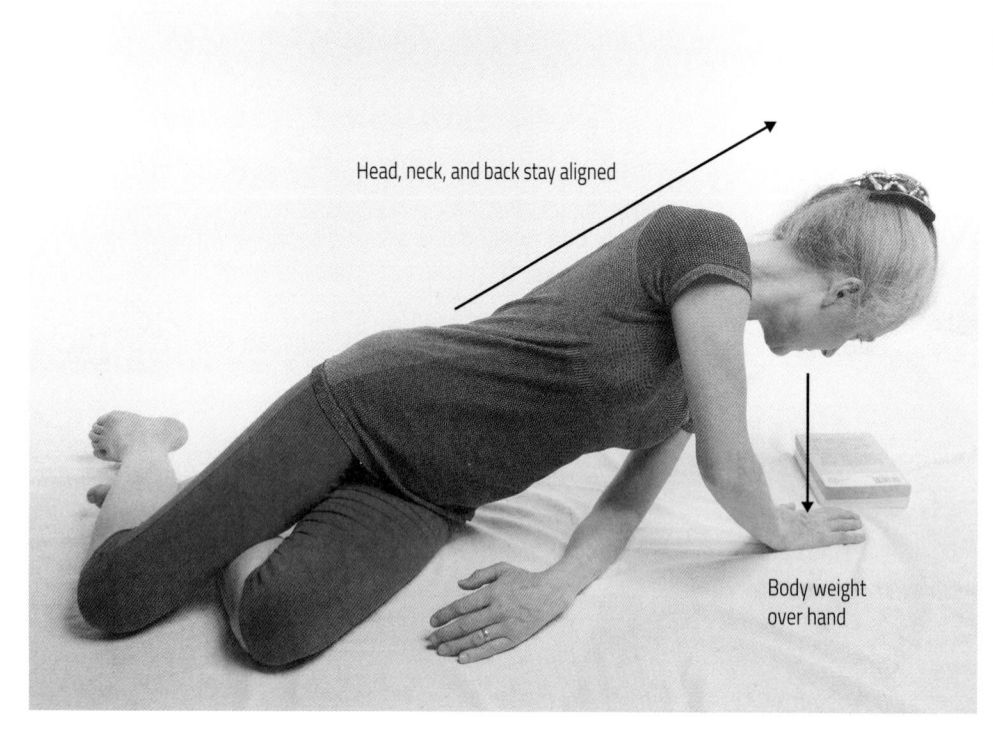

**Figure 4.6**
Rolling out of semi-supine, stages 3 and 4

Head, neck, and back stay aligned

Body weight over hand

- **Stage 5** *Roll onto your knees to come onto all fours. Use your hips to sit back to kneeling, first sitting on your haunches and then kneeling upright.*
- **Stage 6** *Bring one knee forward, so the lower leg is vertical. Tuck the back toes under.*
- **Stage 7** *Let the eyes lead a visual arc down, freeing your neck so the top of the head leads to incline the whole torso forward from the hip joint. When the weight of the chest comes over the front knee and foot, stop, then push the back toes down, send the back of the neck up away from the heels and you will stand up. (Use a chair lightly for balance if you need extra support (Fig. 4.7).*
- **Stage 8** *Take a moment to notice the expansion that you have just found: back lengthening and widening from hips to shoulders, head relaxed on the neck. Look out and see the space around you.*

## What are directions?

Alexander defined a four-step method for changing one's use. We can learn to trust this, like a road-map to take you somewhere you have never been before, whether you believe it to be possible or not.

1. Observe and analyze your current use.
2. Inhibit your usual preconceived ideas of how to move, instead work out what is needed.
3. Give directions – the means whereby the new use will come about: of positive inhibition, preventing the old habits from swinging in automatically, and of positive directions, to bring about a new use.
4. Move, and let the changes happen (Alexander 2011: 165).

Inhibition is a process of stopping habitual paths from being activated, without which nothing new can emerge. Directions are positive, definite thoughts to bring about change. The danger is that we can overdo directions and push the body around. They only work when done from a quiet system, with mind in the brain/body intelligence network, as otherwise there is localized over-involvement and no overall integration of what then happens.

In my training, I overused directions in an attempt to find and engage the up-force. Goldie stopped me doing that, and for several years I did not use

# The fundamentals of awareness and thinking

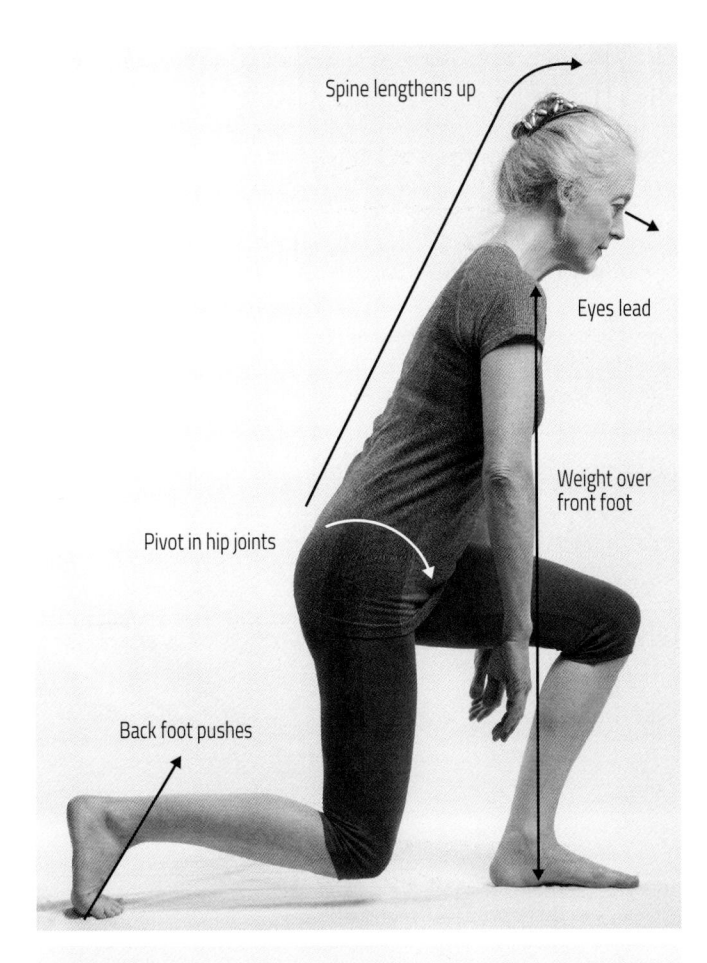

**Figure 4.7**
Rolling out of semi-supine, stage 7

(Labels on figure: Spine lengthens up; Eyes lead; Weight over front foot; Pivot in hip joints; Back foot pushes)

directions, instead inviting connection and intelligence throughout the body. From here, by staying quiet, new patterns of use could emerge (see Chapters 15 and 16). Since then, I have explored many different approaches to directions, summarized here, and we will explore them in detail in subsequent chapters.

1. Directions for opening – the many lines along which the body expands. "You are the core of a big apple," as AT teacher Yehudah Kuperman once told me. By coming to quiet, the body can stop doing the old patterns, and will then expand. We will explore this initially through breath (Chapter 6).

2. Directions for lengthening and widening, expanding the lines of postural support – often along the anatomy trains. These need more specific conscious thoughts, linked to precise understanding of the anatomical pathways.

3. The Initial AT, as redeveloped by Jeando Masoero (Chapter 7), uses groups of precise directions together programmed into the brain for integrated change which can then be taken into dynamic movement.

4. Directions for movement through the extremities – fingers, wrists, elbows, knees, ankles or feet, top of head or eyes, projecting "light beams" or "strings" that lead the body into movement. This is useful for sport or yoga, etc. I often find it helpful to think these not with the leading side – as these are the actively contracting muscle groups which will tend to overwork. Instead, think along the other side, to encourage the antagonistic groups, and so maintain length and balance in the limb or torso.

One can think, say, of sending the knees forward by letting the mind jump to the knee. This is completely different from sending the message from brain to knees through embodied consciousness. Miss Goldie talked of messages getting through, and being patient if this did not happen straight away; it would if one kept projecting the message without expectation.

> Laura had come to learn AT because of hip problems, and was now feeling able to return to Pilates classes. We worked through several of the Pilates moves from an AT perspective, to explore how to bring observation, inhibition and direction into them. One move was to lie on her back with legs outstretched, and lift each leg into the air in turn. Her default was to think of the leading side of the leg lifting, meaning the quads overworked and tummy muscles contracted. Instead, she learned to send a direction down the back of the spine and leg to the heel, sending it strongly away from her horizontally. Her right leg responded by soaring up in the air without imbalancing the torso, but the left leg did not move. For two weeks she simply sent this direction daily, and then, one morning, the messages connected and the left leg also flew upwards.

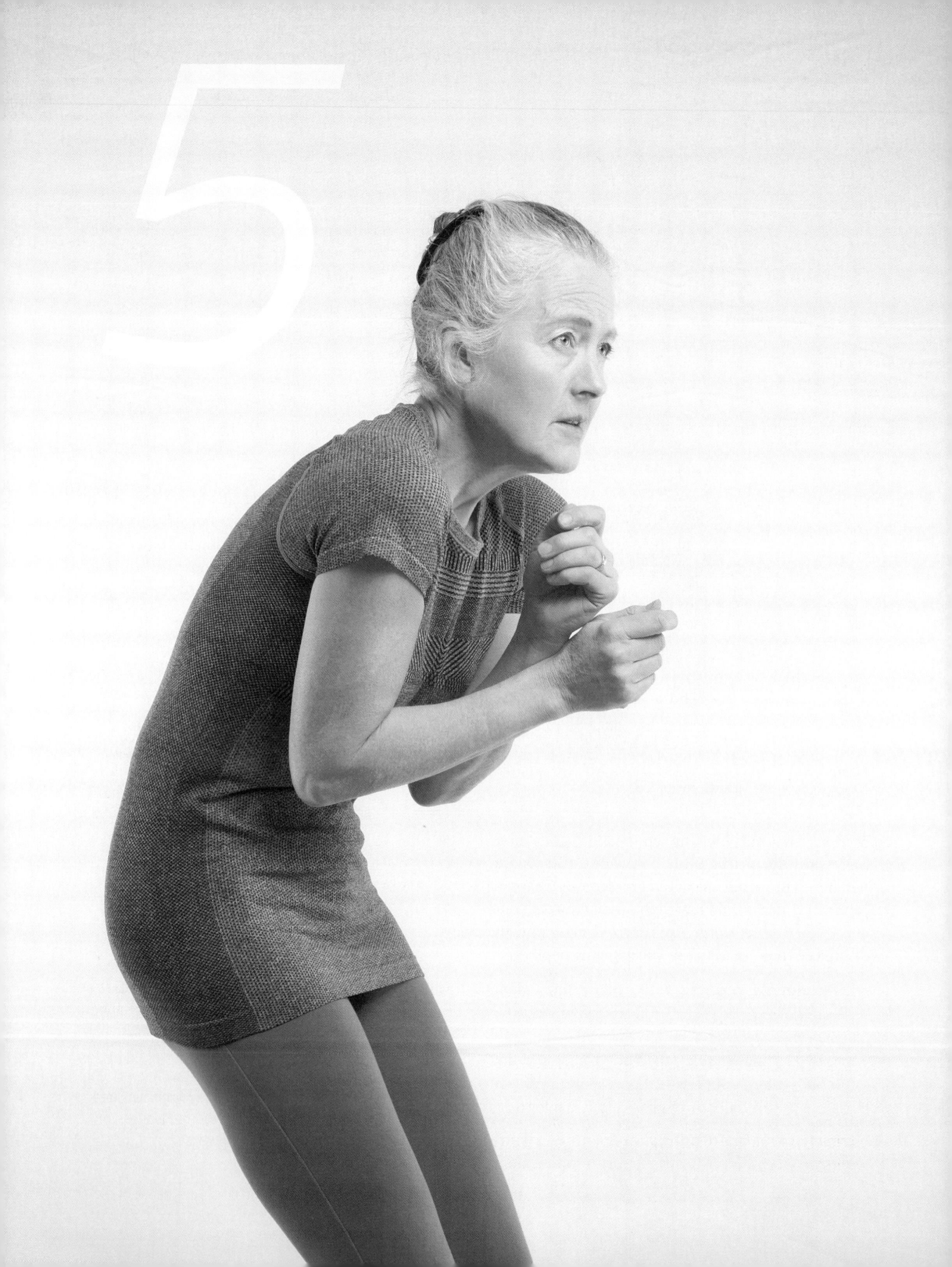

5

# The autonomic nervous system – why we need to work from quiet presence and awareness

*"Come to quiet"* – Miss Goldie

## The three states of the autonomic nervous system

The nervous system has always been understood to play a vital role in Alexander work. Only with a calm nervous system can we observe ourselves, drop unneeded tensions and allow a new muscle balance to come into play. Why is this so? As we will discover, a calm nervous system is crucial for all movement if we are not to injure or distort ourselves over time. This fundamental is so important that it has a chapter of its own.

We flow continually between calm and aroused states. The autonomic nervous system (ANS) has two functions: it regulates our "homeostasis" – the balance of our metabolism – ensuring our organs have sufficient blood flow, oxygen, nutrients, etc. It also regulates our background level of arousal so that we can move from the calm states of resting, self-awareness, socializing, and digesting, mobilize our energy as required for action, and into defensive modes to survive danger – fight or flight (Table 5.1). It was always believed that there are two systems operating in opposition: the resting state, or parasympathetic nervous system (PNS), and the fight/flight system, the sympathetic nervous system (SNS). (Science seems stuck with these ridiculous names: whoever named the fight/flight mode as sympathetic should have been shot at dawn!)

Then, in 2011, the neuroscientist Stephen Porges published the polyvagal theory (2011), which described the ANS with not two but three states in a phylogenetic (i.e. evolutionary) hierarchy. He had discovered there were two distinct parts to the PNS – a modern part and a primitive one. The PNS travels mostly in the vagus. Porges discovered that this emerges from the brainstem in two branches: the

| Table 5.1 The autonomic nervous system | | |
|---|---|---|
| **Autonomic nervous system (ANS)** | | |
| **Parasympathetic nervous system (PNS)**<br>The vagus | | **Sympathetic nervous system (SNS)** in ganglia beside spine |
| Dorsal root: dPNS – primitive | Ventral root: vPNS – modern | Mediated by hormones: adrenaline, osteocalcin, cortisol |
| **Homeostatic balance for normal function** | | |
| Regulates health of organs below diaphragm, especially digestive system | Regulates organs above diaphragm, facial expression, reflexes of sucking and swallowing<br><br>Slows the heart (vagal brake)<br><br>Initiates out-breath | Initiates action<br><br>Initiates in-breath<br><br>Raises heartbeat |
| **Level of arousal for defence** | | |
| *Shut down/freeze system*<br><br>Immobilization for life threat<br><br>Slows heart rate and breathing to below that required for life<br><br>Shuts down digestive system and organs; going into shock | *Safety state*<br><br><br>Diverts blood flow to digestion, peripheral nervous system, extremities<br><br>Allows internal awareness<br><br>Facilitates relationships and bonding | *Fight/flight system*<br><br>Active mobilization for danger<br><br>Activates big outer muscles<br><br>Shuts down internal awareness, digestion, peripheral circulation and extremities |

# CHAPTER five

ventral branch (vPNS) and the dorsal branch (dPNS). The vPNS is the modern myelinated branch (myelin is the fatty sheath around big nerves, which allows for faster transmission of signals). The dPNS is unmyelinated and primitive.

It is thought that the primitive dPNS state emerged 500 million years ago when amphibians and reptiles crawled onto land. If life got tough – too hot, too dry, etc. – the reptile crawled under a rock and the dPNS shut the metabolism down until things improved again – the "freeze" state. Reptiles can do this because they are cold blooded and need very little oxygen when immobile. But for a warm-blooded mammal (or bird), a drastic drop in heart rate, blood pressure, lung action, and temperature is highly dangerous and can kill. So the next level of defense was evolved (400 million years ago) – to mobilize out of danger with fight or flight. Our modern myelinated PNS – which Porges calls the social engagement system – is the most recent, only 200 million years old, and is only found in mammals. It is most developed in primates and particularly in humans, and it allows us to co-regulate – to calm or arouse each other through social engagement (Fig. 5.1).

Because these systems operate below the level of conscious awareness, most people have little awareness of which state they are in, or the triggers that cause switches between states. Much of our work as therapists or Alexander technique teachers is about teaching people to recognize when their system is aroused or shut down, and how to come safely out of those states back to themselves, to the social engagement system and a sense of safety.

## The ladder from safety to danger to life threat

We can envisage these three states on a ladder (see Fig. 5.1):

- When we feel safe, we have our feet on the ground – a ladder is never a very safe place. We feel grounded and secure, the heart rate is low, breathing is gentle, our whole system is relaxed, our muscles are soft and lengthening. In this state, blood flow is diverted to the organs, particularly the digestive system. It is the state in which the body can detox and repair. For humans, it is the place where we feel safe socially – we can make eye contact and relax knowing we are part of our supportive family/social group. But primary to this, we have consciousness of ourselves – self-awareness – as only in the PNS do we have interoception – internal awareness. This is the self-engagement system (Siegel 2007, cited in Siegel 2010: 23).

The next rung up the ladder is where we engage PNS and SNS together for normal life activity. If we have good resilience – a strong link to our vPNS – we can take more on without sliding into overwhelm. Pineau (2018) calls this building our arch – only when the two sides of an arch build equally does the arch stay stable. The greater our resilience, the higher the arch we can build. When the vPNS can go no higher, the SNS takes over and the arch collapses. Many modern people are sensitive, unable to take much on before they reach overwhelm.

- When the arch collapses, the SNS takes over, taking us up the ladder where life becomes increasingly unsafe. There is a network around the amygdala in the limbic system, constantly monitoring incoming signals for danger, safety, or neutral by comparing incoming data with memory banks of past events. This happens below the level of consciousness: Porges calls it neuroception. When a threat is detected, we may move to the next level of mobilization: either anger and fight – our urgent response is often to defend our patch – or flight, the urge to get away. The hormone adrenaline and the stress hormone cortisol are part of these physiological activations: the heart races, the lungs breathe harder, and blood is diverted from the extremities into the big muscles to mobilize for action. It is also diverted from the digestive system which shuts down. If we have gone into fight mode, we may feel angry, outraged, defensive. Our energy is high and hot.

# The autonomic nervous system – why we need to work from quiet presence and awareness

| Life state | ANS state | State of arousal for defence | Ability to relate | Body/mental qualities |
|---|---|---|---|---|
| Life threat | dPNS<br>Primitive PNS | **Freeze**<br>Immobilized<br>Collapsed | Terror or numb<br>Feels absent, dissociated | Unseeing eyes<br>Out-breath dominant/held<br>Muscles floppy or rigid |
| Danger | SNS<br>Hormone mediated | **Flight**<br>Frustration<br>Desire to run away<br>Fear<br>Cold | Aroused emotions<br>Anxious, fearful | Hyper-alert<br>Darting eyes<br>In-breath dominant/held<br>Outer big muscles tensed,<br>core muscles switched down |
| Danger | SNS<br>Hormone mediated | **Fight**<br>Anger, defensive.<br>Hot, energy rises | Aroused emotions<br>Aggressive/defensive | Hyper-alert<br>Staring 'predator' eyes<br>In-breath dominant/held<br>Outer big muscles tensed,<br>core muscles switched down |
| Alert | SNS/PNS<br>Mobilized together | **Engaged** for calm focused activity/action | Normal social engagement | Maintains calm by building arch – coping well<br>High muscle tone<br>Balanced flowing breath |
| Socially engaged<br>Self-aware | vPNS<br>Modern PNS | **Safety**<br>The flow state<br>Rest and digest | Calm presence<br>True empathy<br>Intuitive responses to others | All seeing eyes<br>Balanced flowing breath<br>Balanced muscle tone |

**Figure 5.1**
The ladder of the ANS

> New research shows that osteocalcin, a hormone released by bone, is even more important than adrenaline in mobilizing us for danger. The skeleton is not inert (Berger et al. 2019)!

- If we begin to lose the fight, we go to frustration, fear and flight – the need to get away. The energy is still high, mobilizing with SNS and associated hormones, but we are cold, especially hands and feet.

- Or sometimes we flee first, then turn and fight when cornered.

- Fighting or fleeing cannot go on for ever – the SNS is highly energy consuming. The primitive PNS is our response to life threat. If we are caught, especially if we are pinned down and sense there is no escape, then the final stage is initiated where we freeze and shut down. Giving up, not fighting back, is also protective; this stage is energy conserving. Playing dead can also mean a predator loses interest and lets go, after which you might recover (though you might also die of shock). So the earliest system is still there, to be used in the last resort.

# CHAPTER five

Though these are pictured as discontinuities, they are also on a sliding scale, like accelerating steadily in a car, in which gear shifts bring in another phase and potential. The states can slide into one another, as one part of the system builds and another declines. For instance, in a resilient system, the flow state can continue well into the alert phase.

## Maintaining a balanced life with self-regulation

Porges sees that ideally, the three states are engaged well together in homeostasis – physiological balance – so that we can live in a calm harmonious state.

The dorsal vagus (the primitive parasympathetic, dPNS) looks after the organs below the diaphragm, especially the digestive system.

The ventral vagus (the modern parasympathetic, vPNS) operates above the diaphragm, it controls the connection between face and heart for social interactions.

The sympathetic nervous system (SNS) – the quickener – initiates the heartbeat, but unless checked, it would be too fast.

So, to balance this, the vPNS supplies a "vagal brake" that acts on the pacemaker, slowing the heart. This provides for a quick response mechanism: when more blood flow is needed, say for when we rise from a chair, the heart is speeded by lifting the "brake" and then reapplied when the activity level falls. Breathing also involves both: the SNS regulates the inhalation while the vPNS regulates out-breath. So the heart speeds slightly on every in-breath and slows on the out-breath. No wonder long out-breaths are calming.

### The vagal brake mechanism

This is the process behind "building the arch." It allows us to mobilize more energy as we need it for daily life. When functioning well, the vPNS stays in control as the vagal brake allows us to mobilize more energy while it also inhibits the production of adrenaline and cortisol that would push us over into a full SNS response of fight or flight. We are alert, with all the energy we need to function well, but not reactive (hyper-mobilized) or shut down (hypo-mobilized, energy collapse). *Our stress threshold – or resilience – can be understood as the level of activity and stimulus in which we can maintain the vagal brake and so keep vagal control in a situation.* The ability to return to a calm state from a mobilized one is called *self-regulation*. When the vPNS is in charge, it is called *high vagal tone*.

### *Self-regulation is a learned behavior*

This ability to learn to control the vagal brake, and so keep good vagal tone in more challenging situations, is learned in childhood through good interactions with our caregivers – usually our parents. It is their nervous system which teaches ours, a process called *co-regulation*. The following description of this learning comes from Alan Schore (2003). Babies are highly aware from birth, perceiving and responding to their world. They seek the mother's (or other primary caregiver's) eyes and track them, eliciting a caregiving response of eye gazing, and bonding begins. Now right hemisphere to right hemisphere information exchange can occur. This hemisphere is dominant for unconscious processes and interoception, and is the first to develop. It contains the "non-verbal communication lexicon" of face recognition, emotional gestures, and vocal tone. It is also more deeply connected into the limbic system for emotional responses, and into both the SNS and PNS. These elements weave together as we learn to self-regulate.

A calm baby is aware of its internal needs – hunger, tiredness, etc. – and communicates this with noises and faces, to which a perceptive caregiver intuitively responds with modulated voice. By eliciting the appropriate care, the baby strengthens the bonding and sets the stage for a reciprocal dynamic. By responding to each other's faces with gazing and cooing, the baby can learn social interaction and emotional control. This cooing interaction excites the baby to vocalize more, the adult responds in kind. At a certain point, the adult intuits that the

# The autonomic nervous system – why we need to work from quiet presence and awareness

baby is becoming over-aroused and calms his/her voice again, bringing the baby's excitement levels down too. Then baby and adult then look away briefly before the whole cycle begins again. It is through these highly synchronized rhythmic cycles, which develop into baby talk, then games and play, that a child learns social skills and good communication of needs. They also learn emotional control and how to self-soothe. This process of attachment in the first three years of life constructs the social brain, in which visceral and emotional information from the physical self is related to information from the outside world (Schore 2003).

This is then maintained through safe social interactions, as good friends and family help to regulate each other. (More on this in Chapter 18, working on others.) But if, for whatever reason, this did not happen well, or we experienced trauma, then the nervous system does not learn this capacity. Then we have a very low threshold of resilience before we become angry, want to flee the scene, or shut our energy or engagement down. We also cannot easily return from stimulation to a calm state and get stuck in messy, chaotic, or numb states.

I relate this to the hemispheres and the head/body divide. When the left hemisphere/head dominates, as it so often does in our culture, we are divorced from the body, its grounding, its emotions and feelings, leaving us easily prone to loneliness and anxiety, or numb. Only when the right and left hemispheres are working together but with the embodied right hemisphere leading the show can we function as we are evolved: to be listening to our bodies and each other, and able to pick up on danger cues and respond appropriately without imbalance.

Problems arise when we live in a state of danger or life-threat. Ideally, we all live in the social engagement system, moving easily into mobilized states as appropriate, then returning to the safe state. But sadly, in our modern societies, many of us have been through higher levels of anxiety or trauma from which we cannot get back, leaving us trapped in anger, fear, or numb states.

> Thanks to psychotherapist Deb Dana (2018: 9) for the ladder image, which she envisages hierarchically, with safety at the top. I love the ladder image but prefer to think experientially: it is the belly and the grounding of being that brings stability, and this is at the bottom. The top of a ladder is where you can panic and freeze and need rescuing! It is indicative of how we think in the West – that hierarchies place good states at the top/head, while the ground/body is undervalued. Then safety is construed as being in the head instead of in the body (see Fig. 5.1).

## Bringing the nervous system back to a place of safety

Although many of us left childhood with poor self-regulation and low resilience to stress, it is possible to change this. To my understanding, the nervous system is not organized in a top-down manner as is usually assumed, but is a whole-body network of communication and dialogue. About 80% of vagus nerve signals are from body to brain, while only 20% relay messages from brain to body. This means that we can reintroduce calmness and flow states from many points, to affect the whole system. The key methods for bringing us out of over- or under-aroused states are to work with vision, breathing and voice, and muscle tone, as well as awareness and conscious thinking.

**Breath**. With the vPNS in charge, the breath flows easily in and out of the body. The fight/flight system emphasizes the in-breath. Imagine watching someone cross the road right in front of a bus. You gasp into the upper chest and then hold your breath in suspense – SNS active, then let it out in a long sigh when the person makes it safely to the other side – vPNS active. In the freeze state (dPNS), people can forget to breathe in, or have such shallow breathing it is hardly visible. When we notice that we are interfering with the natural breath, such as holding patterns, we are noticing that we are out of the flow state. If we choose to let go of the holding patterns, this sends a

## CHAPTER five

safety message throughout the body and brain and the system can calm. Deliberately inviting a long out-breath and spontaneous in-breath likewise sends a message of safety.

**Voice.** An embodied, modulated voice – with mid-tones and varying gently in pitch - also sends a message of safety. The ear is tuned for such voices for social engagement – but the SNS screens them out if danger threatens, to optimize hearing growls or rumbles. When aroused or threatened, voices are often raised and become harsh (SNS), or drop and go to monotones (dPNS). By working with voice (or with a calm-voiced therapist), we can come to calm (see Chapter 17).

**Vision.** With high vagal tone, we are alive to both detail and background with spatial perception. The eyes can track smoothly around the visual field. When we are in the SNS, angry eyes can be staring and fixed on the focus of anger, and the background is lost. When fear takes over, the eyes often dart around the background, and the foreground can be lost. In the freeze, the eyes can glaze, seeing very little, and saccadic movements become sluggish. The person is dissociated from the present, their mind elsewhere or nowhere. Peter Grunwald (2010: 130–5) defines three states: presence, over-focus, and under-focus, which I feel equate to vPNS, SNS, and dPNS respectively.

This is why there is such a focus on vision and breath – particularly out-breath – throughout this book. Every time we choose to breathe out fully, rest a moment and let the in-breath take itself; every time we choose to see what is in front of us with depth perception, letting the eyes track gently, we are choosing to return to a place of safety.

**Awareness** is part of this – quiet attentiveness. Only with good vagal tone (the vPNS) are we aware interoceptively: to internal signals of hunger or other digestive signals, to our emotional or physical needs, or to intuitions about others – the quiet voices within us. Once danger threatens, this internal monitoring is shut down in favor of external monitoring. With awareness – maybe with the help of a good therapist –

we can become more conscious of our unconscious neuroception processes, and so take charge of our state.

**Grounding and embodiment.** Becoming aware of our bodies, breathing into the body, all help us to come down the ladder and ground. Grounding, embodiment and safety are the same. When we ground fully, we come home to ourselves. We find stability of being, contentment, confidence – the list could go on.

> While many self-help books talk about getting in charge of your head, and mental illness is likewise seen as being a brain dysfunction, I notice that without grounding, nothing fully resolves. This is a very under-researched area. We need to let go of our obsession with the cranial brain and wake up to the importance of the body and its intelligence.

**Muscle tone** is more complex. I speculate that the vPNS mobilizes the core muscles, our stabilizers, while the SNS activates the big muscles needed for action. (In the shut-down, muscles lose tone and become floppy, or all tense together for rigidity.) In everyday life we want to be mobilized for action yet be aware of what we are doing. Then we have both sets of muscles, the inner and outer muscles together. This is why in every procedure I invite you to start with finding the balanced stance and the whole-body breath, seeing what is in front of you, which finds the inner stability, before we bring in the muscles of activity.

This is also why inhibition – finding the state of quiet within – must always precede direction. Tim Cacciatore and Patrick Johnson (see Chapter 4, lesson 2) see this quiet place, in which the muscles are in a balanced state of responsive tone, as a state of tonic inhibition.

Julien Pineau, developer of the StrongFit system, teaches a new and balanced approach to body building (2018). He also hypothesizes that the internal torque

# The autonomic nervous system – why we need to work from quiet presence and awareness

muscle chains that rotate us inward (he thinks bicep curls, I think cradling a child) are the ones mobilized by the vPNS; meanwhile the external torque chains, the muscles that rotate us outward (think of the pull back to throw a spear), are mobilized by the SNS. We need a balance of the two. He considers that most gyms and fitness classes use pounding music and shouting deliberately to engage the SNS to activate and build the big muscles. But in doing so, they lose engagement of the internal torque muscle chains and their stabilizing balance, creating instability and injury down the line. This idea also dovetails understanding of the vPNS and SNS with observations on primary (inward) and secondary (outward) curves (Nettl-Fiol and Vanier 2011). Primary curves are more internally focused, their gestures include cuddling or hugging, they bring calm nurturing feelings. Secondary curves bring us into action, engaging us out with the world. Even the most intense sport can be done more safely and effectively with balanced muscles and vPNS in charge, as the many top sports people who have used AT can attest.

As we will discover in Chapter 7, most people stand and walk with more external rotation – feet turned out, shoulders and upper back pulled back – suggesting SNS dominance. This fits much of Western lifestyle – many fighting or surviving their way through the day, keeping going with coffee and sugary foods, the adrenaline drip-feeding into their bodies without the benefit of high physical activity that would burn it off, to be followed by collapse onto the sofa at the end of the day. (The long-term risk of this can be burn-out, overwhelm and shut down, with physical collapse – going into the dPNS state.) We will explore re-finding the internal torque of the shoulders and legs in Part 2, and then, how to activate and balance the external and internal torque chains together.

The SNS causes us to overuse our energy. Conscious thinking – the phrase "I can do less" – is useful to invite the body to reduce excess muscular tension and return to more balanced use and calm.

## Recovery by climbing down the ladder

When we are in stressed states, whether fight/flight or freeze, there is no place for processing the emotions involved, and they are stored in the body tissues as tension and molecules of emotion (Pert 1998: 141). A healthy system can debrief these later, perhaps by talking it through with a friend, re-living the emotions involved, and the system returns to safety and relaxation. Dreams are also where we process what happened during the day, restoring equilibrium (Walker 2017). When our systems cannot re-set themselves, we are stuck up the ladder and need help. A skilled therapist leads us safely to re-encounter this distressing state, and to stay present to the body's response, so that our experience can be integrated.

If we soothe the system without encountering the emotions hidden below, we are trying to jump from trauma to calm. There is a danger to using relaxation or calming methods of any type, including meditation or AT work, as anesthetic. To do so simply traps one in needing to, for instance, meditate for longer, or repeat directions more often, to keep the scary stuff hidden. Instead, working to reawaken the vPNS with quiet awareness, allows the body to process and become aware of the emotions held in your body that were not felt at the time. It is safe to let these happen, simply observing the sensations, however strange, and watching them process through and pass.

This is why coming to quiet can take courage. It is why we can have to be very firm with ourselves that this is what is needed, although it may not feel safe to do so. It is always safe to bring in more vagal tone, to ground, to embody, to listen within. You may need to work with a skilled therapist to build confidence in this before you can do it alone.

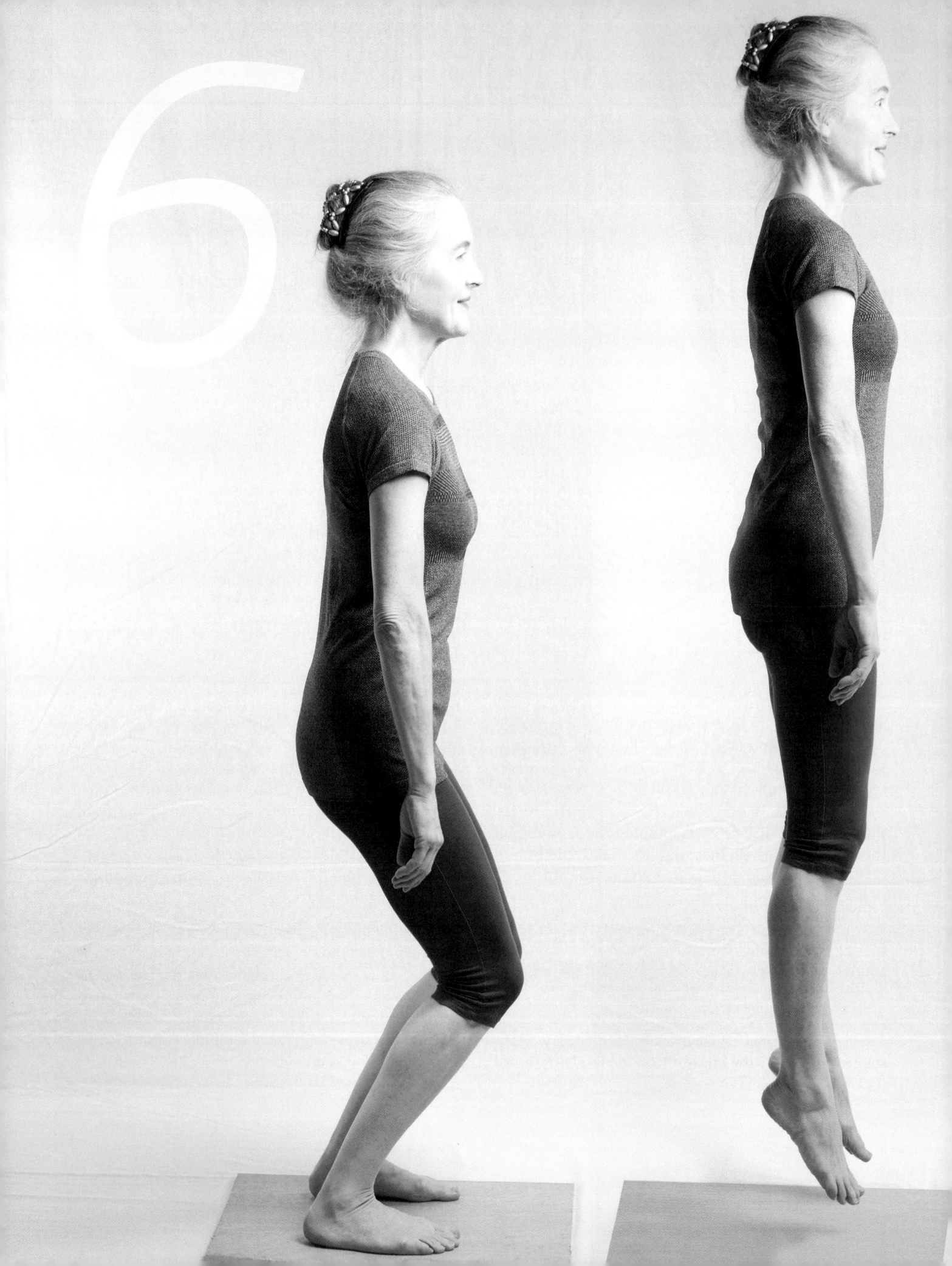

6

# Finding the innate movements of breathing and walking

## The evolution of our movement, finding the buried patterns

For movement to be coordinated, there must be an integrating mechanism. Alexander thought he had discovered this in the head-neck-back relationship and he called it the primary control. Following the scientific thinking of the 1930s, he located this firmly in the brain.

The assumption has always been that the brain controls everything we do. But how was movement controlled before there was a brain? Very primitive animals had neither brains nor spinal cords, but did have the very first nervous systems. These were "reticular nerve nets," a wide-spaced net of interconnecting nerves serving the whole organism, which evolved to provide organization for some of the first multicellular animals, such as hydras. They communicated sensation from the outside world and organized digestion and movement as a peristaltic wave down the body of the animal (Damasio 2017: 59).

*There was whole-body organization and coordination, long before there was a brain*

We even still have a reticular nerve net ourselves, in the enteric nervous system – the belly brain. Some call this the second brain as it has even more synaptic connections than the head brain. But from an evolutionary perspective it is the first brain (Damasio 2017: 60) and is probably doing much more than we currently know.

As evolutionary complexity progressed, heads were developed, with vision sensors (eyes), a mouth with taste and smell; and the spinal cord running the length of the body. Digestion continued to be organized through the peristaltic wave from the mouth, down the digestive tract to the tail. Initially bodies were unsegmented (like roundworms and leeches), then segmented (like earthworms or insects), to allow further control of each segment. We still show segmentation – think of the spinal vertebrae and their emergent nerves, each serving a portion of the body.

Picture a centipede moving towards food, its many legs rippling along under it, in waves of movement down the animal. The stimulus to move is initiated from the head and conveyed down the spinal cord to give a whole-body action. But what controls the action of each leg, and what organizes the pattern of leg movements to make a wave? Rather than the brain controlling these, there are mini-reticular nerve nets at each point, like little computer circuits, that control the locomotion locally. These are called *central pattern generators* (CPGs).

CPGs create oscillating rhythms by alternating excitation (allowing a nerve to fire and bring about movement in a muscle) and inhibition (to stop the nerve firing). They were first identified by Graham Brown in 1911, but were not picked up on till the 1960s. Since then they have been found in all invertebrates and vertebrates studied. They provide the rhythmic generators for many functions such as breathing, swallowing, peeing, and of all types of rhythmic movement: walking, running, swimming and flying, bouncing, chewing, shaking and scratching. For animals such as the centipede, with 15–150 segments, each with a pair of legs, CPGs within each segment control the alternation of flexors and extensors in each separate leg by inhibiting each in turn. Spinal mini-circuits and CPGs also coordinate between segments to pattern the wave of action both across and down the body – quite a feat (Orlovsky et al. 1999). (I don't know whether centipedes have been studied directly, but certainly lobsters have, with their five pairs of legs.) CPGs are the basic building blocks of movement, and they are not in the brain.

> Thomas Graham Brown was the junior colleague of Sir Charles Sherrington, discoverer of the reflex arc and proprioception. Reflexes were the hot topic of the day and Sherrington was famous for his discoveries which explained so much about the organization of posture, and which he presumed also controlled locomotion.

# CHAPTER six

> Brown's apparently competing theory for how locomotion was organized was ignored; he left science and became a mountaineer. In 1961, Donald Wilson identified CPGs while investigating how locusts generate rhythmicity to fly. Brown's findings and proposed mechanisms were then rediscovered and explored as many others joined in this research in how movement is controlled (Berkowitz 2016: 83–92; Prochazka and Yakovenko 2007: 257).

The complexity continued. Fish developed a bony spine around the spinal cord, but the basic pattern of side-to-side traveling waves of movement down the animal continued (Grillner 1996). But now there was more power generated at the rear of the movement wave, so that as the tail drives the fish forward, the head stays still. This both increased streamlining for efficient movement and also stabilized the navigation systems – you don't want your eyes and other head sensors thrashing about as you navigate or bite at food.

When reptiles colonized land, limbs were developed, but they were added on to the original patterns, which were simply modified – the hind legs still had the driving power. Mammals added dorsiflexion – an up-and-down wave (think dolphins leaping, versus sharks swimming) – but under this complexity, the original patterns generated by CPGs were not lost. (We will explore this conservation of ancient systems in our own locomotion in Chapter 11).

While patterns in the spinal cord were retained, the brain developed as evolutionary complexity leapt exponentially in mammals, with their warm blood, social structures, and care of the young. To control all this, the brain was remodeled and enlarged, with a much bigger neocortex and a bigger cerebellum. These enlarged again in primates and even more so in early humans as social structures, communication, planning, and spatial awareness were increasingly developed, and brachiation gave way to bipedalism and tool use. In *Homo sapiens*, our own species, language and thinking added a whole new dimension of complexity, as we unlinked thinking and action. This allowed our thoughts to take journeys into virtual reality and envision completely different possibilities for ourselves. The rest is history, not evolution, as we became able to separate ourselves from our biological roots. But herein lies the problem. We need to return to a better linkage between the two.

So evolution in vertebrates moved from simple forms to increasingly complex ones, while conserving developments that worked. In the brain, as new structures were developed, feedback loops always linked them to the core structures and to sensory and motor components (Eilbert 2014).

*We are complex, multi-layered beings, but the original layers are still there in our nervous systems, often overlooked or forgotten, and can make life easier if we let them!*

## Lesson 1   Natural breathing – finding the natural expansion of the torso

This is a big chapter, on which many other chapters will build, so please take time to explore it. Our cultural understanding of breathing is that to improve its functioning we need to alter it directly, using instructions for muscular actions such as "puff out the belly," "expand the chest," etc. Here you will learn to get out of your own way so that your body shows you how to breathe. It explores the linkage of balanced muscle use and the calm nervous system. This is the preparation for engaging balanced muscle patterns of the body, which will build up to more complex tasks as the book progresses. Lesson 2 introduces the crucial deep stabilizing muscles of psoas and pelvic floor, which will be further explored in other chapters.

### *My breathing story*

I screwed up my own breathing at age sixteen, learning yoga breathing from a book. In retrospect, I was probably already tense and breathing poorly, but did not know it. Then in my first term at college I got so

# Finding the innate movements of breathing and walking

tense one evening while working too long on an essay that I had a hyperventilation attack. It was extremely frightening, and left me paralyzed on the floor, straining for breath. Fortunately, a friend came around and ran to phone the college nurse. She returned some minutes later with the advice: "Just tell her to stop breathing and it will all calm down." And so it did. But for many years, I could not think about breathing without hyperventilating and going into fear.

My first teachers in the technique never mentioned breathing, and neither did my training school. Occasionally I remember some teacher mentioning breathing and myself telling them firmly to back off. I was very happy then that breathing was not a major part of the technique! Later I was aware that Goldie would get my breathing going very differently but I did not know how. It was Miss Sage, the ninety-year-old Bates natural vision teacher, who one day grabbed me round the ribcage and expostulated: "None of you Alexander technique teachers know how to breathe. You do it like this!" She showed me that the floating ribs should go in and out, rather than the chest go up and down. This was a revelation and it made life a lot easier for the few weeks I remembered it. (This was 1990. The AT community has progressed hugely in reintegrating breathing since then, with teaching such as Jessica Wolf's *Art of Breathing* and many other wonderful teachers working with voice.)

Then I did a weekend workshop with John Hunter, on facilitating our natural breathing. He too had been pondering on what Goldie was actually doing, and also had been exploring the natural breathing mechanism with opera singers. He gave me the basic inhibitory tools, introducing me to the magical world of letting my respiratory system alone and discovering what happens next. Since then, I have been fascinated by breathing; it is a lifetime's journey of discovery.

## Breathing is misunderstood

At university I learned about the rib muscles: that the external intercostals pull the ribs apart from each other, lifting the ribcage, while the internal intercostals pull them down again. You can feel this for yourself. Breathe in by deliberately lifting your ribs. Then using equal effort, use your rib muscles to breathe out again. Such antagonistic action is a classic model of how muscles work. I consider it a description of overuse, but so common it is deemed normal physiology. I suggest it is because the muscles are overworking that we can feel them.

Most methods that teach people to breathe (most yoga streams, most relaxation methods, Buteyko, fitness work, etc.) are over-using breathing muscles. (My Viniyoga teacher tells me that the current method taught as yogic breathing – breathe in by pushing the belly out, next expand the ribs and then lift the chest, and reverse it all to breathe out – was a Western invention in 1970s.) People learn to push their bellies in and out, or "support the diaphragm" by tensing stomach or belly, and to expand the chest, in the belief they are breathing deeply. Or to exhale fully they learn to give huge, releasing sighs. All this is pulling the delicate balance of the respiratory mechanism in all directions, and in doing so, completely preventing the beautiful natural mechanism from flowering into being, with corresponding benefit to our whole structure and psyche. Imbalanced breathing is rife: in the world of sport; for opera singers, who can suffer greatly from the strain placed on their breathing mechanism; with asthmatics, obviously; and in virtually everybody suffering from tension or stress.

## *Seven advantages to re-establishing natural breathing*

Natural breathing gives us more than a good oxygen supply.

1. It is a superb tool for exploring coming to quiet, to find the "state of tonic inhibition" (see Chapter 4, lesson 2). Tense, imbalanced breathing is the breathing of an unquiet nervous system, whether in fight/flight or freeze mode. Balanced natural breathing brings in (or is brought in by) the parasympathetic nervous system.

# CHAPTER six

2   It massages the organs, and is health promoting.

3   It brings us into our volume, our quiet center, in which we are present both to our internal and external environments.

4   I see it as restoring the natural balance of muscles: from alternating concentric contraction with passive lengthening – the classic image of antagonistic muscles pairs, to responsive, integrated action with dynamic modulation of postural tone, in which breathing is part of postural support.

5   Like catching a ball from a non-doing place (see Chapter 15), it is an activity where we can experience completely getting out of our own way. From this we can observe our own natural balance of muscles in action.

6   It is the fastest way I know of opening out deep tensions in the spine and torso generally. It enables us to access the core muscles, to access the very depths of the torso and also the very top, and to access the natural strength of the body as muscles come into balance.

7   It balances the spirals of movement – the external rotations (in-breath) which tend to be dominant, and bring the internal rotations (the out-breath) more into a primary role.

8   Because breathing is cyclical, we can completely experience our bodies in dynamic and ever moving balance, even while we are holding still.

## The path back to natural breathing

We will navigate a path back to natural breathing in several stages.

For full video tutorials, talking you slowly through all these explorations, with trouble-shooting suggestions, see inside the front cover.

### Exploration 6.1   Observing the breath

**Stage 1:** Get out of your own way

- *The first and key step, is to stay out of the way of your breathing and use spatial awareness. Bring your mind to the brain and look out with depth perception and peripheral vision.*

**Stage 2:** Observing what is happening

- *Let the awareness of your breathing float up to you as you look out at the world. Gently notice:*
- *Can you hear your breathing? Is it through nose or mouth?*
- *Where is it in the body: belly, pelvic floor, chest, ribs, back?*
- *What direction is it moving in: up/down, down/up, sideways, expanding forwards, expanding the back?*
- *Is it fixing or straining at the top or bottom of the breath (the breath end-points)?*
- *Which is longer, the in-breath or the out-breath? Which is easier?*

> I think that breathing was abandoned as a direct part of the technique simply because these fundamentals of getting out of our own way were not articulated; many teachers decided it was better to leave breathing to sort itself out. Even teachers such as Goldie who worked with breathing did not usually teach it.

### Exploration 6.2   Exploring false ways of expanding the lungs

Have a go at all these to see what you or your pupils are up to.

*Draw breath in by:*

- *pulling up the collarbones and shoulders*

# Finding the innate movements of breathing and walking

- *lifting the chest, arching and narrowing the back*
- *using the intercostal muscles to force the sideways breath*
- *pushing the belly or solar plexus in and out (you can do these sharply to make a sniffing sound).*

Singers are often taught some of these to "support" the breath. They may also be taught to expand the chest hugely, or to keep the back expanded while breathing out, which can create a lot of stiffness. The full natural support to the breath we will learn here is completely sufficient to support the breath for a big tone, with no additional in-breath needed either.

### Exploration 6.3    Noisy breathing and mouth breathing

- *There are a multitude of muscles over the nose; when these are tight, breathing becomes noisy or must happen through the mouth. Think "I can do less with my nose."*
- *Relaxing the nose can free up constrictions, even with a cold or mucus. Many mouth breathers find they can breathe through their nose with this.*
- *It can also help release the holding at the top of the breath – see exploration 6.4 below: holding tension in the face is linked to holding the top of the breath.*
- *Free the jaw to help these: "I let my lower back teeth drop away from the upper back teeth, and let the upper back teeth float up and off the lower back teeth."*

Some people take an in-breath in two stages. The first part fills easily, but they then strain for more breath, out of some belief that this is needed to fill their lungs fully. People with compromised lungs, such as after lung surgery, often feel they need to do this to get enough air. This second part of the breath simply is not needed if one uses the breathing mechanism correctly.

### Exploration 6.4    Stopping or straining the breath

- *If you are straining the later part of the in-breath, choose not to do that later part. Think, in the brain: "I can breathe out now" after the "easy" half, and before you commence straining the breath.*
- *If you are stopping (however briefly) at the top of the breath, you can choose not to do this. As you approach the top of the breath, think in the brain, "I can breathe out now." Likewise if you hold the bottom of the breath: "I can breathe in now."*
- *If at any point you start going dizzy, it is likely you are doing too much, and hyperventilating. To come out of this, think "I can do less with my breathing."*

If you now feel you are not breathing enough it is usually faulty sensory perception, often because we are using so much less effort, which feels wrong. If your fingernails are not going blue, you have enough oxygen! I suspect there can also be panic in the system because long-held tensions in the respiratory musculature are being released. These may have been put in place years before, such as during an unsafe time at school. Your body does not know that it is now safe to release these old tensions, and so the stimulus it sends to breathe more is aimed at putting the tension back, by asking us to strain.

### The breath is linked with the nervous system

There is no place for holding the end of the in-breath. Breaths are like waves in the ocean. A wave flows in and it flows out again, it only stops on the shore if it freezes. But when a wave has withdrawn, there can then be a pause until the next wave comes in, so a pause at the *bottom* of the breath is not inappropriate.

The pause at the top of the breath is often a manifestation of anxiety. Think of watching somebody cross the road too close to a bus. Our response is often to draw in the breath high into the chest and hold it there until the person is safe, when we let it out with a sigh. This illustrates how the in-breath is linked to the sympathetic nervous system, the fight/flight response, while the out-breath is linked to the parasympathetic nervous system, the rest and digest system. (This is why out-breaths are emphasized for childbirth, or any situation requiring calm. It also would explain

# CHAPTER six

why a hold at the top of the breath links to tension in the face – which also indicates an agitated nervous system.)

In contrast, some people simply do not breathe, they get to the bottom of the out-breath and forget to breathe in. This one, I suspect, is linked to the freeze mechanism.

> I worked on breathing with a pupil with scoliosis. The sideways displacement of her upper torso was quite marked, so that one side was effectively unsupported by the hips and legs. She was unconsciously using breathing to lift the ribs on this collapsed side and then would hold the top of the breath in a clear attempt to stabilize it before then having to collapse it down again on the out-breath. This looked like hard work! When we restored natural breathing her torso became much more self-supporting on every part of the breath.

## Anatomy of respiration

There are twelve pairs of ribs, which articulate with the thoracic vertebrae to allow the movement of breathing:

- 1–7 are the true ribs, attached to the sternum by short cartilages, so with limited flexibility
- 8–10 are the false ribs, that join together with flexible cartilages to form the costal arch
- 11 and 12 are the floating ribs, with greatest flexibility of movement.

The diaphragm muscle is attached round the base of the ribcage, with deep roots attaching onto the vertebral column. The body of it is flat, and makes a "plunger," creating a vacuum when it contracts and pulls down, making the in-breath that pulls air into the lungs. On the out-breath it domes up as high as the 5th rib.

As the diaphragm moves *down* on the in-breath, the ribs go *up* – like slightly lifting a bucket handle – and *descend* again on the out-breath as the diaphragm travels *up* again. This continual movement massages the internal organs: down and wide on the in-breath, domed up again on the out-breath. This displacement extends right through the torso to the pelvic floor, and widens the whole back, on every in-breath.

The lungs extend above the collar bones. The fully extended and fully deflated states of the lungs are shown in Figure 6.1 – they never deflate below 40%, or they would collapse. There is more lung tissue in the back than the front.

### Breathing movement patterns

Many people breathe with an up/down direction, maybe with chest and /or shoulders rising on the in-breath and collapsing on the out-breath; or the upper back rises and sags on and off the lower back. Here we are, attempting to maintain an upward flow against gravity at all times, and yet every breath sabotages this! Another pattern is for the chest to be quite fixed, with only the belly breathing, expanding forwards on the in-breath.

In both these patterns there is likely to be little or no movement across the solar plexus area, which includes the diaphragm and floating ribs. Instead, the breath is pulled in by external muscles – the intercostals of the ribs, belly muscles, scalenes of the neck, etc. With so many other muscles in play and "doing" the breathing, the diaphragm, an involuntary muscle, is partially disabled – it cannot fully breathe out, and so cannot properly initiate the in-breath. This creates a lot of tension through the whole system.

### Exploration 6.5  Restoring the action of the diaphragm and floating ribs

- *Breathe out gently, and rest at the bottom of the out-breath. Do not breathe in again until absolutely necessary. Keep looking out, stay out of the way. When you have to, allow the in-breath to happen and see what happens.*

# Finding the innate movements of breathing and walking

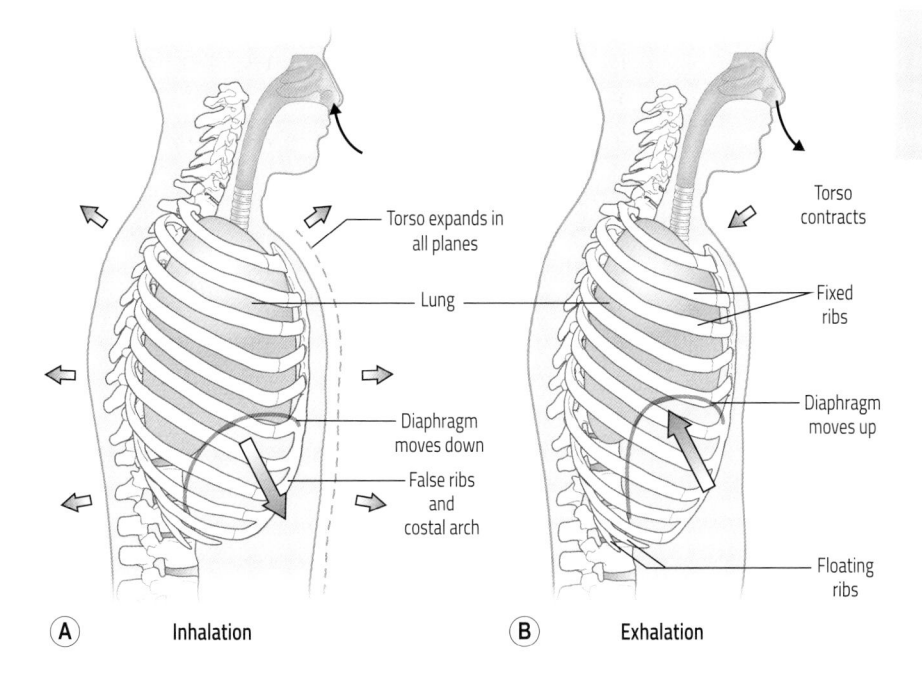

**Figure 6.1**
Movements of the chest and upper body with breath: (A) breathing in; (B) breathing out

(A) Inhalation — Torso expands in all planes; Lung; Diaphragm moves down; False ribs and costal arch

(B) Exhalation — Torso contracts; Fixed ribs; Diaphragm moves up; Floating ribs

- *Do not hold the top of the breath, or strain a longer in-breath, but immediately allow the full out-breath, and rest again at the bottom. Again wait till you have to breathe, and then allow it to happen.*

- *Continue doing this, gradually shortening the length of the rest on the out-breath, by thinking in the brain "I let myself breathe in now." You are allowing the body to revert to a breathing form closer to the natural breathing.*

- *Use your hands on your floating ribs if needed to cue the body where they are. Invite them to recoil elastically away from each other on the in-breath, and if needed, gently press the lower ribs together on the out-breath to encourage them to drape downward again.*

You may notice the following:

- *The floating ribs are now moving sideways freely, springing outwards on the in-breath and draping in and slightly down on the out-breath.*

- *The lower back has come into play in the breathing.*

- *The in-breath now takes much less effort, being now an elastic recoil action to the out-breath. I call this the springy in-breath.*

- *The in-breath may be shorter than the out-breath. Your out-breath may now be fuller.*

**Video link for exploration 6.5**

### First brain teaser

*Think out (of the floating ribs) on the in-breath, and in (of the floating ribs) on the out-breath.*

This may feel very different from where you started. It may even feel scary, or unreal. But see if it also feels free and natural! Reassure yourself, if necessary, that this is safe. Also there is no right answer.

Semi-supine is a great position in which to work on breathing, or do it at night in bed. Because my breathing was so skewed I could initially be lying still for a long time till eventually I would manage one non-doing breath. I also often walked with my hands on my floating ribs to come present there, without which

# CHAPTER six

the middle of my body was often simply absent and contracted. One day after six months I woke and found that natural breathing was just happening. Most people get it a lot quicker than I did!

### The in-breath can be the easy one

We think of the in-breath as being the breath that takes work, while the out-breath is a letting go. But this way of breathing is actually *straining* alternated with *collapsing*. Consider that in speaking or singing, the out-breath is the one on which the work is done, while the in-breath needs to be speedy and efficient. In swimming, the same is true where the head is mostly under the water, breathing out in a sustained fashion, followed by lifting the head briefly with a fast, efficient in-breath.

In natural breathing there is no collapse, instead both the in- and out-breaths are an important part of sustaining body tone and alignment. They both involve appropriate work, as the oscillation of the CPGs recruit alternating muscle patterns.

### Allowing the rhythmic control of breathing with central pattern generators (CPGs)

- CPGs are little "programs" in the brainstem or spinal cord that generate a repeating signal at a constant frequency to coordinate any rhythmic motion in the body, such as walking, swallowing, breathing, blinking.

- They are *localized*: for example, walking CPGs are in the lower thoracic and lumbar regions of the spinal cord, while CPGs for breathing, or rhythmic tongue movements for swallowing are in the brainstem region.

- *They can work without input from sensory, other motor, or higher brain functions.*

> There is a crucial difference between the CPG model of motor control and the reflex model of Charles Sherrington. In the reflex model of – say – a fish swimming, one side of the fish contracts, which bends the fish's body laterally, causing the muscles and skin on the other side to be stretched. This is picked up by stretch receptors, which feed back their sensory information in a reflex arc into the spinal cord, which then stimulates the muscles on that side of the body to contract, thus causing a stretch on the first side, and so on. This would indeed cause an alternating pattern of contraction to occur, though it would be neurologically slow. However, these rhythms of movement can be generated without sensory feedback producing a much more versatile situation that is always ready for action (Grillner 1996); sensory and proprioceptive information then input via the brainstem to modify the movements as needed for current metabolic or kinematic requirements (Grillner et al. 2008). See Rosenbaum et al. (2007) for a full list of problems with the reflex model.

- *They provide the building blocks of movement.*

- Because each CPG is composed of smaller patterns, down to simple units of movement, they can be *flexible* and *versatile*, using different combinations in different circumstances.

While CPGs are always working, in poor posture there seem to be factors preventing them functioning optimally. These could perhaps be cortical overlays of learned habits, or compensatory patterns because some or many muscles are out of play and so muscles must be used that are not the best fit.

I suspect that most people are complicating their moving or breathing patterns because they are over-involved with their action, trying to control it, whether consciously or unconsciously. This involves cortical brain patterns – using phasic muscles when tonic, innate hindbrain patterns is what we were evolved to use. This is like management getting over-involved when the problem can be sorted at ground level.

When we "stay out of our own way," we are booting management back to head office, but leaving the

# Finding the innate movements of breathing and walking

office door open – spatially aware of the world outside us. (Remember "the boss in the office" from Chapter 4, lesson 4). Then we stop feeling into controlling the action and give it the space and permission to do itself. We are letting right hemisphere/bottom-up processes lead rather than left hemisphere/top-down processes.

By waiting at the bottom of the out-breath, we are choosing not to let these unhelpful habits of respiratory movement patterns, programmed in the cortex, come into play. But the body will not let us oxygen starve; it is continually monitoring our oxygen levels and needs, along with acidity levels in the blood (indicating $CO_2$ levels). When we get out of the way, these feedback pathways can be fully autonomous again, enabling the CPGs and other spinal microcircuits in the brainstem and spinal cord to recruit the muscles needed. Then the diaphragm comes fully back into play, with its rhythmic action, and alongside this, all the other muscles of the torso work in adaptive tone.

You may notice that as you find your natural breathing, you also come to quiet, your eyes focus, you become more spatially aware and embodied. We are self-organizing, whole-body, networking structures, so that working with one fundamental will often bring all the others into play.

When natural breathing is happily looking after itself, and we are just watching it, it is like sitting on a beach watching the waves roll in and out, every one of them different, and each an appropriate response to that moment. There is a continual gentle oscillation of movement throughout the entire torso, in which every muscle is involved and every joint too, including all the little joints of the spine, as the whole torso expands and contracts, lengthwise, sideways, and front to back. The diaphragm drives the movement, creating a vacuum at the base of the lungs, which draws air into the lungs. This expands the lungs like balloons, and the ribs ride on the lungs' expansion like corks on a wave. The spine curves out and back, the sternum gently lifts and falls, the pelvic bones move apart and back. (For a beautiful depiction of this, it is well worth watching Jessica Wolf's *Art of Breathing* DVD.) The muscle tone is readjusted continually so appropriate tone is maintained for every micro-positional shift.

"All of the spinal column's 186 joints are involved in every movement of the body. This is especially well demonstrated in breathing, which is not generally thought of as a 'movement'" (Schultz and Feitis 1996: 29).

### Exploration 6.6    Expanding the whole torso on every breath

Once your breath is expanding sideways with free movement of the floating ribs, organized to a greater extent by the CPGs rather than yourself, you are ready to take it lower. This is gentle, subtle, non-doing work; you will need to stay out of your own way. Be patient and allow it to take the time it takes, maybe over several sessions.

- *To encourage the diaphragm back into full action, invite the in-breath to be initiated near the base of the sternum but deep inside the body, in the diaphragm itself. Wait until it does itself, it may be a very new sensation: the subtle sense of the diaphragm "plunger" moving downward on the in-breath and the ribs simply riding on the breath.*

- *Allow a full out-breath, then rest there longer than you would normally, and then longer again. Stay out of your own way – looking out, etc. You may notice the in-breath then deepening down the body, and widening the lower back. You can also gently invite it to move downwards.*

- *If it does not descend, bring your consciousness to the "block point" and wait there, gently, and a bit longer again. When the in-breath comes, you may find the block dissolves, and takes you a little lower. This process may need repeating till you reach the pelvic floor.*

- *Observe the breath deepening down the back, until the whole lower back is widening with the in-breath, and until it includes the pelvic girdle, expanding and contracting with the breath. You may also notice the pelvic floor descending on the in-breath and rising again on the out-breath, mirroring the action of the diaphragm.*

- *If you have a deep curve in your lumbar spine, then it may be hard for the spine here to widen. It can help to think the*

# CHAPTER six

*anterior superior iliac spines (the frontal knobbly bumps of the hip bones), moving back to open the lumbar spine and allow the widening there. (More on this in the next chapter.)*

The awareness of widening on the in-breath can then be brought up the body to the upper back and shoulder blades. Can these areas fill with air without lifting?

Second brain teaser

The breath wave moves:

- down and wide on the in-breath (right down to the pelvic floor)
- up and in on the out-breath.

I do find this to be the quickest way of opening up the lower back so it is worth persevering to find this. Rome was not built in a day – it may take a few sessions to reach the pelvic floor. We are so habituated to thinking and feeling the wave of the in-breath going up, so this can be very foreign concept.

I also find this the quickest way of re-integrating the legs with the torso. Once the pelvic girdle comes alive with this dynamic breathing you might notice your legs feeling less stable. This is a good thing! As the core muscles re-engage the big muscles are enabled to let go, which confuses our faulty sensory perception for a while.

## How muscles work – old understandings and new beginnings

With natural breathing we enable a new relationship with the body – not "doing" anything, just letting it move in a dynamic modulation of tone. By working from the inside, this widening breath gently opens out the tense muscles of the back – especially the lower back – and brings them into dynamic play. This brings strength and resilience to the lower body, which otherwise has little to support its width. This in turn gives the upper body something substantial to rest on, so the shoulders can relax.

I see this as a different model of muscle action. With imbalanced use, we are often over-using "concentric" muscle contractions, where the muscles shorten as they work. But there are two other types of muscle contractions that many people have never heard of: eccentric and isometric contractions.

## The three types of muscle contraction

Muscles exist to contract. Each muscle consists of a bundle of smaller muscle fibers, each with its own motor nerve, all wrapped in a sheath of connective tissue. When the nerves to the muscle are stimulated, they cause the muscle to contract, and in the standard picture, they shorten and fatten, like a mouse. (The word muscle derives from the Latin for mouse).

Telling someone to relax is meaningless at the neurological level, there is no nerve stimulation causing a muscle to relax. At school, I learned that muscle relaxation happens passively when its opposing muscle contracts and pulls the first muscle long again. Muscles are understood to work in phasic pairs of flexors and extensors, such as biceps and triceps (in the upper arm), quads and hamstrings (in the thigh). That is why after hunching over a desk for hours, we roll and rotate our upper bodies and arms back and stretch the chest – we are trying to utilize the opposing muscles to undo our scrunching.

But from Chapter 3, lesson 4, we have another picture of how muscles work in an integrated body: where *all muscles are working* in a balanced framework, holding tone as stability and movement occur together. Even as a muscle contracts there are *lengthening forces on it*. To bring about the changing relationships of movement, some will be contracting more at any given time, while others are lengthening as they work, but it is always within this balanced framework. How does this work?

Muscle can contract in one of three ways: concentric, isometric, and eccentric (see Fig. 6.2).

# Finding the innate movements of breathing and walking

Find these experientially:

### Exploration 6.7　The three types of muscle contraction

- Bend your lower arm up towards you with empty hand. You are using the biceps of the upper arm in a concentric contraction, while the triceps at the back of the upper arm is extended.
- Now let your hand and lower arm drop again; this is a passive opening of the biceps, initiated by the triceps.
- Now pick up any heavy object you can hold with your hand palm upward, such as a large book.
- Bring it up toward you as before. Be aware of the biceps working as it makes a concentric (or shortening) contraction – it becomes bunchier.
- If you then hold that object in the air, the muscles are neither lengthening nor shortening, but they are clearly working. This is isometric (or same length) contraction.

Now lower the object slowly. Be aware of the biceps working as it extends. This is an eccentric (or lengthening) contraction.

You might notice you have more strength and control when putting the object down than when lifting it. It was first noticed in 1882 that stretching a muscle while contracting gave a much greater force, and also has more stability.

*My hypothesis is that with this work, we are learning to inhibit the overuse of phasic muscles, activated from the cortex, and use the self-organizing hindbrain pathways more. These evolutionarily older pathways operate unconsciously, and allow more efficient and adaptive tonic patterns, which bring more stability and balance. Then only the phasic muscles needed for a precision task need be employed, giving greater coordination, as background stability is maintained through dynamic modulation of postural tone. The scientific language I am using to express this comes out of Cacciatore's work (2014). See Cacciatore, Johnson and Cohen (2020) for a more detailed review of this.*

Phasic muscle contractions, activated from the cortical brain, have been most studied because, being mostly surface muscle contractions and usually more

**A** Concentric　　　**B** Eccentric　　　**C** Isometric

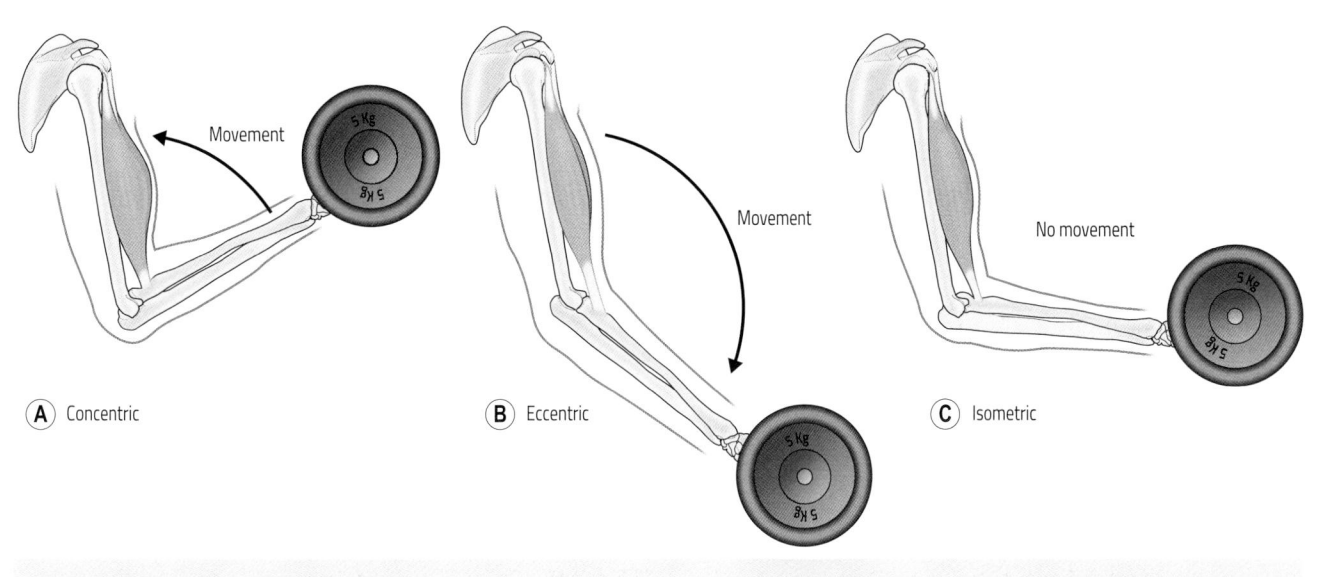

**Figure 6.2 A, B, C**
Three types of muscle contraction

# CHAPTER six

intense, they show up well on EMGs. Tonic contractions are much less understood. They are hard to detect with EMGs, especially in activity as electrodes must be inserted deep into the muscle. Large forceful movements, such as ball throwing, show triphasic contraction patterns: the throwing muscle – the agonist – works to accelerate the arm, the antagonist brakes and stabilizes it, then the agonist works again to prevent reverse thrust. Without phasing these, the opposing muscle would be ripped apart. But all muscles can work phasically or tonically, it depends on what input they receive. I wonder whether martial artists train movements so slowly over years so that they can maintain tonic contractions even in huge forceful movement, to achieve their huge levels of stability and power together. This is not known. However, AT teachers could maintain responsive movement and extensor activity even when asked to attempt to stand more quickly than is possible, whereas controls could not (Cacciatore et al. 2014).

## Lesson 2   More breathing explorations

### Exploration 6.8   Letting go of face or throat tension in natural breathing

- *While allowing natural breathing, integrate the head and neck with the body, by visualizing "liquid light" flowing through.*
- *Explore seeing from back of head and neck, to take pressure off the front of the throat and face.*
- *See the breath circling in/out through the frontal sinuses and the back of the head and neck.*

### Support for the torso on the out-breath – eccentric contractions at work

### Exploration 6.9 Tone and support from the ribs on the out-breath

- *If the breath rushes out, especially as the out-breath begins, think of letting the ribs release towards each other more slowly; they are working against the air pressure inside.*

Think of a parachute descending slowly from the sky: if there was no air pressure within, the man would plummet down.

**Video link for exploration 6.9**

### Exploration 6.10   Imagine the out-breath going up, and out through your eyes

Our tendency is to think down and inward on the out-breath, to lose the world and retreat slightly into oneself. Although the classic tendency is to sag forward in a slight slump on the out-breath, some people sag backward slightly on the out-breath.

- *Look out at the world on the out-breath, and imagine the breath also exiting through the eyes. (This is not as daft as it seems, as there are sinuses through which breath circulates through the cheek bones and sphenoid bone, while the frontal sinus is above the eyebrows.)*
- *This orientates the out-breath outwards, forwards, and upwards, and encourages the natural return movement up of pelvic floor, guts, and diaphragm. You may notice your spine lengthening and feeling supported.*

**Video link for exploration 6.10**

### Take the breath lower still – breathing from the pelvic floor

#### Anatomy

The pelvic floor is the muscle layer inside the pelvic girdle (Fig. 6.3). One set of muscles – the pubococcygeals – run front/back, from pubis to coccyx, while

# Finding the innate movements of breathing and walking

others run at various angles from side to side. Between them they make another "diaphragm" which, when toned (rather than clenched or flaccid), mirrors the thoracic diaphragm in expanding downwards and widthways on the in-breath and coming back up and in again on the out-breath.

### Exploration 6.11   Allow the movement down and up of the pelvic floor

- *To experience this, stand in alignment, or it can help to go into a flat-footed squat (maybe hanging onto a door handle) or in child's pose (see Fig. 14.4A).*
- *To bring awareness and sensation down into this often unfamiliar region, initially you may need to send the breath down into the pelvic floor. Then take the mind to the brain, look out and let it happen, noticing the slight movement in your peripheral awareness.*
- *Notice the widening on the in-breath as the whole pelvic floor domes and expands.*

Philip Shepherd observes (2017: 270–3) that the resting position of the pelvic floor is neutral, from which it domes down for the in-breath and domes up on the out-breath. So it has two active, toned positions, with the neutral position between. To initiate either the in- or the out-breath, the pelvic floor releases into movement. The perineum (slung between the sitting bones, and the torso's lowest point) also moves with the pelvic floor. When these areas participate fully in breathing, the breath ripples down into the legs.

### Exploration 6.12   Breathing in through the pelvic floor and perineum, and out into the legs

This exploration comes from Philip Shepherd's Radical Wholeness workshop (www.philipshepherd.com). It seems anatomical nonsense but it works, because to imagine this seems to bring us out of over-involvement with the nose and lungs, and allows the lower body to initiate the whole-body breath. Try it running – it is dynamite!

- *Stand in alignment.*
- *Imagine the breath coming in through the perineum and circulating through the pelvic bowl.*
- *Let the out-breath go down the legs to the feet like water down drainpipes.*

### Exploration 6.13   Support for the lower body on the out-breath – finding the psoas muscle

If the out-breath is unsupported, the organs sag downward. While the belly muscles form the front and sides of the abdominal cavity, the back wall is formed by the psoas, iliacus, and quadratus lumborum muscles (see Fig. 6.3). The base is the pelvic floor, while the ceiling is the diaphragm. The top of the psoas major and the roots of the diaphragm both insert on the lumbar spine, and their fascia intermingle. A supportive out-breath draws the organs back and up into the abdominal cavity along the line of the spine, and engages the lower back and core muscles.

- *Lie in semi-supine, knees pointing toward the ceiling. See the ceiling with spatial awareness, then invite in your awareness of your breath. Put your hands on the base of your belly, and invite the breath to happen right to (or from!) the base of the torso.*
- *Notice that on the out-breath the belly naturally falls with gravity back towards the spine. Observe whether you have other pulls and tensions happening in the belly wall, and gently invite them to disengage, until only gravity is doing the work. Likewise allow the in-breath to look after itself.*
- *Now take your consciousness a little deeper, to the belly wall. Let the belly muscles fall back from right inside the pubic bone, towards the spine.*
- *Take your consciousness deeper still, and invite the organs here – the bladder, sex organs, and lowest parts of the guts – to fall back to the spine on the out-breath. Allow them also to be drawn up along the spine, following the diaphragm moving up on the out-breath. Then on the in-breath, they move down with the movement of the pelvic floor (Fig. 6.4).*

On the in-breath the organs are moving down and wide and a little forward, on the out-breath moving back and up along the spine.

# CHAPTER six

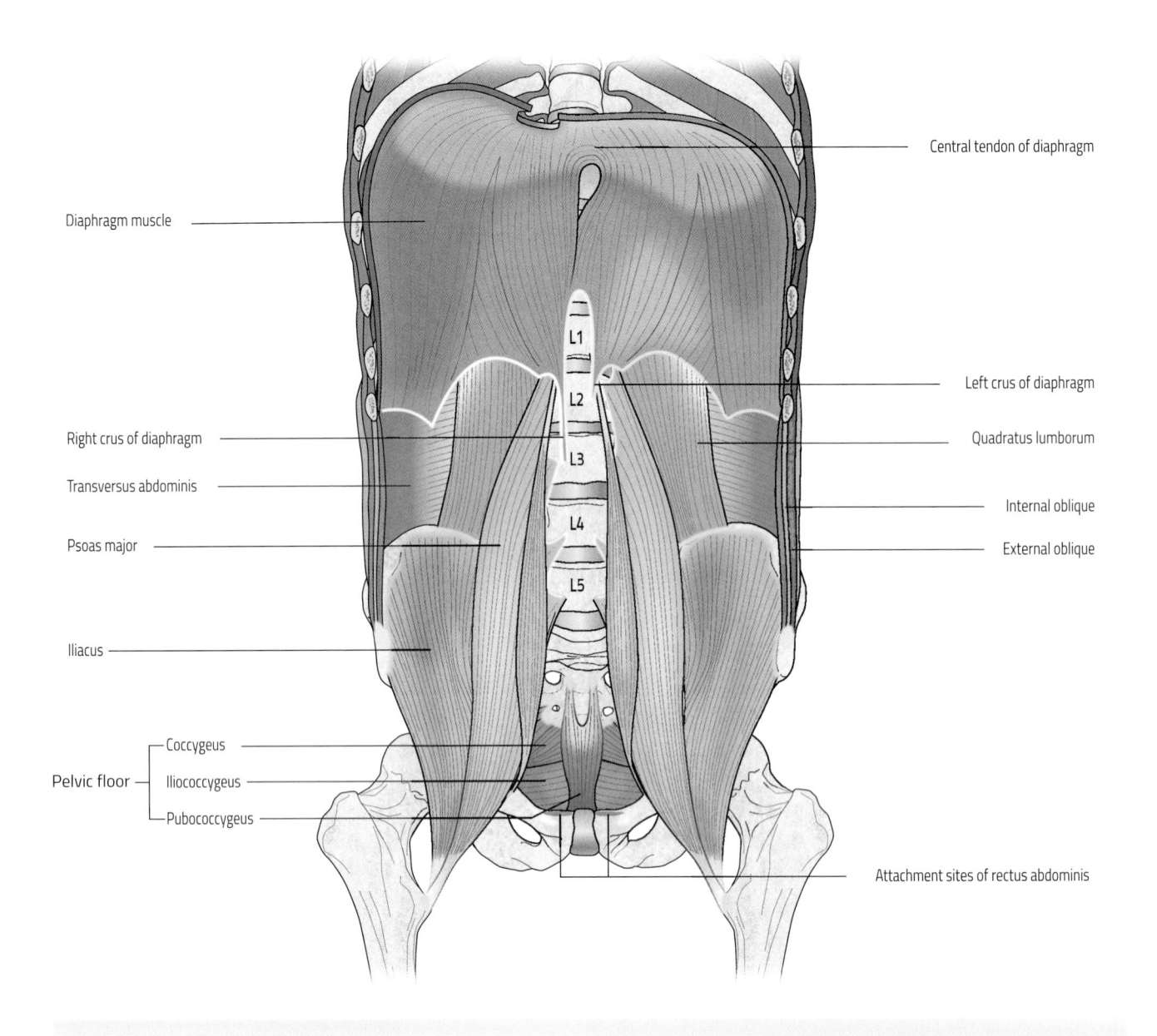

**Figure 6.3**
Muscle groups that form the abdominal cavity walls

Notice that the back is flattening onto the floor, as the psoas and erector spinae lengthen on the out-breath. Invite them to maintain this length on the in-breath. Notice also that the thighs lengthen up and out of the hips as this happens, and the quads on the front of the thighs lengthen as the psoas releases and tones. Don't worry if you don't get all this straight away, there is a lot going on here which we will revisit in subsequent chapters.

- *Now gently engage the pubococcygeals (see Fig. 6.3) by thinking to draw the pubic bone forwards; you will notice the pelvis tilt forwards slightly.*

- *Retain this gentle pull as you continue to draw the organs back and up along the front of the spine on the out-breath. Does it add more lengthening and stability?*

# Finding the innate movements of breathing and walking

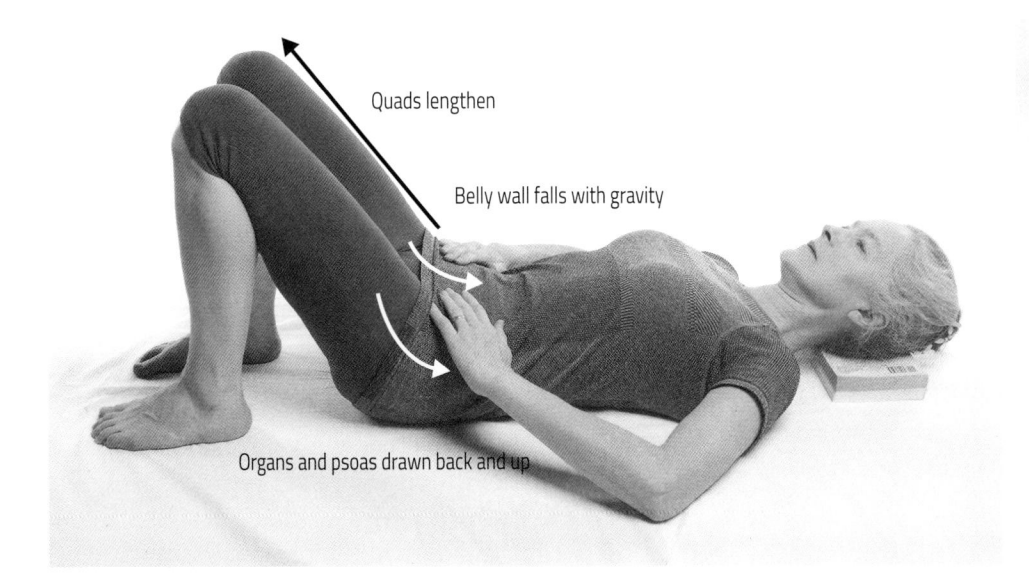

**Figure 6.4**
Finding support for the lower body with the out-breath

Quads lengthen
Belly wall falls with gravity
Organs and psoas drawn back and up

- *Notice that the psoas and pubococcygeals work in opposition to each other to create lengthening.*

Video link for exploration 6.13

These explorations tone the core muscles without the strong tightening moves so often encouraged by Pilates classes or Kegel exercises. A tight muscle is not free to respond to the activity required in the moment; we need toned core muscles, not tight ones.

### The thoracolumbar fascia – the flow of mechanical information throughout the whole-body

With natural breathing, one can find a sense of the whole-body expanding and contracting, the coordinated movements ebbing and flowing as effortlessly as waves on a beach. With time, the mechanotransduction of the breath waves can be sensed right through the limbs to the fingers and toes, and into the skull. I think the thoracolumbar fascia can give us another sense of how the whole structure all links up.

The latissimus dorsi muscles do not attach directly to the spine, but onto a diamond-shaped sheet of tough, elastic fascia that itself is attached to the spine (Fig. 6.5). This is the posterior layer of the thoracolumbar fascia, to which the gluteus maximus also attaches. Fascia does not have set start and endpoints as muscles do; it is a continuity that connects everything to everything. Figure 6.6 shows the abdomen at the mid-lumbar level, where the thoracolumbar fascia is in three layers. The outer, posterior layer is the sheet to which the latissimus dorsi muscles attach. Below this are fascial pockets of middle and anterior layers that envelop the erector spinae (and the smaller multifidus), quadratus lumborum, and psoas muscles respectively. These fascial layers then join at the lateral raphe and divide again to continue between the belly muscles in a circle of elastic connectivity. The vertebrae are also caught in this continuity of flow, their ligamentous and tendinous attachments stretched with every breath. This gives us continuity front to back.

Through the latissimus dorsi muscles and gluteus maximus, there is connectivity to legs and arms, and by connecting to the fascial attachment of the trapezius, links also to the neck and head. Through fascial links, the breath ripples through the whole-body.

# CHAPTER six

## Lesson 3  Finding our emergent rhythmic movement – walking and bouncing

> I was told this story of a young AT student's one and only lesson with Miss Goldie. She showed him into the room where he stood in front of the chair, then she excused herself and went out of the room. He continued standing, and when she came back she looked at him curiously, walked all around him, and asked: "Young man, what are you doing?" He replied: "I'm grounding myself, Miss Goldie." "Grounding yourself? You look like the Bank of England!"

Many people use their legs for support in this way, not regarding them as part of themselves. For a long time in my lessons with her, Miss Goldie was trying to show me a different way with my legs, but I was not understanding. One day in desperation she said, "I shall just have to put you on the table." In that turn she showed me that legs connect up to the body. She had often told me that my legs were dragging on my back and weakening it, and in that session, she showed me how to reverse this.

Sometime after that, I walked down the street after my lesson and discovered, with an astonishment I can still remember, that my knees were releasing up and forwards from my hips so that I felt like a one of those beautiful dancing Lipizzaner ponies who

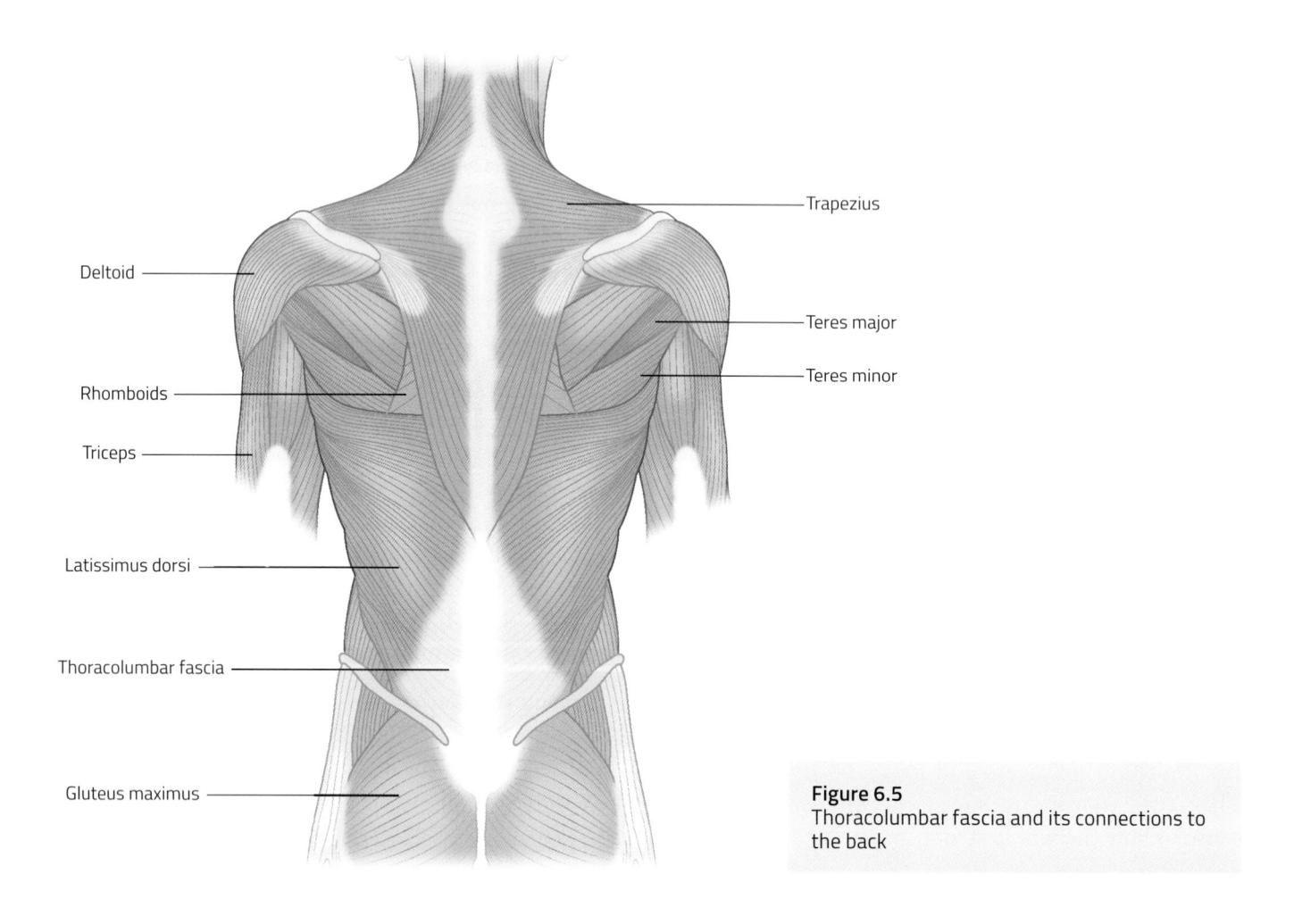

**Figure 6.5**
Thoracolumbar fascia and its connections to the back

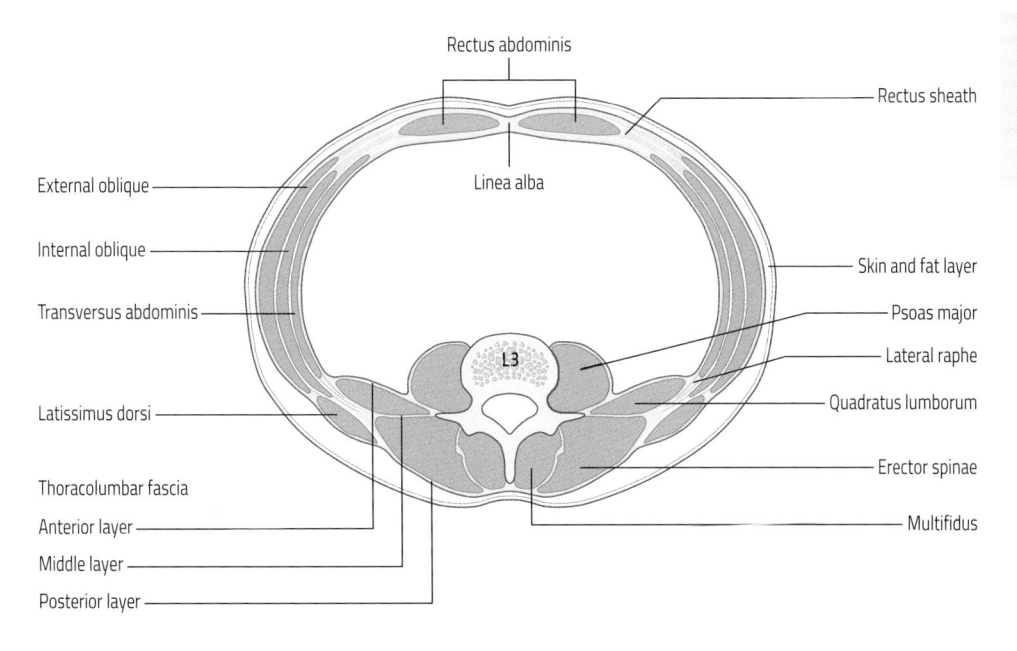

# Finding the innate movements of breathing and walking

**Figure 6.6**
Horizontal section through the abdominal region, showing front to back connections of the thoracolumbar fascia

lift their knees as they dance. I hoped fervently that nobody was looking – it was one of those "I must look so weird" moments such as I hadn't had since I first began lessons. There were other procedures with legs also that at the time I simply did not understand. It was years before I put it all together and began to discover what she was after. Most of us stand too heavily on our legs, with little springy tone in them. It feels relaxed, but parts of the body are collapsing into each other. Miss Goldie showed me our possibility is to be lighter and springier, connected and integrated.

Thinking up the back of the legs to the sacrum (exploration 3.12) came from this understanding. Have a go at engaging everything we've done so far, and see whether you are already walking differently.

## Exploration 6.14  Let yourself walk using the fundamentals

- Find your balanced stance – feet hip-width apart, equally balanced on both legs.
- See forward (the eyes tracking the scene gently) with the head balanced ("roll your raindrop" as needed).
- Invite your depth perception and peripheral vision, seeing from the back of the head and including yourself in the scene.
- Keep your mind in the brain and an awareness of your whole-body.
- Lift one heel and lower it slowly, thinking up the back of the legs to the sacrum. Do this a few times.
- Let the out-breath be full, and rest there till the springy in-breath does itself from the diaphragm and floating ribs. Allow your natural breathing, if possible, right to the pelvic floor. You may notice the legs destabilize a little as the muscles round the hips begin to rebalance.
- Then keeping spatial awareness, internally and externally, let your eyes be drawn to a point in your room. Let yourself walk towards it and notice what happens.
- Did you allow something different to happen? Do your knees release forward into movement more than before, so that the hips are not over-involved?

"I just focus on keeping my "raindrop" rolling, and seeing where I am going, trusting to my lower quadrant to see the ground sufficiently, and let the magic happen below in my body and legs. I can now walk freely for the first time ever!" as one pupil put it to me recently.

# CHAPTER six

*Stopping without stopping*

Think of how people walk to a bus stop. Their movements maybe upright and lively, but on reaching the bus stop, they sink into a "jammed" pose. Perhaps they collapse down on one hip, or push the hips forward, maybe with folded arms. It looks and feels relaxed, but is held rigid by some strong tensions that become apparent if you pay attention. Those of us who know better than to slump like this may still be settling down into the legs. Whether we "jam" or only settle, the legs have "stopped," and have lost consciousness and tone.

### Exploration 6.15  Stopping without losing tone

- Walk again, then stop and notice if you let go of some of the tone you have been holding. Do you collapse down a bit, or shuffle your feet to a firmer "standing stance"?
- Notice that from this stopped place, it takes effort to begin walking again, as muscle tone needs to be re-engaged. You need to "crank yourself back into gear."
- Bring back your "up" lines, "raindrop", free breathing, etc., whatever has been lost, and walk again. Is it easier again? Now stop again, and this time, see if you can do so without letting go of tone. It may feel very unfamiliar!

## Bouncing on the spot

If you can bounce, you are demonstrating the elastic energy storage and springy recoil of a well-functioning body. Up to 50%, or even more, of the energy expended in movement is recovered when these mechanisms are in play (Lindstedt et al. 2001). This is worth having! It is a lack of springiness that often makes us feel old.

So often, when we bend our knees we sink into the movement. In doing this we release muscle tone and compress our joints, which dissipates the elastic energy stored in tendons, ligaments, and muscle, without which we must struggle to get back up again.

The quality of holding tone we employed above is what we need for bouncing.

### Exploration 6.16  Starting to bounce

- Trace a visual line towards yourself so that your head nods forward a little and allow yourself to find the fundamental bend in your hips and knees and ankles (exploration 4.15). But this time only go a little way and invite the torso to stay vertical. Do not let the weight come off your heels.
- If the up-line between your heels and your crown is still active (do not let your head fall back!), then you have put a stretch on your Achilles tendons and calf muscles, and even hamstrings and erector spinae, which you can immediately release to bounce you up again. Thinking an elastic string between your crown and the ceiling can help also. Once up, immediately allow the natural bend to happen again, and then let yourself oscillate between bending and straightening – which is bouncing. Maybe say "I can do less" or "I am not bouncing" and notice what happens. You are letting your muscles adapt responsively to the movements.
- Initially, leave your heels on the ground, but as your bounce discovers its spring momentum you may find that your heels start leaving the ground as you go upward, until your whole foot is bouncing up into the air. You are using the CPGs of locomotory movement (Fig. 6.7).
- If you have lost touch with your bouncing pattern, find it again in four stages – bend, straighten, lift onto toes, come back to flat, bend again ... then in two movements – lower heels → bend; straighten → release up off heels, until the bounce movement self-organizes.

Could you bounce? Or did you not know how? While many people will find a bounce pattern immediately, others will need to reawaken the adaptive muscle patterns we need. In a well-functioning body, the CPGs coordinate the oscillating muscle patterns so that we naturally alternate bending the knees with springing up again. For this to happen, we have to

# Finding the innate movements of breathing and walking

allow our muscles to operate responsively. When we have lived for years in a co-contracted state, in which we probably organized any new movement patterns consciously, this can take some adjustment.

*Springiness happens when elastic resistance is paired with adaptive muscle tone, so that the body can utilize the elastic recoil.*

Greater overall muscle resistance on its own is not efficient; it produces stiffness across joints – co-contraction. Elderly men were compared with young men while treadmill walking, and oxygen use was monitored to observe how much energy they expended, along with

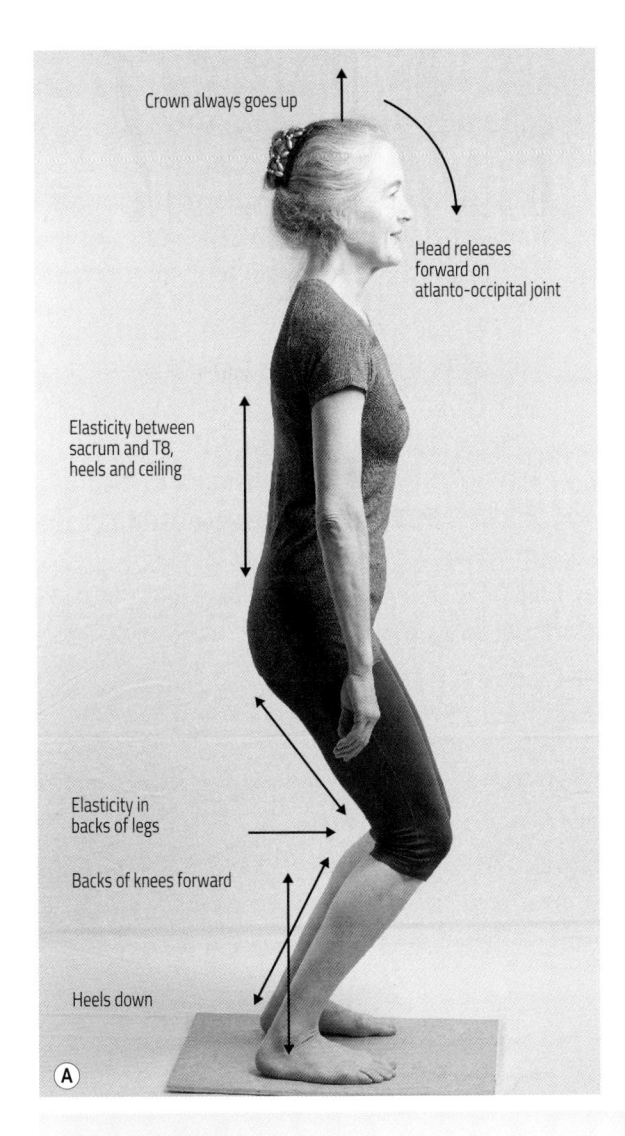

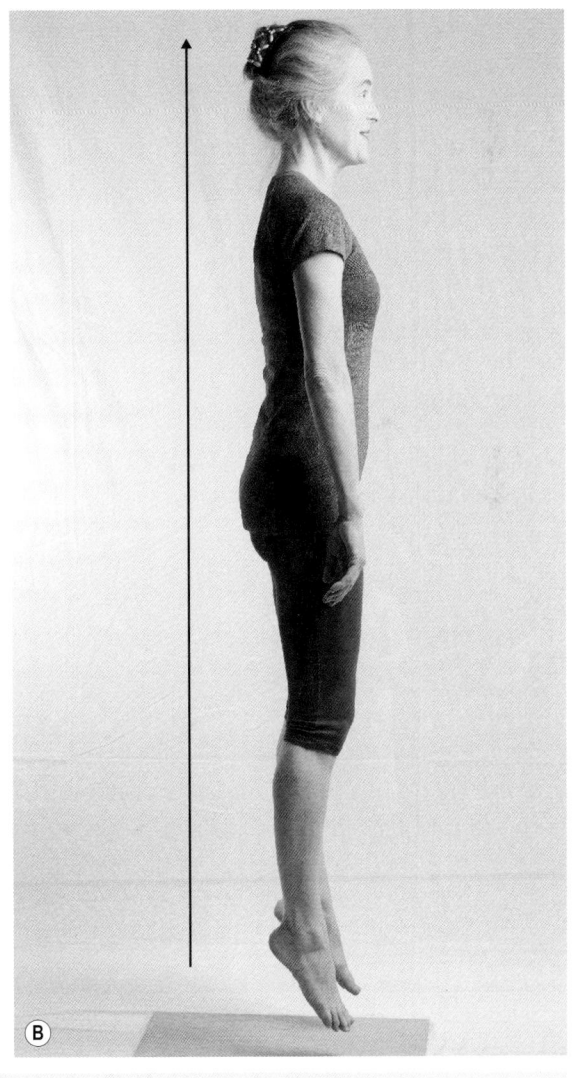

**Figures 6.7 A, B**
Bouncing. (A) Elastic energy stored as we fold without shortening; (B) Elastic energy released helps to spring us upward

# CHAPTER six

> other factors. The older men used more energy to walk and researchers concluded this was from their greater stiffness from co-contraction, which was probably engaged for greater stability (Mian et al. 2006).

We will explore more bouncing in subsequent chapters, as it is a great test of how well we have brought our alignment and springy adaptive responsiveness back into play. So, don't worry if your bounce isn't up to much yet.

Find your current personal rhythm in this. If you bounce too slowly it becomes labored as you lose the moment of springy recoil, while bouncing too fast can be uncomfortable.

## More on CPGs – the building blocks of movement

- CPGs have been shown to be in all animals, including humans.
- Because CPGs are rhythmic, they provide the basis for springiness in movement.
- Each CPG is composed of smaller patterns, down to simple units of movement, so they can be flexible and versatile, using different combinations in different circumstances. They provide the building blocks of movement. This subdivision into smaller functional units means that the same basic circuitry can be used for jumping, bouncing, walking backwards or sideways, or hopping, etc. (Grillner et al. 2008).
- This close group of synergists are all directionally related, so that when they are activated they will move the limb or part of the limb in a well-defined direction, an arrangement that also gives accurate information to the CPG about limb position. This information then allows the motor cortex to construct an accurate picture of the type and the direction that the movement should take.
- CPGs are predictive. The sensory information interacts with them and modulates them, but the movement patterns themselves are innate. This means the higher brain can get on with modulating and directing movement, with guiding the body, but it does not have to control the *mechanisms* of locomotion or movement.

# Part 2
## Linking Brain and Body with Explorations of Physical Integration

7

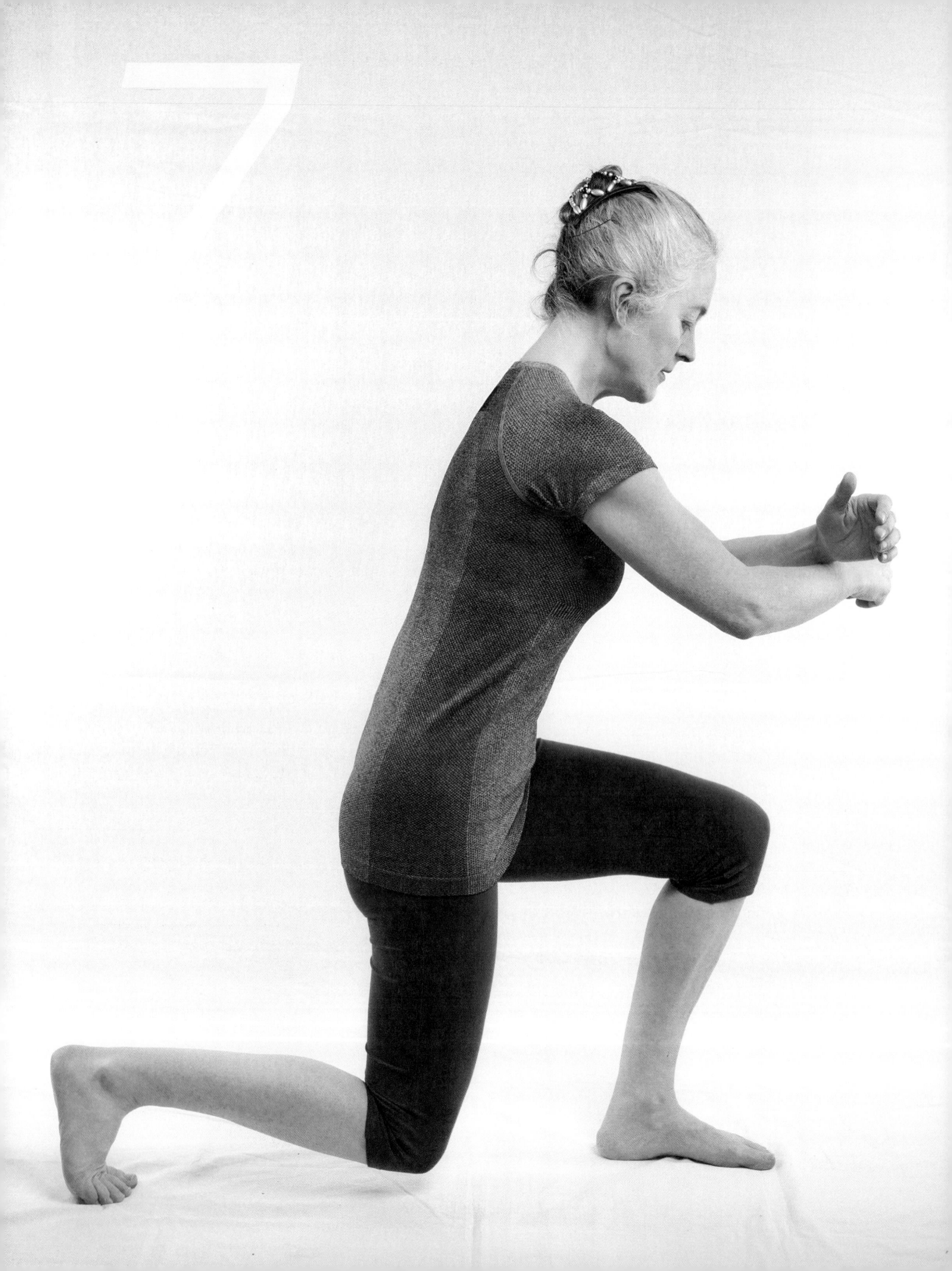

# The Initial Alexander technique, and a new model of postural alignment

## Introduction to Part 2 – exploring Miss Goldie's model of the structural body

> As you dive into Part 2, your body may take time to find all the new body geometry and adjust to it. Do alternate with Part 3 chapters as needed, to balance inhibitory and directional activity.

Miss Goldie's model of the Alexander technique was very different from anything I had encountered before, with different ideas of inhibition and direction and of how the mind and brain were to be used. She seemed also to have a different model of how the body is structured, with unfamiliar working procedures which were precise and had clear goals that often I did not understand. While others talked much of her work on the brain and inhibition, no one else seemed interested in analyzing the biomechanical aspect of her work, which I first wrote about in 2004 (Easten 2004). I pondered on it for years, but many questions stayed unanswered.

In Part 2, we mostly explore my understanding of her model of body structure and movement. We begin with the torso and progress through hips and legs, then shoulders and arms, to walking, the hinging of the torso on the legs for chairwork, the upper body, and finally the head and neck. While what follows involves a lot of physical exploration and play, this is only a starting point. *The aim always is to wake up the brain/body links from which we can bring much more clarity to directions and thinking, and understand more deeply what we are attempting to do.* Direct physical work was always frowned upon within the Alexander technique. However, the modern world moves fast and a few simple physical experiments can get things moving quickly and easily. This approach will be familiar to many current AT teachers.

However, in this chapter we jump straight in with some different work. While this also aims to connect brain and body, it particularly aims to activate and rebuild myofascial elastic resistance and responsiveness, which bring increased springiness and strength.

A few years ago, I encountered the work of Jeando Masoero, a French AT teacher. He had been studying Alexander's books for decades, pondering the origins of the technique, and was puzzled by continual contradictions within them, as if there were two different techniques being described. He, like others, was then intrigued by the discovery of Alexander's 1902 business card, in which he had advertised himself as a teacher of the Delsarte method of breathing. Delsarteism is still known in the USA, popularized initially by Gertrude Stebbins (1885). It instructs readers to spend long hours in front of mirrors, which we know Alexander did, so some have assumed this is what he read. But Stebbins's approach brings about changes through somatic feeling and physical release, rather than thinking and directing.

In 2009 Delsarte's original writings were published in French for the first time, and Masoero was poised to read them (Delsarte 1854; Gauthier 2011). He found a mosaic of clues from which he deduced Delsarte's methodology for physical change, and that explained the contradictions in Alexander's writing. Through these, linking to another mosaic of clues in Alexander's books, he has hypothesized some origins of the technique. Alexander's understanding was remarkably complete early on, but his descriptions, interpretations, and teaching methods evolved over nearly seven decades. While there are always unifying strands, there are perhaps not two techniques even, but three or four. To understand the technique fully, we need all of these.

> **AT info:** François Delsarte (1811–71) had been a gifted singer, but formal singing training had damaged his voice. He became a keen observer of people – both of living and dissected bodies – and through this worked out how to heal his problems. He taught his "gestural training" to give singers and actors real control of emotions they were communicating on stage through their bodies and presence. Though known as the voice doctor, he was not interested in the healing element of his work. His student Steele MacKaye took the work to the USA, and Stebbins was his pupil.

# CHAPTER seven

> Hidden in Delsarte's writings, Masoero has found many elements of Alexander technique. Delsarte had developed a method in which you could learn to work from plans and coordinate them to bring your torso back into alignment: "To be the architect of your own building," as Masoero describes it (Masoero, workshop in Ennis, Ireland, October 2019). Delsarte's central ideas include the concept of faulty sensory perception, the law of opposition and the law of extension. He saw the body as only an instrument of the mind. Only lengthening can be trusted, and this is brought about by constructive conscious control. To bring about change, you were to understand and memorize the directions, and work industriously in front of two-way mirrors with strong physical work brought about with thinking, until you saw the desired results.
>
> How had Alexander learned this work? His acting teacher of 1898, James Cathcart, had worked alongside Steele MacKaye in 1873, and so presumably taught this (Staring 2005: 248). Masoero has also uncovered that Delsarte had trained his brother Camille (1817–77) who then emigrated to Tasmania and Australia in 1851. He presumably taught many of the stage community of the day with whom Alexander would then mingle and learn, possibly including Edith – Alexander's future wife.

I worked with Masoero for a year, via an online application. It is very different work, applying strong, precise pulls to one's own body, using conscious guidance and control. Once these are understood and the brain/body links are there, they are applied in groups, programmed from the brain.

But Initial AT is not just about pulls, but about *experiments* in movement. While Alexander used mirrors, Masoero uses video, to judge the result of each experiment of constructive guidance. Then, where needed, one can change the program and have another go. This is real self-exploration. This aspect was not in Miss Goldie's work; however, the discovery process she taught me is described in Part 3.

Many AT teachers, especially experienced ones, have initially recoiled from the physicality of this work, as I also was tempted to do; it seems so opposed to our current methods. I chose to stay with it because the directions and strong pulls Goldie applied to me in my lessons were evidently the same as Masoero was instructing me to bring about for myself. It explained to me all the contradictions between what I had been taught by my modern AT teachers and what Goldie (and other first-generation teachers) were doing. Masoero calls it building a new body geometry, and to me, it is building the different body structure Miss Goldie's work aimed to find, only this time with clear instructions. Whether or not this is exactly what Alexander was doing, Masoero has given us a missing link.

On the first training course, directions were employed more dynamically than they are today, with many strong self-work procedures that were watered down or lost within a few years. These included the cigar box procedure and self-supporting back in the chair, going up on the toes and the mantelpiece game, the wall game, and lifting yourself back in the chair, alongside the better known procedures of whispered Ah, hands on back of chair, "monkey," chairwork, and squat. These were the vehicles through which Alexander taught the pulls and through which Goldie taught me. "By physical culture methods you do not get the desirable antagonistic [muscular] pulls" (Alexander 2015: 172). He must have done these for himself originally to bring about lengthening – for there was no one else to do it for him. Masoero teaches them in a deconstructed way, invaluable for real understanding. However, we do not know Delsarte's actual methods that Alexander might have learned.

The first-generation teachers I encountered were wickedly strong and *when needed* could apply huge pulls that were often uncomfortable. The technique has become increasingly gentle with hands. I suspect this is partly because without these strong pulls, we no longer have the full dynamic lengthening that brings in such integrated strength with precision of action. The lengthening pulls proposed, if used correctly, can

# The Initial Alexander technique, and a new model of postural alignment

bring this back in. It also enables teachers to be less reliant on colleagues for the maintenance and development of their use.

I encourage all teachers (and everyone else) to give a trial to each set of pulls, not just once but daily over a couple of weeks. My observation, and that of many of my pupils, is that initially these pulls feel strenuous and strange, as one works to traction deep, habitual tensions and imbalances. But they become normalized, often within a week to a fortnight, when the lengths readjust. (Deeply stuck muscles will take longer.) I observe that the graph of change is often non-linear: nothing happens for days then at a certain point the change happens and is done. This is why this initial stage can be short term. Once the lengthening and integrating change has happened it takes less work to maintain, though the directions still need activating regularly. It is then up to you how you use it, whether by instructing pupils to do likewise, or whether, as Alexander then did, you use it to inform and strengthen your own use to bring about the change non-verbally in your pupils, or a mixture of the two.

I am starting Part 2 with this more challenging material for two reasons. It complements the breathing work of the previous chapter, opening the torso strongly so that the breath can access all areas. But more fundamentally because the torso is primary to the limbs, so that it paves the way for the other chapters. The first self-stretch includes a move that Goldie and many other senior Alexander teachers did on me regularly, namely a pull to the elbow.

## The seven steps to a new body geometry

(FACTISPAL for those who like acronyms)

1. FIND the joints and muscles involved and play physically with what they do and their directional pulls.
2. This ACTIVATES the muscles and
3. re-CONNECTS the links between brain and muscle, waking up the brain maps.
4. Then THINK it. Use constructive conscious control (CCC) from the brain to apply strong, precisely aligned pulls which awaken functionally inactive muscles. This is reparative work and needs doing systematically for several weeks or even months, until change happens. We use brain programs to INTEGRATE these pulls into larger and larger groups, as more of the structural body is linked up and the process becomes subtler.
5. We can then connect these to our SPATIAL PERCEPTION, with our expanded field of awareness.
6. ALLOW it. As the muscle lengths readjust, the pulls from our CCC (stage 2) feel "normal" and become much more subtle and non-doing as they tone and realign us.
7. LIVE it. With time, we can notice that the new alignments happen by themselves, especially when we are using the inhibition, spatial awareness, and focused thinking of Part 3 of this book.

## The five stages to Alexander's path of discovery

### 1869–84   The problem

Frederick Matthias Alexander was born in Tasmania. He was premature and suffered recurrent breathing attacks. His initial search in 1883 was for solutions to voice problems that developed when he took professional acting classes. He later claimed (1985, ch. 1) he sorted these problems unaided, as if the colonies were a cultural desert. Research by McLeod (1994), Evans (2001), Staring (2005), Murray (2015), and Williamson (2015) shows that a wealth of ideas was available alongside Delsarte work: he drew on books of natural elocution, explored different methods, and worked with natural elocution teacher Fred Hill (Evans 2001: 96). Murray, Williamson, and Masoero consider that Delsarte work was part of his cure, though it is possible he added this later. In only eighteen months the problems were sorted, and he became a professional reciter and teacher of natural elocution and public speaking.

# CHAPTER seven

### Stage 1: 1894–1908   The natural breathing and voice teacher

Alexander first taught breathing as part of "natural elocution," to strengthen and build the voice. In this period, although the work was educational, he saw his technique as physiological, and curative for many health problems because it encouraged the correct placement and massage of the organs. His brother A. R. and sister Amy soon worked alongside him.

In 1904, Alexander moved to London, still only teaching natural breathing. There he encountered new ideas and slowly developed the theories and concepts we know as Alexander technique. AT teachers later assumed these were entirely his own, but the research shows otherwise; many are Delsarte concepts. However, this does not make him any less remarkable. Western culture then lauded the self-made man and Alexander chose to generate that myth. But no one is self-made: all great thinkers have drawn on the ideas of others to evolve their own approach. What matters is the depth of understanding he found with the material he drew from.

First he found the philosophy of William James and ideomotor theory, with the concept that one needs to "inhibit" to gain a moment of choice, from which a new reasoned action can be set in motion (Murray 2015: 37). The concepts of antagonistic action, mechanical advantage, then kinesthesia appear in his pamphlets (Alexander 2015). In 1918, Alexander told the philosopher Horace Kallen that William James and Delsarte were sources of his technique (Murray 2015: 37).

### Stage 2: 1908–14   The Initial Alexander technique

In 1908, a new phase began, focusing on rebalancing the muscle patterns of the whole-body through consciousness and directions. Alexander's first book, *Man's Supreme Inheritance* (MSI) (Alexander 2011, first published 1910), is the book of this period. Careful reading reveals a more complex directing of parts of the body than later on, with the pupil doing the brainwork to bring about change for themselves. Alexander dictated orders that the pupil was to recite and gave guidance with his increasingly sensitive hands. The torso and organ health are still the primary focus, with the head and neck secondary. Breathing was still sometimes seen as primary and at other times as tertiary: consciousness (the primary) affects the use of the muscular mechanisms (secondary), and natural breathing is then a result of good use (tertiary) (Alexander 2015: 92). He increasingly realized the need to be indirect, to reduce pupils' interference with their preconceived habits.

Alexander had always taken the head up to lengthen the spine, as did many other breathing teachers. But in 1908 he began to understand the importance of head leading forwards and up (Staring 2005: 128). Irene Tasker recalled: "In those very early days (1913) … his manner of teaching was entirely different from what it became in the later years." She also recalled his frustration when pupils could not do as he asked, and how he would scold her fiercely (Tasker 1978: 10). Others recall him and A. R. shouting orders at pupils.

### Stage 3: 1914–25   Hands-on work begins

About 1914, Alexander realized that his hands conveyed his own use to the pupil. Now the focus changed: pupils recited their orders while he gave them the new sensory experiences that they could then bring about for themselves at home. He rewrote MSI (1918), emphasizing that you need a teacher – you cannot do it for yourself.

Ethel Webb and Irene Tasker (Montessori trained) became teaching assistants. He and A. R. gave main lessons to pupils, then the women gave a lying-down lesson on inhibition (Tasker 1978: 14). Through them, he worked with Esther Lawrence, head of Froebel education (who brought Goldie along in 1927) and John Dewey, philosopher of education. The emphasis of the work now shifted to being purely educational, and "clients" were now "pupils." The "means whereby" a task is carried out – a key element in progressive education – was introduced.

Alexander's second book, *Constructive Conscious Control* (CCC) (1987, first published 1923), has much

# The Initial Alexander technique, and a new model of postural alignment

detail on consciousness and thinking; it was Miss Goldie's favorite book. I believe the physical aspect of her work was also rooted here. In CCC the torso and breathing are still important, but organ health is no longer mentioned.

### Stage 4: 1930–45    Primary control and the modern AT

In 1925, Alexander was shown the new work of Sherrington and Magnus, of central control of an organism through the head and spine. He realized he had already been working with this for twenty-five years (Alexander 2015: 141). He began to revise his theories again, culminating in his third book, *The Use of the Self* (UoS) (1985, first published 1932). Chapter 1 is called "Evolution of a technique" and convincingly describes his discovery of the primary control mechanism, and how he did it alone. From what is written above, one can understand why researchers now consider that this account is at least partially an invention, as the original focus of the work was on rebalancing the primary movements of the torso for improved breathing mechanisms and general health, not on the head-neck-back balance. He later rewrote MSI once again (1946) and also CCC (1955) to include the new concepts. No wonder the books get confusing! "Primary Control" brought in much simpler directions. Any reference to breathing or organ health is gone. This coincided with the first training course and became the modern AT; the rest was forgotten, and Goldie, Whittaker, and others were angry at this. John Skinner, first generation teacher and close friend of Goldie, told interviewer Edward Owen that "US is a terrible book – falsifying what happened and misleading to many who read it" (unpublished interview, via Jean Fischer). However, I prefer to see it as another stage in his evolution of the work, and we will explore and integrate it in Chapter 14.

### Stage 5: 1945–55    Final years

In the last years, Alexander could work while distracting his pupils with chat, not asking them even to think for themselves, and his temper was the better for it (Westfeldt 1985: 61)! He withdrew more from his training school and only those close to him really heard his thoughts. His last book, *Universal Constant in Living* (1941), adds nothing new to his ideas.

Alexander prospered with his "self-made man" myth. How else would such an uneducated man from the colonies have made such a splash in Edwardian England? He reinvented himself and his technique regularly with the excitement of new discoveries, and in the spirit of progress of the time, negated what had gone before as inferior. He covered up his family convict background, the sources he had studied, and the progressive stages of his work. His family must have been loyal co-conspirators all the way through; his sister Amy's daughters, Marjory Barlow and Joan Evans, his secretary, knew none of it when later interviewed extensively. Today we see family secrets as shameful, but the Victorians saw them as the glue that bonded a family (research cited in *Stephen Fry's Victorian Secrets*, www.audible.co.uk). This must have been true for the Alexanders, keeping their family afloat in a new land.

Alexander said "Anyone can do what I do, if they will do what I did. But none of you want the discipline" (Alexander 2000: 76). He gave UoS as the path to follow. We now know it was not the path he took, and he must have been using all stages even then to look after his own use. This is not to call him a liar; instead I presume he felt his students would not understand the complexity. Teachers knew that the work had evolved but were given to understand that the present work was all they needed; the vast degree to which the work had changed was not known. Since stage 4 is the dominant method now taught, no wonder the early teaching protocols, such as whispered Ah and hands on back of chair, can seem so mysterious. In this book we are working through all the stages Alexander took, from breathing, to Initial AT, using the mind constructively to bring about change, to integrating primary control, and finally to using energy and decisions alone. We also look at using hands as Alexander did in Chapter 18. Then we

# CHAPTER seven

can discover how to bring about all stages of the work for ourselves and our pupils, as he used to look after himself throughout his life.

## Lesson 1  How well is your body aligned with gravity?

### What anatomical paradigm are we working to?

Erika Whittaker (who was on the first training course), once told me about sitting in a concert, while in front of her a young man sat bolt upright on his chair, his legs firmly to either side, hands upside down on his thighs. She said "I knew he was an Alexander teacher, and I spent the whole concert wanting to give him a push." She saw that his upright stance was fixed.

People often come to Alexander technique with what they call poor posture, by which they usually mean a slump. When, through lessons, they can maintain an upright stance while sitting, the job seems to be done. But often they are now in a subtler reverse curve, with a fixing across the lower ribs to hold the overly upright spine. When I first went to Goldie, after six years of Alexander work and proud of my upright spine, she undid this fixing and collapsed me. Then she worked to integrate my system for stability with mobility. Just as there are two distinct paradigms of anatomy (Chapter 3, lesson 4), so there are two distinct models of postural alignment, and we need to understand them to be clear which we are working with.

### The standard model of "correct" postural alignment – the noble (or plumb line) posture

The ideal Western posture of chest raised, chin up, shoulders back, and feet turned slightly out goes back to Ancient Rome and Greece. It is the posture in which kings and nobles always had their portraits painted. In singing and acting circles it still is called the noble posture because it commands attention, and opens the chest to breathe more freely. It is assumed to be the posture we are meant to have and so its biomechanics have been worked out: a plumb line that should run from the crown down through the head/neck joint, then level with the center of the shoulder, hip, knee, and ankle joints, and through the arch of the foot to the ground.

Postural advice to attain this can include pushing the shoulder blades together, keeping an arch in the lower back, and pulling the head and neck strongly back. (An Internet search for "good posture" will find many sites recommending this, such as Medline Plus 2020.) To bring about these changes requires pulling on the superficial musculature. The underlying postural muscles are shifted from one pattern of imbalance to another. This is why we don't like the word "posture" in Alexander technique (Fig. 7.1).

This cannot be how we are evolved to stand. If we consider the curve patterns (Chapter 3, lesson 4) we can see that secondary curves and external torque chains are dominating. My sense is that this posture was developed to distinguish the nobles from the peasants, a posture conveying respect, aloofness, and reserve. To hold these curves requires fixing; this is a stiff posture from which one must *make* the body move and continually work to find flexibility.

### Natural posture and the unity line

Delsarte disliked rigid stage presence; he was seeking flowing natural movement that conveys an authentic presence on stage. He saw how nature unfolds and folds, like flowers, from the center outward, in a balance of curve patterns. From his anatomy studies he realized that for the larynx to be free to work fully the muscles must all be in tensioned balance, for which the bones must be aligned with gravity.

We do not know Delsarte's precise method to achieve this balance. But from photos (Fig. 7.2) and from clues in his books, Masoero believes Alexander was using a "unity line" as a reference frame to integrate the body: a vertical line up the front of the body, on which the instep, anterior superior iliac spines, costal arch, top of sternum, and base of the ear are all aligned. The back is straight between the sacrum and eighth thoracic vertebrae (T8) between the shoulder

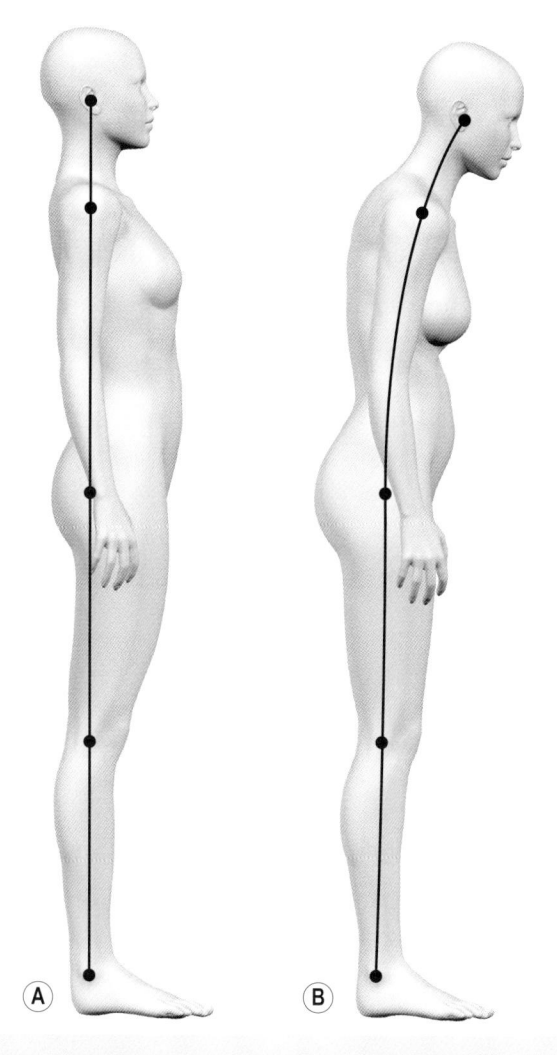

# The Initial Alexander technique, and a new model of postural alignment

**Figure 7.1 A, B**
(A) Over-straightened, "correct" posture; secondary curve dominant. (B) "Poor" posture; primary curve dominant

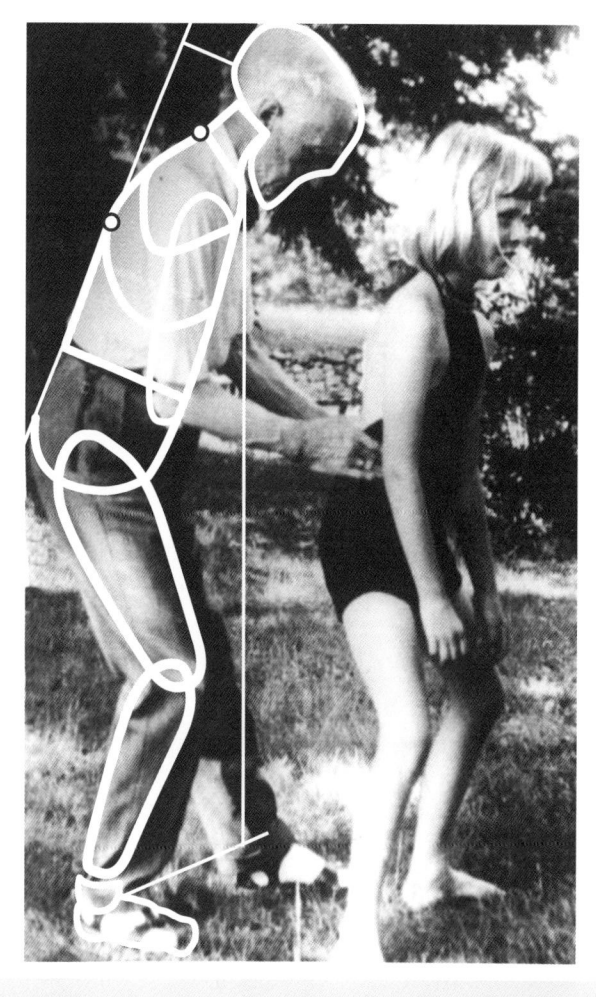

**Figure 7.2**
Masoero's understanding of Alexander's body geometry while working. Photo courtesy of the Walter Carrington Educational Trust © 2020 (www.constructiveteachingcentre.com). Graphics following Jeando Masoero

blade tips, and from there the head, neck and upper spine come forward and up. This then truly allows the head and vision to lead the movement. The shoulders sit slightly in front of the unity line, with the arms hanging vertically, palms facing backward (Fig. 7.3).

I recognize it now as the form that Miss Goldie's work brought about in me. No wonder I was puzzled at the time. Goldie did not explain the difference; I doubt she could have done. Alexander, who never studied anatomy, rarely defined his new anatomy precisely and left us very imprecise directions. But Goldie's work was precise (as I am sure was Alexander's), and so is this work.

Using modern biomechanics and keen observation, Katy Bowman has also reached the same conclusions (2017: 226–7). Masoero has also studied Bernstein's work. Good yoga and martial art teachers also often teach the same alignments. This suggests that this is the optimal alignment of the body, discoverable by anyone who pays detailed attention to how the body moves.

# CHAPTER seven

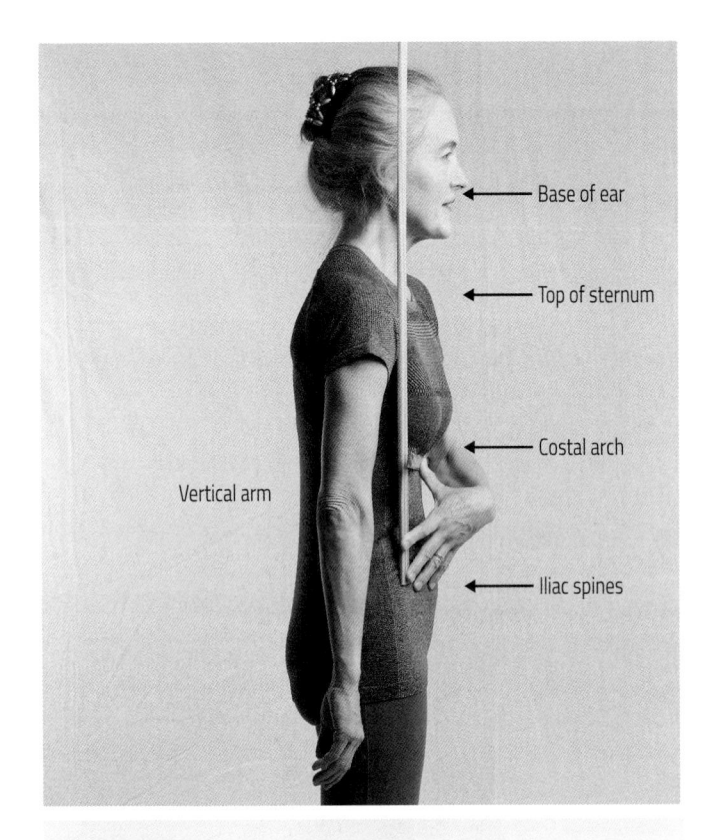

**Figure 7.3**
Points connected vertically by the unity line

(Labels on figure: Base of ear, Top of sternum, Costal arch, Iliac spines, Vertical arm)

In this form, internal and external torques and curves come into balance, the body self-organizes and alignment with gravity happens. The organs are optimally supported and the nervous system calms, which then makes inhibition work easier.

> **A note on the illustrations in this book**
>
> I am presenting a new model of body geometry here, for which there are currently no skeletal images available. The illustrations in this book fall into two categories: the Anatomy Trains® images used throughout are redrawn from Myers's images, which use the standard anatomical model. In the other illustrations, I have attempted to portray the probable skeletal arrangement that underlies the new model of optimal alignment. These can only be speculative until research is done on this.

## Finding the unity line – points you will need

We first need some precise anatomical definitions (Fig. 7.4). Take a few minutes to find the points listed below.

**Iliac spine:** (technically, the anterior superior iliac spine) – the *front* projection of the hip bone. (The iliac crest is the highest point of the hip bone, at the side.)

**Top of the sternum:** where the sternum (breastbone) meets the clavicles (collar bones), at the **sternoclavicular joint**.

**Costal arch ribs,** or **ribs**: the area indicated is where the ribs project furthest forwards at the front. These are the 8th ribs, inserting at the back onto the 8th thoracic vertebra, T8.

**Instep**: the top of the instep, where it meets the lower leg bone.

**Shoulder**: the front of the shoulder. This is actually the top of the humerus (the upper arm bone).

**Elbow**: the tip of the elbow.

**Middle of wrist**: just below the face of a wristwatch.

**Sacrum**: the fused section at the base of the spine, part of the pelvic girdle.

**Sitting bones**: the lowest projections of the pelvic girdle and the very base of the torso.

**T8, the 8th thoracic vertebra**: lies between the lower tips of the shoulder blades.

**RBAP, rib at the back of the armpit**: part of the 4th or 5th rib.

### Exploration 7.1  Assess your own alignment

Exploring your own body geometry needs a little equipment.

You will need two long, straight poles or sticks, one at least 3 feet long (1 m), the other about 18 inches (0.5 m) long. You can use rulers, bamboo canes, wooden trim, even a floor brush or mop handle will work.

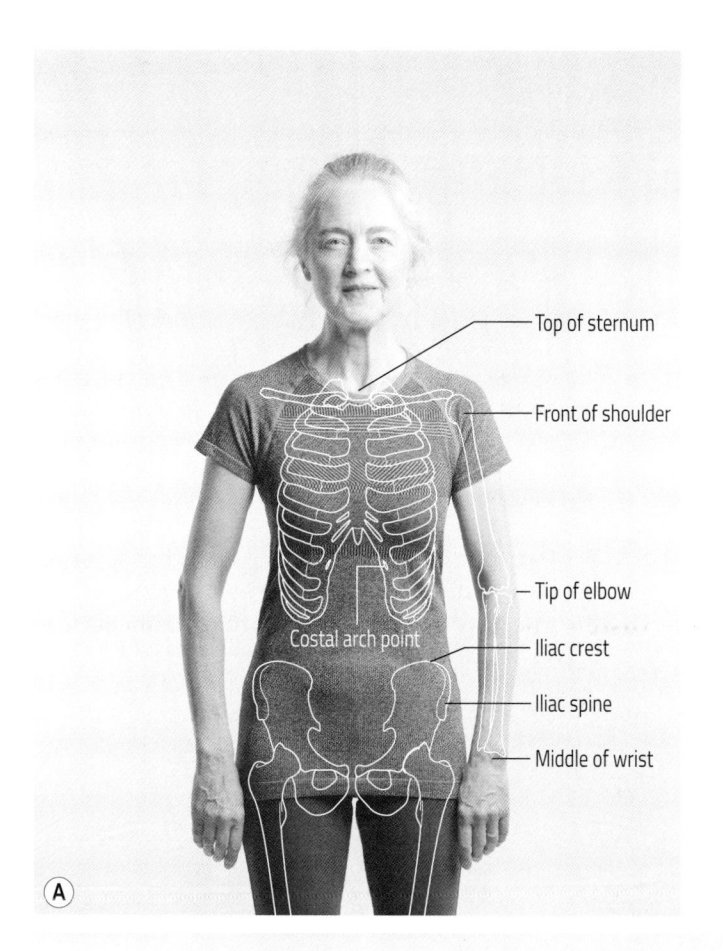

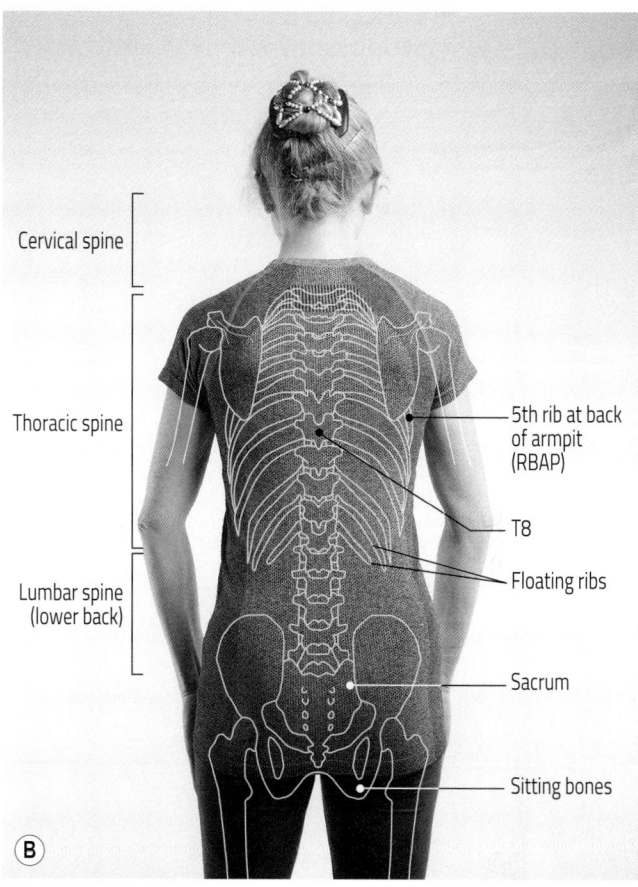

# The Initial Alexander technique, and a new model of postural alignment

**Figure 7.4**
Body geometry points used throughout book. **(A)** Front; **(B)** back

You will also need a mirror, mobile phone, or camera. It is easier with a helper, but perfectly possible on your own. Be as accurate as you can: check your verticals and horizontals carefully and measure with a little stick or your fingers. I suggest you write down your measurements and chart your improvements as you work through the book.

**Video link for exploration 7.1**

1   Is the top of the sternum (breastbone) behind the unity line?

- Place the long stick vertically on your iliac spine as in figure (Fig. 7.5). With your other hand, place the short stick horizontally across the top of your sternum. By nodding and turning your head (using atlas and axis joints only! (Chapter 3 , lesson 3)), see whether there is a space between the crossing point of the two sticks. This tells you how far the upper torso is behind the hips. Alternatively, though rarely, it could be in front. If so, by how much?

2   Are your costal arch ribs on the unity line?

- Use the long stick vertically from the iliac spine as before. Now place the short stick horizontally across your costal arch (Fig. 7.5). Is there a space between the crossing point of the two sticks?

# CHAPTER seven

3 Do you have a lumbar arch?

- *Place the long stick vertically on your sacrum, so the top lies between your shoulder blades. Is there a gap between your lumbar spine (lower back) and the stick?*

- *If there is a gap, are you aware your back is in an arch? Feel it with the flat of your hand. You can also assess the angle of the sacrum line (Fig. 7.5) which will reflect the lumbar curve.*

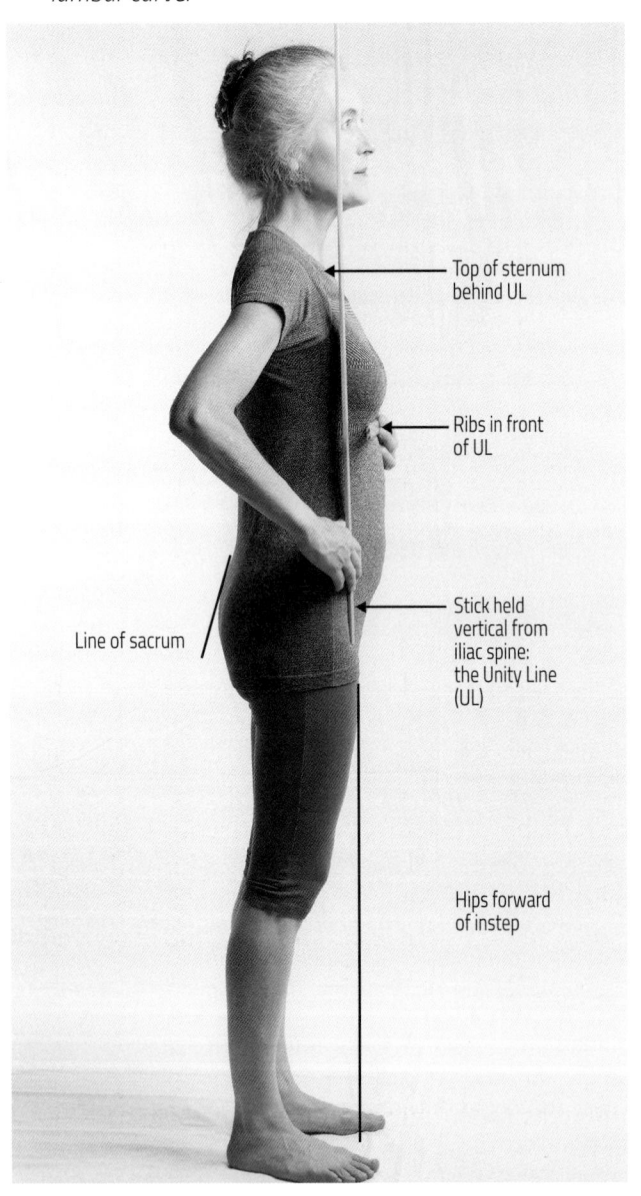

**Figure 7.5**
Assessing geometry of upper body, hips and sacrum line

Labels: Top of sternum behind UL; Ribs in front of UL; Line of sacrum; Stick held vertical from iliac spine: the Unity Line (UL); Hips forward of instep

- *If there is no lumbar arch, does the stick touch the spine between the lower tips of the shoulder blades, or only below this point? How much lower?*

4 Are your shoulders behind the unity line?

- *Place the stick horizontally on your top of sternum. Are your shoulders behind the top of sternum, in front, or on the same plane? If your shoulders are behind the stick, are they equally so (Fig. 7.6)?*

5 Do your upper and lower arm hang vertically (see Fig. 7.6)?

- *Photograph yourself side on.*
- *Is the upper arm vertical, or inclined forward or back?*
- *Is the lower arm vertical, or inclined forward? How far?*
- *Where do your palms face – backwards, towards your sides, or forwards? At what angle?*

6 Are your hips aligned over your feet (Fig. 7.5)?

- *Place the long stick down vertically from the iliac spine to your feet. Stand upright to place it, then look down to see where it touches the foot. How far is it from the instep point?*

7 Observe the placement of your feet

- *Do they point straight forward, turned inward or outward? They may be different.*

> Be aware of your critical voice. If you are discovering, as even many experienced professionals will, that you are not perfectly aligned with gravity, can you handle these discoveries as interesting? Just say hello to what you find and carry on being an enquiring explorer.

## What did you find?

Most people stand with the back slightly arched (secondary curve dominant), with shoulders behind the unity line – including many Alexander folk and bodywork teachers. This backwards slant of upper body and shoulders would pull the body over backwards if there were no counterbalance. Many people

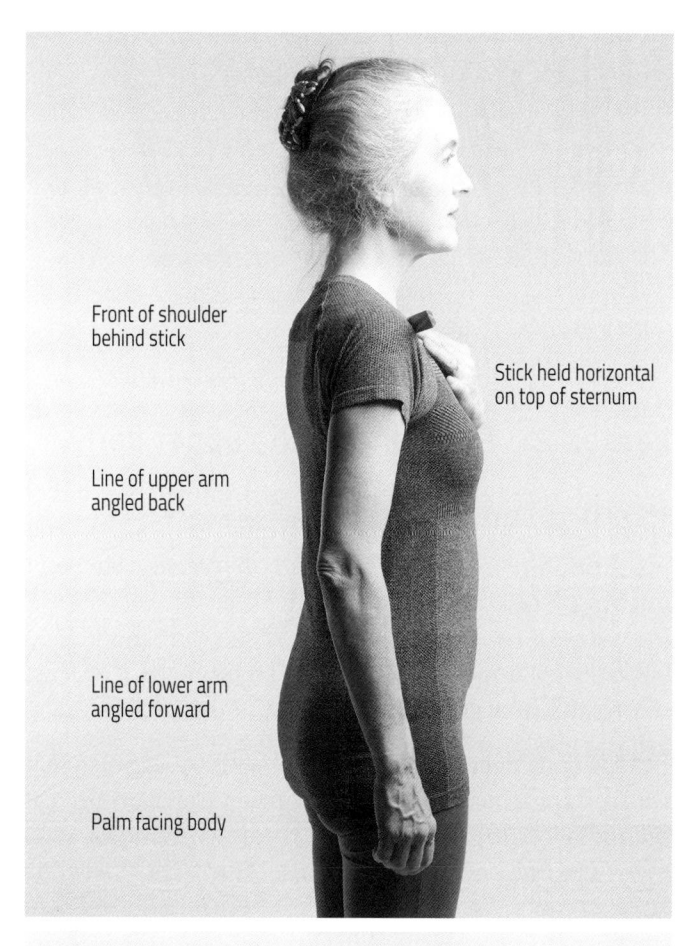

# The Initial Alexander technique, and a new model of postural alignment

**Figure 7.6**
Assessing body geometry of shoulders and arms

(Labels on figure: Front of shoulder behind stick; Stick held horizontal on top of sternum; Line of upper arm angled back; Line of lower arm angled forward; Palm facing body)

push the hips forward for this reason. The hands and lower arms also hang forwards to counterbalance the backward falling shoulders, resulting in a permanent angle at the elbow.

There are many other patterns to be seen. Some have a pronounced pelvic tilt and lumbar arch (maybe with knees locked back – think of "pert little girl" posture); others have the shoulders and neck slumped forward with rounded spine, or pushed forward with an arched spine.

Explore this further by gently increasing this backward falling of the upper body onto the lower body, letting the shoulders also fall back further. Where does it put pressure? What compensations do you need to make? Even though different people will be making different compensations, there is an overall pattern at work, suggesting why lower back problems are so commonplace. Not only is this area carrying too big a lumbar curve from the pelvic tilt, but also the weight of the upper body is not self-supporting, and instead is falling onto the lumbar spine, causing imbalanced compression.

We want each area of the body to be self-supporting by holding tone. Instead, areas (or more correctly, volumes) of the body are flopping onto other areas, and the shoulders and neck are then overcompensating to hold the structure from collapsing completely.

### Bringing about anatomical change for yourself – the Initial AT

In modern AT, a teacher will make changes for you and may employ some strong pulls to your body to do so. Certainly, Miss Goldie did! But Alexander had no one to do this for him. In Delsarte's method, you made the adjustments yourself, and Alexander must have done this initially for himself. For the remainder of this chapter, this is what we will learn to do for ourselves.

If you simply apply huge pulls to your own body, such as to pull your belly in or shoulders back, it only serves to increase the tensional load on the body and further imbalances it, tightening across the joints. The difference here is that the pulls are applied only at precise points, and in precise directions, that act to *undo* the torque and curve patterns taking us off-balance. These pulls then act to free joints and increase length and tone of muscles. Initially one may need to apply strong pulls to get things going, as muscles may not have worked for a long time, and may be opposed by strong tensions of over-working muscles which you are in effect tractioning. But in my experience, tight areas soon lengthen in response to these pulls and muscles re-engage.

For myself, by using these I can now do movements requiring upper body strength in yoga and gym exercises that were beyond me before; and when dancing

# CHAPTER seven

I can isolate areas of the body for precise, fluid movements that before eluded me. The same is happening for my pupils, who include sports people and athletes, and who are often very excited at the benefits these moves bring, once they are understood. So please give these strange moves a go, and see what you discover.

Once the pulls are understood, we can learn to activate them in groups, organized from the brain, so they integrate into the whole. Although the pure AT process would ask us to find these directions and body/brain links only through thought, it will hugely quicken the process to play anatomically first.

> **How we use our muscles affects their physiology and health**
>
> All body tissues are responding moment by moment to the mechanical forces acting on them – for better or worse. *If a muscle is working in alignment, then its fibers are being stretched repeatedly in the correct direction of pull, causing them to strengthen.*
>
> The blood supply is also responding to the current situation. Blood is diverted constantly to the tissues currently needing it: to the big muscles while running, the digestion while eating, etc., *oxygenating, nourishing, and carrying away waste products*. For muscles, it is drawn in by their contractions. For those people in Borneo, over the course of a day, varied and continual movement would bring all the muscles into play in turn, strengthening and nourishing them.
>
> But bodies are economical. *When a muscle is not used for some time, these two factors cause profound change.* Without the stimulus of properly aligned stretching along its fibers, the fiber alignment becomes chaotic. Compare the aligned fibers of hair that is brushed daily with the chaotic fibers of dreadlocks. When these changes occur, the muscle is no longer transmitting weight and tension; it becomes isolated from the mechanotransducting flow of the body. The surrounding muscles then must work harder to compensate, putting extra strain on them.
>
> When lack of use means that blood is not drawn into the muscle, the ever-responsive body removes muscle mass and capillaries from it, to use the materials elsewhere. Such muscle is then inadequately nourished or cleansed and becomes deoxygenated. This also affects regeneration as muscle fibers are replaced by connective tissue, further gluing up the muscle function (Bowman 2017: 1–76).

## Lesson 2    Rebalancing the upper body

When I was seventeen, a new girl joined our ballet class. Our old teacher was fulsome in praising her posture: "She is so upright, look at her, girls," she kept gushing. The class were puzzled. Since we were standing side-on to this girl, we could see that she leaned back in her upper body at quite an angle. But at least she wasn't in a slump like the rest of us!

This confusion of leaning back with upright is what we are exploring here: the assumption that a dominant secondary curve is correct. What did you find in your own exploration? Is your "top of sternum" behind your "iliac spine"? Are your shoulders behind your "top of sternum"? I was alarmed to discover that this was my pattern when I first worked with Masoero. Figure 7.7 is a photo I did some years ago, when giving workshops locally on walking in high heels. (And great fun they were too!) At the time, I was so pleased with this picture. Now – with new knowledge – I observe my backwards-leaning upper back, pelvic tilt, lumbar curve, and backwardly pulled shoulders with palms facing the body. So here's a new picture! (Fig. 7.8).

### *Upper body anatomy play*

> ### *Exploration 7.2    The effect of primary and secondary curves on the upper body*
>
> In exploration 3.13 we played with going between a full primary curve and a full secondary one. Do the same now, but with the torso only:

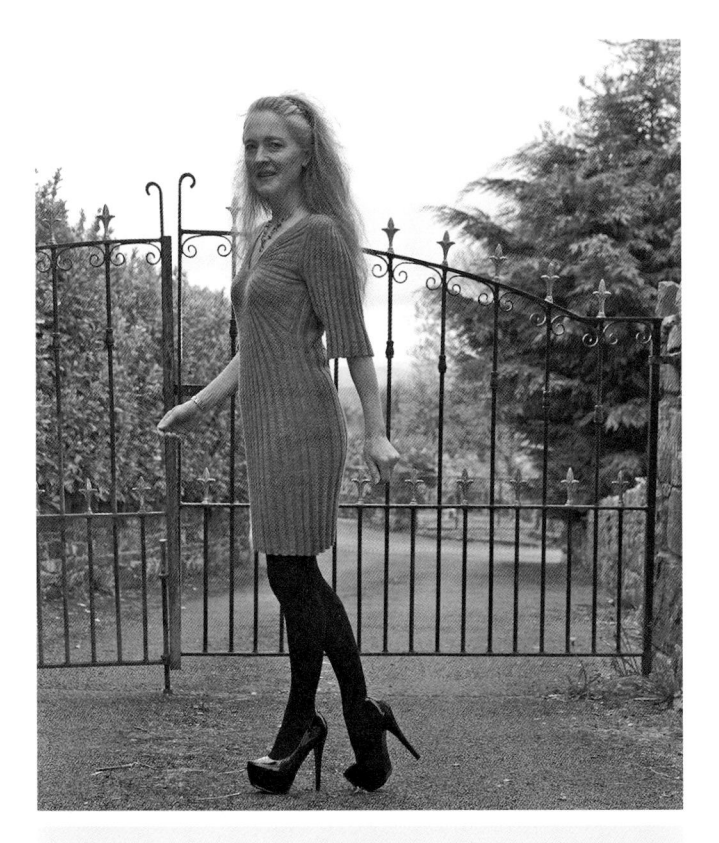

# The Initial Alexander technique, and a new model of postural alignment

**Figure 7.7**
High heels, 2013

- *Primary curve: collapse the chest so the shoulders round and pull you into a slump.*
- *Secondary curve: pull the chest upwards and the shoulders backwards until there is an arch in your back.*
- *Do this now with a pencil vertically along your breastbone and notice how it lifts and drops at the base when you lift and drop the chest in this way. Explore the chart in Table 7.1 for yourself.*

## Explorations to find the neutral balance of the unity line

Note: Though I only discuss undoing a secondary curve, the same moves are needed for dominant, primary curves. These moves all widen and lengthen the back, whichever way it is curved. (See p. 214 for more on this.)

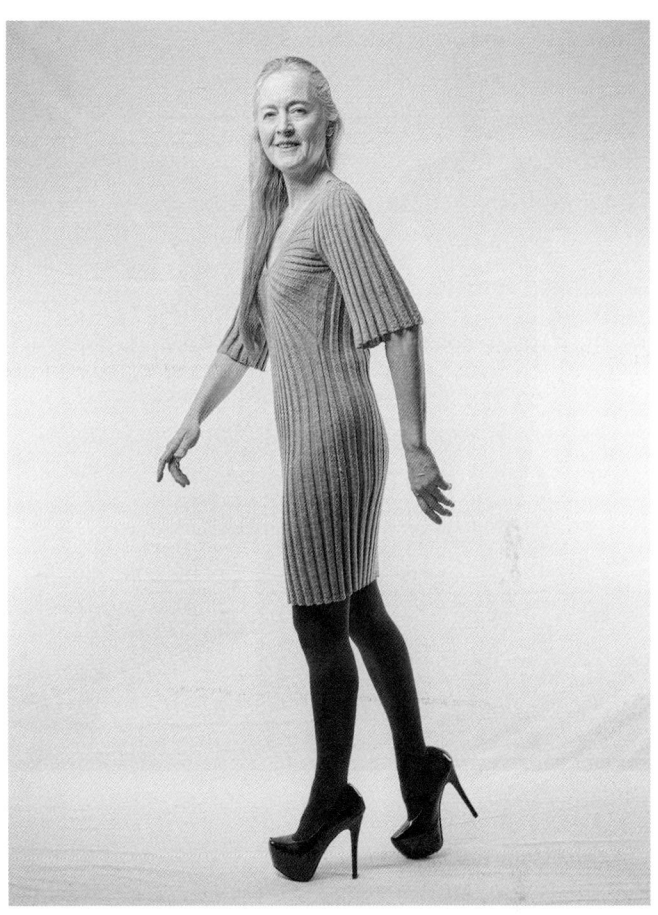

**Figure 7.8**
High heels, 2020

### Exploration 7.3    Find your sternoclavicular joint

- *Move one shoulder back and forward while touching the top of the sternum where it meets the clavicle.*

### Exploration 7.4    Widen by using the elbow as a lever on the muscles of the back and shoulders

Video link for exploration 7.4

## CHAPTER seven

| Table 7.1 'Good' posture versus slump | |
|---|---|
| **'Good posture' (secondary curve dominant) produces:** | **Slump (primary curve dominant) produces:** |
| Chest expanded and lifted | Chest collapsed and narrowed |
| Shoulders push back | Shoulders rounding forwards |
| Sternum raised at base, angled upward | Sternum dropped |
| Back narrowed | Back widened but rounded |
| Breathing restricted in the back | Breathing restricted in the front |
| Body shortened in the back | Body shortened in the front |

- *For these moves, refer to Figures 7.9 (back view) and 7.10 (side view). Explore a strong outward and forward rotation of your elbows (pull 1a), to pull the shoulder blades wider apart (pull 1b), and forward (pull 1c). Pull them downward also so the shoulders do not lift.*

- *How is your breathing now? Is it freer across the back? (We are using the deep back arm line (Fig. 9.2).*

- *Repeat this with hands on thighs. If the hands shift up, your shoulders have gone up.*

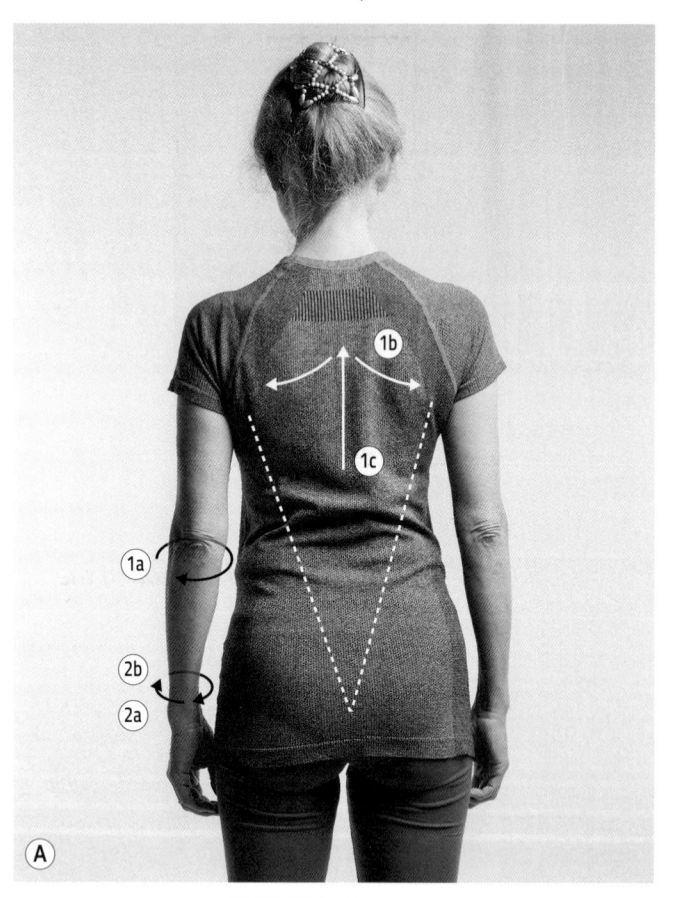

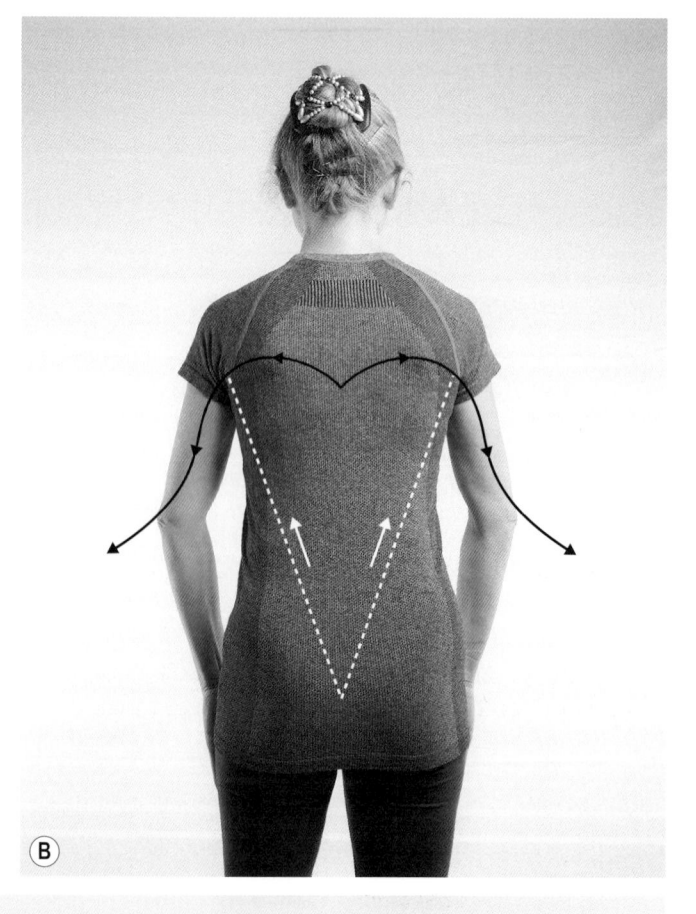

**Figure 7.9**
Widening and lifting the upper body by using the elbows as a lever. **(A)** Pulls required to shift out of "noble posture": (1a) pull the tip of the elbow forwards, outwards and downwards, allowing the shoulders to follow; (1b) widening the upper back; and (1c) pulling it forward and up; (2a) pulling the wrist back; (2b) so the thumbs come to the side of the thighs. **(B)** New body geometry

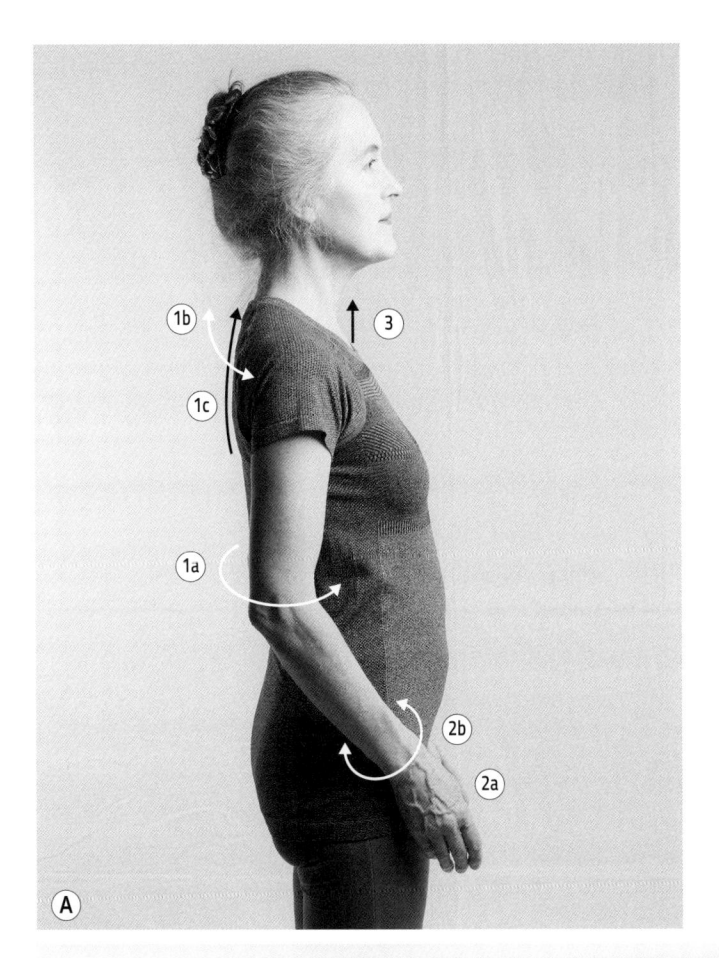

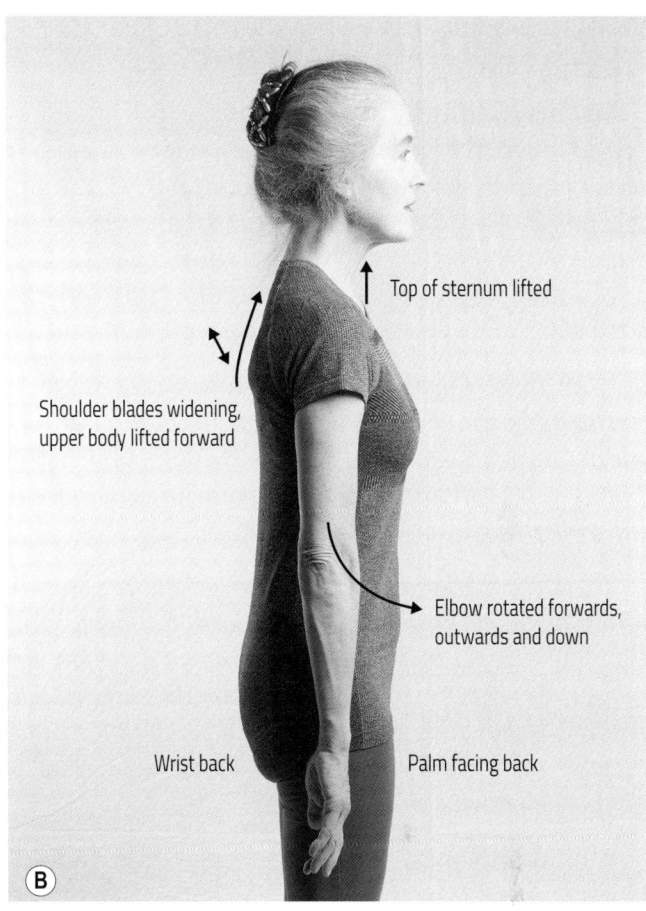

# The Initial Alexander technique, and a new model of postural alignment

**Figure 7.10**
Programming a change in the upper body. (A) before, with pulls needed (refer to text); (B) after

### Exploration 7.5    Find the vertically hanging arm

When the shoulder comes forward with the elbow, the lower arm rotates also, and probably moves forward.

- *Draw the middle of the wrist back, (2a) so that the thumbs touch the thighs and the palms face backwards (2b).*
- *Notice that if the little fingers lead the elbows round, the shoulders comes forward but are rounded in. Instead, lead with the elbows, and if needed, counter-rotate the little fingers a little, so the palms face backward, while the elbows stay out. This opens the side of the upper chest.*

### Exploration 7.6    Lengthen up from the top of the sternum

- *Notice the difference between lifting the base of the sternum (which sticks the chest out), or lifting the top of the sternum (which brings the chest up, but does not change the angle of the sternum). It can be easier to find this small move while breathing in. (Compare Fig. 7.10A, pull 3, and Fig. 7.10B.) Think these upward pulls right from the sitting bones.*
- *By sending the heels down firmly, the whole-body does not rock forward with these movements.*

## CHAPTER seven

- *Notice also whether you tense your neck or face; can you leave them alone as you make the pulls?*

You may find you resist these pulls, which are working to undo the imbalance of secondary curves. It feels culturally wrong to give more dominance to the primary curves, for just as we confuse the secondary curves with being upright, so we confuse a neutral balance with slumping. Checking your unity line with the stick will show up faulty sensory perception in this.

With these moves we are working many muscles, particularly the serratus anterior muscle, whose postural tone holds the scapula forward and in against the ribs (Fig. 7.11). Its functional movement is to stretch for something just out of reach, or for punching.

*Stretch your hand forward. Do you notice the side of the body working? Now let the arm fall again and the shoulder fall back. The inner edge of the shoulder blade may now protrude – a clear sign that this muscle is slack. If they were to stay slack, then the rhomboids, between the shoulder blades, would become shortened, further narrowing the back.*

While, with these moves it may feel as if you are twisting your arm, in practice you are finding the oppositions to *untwist* the imbalanced spirals of the arms.

These three pulls aim to bring both upper body and shoulders further forwards over the center of gravity, while not sinking the sternum down, or compressing the chest. Play with these movements individually for a while until you are certain you understand and can physically do them. If the upper body is not yet lifting forward with the shoulders, it is because the lumbar curve is still too tightly held. We will come to this shortly.

### Exploration 7.7  Removing unnecessary tension by checking that other body areas remain uninvolved

With the precise pulls of Initial AT, it feels as if one is introducing huge levels of tension to the body. You can easily check the appropriateness of this, firstly by exploring whether the joints are still mobile.

- *Check your arm mobility before applying the pulls, e.g. by taking your arm above your head. Now apply the pulls and check again. Is there a difference?*

Where tension is applied across joints, the result is stiffness in the joints and the body overall. Where it is applied correctly, it increases active mobility of joints, tone, and strength together. You can also check whether you have involved other areas of the body inappropriately.

- *Wobble your knees back and forth, then continue this while making each pull in turn. What changes?*
- *Do the pulls again, but this time wobble your head on your neck, then waggle your fingers.*
- *Repeat the above, but now use THINKING to leave the knees free as you make the pulls.*
- *Repeat for the head/neck, and for the fingers.*

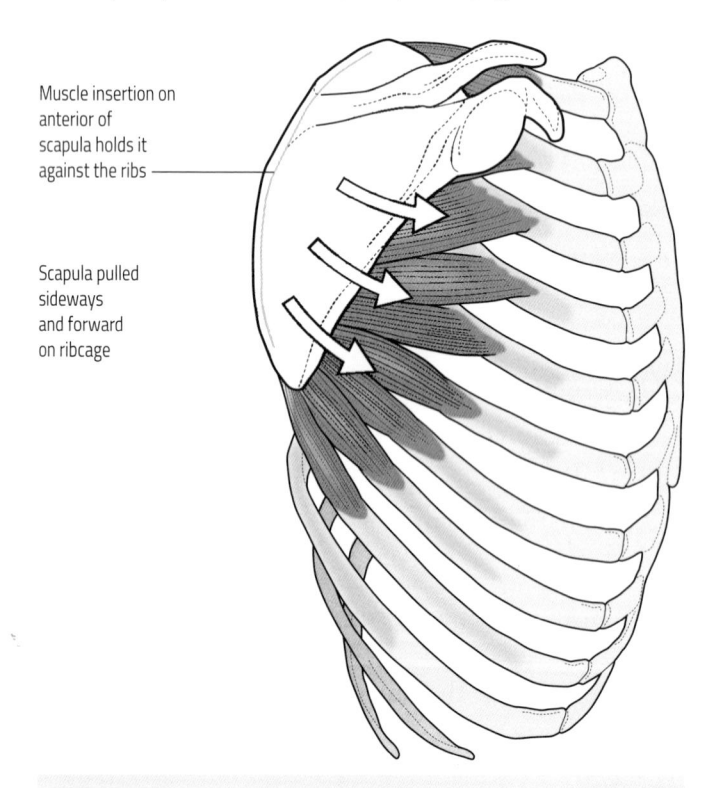

Muscle insertion on anterior of scapula holds it against the ribs

Scapula pulled sideways and forward on ribcage

**Figure 7.11**
A toned serratus anterior holds the scapula in place

# The Initial Alexander technique, and a new model of postural alignment

People often notice that there is now more sense of flow in the pulls, less of tension. We have isolated the pull to the muscles involved, so that the rest of the body is free to breathe and move.

## Lesson 3    Making an integrated change

### Giving directions all together, one after another

Notice that if you do each movement in turn, there is no integration between them. This increases tension in the system, as well as tensing our brains to remember all of it! Delsarte realized that the body was too complex to control by our conscious action, and Alexander understood the importance of this.

For default settings to alter, changes must be made from the brain. We also need to do them all together, so they integrate with each other and the rest of the body. No muscle acts in isolation. Groups of muscles are recruited together, which balance each other, opposed by other groups, and always within the overall organizational balance. The three moves we have just learned are in balanced opposition to each other.

Directions "form a co-ordinated series of acts to be carried out all together, one after another." Alexander uses this phrase in *Use of the Self* (Alexander 1985: 64), but it is Delsarte who explains it. "What constitutes the weakness of articulated speech is that it is successive (one after the other). How many things must you write to describe a sentiment? A unique gesture will say it (altogether)" (Porte 1992: 103, translated by Masoero). If one thinks directions in a feeling way (with the left hemisphere, trying to control the situation), three is about the maximum number one can hold and work with at once. But directions given from spatial awareness have a different quality. By staying out of the way and letting the brain sort it out (the exploratory, three-dimensional, right hemisphere/whole-body intelligence), one can have maybe ten or twelve directions going on simultaneously. The more directions used, the subtler it becomes, as more muscle systems are integrated together. Delsarte called this the law of dynamic wealth: the more joints are involved in a gesture, the better its poise and expressivity (Stebbins 1885: 24).

Alexander did not have the metaphor of a computer to explain how the thinking of inhibition and directions are separate from the doing of the act. Nowadays, we know that to send a rocket to the moon, first you must *reason* the program out in all its component parts, then *write* it onto a silicon chip. Only then do you *connect* the silicon chip to the rocket for it to *run* the program, and it organizes the firing of the rocket.

That is precisely what we will do here: to work out, by reasoning, the complete program we need to write, then program it into the brain/body intelligence – our on-board computer. We need to know that there is a connection to the physical body, but not let it affect the body until we run the program. We can then observe what happens, and use reasoning to modify our program if needed. Alexander called this conscious guidance and control. We use spatial perception to stay out of interfering with the body as we run the program.

### How do we envisage the projections of directions?

Projecting directions instinctively involves a visual component, but we cannot see our bodies as we do this. Delsarte's solution was to project directions to his own reflection in the mirror (Stebbins 1885: 25). In *Use of the Self*, Alexander tells us he uses mirrors, but then comments that this is a trap because one cannot take a mirror everywhere one goes. He writes of "projecting his directions," but does not add "to my reflection," though he must have started this way. Delsarte also drew illustrations for his pupils to use. Alexander never did this but you could use the photos provided here for this purpose. Or you can imagine a body in the air in front of you.

But longer term, we need to trust our brain/body intelligence. The brain maps know where all the body

# CHAPTER seven

points are, particularly if we've had a good play to find them. Trust the "emails" to get through, and stay out of your own way! If you have difficulty with this, explore catching a ball with non-doing (Chapter 15).

### Exploration 7.8  Practice programming – opening the palm of the hand

It is easier to learn brain programming with the hand, as we can watch the process as it happens. Many people's hands are habitually contracted, so this is also a useful process.

1   Reasoning the program that one needs to write.

Initial Alexander technique always defines the precise points where directions begin and where they go. These are often the origins and insertions of muscles. (Fig. 7.12)

2   Physical exploration to understand the directions.

*I pull the base of the thumb away from the base of the palm.*

*I pull the base of the thumb away from the base of the third finger.*

*I pull the little finger away from the base of the thumb.*

Explore each directional pull individually to ensure your brain understands their purpose.

3   Separating thinking from doing.

- Find your spatial awareness: bring your mind to the brain, see your surroundings with depth perception, then include the space to your hand.

4   Programming the brain.

- *Once you understand the directions, program your brain by saying them one after another. Say them out loud (if possible), from mind in the brain being aware of their meaning.*

5   Inhibiting any response.

- *As you program the brain, do not make any response from the hand – watch it to check. See the space between you and your hand, to help you let go of responding. Don't go into the body by feeling and checking out what is happening – stay in relation to space and awareness of your activity.*

6   Running the program.

- *Count 1-2-3 out loud, leaving about a second between each count. (Don't be tempted to go slower.) The movements of the hand are all to happen together, starting on 1 and finishing on 3.*

- *As you count, MOVE! Open your hand according to the directions you have just spoken. Counting out loud helps you ensure precise start and end points to the pulls. It also keeps your mind involved with the counting, and uninvolved with your hand, which will probably feel wrong. Allow the brain to sort the hand.*

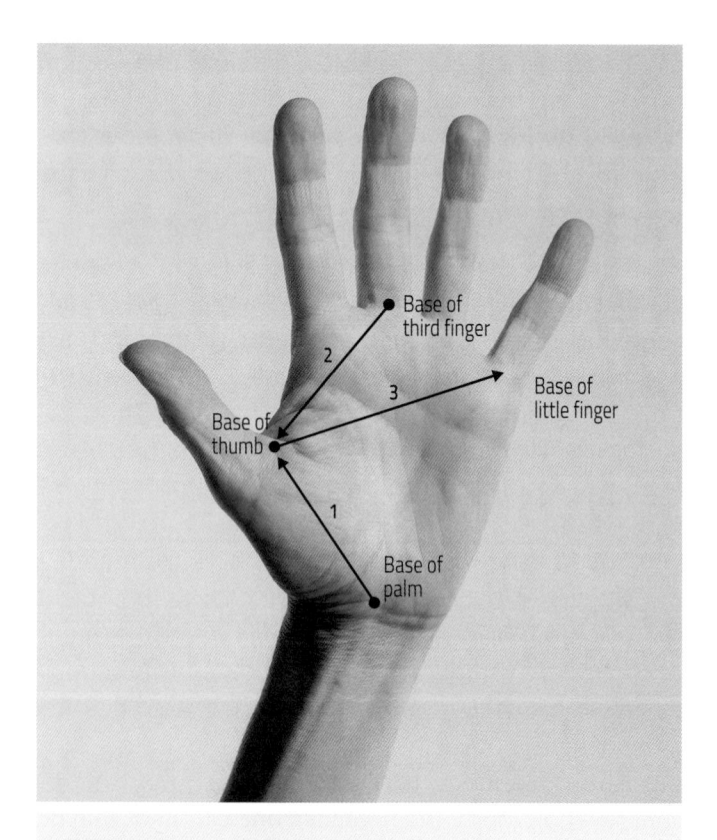

**Figure 7.12**
Program for opening the palm of the hand

# The Initial Alexander technique, and a new model of postural alignment

- *As you move, keep watching your hand objectively – across the space with spatial awareness.*

7   When the movements are done, stay with it.

- *Do not immediately slacken off the tension. Now can you do less – reduce the tension but without the hand closing again?*

8   Checklist – what did you observe?

- *Did you make the movements altogether or one after another?*

- *Did you start moving before you started your count?*

- *Did you continue moving after the count of 3? Or slow down for the third one (1-2------3)? If so, you have gone into feeling the movement, perhaps feeling that one movement wasn't enough.*

- *Was the movement smooth throughout the count, or did the speed of movement change?*

- *Did you do a full movement, or only a little bit? We are applying real force to maximize the movement. Count another 1-2-3 and move again – was there further to go? Repeat this until you cannot go any further out. This is how much stretch we are after!*

9   Alter the program if needed and repeat.

- *Include more thoughts in your program as needed, such as "Stay more out of the way," "allow the movements happen together." Keep having a go until you can start on 1, stop on 3, with movements smooth and integrated throughout.*

Pointers:

- *You are staying out of the way and letting the brain do it. We want the directions to take root in the brain and then work together "like a chord" – as Delsarte said. (A chord is three or more musical notes played simultaneously, like on a piano.)*

- *Once you know the program, you do not have to say it each time, but simply to count 1-2-3, and move.*

- *Always give instructions to your brain in the first person – we internalize it more easily. Saying them out loud goes through different pathways to thinking them only, and will be more effective, and you have to be clear in what you say!*

> **Video link for exploration 7.8**

### Exploration 7.9   Adding a deeper inhibitory process to these directions

Once you can run this program with ease, have a go at adding these thoughts before running the program.

- *Bring your mind to the brain.*

- *Find your expanded field of awareness – use depth perception, peripheral vision, seeing from the back of your head.*

- *Allow the out-breaths to lengthen, and the in-breaths to be a springy response.*

- *If you can, let the breath deepen down the body till your whole torso, including your pelvic girdle, is gently widening on each in-breath, and coming in again on each out-breath.*

- *With long out-breaths, let the ribs drape downwards, then let the in-breath happen from deep within you, so the in-breath does not arch the ribs up again, instead the whole back expands gently.*

This natural full body breathing allows you to find spatial awareness with your body, and re-establishes a connection between the brain and body. (If you cannot manage full natural breathing yet, do not worry, just keep having a go.) Alternatively, you could run "liquid light" through you to bring the whole-body into play.

- *Then run your program for opening the hand. Is it different? More or less fluid? Are you less involved with the hand, but can still make a strong move?*

# CHAPTER seven

*Exploration 7.10   Programming a change in the upper body*

**Video link for exploration 7.10**

1   Reasoning the program that one needs to write.

- *The first time you do this, use the pulls given here. With experience, you can change the program as you need.*

2   Physical exploration to understand the directions.

- *Repeat the anatomy play from lesson 2 to find the pulls, activate muscles and connect the brain to what is happening.*

3   Separating thinking from doing.

- *Find your expanded field of awareness and full embodiment as above.*

4   Programming the brain.

Think/speak the following directions, using spatial awareness:

- *Feel the body wanting to respond, but don't go there. Or play with looking in a mirror and projecting the directions to your reflection.*
- *Alternatively, play with thinking "emails" that you trust to connect.*
- *The key is not to think the directions in the body itself.*

Figures 7.9A and 7.10A above show the directions to use, numbered rather than labeled, to give a challenge to memorize them. Alexander was firm about the need to memorize the core directions so one could use them in daily life.

*I pull the tip of the elbow outwards and forwards to the unity line, allowing the shoulders to follow (1a), widening the upper back (1b) and pulling it forward and up (1c).*

*I pull the wrist back (2a) so the thumbs come to the side of the thighs (2b).*

*I pull the top of the sternum up away from the sitting bones (3).*

*I send the heels down firmly.*

5   Inhibiting any response.

- *Inhibit/stop any movement from happening yet.*

We want the directions to take root in the brain and then work together.

6   Running the program – move!

- *Count 1-2-3 to measure two seconds, and during this time MOVE your body following the directions.*
- *Do let your shoulders follow the elbows forwards (and wide), so that the arm rotates and your palms now face backwards. (Relax your hands.) This is the natural position for the hands.*

7   When the movements are done, stay with it.

- *Do not immediately slacken off the tension.*

8   Observe what happened.

- *Firstly, use the check list for opening the palm of the hand in exploration 7.8 to assess how you did at coordinating the program.*
- *Then observe what changes you made, preferably using a video, mirror or stick.*

   *Do your arms hang vertically, or nearer to vertical?*

   *Is your top of sternum now closer to the vertical above the iliac spine?*

   *Did your shoulders move further forwards, or backwards?*

If it did not work, or not enough, have another go! Let those shoulders come forward with the elbows! Let real movements happen!

9   Alter the program if needed and repeat.

- *Run the program several times until you can memorize the directions, and you can run it smoothly, doing all three pulls together.*

# The Initial Alexander technique, and a new model of postural alignment

- *Can you see (or measure) a change in your alignment?*

10 Check that other body areas remain free as you apply the pulls.

- *Use exploration 7.7, first wobbling knees, neck, fingers to check they stay uninvolved, then thinking to leave them alone. You can then incorporate these inhibitory thoughts in your program as needed.*

## Emergent movement

It may feel stiff and unnatural initially – I felt like a guardsman for a week! But a good test is to try a bounce (exploration 6.16). If you have brought the upper body forward, you may notice a real difference. Bouncing with the upper body leaning back places huge stresses on the lower back, and many people will instinctively not want to do it. Once it comes forward, and the springiness of the spine begins to come back into play, then bouncing becomes a natural movement once again.

## Three anatomical surprises

- *Shoulders don't go back, they go forwards.*

    Pupils are always confused initially by this move – we are so convinced by our culture that shoulders should be back. But check out some sports heroes (especially Lionel Messi) – often their shoulders are widening forwards. Sports people cannot pull back from the game: they need to be ready to spring forward into action at any moment. The head cannot lead forward and up if the shoulders and upper body are pulling back. Figure 7.13 shows Alexander taking shoulders forwards and wide, opening the pupil's upper back.

- *The palms of the hands face backwards, not sideways into the body.*

    At this idea, pupils exclaim: "but I feel like a monkey!" To which I reply: "But you are a monkey …", which makes them laugh. It is not something which modern people contest. However, Western

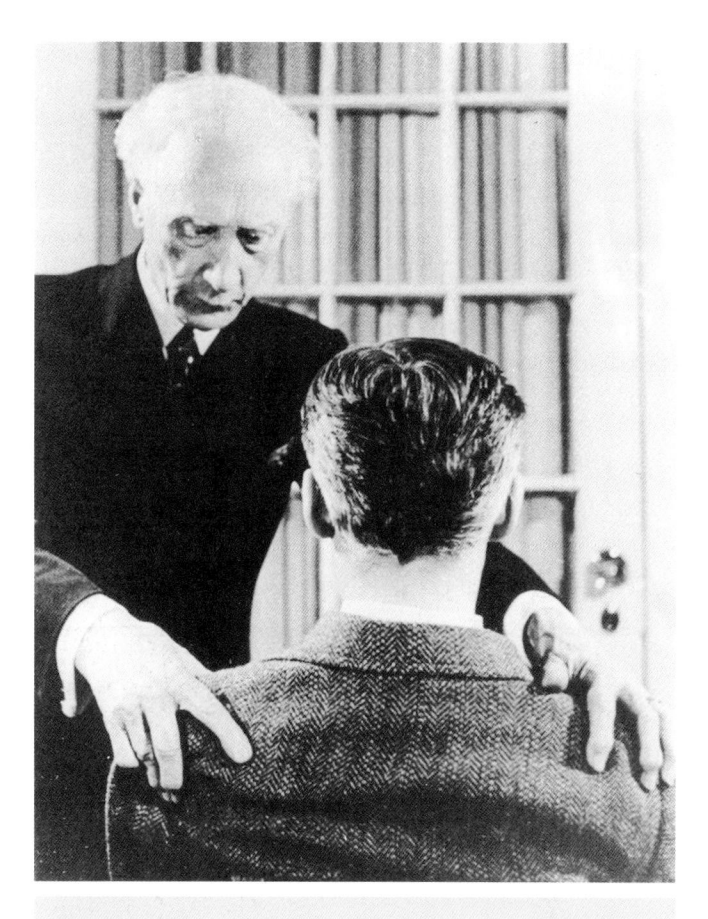

**Figure 7.13**
Alexander teaching, late 1930s. Courtesy of the Walter Carrington Educational Trust © 2020 (www.constructiveteachingcentre.com)

European civilization was determined to distance themselves from animals; the old nobility would not have liked this position of the hands at all. In the past, women in UK and Ireland were even encouraged to stand with the palms of the hands facing *forward*. Try it – it is a frighteningly exposed position, but it certainly puts the shoulders back and lifts the chest! To Alexander, that palms were facing back was a test of good coordination (Alexander 2011: 239).

- *The bulk of the lungs should be behind the arms, not in front.*

# CHAPTER seven

This is obvious once you try it, there is so much more room for the breath with the shoulders widening forward. The bulk of the lung tissue is at the back, not the front of the body. Breathing from the back of the body stops the catch in the throat at the top of the in-breath, particularly when exercising. Alexander specified this also (2011: 218).

This has also benefited my heart. Since late teens I have had frightening tensions and wacky pulses in my heart on walking up hills – most frustrating as I loved hill walking. Doctors could find nothing wrong. But now I discover that when I keep my shoulders forward, my back opens, and these symptoms stop.

## Lesson 4 Rebalancing the lower body

Many people stand with the pelvis on an anterior tilt, i.e. angled forward at the top. This holds the lumbar spine in a curve. We will explore the forces on the pelvis, to find the directional pulls needed to bring it more vertical. Then we will integrate the pulls.

### Anatomy play for the lower body

### Exploration 7.11   The sacrum line

- *Put the short stick on your sacrum pointing down to your coccyx (Fig. 7.5). Is it vertical or at an angle?*

### Exploration 7.12   Exploring "tuck your bum under"

To open the curve in the lower back (Fig. 7.14A) many methods, such as dance and fitness classes, instruct you to "tuck your bum under." Try this – notice the pelvis angle changes and the arch in the back flattens. But the sacrum goes down, and the knees may even bend. If we tilt the pelvis forwards and down like this, it tucks the bum under but sends the body down and makes the legs heavy. This is not what we are after (Fig. 7.14B).

So to oppose this:

- *Take hold of your waistband with two hands front and back, in the midline. If your pelvis is on an anterior tilt, the front hand above the pubis will be lower than the back hand above the sacrum. Pull on the front waistband to pull the pubic bone up, but pull the back hand up also to prevent the back from going down (Fig. 7.14C).*

To find this by internal directions, think up from your feet to your sacrum.

### Exploration 7.13   Think up from your feet to your sacrum

- *Lift one heel, then gently send it back to the floor thinking up from the back of your heel to your ankle, up your lower leg and calf, up the back of the knee, up the length of the thigh, up and across to your sacrum.*
- *After the upper body adjustment, you may also be able to take it further, up your lumbar spine, up your thoracic spine to the 8th thoracic vertebra, which is between the lower tips of your shoulder blades (Fig. 7.4B). Repeat on the other leg.*
- *Do this a few times. Do your legs lighten? Does it send your torso up?*
- *Now, while standing on two legs, sending your heels down, use embodied awareness to find these up-lines.*

### Exploration 7.14   Explore your iliac spines and the transverse abdominals

The transversus abdominis fills in all the spaces between pelvic girdle and ribs, and between the rectus sheath at the front and the thoracolumbar fascia at the back; its fibers are predominantly at the sides of the body (Fig. 7.15). This means that when it contracts, it will squeeze the lower torso into more of an oval, flatter from front to back (Fig. 7.16). Since the lower part is attached to the iliac spine, crest, and pubis, this action will rotate an anterior tilted pelvis upwards and back.

- *Find your iliac spines (Fig. 7.4A) and rub them to cue your brain.*

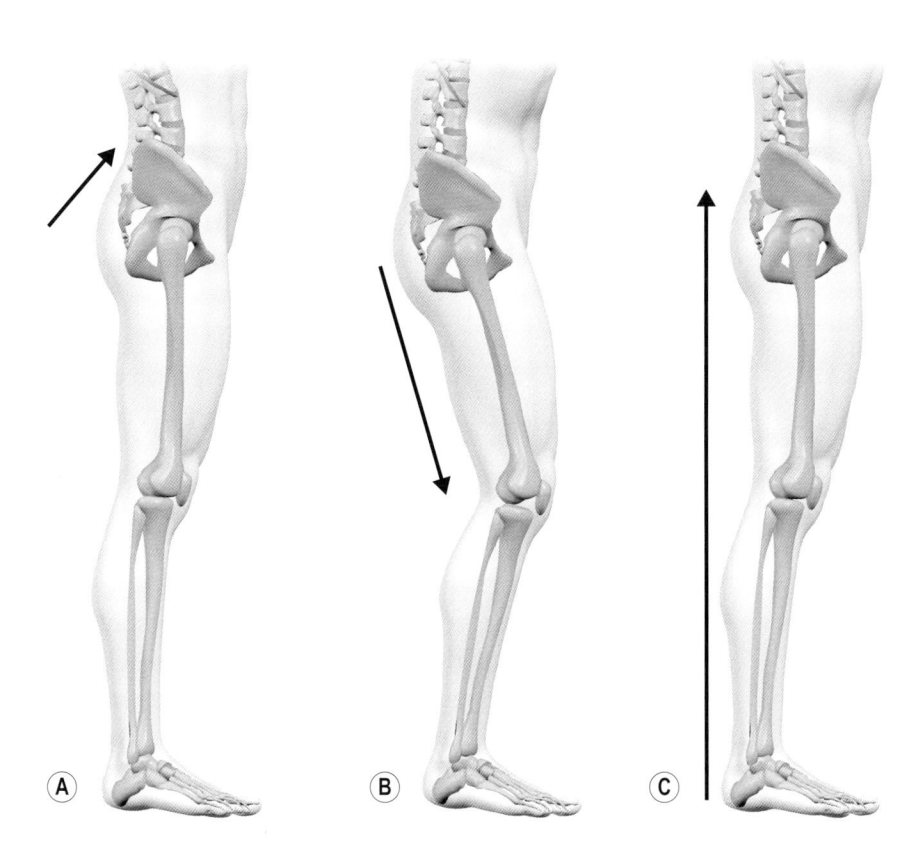

# The Initial Alexander technique, and a new model of postural alignment

**Figure 7.14**
(A) Pelvis tilted forward at the top (anterior tilt) arches lumbar spine. (B) Backside tucked under (posterior pelvic tilt), sends knees forward and bent. (C) Optimal balance of pelvis

- *Engage the transverse abdominals by pulling your iliac spines back in space, from the inside. It can help to put hands on your belly and stroke outwards (Fig. 7.17A, pull 4, ; 7.17B), and to have your back against a wall.*

    You are now working from the top of the pelvic girdle, instead of the bottom, and using very different muscles. You may notice your belly flatten out sideways, while your lower back also widens and flattens. (We will do this sitting in exploration 10.9, which can be easier.)

- *Now think up from your heels to sacrum as you send the iliac spines back in space. How does the pelvis angle change? Does it lengthen the back?*

**Video link for exploration 7.14**

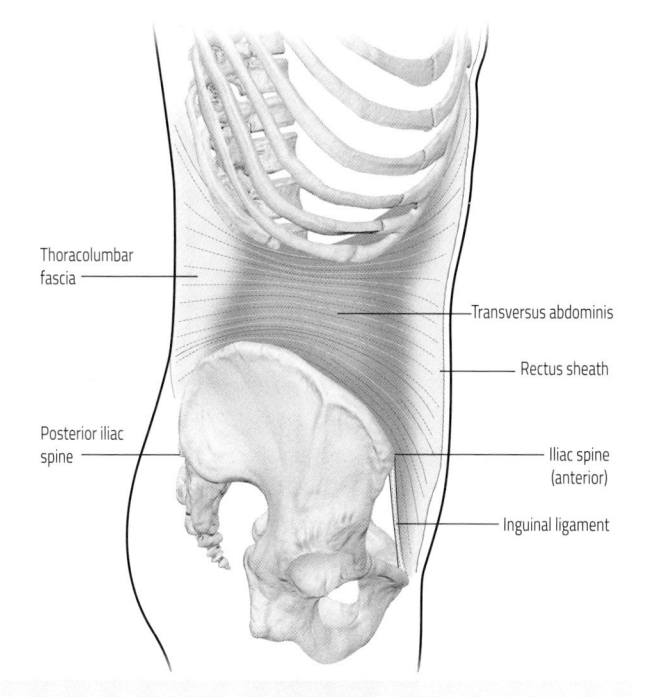

**Figure 7.15**
Transversus abdominis

# CHAPTER seven

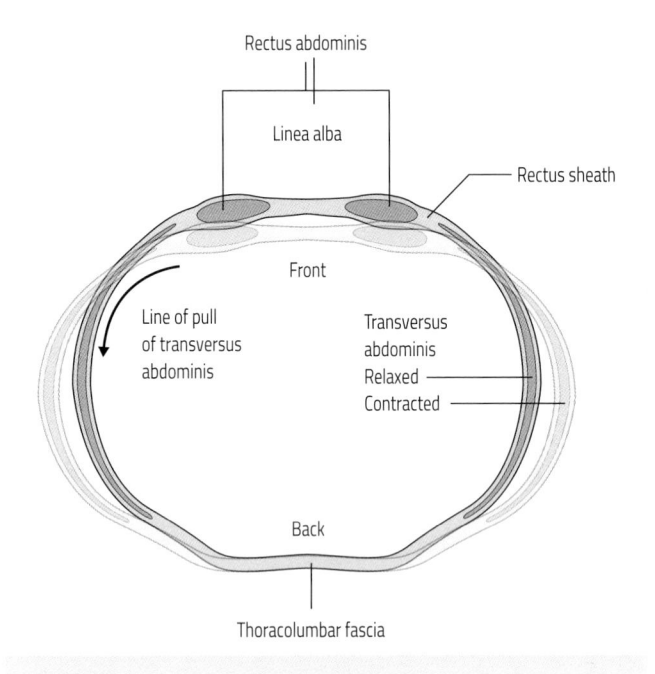

**Figure 7.16**
Cross-sections of abdomen above iliac crest. Action of transversus abdominis widens the lower body and flattens the belly

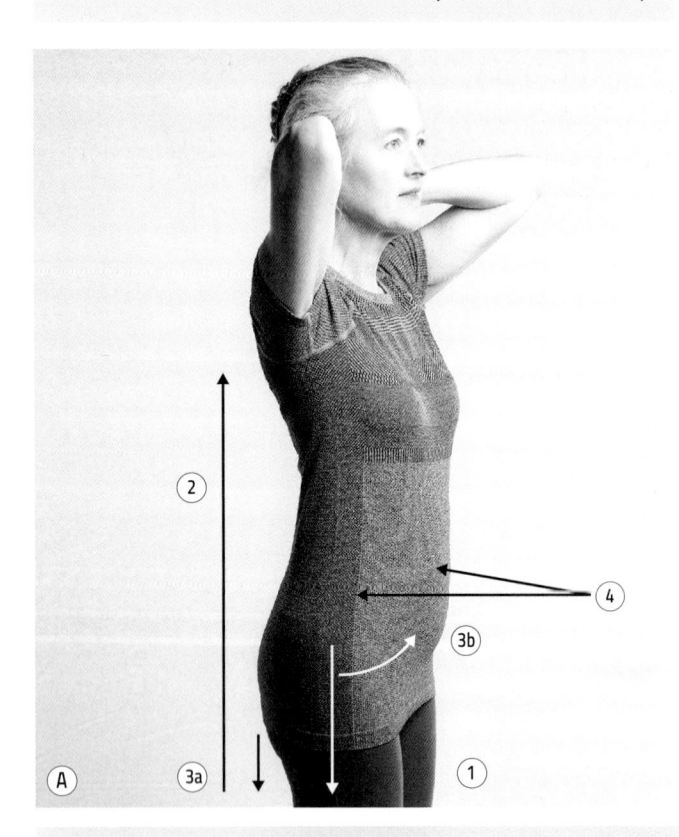

## Tone in the hamstrings

People often say their hamstrings (the huge muscles at the back of the thighs) are tight. The hamstrings are part of the superficial back line of the body, the extensors that keep us upright (Fig. 3.21). If we cannot touch our toes, it is because the *whole* of this line is shortened, co-contracted along with many other muscles in an effort to restore stability. With the shortening of the whole-body system, the adaptive responsiveness is lost, then all muscles must use more contractive force to move us, creating further tightening.

But sitting for prolonged periods from early childhood puts the hamstrings and gluteal muscles into a slack state for hours at a time, while the quads are shortened. This results in slackened, switched-off hamstrings and gluteals, and overtightened quads. When we return to standing, this imbalance then tips the pelvis into anterior tilt. We need to wake up the hamstrings.

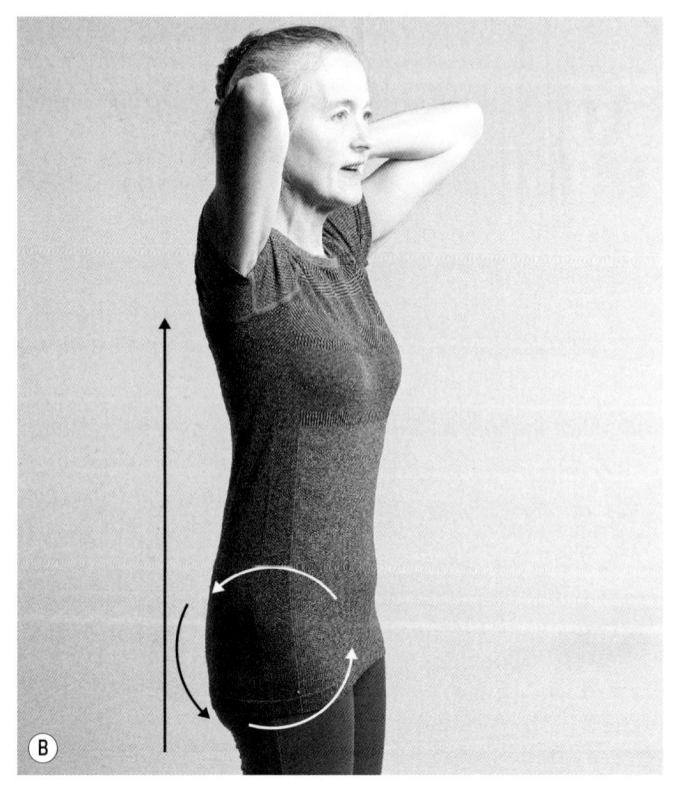

**Figure 7.17**
Programming a change in the lower body. (A) before (refer to text); (B) after

# The Initial Alexander technique, and a new model of postural alignment

### Exploration 7.15   Anatomy play

Hamstrings run from the sitting bones, the lowest point of the torso, to the tops of the lower legs just below the knees (Fig. 3.21). As with many extensor muscles, they have very little sensation, so you may need to play around to find awareness of them.

- Push your fingers in below your bum crease, and feel for the hamstrings working.
- Keeping your knees straight, let your torso fall forwards from the hips. The hamstrings will lengthen passively, and the pelvis may tilt (Fig. 7.18).
- To come upright again, activate your hamstrings by pulling your sitting bones towards the back of the knees. Now keep the pull going as you tip forward again – you may notice you have much more control of the movement.
- While standing, notice that when the hamstrings are not engaged, it lets the pelvis tilt forwards at the top. Think to engage the hamstrings, by pulling the sitting bones towards the back of the knees, and notice how it pulls the sacrum more vertical (Fig. 7.17A, pull 3a, and Fig. 7.17B).

Instead of releasing the pelvis, we need always to keep tone in the hamstrings.

Note this is not the same as squeezing the gluteus maximus (the bum cheeks) together, which narrows and constricts the hips. When the hamstrings engage, the hips stay widening and free to move.

### Exploration 7.16   Engaging the pubococcygeal muscle

In exploration 6.13, we practiced pulling the pubic bone gently forward to engage the pubococcygeal muscle – the front/back muscle of the pelvic floor (Fig. 6.3).

- Do this now standing, and observe that it stabilizes the very base of the torso in vertical tilt. It also supports the move of sitting bones to back of knees (Fig. 7.17A, pulls 3a and 3b, and Fig. 7.17B).

### Exploration 7.17   Making an integrated change

- Find your spatial awareness, finding your relationship to the external world and your internal awareness together.

A.   Think the following directions, from mind in the brain (pull numbers relate to Fig. 7.17):

- Feel the body wanting to respond, but don't go there; or project the directions to a mirror or image. Alternatively, think "emails" that you trust to connect.
- Inhibit/stop any movement from happening yet.
- Keep the knees straight throughout.

  *I send my heels down (1).*

  *I send an up-line up my legs to the sacrum and then T8 (2).*

  *I pull the sitting bones to the back of the knees (3a), and pull the pubococcygeals gently forward (3b).*

  *I pull the iliac spines back in space (and widening) (4).*

B.   Move, keeping the knees straight and torso erect:

- Count three seconds 1-2-3, and during this time move your body following the directions. Yes, move yourself! Real work is being done here, it may feel stiff, awkward, wrong, tense…

C.   Observe what happened.

- Reassess your sacrum angle. Is it more vertical? Is your lumbar curve flatter?
- Check that other body areas remain free as you apply the pulls, as with the method in exploration 7.7.
- Run your program again, then try a bounce.

> **Video link for exploration 7.17**

# CHAPTER seven

> **What is an over-straightened spine?**
>
> Masoero suggests that our backs should be almost straight from sacrum to T8. He points out that the lumbar vertebrae have spinous processes of different lengths, the curve of the vertebral column is *inside* the body. (Though I assume the degree of natural curve will vary between individuals.) I suggest that bouncing is a great way to check you have not over-straightened your spine. If the spine is functioning well, it will be springy and bouncing is fun. If the spine is over-straightened it will be rigid, making bouncing uncomfortable and jarring. (Try forcing it straighter to confirm this, but be careful!) Use this to see how straight your spine wants to be today.

## Emergent movement – finding stability from hamstrings as we kneel down

### Exploration 7.18  Anatomy play

- *Release your hamstrings as you tilt forwards, while letting your knees bend. You will notice your ankles also bend. To stop ourselves falling we then must grip with the quads (the big muscles at the front of the thighs). This puts huge forces through the knees (Fig. 7.18; compare Fig. 13.3).*

- *Step forwards as you would normally to kneel on your back knee, then come up again. Notice whether you feel stable in the movement, and how much the quads must work. It may be easy to drop down, but hard to get up again.*

When hamstrings, knees, and ankles all release together, it results in heavy movement. We do not want to release the muscles and joints in this way; we need to find a different way of bending that holds tone.

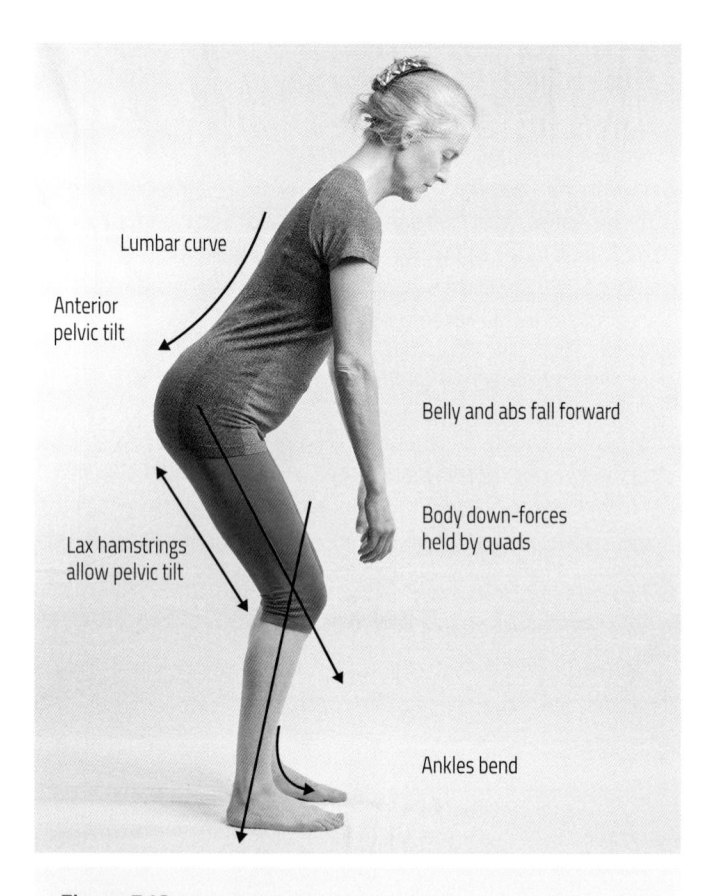

**Figure 7.18**
Releasing hamstrings, knees, and ankles when tilting forward

### Exploration 7.19  Toned hamstrings help us stabilize without gripping

- *Prepare by engaging your muscles (see pulls 1–4 in Fig. 7.19).*

  Keep the knees straight.

  *I send my heels down (1a).*

  *I send an up-line up my legs to sacrum and T8 (1b).*

  *I engage my hamstrings by pulling the sitting bones towards the back of the knees (2).*

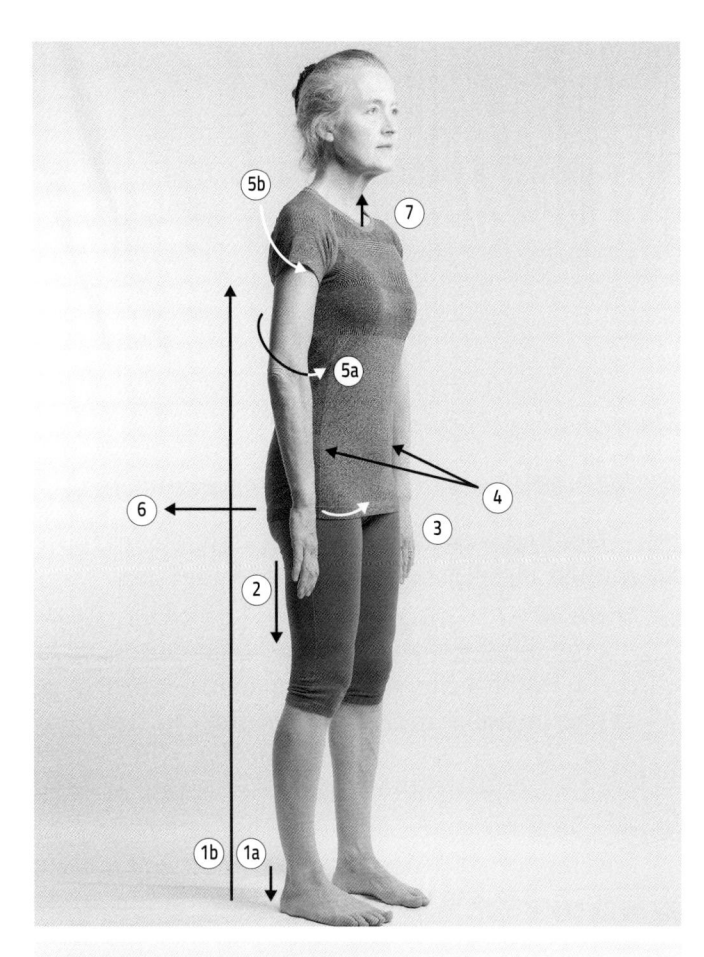

# The Initial Alexander technique, and a new model of postural alignment

**Figure 7.19**
Integrating upper and lower body

## Lesson 5  Lengthening the back from top and bottom

Any curve in the lumbar spine shortens the back. To lengthen the back, we need to work from both ends together: bringing the shoulders forwards to straighten and lift the upper spine, and opening the lumbar curve by reducing the tilt of the pelvis.

### Exploration 7.20  Thinking up from heels to T8 for extra lift

- *Find T8 (the eighth thoracic vertebra) between the lower tips of your shoulder blades. Give it a rub with a hand behind your back to wake up your awareness of it.*

*I pull my pubococcygeals forwards (3).*

*I pull my iliac spines back in space and wide (4).*

- Count 1-2-3 as you move, keeping the knees straight and the torso upright.
- Holding all this tone, particularly keeping the hamstrings engaged and the iliac spines back, count 1-2-3 again as you step forward and kneel on the back knee (Fig. 7.20).
- Notice how you may easily lose focus and release the hamstrings. From your brain, remind them to engage, engage, engage, engage ... and then not to release when you have reached the floor, but keep engaging ... and all the way up again too! Is it more stable? More coordinated? Lighter? Easier to get back up?

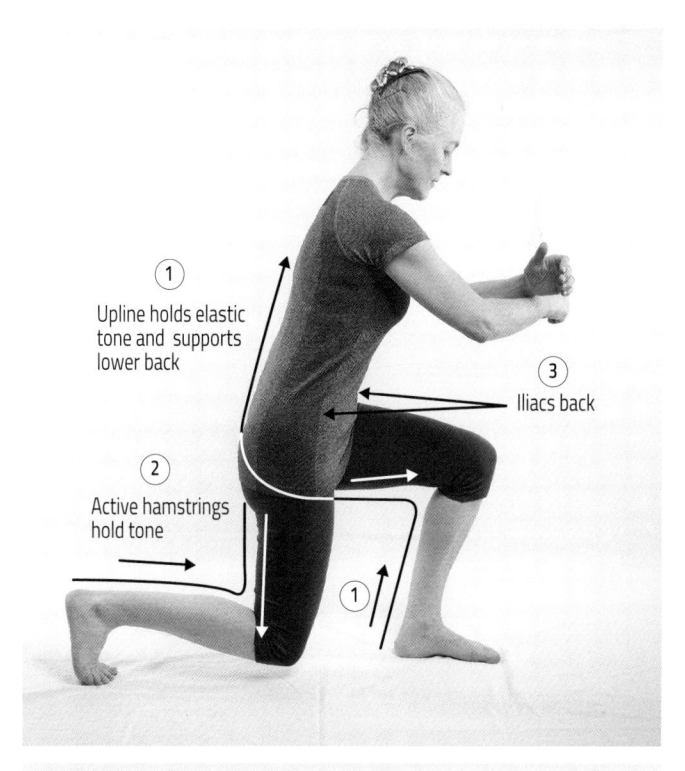

**Figure 7.20**
Keeping hamstrings (and other extensors) engaged while kneeling

# CHAPTER seven

- *Think up from heels to sacrum to T8 – it helps to bounce as you think it.*
- *Now reverse this as a pull: I pull T8 up away from the sacrum and from the heels.*

Notice that this helps to lengthen the spine. When the spine is fully lengthened, the line – sacrum to T8 – will be straight. You may notice that it also lifts the upper spine forwards from this point, and so tilts the ribcage on the lumbar spine. We will return to this in later chapters.

### Exploration 7.21  Integrating the upper and lower body – thinking seven directions at once

We are integrating the pulls for the upper and lower bodies. Explore each direction separately if needed, then trust that your brain knows the destination and intention of the directions. Keep your spatial awareness going and trust your brain to sort it. Speak the directions if possible. Do this while inhibiting any response, and then count 1-2-3 while you make the movements and see what happens (Fig. 7.19).

Keep the knees straight throughout. Refer to Figure 7.19 for pull numbers.

*I send my heels down – and an upline to the sacrum and T8 (1).*

*I pull the sitting bones towards the back of the knees (2).*

*I gently pull the pubococcygeals forwards (3).*

*I send my iliac spines back in space and wide (4).*

*I pull the tip of the elbow forwards and outward (5a), allowing the shoulders to follow (5b), widening and lifting the upper back.*

*I pull the middle of the wrist back to the unity line (6).*

*I pull the top of the sternum up away from the sitting bones (7).*

Rome was not built in a day. This is an experiment and may not work first time, so keep having a go, preferably daily, until it comes together.

### Exploration 7.22  Emergent movements

- *Use all seven directions before bouncing and kneeling on the back knee. For each, speak the program, use a 1-2-3 to engage your muscles while standing upright, then give your 1-2-3 again as you make the movement.*
- *For your bounce: think of the spine from sacrum to T8 as connecting to floor and ceiling with elastic strings (Fig. 6.7A).*

**More anatomical surprises**

- *We need always to keep tone in the hamstrings.*

  Holding increased tone feels so wrong to those trained in releasing any and every tension. I was taken aback when Miss Goldie stopped me releasing my shoulders and insisted I hold more tone in them. But if she increased tone in my hamstrings, as she probably did, I was not directly aware of it. Initially increased tone can feel stiff. Check whether this is faulty sensory perception at work by checking your mobility in an action such as kneeling or squatting. If you are stiff you will be restricted in your movements, from tension *across* joints. If you are mobile, you have toned the muscles *around* joints, building strength, mobility, and coordination together. You can also check with your breath: if you cannot breathe freely to the base of the body then you are holding tension.

- *The back should be straight between the sacrum and T8 – the curve of the spine is inside the body.*

  This is different from the over-straightened spine warned against on physio websites and which, I have noticed, is feared by some AT teachers. If you can bounce, the spine is springy, not over-straightened. On starting AT I noticed that women and men from the Far East have straighter torsos and rarely have the pronounced lumbar curves and lifted chests of the West. As my own body released some of these I felt it humbled me, down from my "refined Western superior person" position to become simply human. Although disconcerting, it was also a relief.

# The Initial Alexander technique, and a new model of postural alignment

For me, the straightened spine has accessed strength I previously only dreamed of. Compare the high heels photos (Figs 7.7, 7.8). The recent one is stronger looking, more grounded. It's more modern too, as finally it is becoming preferable for women to have strong, grounded bodies.

- *The head is forward and up from the body from T8.*

Contrary to what one might expect, the head is not balanced directly over the body, but is slightly in front of it. As we saw in exploration 3.8 the center of gravity of the head is both forwards and up from the pivot – the atlanto-occipital joint. With more weight in front of the pivot, the head wants to nod forwards from this point, and because it is also set higher than the pivot, this exerts an upward pull on the erector spinae, the muscles that lengthen the spine. Hence, when the head goes forwards and up, the back lengthens up and off the legs and the body opens into expansion. This is why we are not solely stacked from the ground up, as standard thinking would have it.

But within the AT world there are different understandings of the head placement. On my own training we directed our heads to go as "up" as possible, and I understood that the ideal was to need no book under the head when in semi-supine. Later, I noticed that senior AT teachers often had heads that were further forward from the body, and looked much more relaxed and grounded, which puzzled me. Goldie's head was certainly forward from her spine and on my only lesson in semi-supine from her she gave me quite a pile of books. In the photo from the first training course (Fig. 7.21), Alexander and all his students clearly have heads going forward and up from between the shoulder blades. He called the top of the thoracic spine the "hump," and was clear that in wall work it should be coming away from the wall while the lumbar spine flattens (Robert Best 1930, cited in Murray 2015: 169). It was Pat MacDonald who switched the focus of freeing the neck to the atlanto-occipital joint (Barlow 2002: 81).

I have heard it said that only children up to the age of six have the head directly over the body; after this it moves forward from T8 – the point from where the thoracic curve slopes forwards. This may be part of the spinal curve changes that occur through childhood as head and body change their relative sizes. Bowman pictures this connectivity of upper thoracic and neck spine clearly (2017: 227). She calls it "ramping the head" (though she works physically and locally to bring about change, rather than seeking whole-body change integrated through the nervous system). This is not the same as forward head posture, such as text-neck, which comes forward and *down* from vertebrae C7 and T1 (see Fig. 3.13 and 14.2).

- *We are stable on our feet.*

There is a line of thinking within the technique that with offset centers of gravity down the body and free joints we are always poised to topple into movement. When the focus of work is on release and free joints, but not on building resilience,

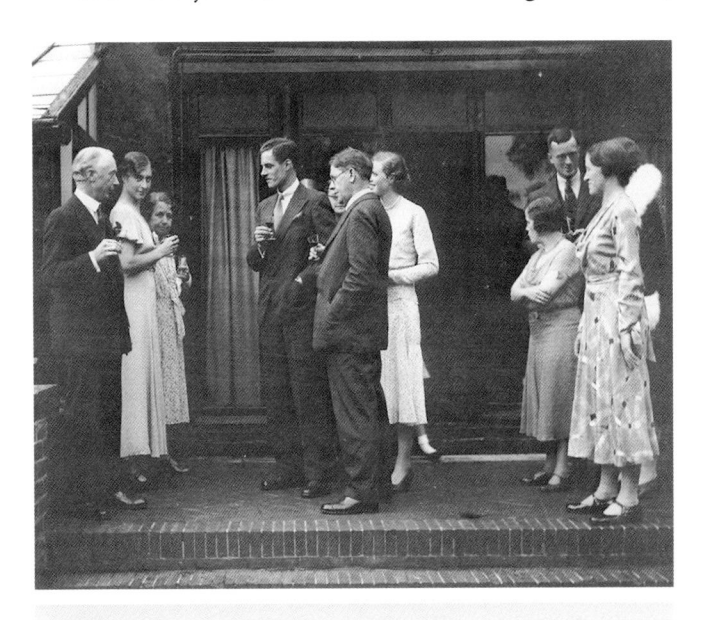

**Figure 7.21**
The first training course, circa 1931–4. F. M. Alexander is on the left. Courtesy of the Walter Carrington Educational Trust © 2020. (www.constructiveteachingcentre.com)

# CHAPTER seven

integration, and strength throughout the body, there will be much more instability and "tottering." But when one works to increase tone in the system, there is much more stability. The body is indeed poised to go into movement at all times, but with deliberate intent and toned movement, not through release and toppling.

### This new anatomical model is work in progress

This is very new ground and needs some real research: both officially, and on ourselves and our pupils. I would invite everyone not to dismiss it without playing with it first – I've observed it usually proves itself if given a chance. Posture and body geometry have been very little studied, even in the AT world where the sense of it is highly developed. The noble/plumb line posture as a paradigm has held total sway until very recently; Bowman's book (2017) is the first I know of to put the new paradigm in print for the general public; I believe this book is the second. We need to find parameters we can define, so that we can compare what we are doing. While the Alexander world in general shies away from such definite statements, without them we are as woolly as everyone else. We will explore more of the new model in subsequent chapters.

### Are we aiming for perfection?

Alexander work can attract perfectionists and this work may especially do so, with its apparently set goals. The unity line is an ideal, but *any* progress towards it will bring benefit. We all start from different points and are on our own discovery path. While my own body is much more aligned as a result of this work, the astute will spot my remaining asymmetries in the photos. Our real goal is not perfect posture, but the benefits that come with improved alignment.

### Wakening our springy responsiveness by finding positions of mechanical advantage – a state of dynamic balance

Why are we creating these pulls that feel so bizarre and tense?

1 *We are finding the flow of dynamic balance.*

   These pulls are working to rebalance the curve and spiral patterns of the body, so that muscular forces acting on both sides of the body are equalized, aligning it with gravity. You may have experienced more fluid bouncing or kneeling movements after using these active directions.

2 *Correct alignment takes the pressure off our joints, preventing damage.*

   When your spine is properly aligned, pressure is equally distributed across the vertebral discs, allowing smooth transmission of compressive forces. When the spine is curved incorrectly, the pressure is focused on smaller areas, causing stress to the tissues and possibly trapped nerves. The tissues respond to this pressure by building up bone or fibrous tissue to spread and hold the load, potentially causing damage to the vertebrae. When pressure is again equalized, this has a chance to stabilize or reverse. Pressure on nerves can also be released so that pain reduces or stops.

3 *Building the elastic resistance of our muscles for strength.*

   A common misconception is that muscles exert more force only when they shorten. Now new research finds that when muscles overstretch, they can *either* relax, *or* they can hold tone and build elastic resistance. Think of a weak spring made of thin wire which will recoil after a small stretch but is easily over-stretched. It has now lost its elasticity and cannot contract back again. Most people's muscles have very little elastic power, so when over-extended they have no power to pull back again. Then think of a powerful spring made of strong wire, and with many coils. When you pull the ends apart it will resist, and you cannot over-stretch it. When you let go it will pull back powerfully. This is what we want for our muscles, a powerful natural springiness that comes about each time the muscle is stretched.

# The Initial Alexander technique, and a new model of postural alignment

Ideally, when we are moving, a whopping 50% or more of the energy of movement is provided by this passive springiness. For instance, the arch of the foot is a spring. As the weight comes onto each foot, the arch of the foot is stretched and springs us back up again. Flat feet don't do that and walking becomes hard work. This is why a healthy foot does not need arch supports.

How is this muscle springiness generated? Scientists are now discovering that when you go past the disengaged point, *if you maintain tone in the muscle*, there is still a small electrical charge in it, enough to make the muscle fibers behave in a different way. They attract calcium and create great resisting bonds, like a mechanical spring. These apparently over-lengthened yet engaged muscles are the strongest of all. They are also the springiest, being the most elastic, and so the most energy efficient also. This was first noticed in 1882, and in 1932 it was found that eccentric contractions used less oxygen than concentric ones (Lindstedt et al. 2001). Methods have only recently been developed to study this.

Fascial elements, particularly tendons and ligaments, are "stiff springs" – acting as a protective layer if a muscle is over-stretched. The big tendons, such as the Achilles, contribute hugely to power in movement through being stretched – which presumably happens more when muscles are working eccentrically.

## Using active stretching as you move – rebuilding your elastic resistance

The common habit of releasing muscles (which we call relaxing) causes them to lose their tone and elastic resistance. It takes work to rebuild this, and unfortunately it can hurt! Think of a couch potato, whose muscles will have little tone. If one day they take a walk in the mountains their apparently over-taxed muscles will probably hurt – a lot! Downhill will be hardest, where springiness is crucial against the greater impact from hard ground. Their sore back and legs will probably convince them to stay home in future, and the little tone gained in the muscles would soon be lost. However, if this person persevered, their springy muscle tone would resume natural function.

Both posture and movement require effort, but not the forced effort we are accustomed to, which causes imbalance. They require a maintenance of tone. By using these pulls to restore a balance of antagonistic relationships, over-lengthened muscles can re-engage and muscles that are over-contracted can lengthen. As we maintain tone in this, the elastic resistance and adaptive responsiveness of the muscles is reawakened. Then all this effort pays off for us in increased lightness and freedom and ease of movement.

But it is not just a physical effort required, as tone requires embodied consciousness. When one pays attention to tone in, say, the hamstrings while walking or moving it can be alarming to discover just how fast we switch the tone off. When tone is reduced there is insufficient elastic resistance or responsiveness and we become heavier and less efficient. The same thing can happen when we are self-absorbed – "off in our heads" – and lose relationship with the world.

### Exploration 7.23    Playing with walking

- *Release the hamstrings and let the iliac spines come forward; you will notice the lumbar spine sag forward and movement will be heavy. Then think iliac spines back and hamstrings engaged; the back comes back and the movement lightens. You might notice your stride shortens as the walk is "more underneath you," meaning you are staying better aligned and so have more lift.*

- *Now keep walking but go off somewhere in your head – what happens to the springy tone?*

- *Play then with bouncing rhythms. Keep aware that you are bouncing between your crown and the heels, as if you were bouncing on a piece of elastic, with your weight and spring happening through the balls of the big toes. Notice that if you think "iliac spines back" and keep the hamstrings engaged it gets easier, both because you are better aligned and because the "springs" of the muscles are stiffer and so hold more elastic energy.*

### Muscles as shock absorbers

Muscles act as both springs and compressible shock absorbers. A muscle that is stretching and eccentrically contracting can better absorb the mechanical energy of landing – the shock absorption. This energy is then released again as heat and springiness. A muscle that is already shortened will not have much compressive ability. For maximum efficiency, we want more energy released as springiness and less as heat. This instinctive understanding is often played out in films. For *Lord of the Rings* fans, think of the elf Legolas and Gimli, the dwarf, jumping off a high structure and running. The long slender springy elf will land easily, spring up and run lightly, while the short stumpy dwarf grunts as he lands, winded and shocked with the impact, and then runs with great muscular effort. There are similar pairings made in many Disney cartoons.

> *Exploration 7.24   Bounce speed*
>
> - Play with this by observing your bounce speed. Notice that you will naturally find a bounce rhythm that is optimal for your weight. Now alter the rhythm. Try bouncing very slowly, and notice how much harder it becomes as spring is lost.

Elastic resistance is timing dependent: the stretched tissues acquire potential energy that if not used quickly will be lost as heat instead. Play with this coming down a hill – plod, plod, plod. Very often that is when the knees really start to hurt. By increasing tone and inviting adaptive responsiveness (thinking up from heels to sacrum as you land), the landing is lighter and springs up again more easily. Bouncing downhill is easier still!

### An evolutionary perspective

When muscles are working eccentrically, over longer lengths, they are accessing greater force for less energy expenditure. I presume this is how we were evolved to function. Modern athletes are made to consume ridiculously vast amounts of food daily to fuel the power output of their bulked-up muscles. The best-selling book *Born to Run* (McDougall 2009) describes the ultra-running tribe in Mexico, the Tarahumara, who regularly run distances of 100 miles or more for fun. On YouTube videos of them, I have seen a Western commentator puzzled as to where such a runner was getting the 20,000 or so calories needed to run this far. But so-called primitive societies are often under-nourished as food is scarce. I speculate that if these people are running with springy responsive efficiency, they will need far fewer calories.

I wonder if the Western fitness obsession with burning maximum calories (desirable in today's overfed society) is in conflict with optimally efficient movement? I even wonder if Western fitness trainers are deliberately targeting muscle action that is intrinsically inefficient. There is much research to be done here.

## Lesson 6   Integrating directions within the expanded field of awareness

Another way of experiencing spatial relationship is through a sense of time. To quote Delsarte:

"The gesture is composed of movements, and the movement of time. The wealth of a gesture is proportional to the number of its agents, each agent revealing a function … the more joints a gesture brings into play, the more its wealth and power.

"Every movement is proportional to the mass moved, i.e. the big agents move slowly and the small ones move fast. Hence each joint produces a particular rhythm in the gestural harmony and necessitates a special study in this perspective" (Delsarte 1854, translated by Masoero).

> *Exploration 7.25   For integrated movement, the relative speeds of spatial change are different for each body point*

Movement has a flow to it that we can experience most easily with music: the length of a sung note can be short (dah) or long (daaaaaaaaah).

# The Initial Alexander technique, and a new model of postural alignment

- *Extend your hand up and out to the side while singing a long note. Do you have more of a sense of the flow and continuity of the movement?*

- *In music, different instruments often play at different speeds. Extend your hand again, this time turning your head. Compare moving head and hand at the same speed, or letting the hand move faster because it has further to travel. Is there a difference?*

This is another way of thinking about oppositions within movement.

"Music creates a structure of spaciousness into which we can slip. That structure is hidden in everything, and we need to attune to it" (Philip Shepherd, in conversation).

- *Play again with your eyes leading the body into sitting (exploration 4.16).*

- *Try tracking the visual arc at the same speed as your sitting bones move backwards. You probably came a long way back in the chair but arched your back.*

- *Now let your eyes track quickly, as they have furthest to travel, while the iliac spines lead back more slowly, and the sitting bones slower still. Play around with relative speeds until your back stays aligned and the movement is stable.*

- *Play again with kneeling, bouncing, or the basic pulls with these spatial concepts, and see what you discover. If you video your experiments, observing the effect on your lengthening and widening, then adjusting your program to try again, you will be learning to write your own programs, and truly using Alexander's process of constructive conscious control.*

8

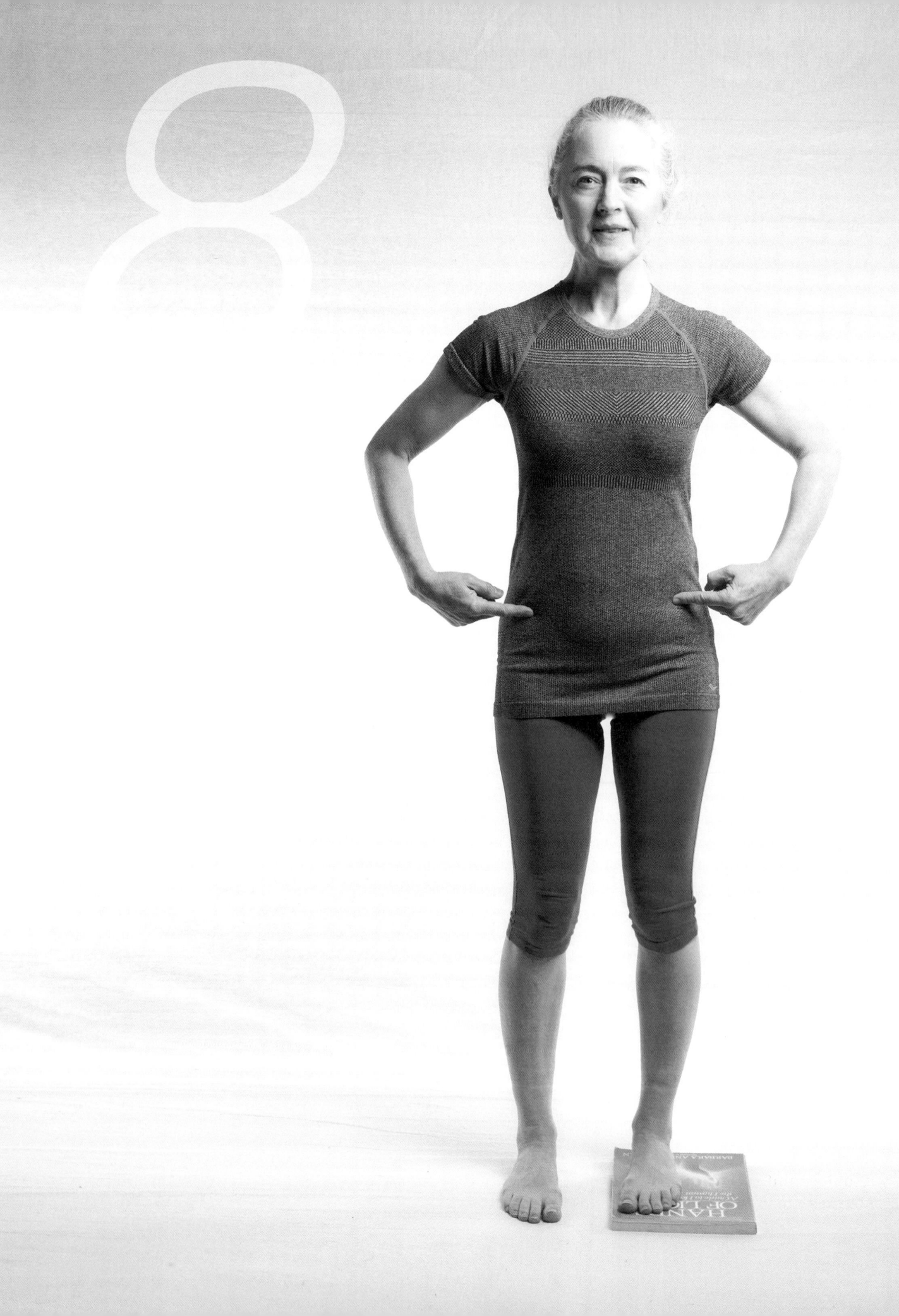

# Single leg balance

## Lesson 1  Introduction to balance

Balance is more than a physical phenomenon. In Africa, there is a tribe called the Anlo Enle, who only define one sense, that of balance. Balance to them is everything, and all a child's education is about promoting good balance. Physically they need balance for carrying water pots, etc. But then there is emotional balance, mental balance, balance in relationships ... Balance is not a one-dimensional activity. In this chapter we will look at many aspects of physical balance, how it works, and why it needs practice. As (hopefully) your physical balance improves you may also notice some other aspects changing: like an increased sense of stability of self, that you are not "knocked off balance" so easily.

*For optimal standing balance, the parts of the body need to be aligned with gravity.* That we can stand despite being off-balance is due to our complex muscle and fascial oppositions of spirals and curves, designed to hold us, briefly, at all sorts of odd angles. Problems arise when we live in these imbalances and the body must adapt and strengthen to withstand the new down-forces involved.

In order to walk, we need to be able to balance on one leg. Without that ability, we need a walking stick or frame to balance us as we swing the free leg forwards, before placing it and transferring our weight. Then this leg must support us alone, as the other one swings forward. It is easier to do this in motion, like a sailor, as the motion itself helps stabilize us, so most people do not consider this until they can no longer walk unaided. But why wait till trouble strikes? A single leg balance while stationary is a real test of our alignment, muscle tone, and joint stability, and by practicing it, can help develop better alignment.

But practice alone is not enough. As a child and young woman, my balance was poor. Despite twice-weekly ballet classes, I could never stand on one leg with the ease of the other girls or pirouette without spinning out of control. Ballet teachers instructed me to tighten my hips, leg muscles, belly muscles ... all of which made me more tense and less able to balance.

After my first seven Alexander lessons I returned to my ballet class and discovered, to my total amazement, that I could balance and pirouette. When the teacher gave instructions to pull up, pull in, etc., I quietly thought "no" and let my joints stay free, rather than locked as I had always been instructed. Within a year, an old ankle injury that had left me unable to do *pointe* work had healed. When *en pointe*, there is nothing to rely on except balance through one's axis. Now I found I could do this on one leg, with loose knees. Our first balance experiments will follow the work we did in Chapter 3.

Breath work over the years has also helped my balance. It embodies us, enlivens the torso muscles, and brings in the parasympathetic nervous system, which activates the core muscles that stabilize us.

In my lessons with Miss Goldie, she would often work with me while standing on what seemed a very simple procedure – to allow one knee to bend forward, then to lift the foot out to the side and place it down, without displacing the hip or torso. Then to bring it back in again in the same way. It was ridiculously hard! I would always tilt one way or another, and get told off, with, of course, no explanation of what we were trying to achieve. Eventually I got it, but how? I ruminated on this for over twenty years and slowly discoveries and insights happened. Key to these was understanding the importance of the sesamoid bones under the balls of the big toes, the hip stabilizers, and the lower belly muscles. These brought increased tone and ever better alignment, increasing my balance still further. I now have balance and coordination that I simply never had as a young woman.

No discussion of balance should miss out the vestibular organs, often known as the balance organs. In lesson 2 we will explore our cardinal directions, and how to wake them up.

# CHAPTER eight

### Exploration 8.1    Some trial balancing

How is your single leg balance now? As always, we will start with observation and awareness.

- *Try this with shoes on and shoes off, on or off carpet. We need to balance in any situation.*
- *Balance on one foot and count the seconds till you fall over: less than 5 seconds? You have work to do. 5–10 seconds? Not bad. 10–20 secs? Jolly good. Over 20 seconds – fantastic. Now try on your other leg.*
- *How was your balance? Was it truly stable, or did you wobble? Even good balancers will wobble eventually, until balance is lost. Notice whether repeating the task improves it.*
- *Now try with your eyes shut. Yes really. Did you notice a marked worsening of your score?*
- *Keep having a go, with eyes open or shut, according to your challenge level. Notice whether you are "end-gaining" – being so focused on getting a better score that you have forgotten about how you are bringing it about. Does this make it worse?*
- *Now observe yourself in a mirror, or video yourself, as you come onto one leg. One needs to shift the weight somewhat onto the supporting leg, but do you make a small shift or a big one? What happens to the supporting hip? Is it now slumped or displaced?*

### Exploration 8.2    Use your learning so far

- *Stand on both legs, heels vertically under your hips and with free knees, think up from your heels, up the back of your legs. Bring your mind to your brain, and include your sense of your body as awareness not feeling.*
- *See the whole visual field before you, with peripheral vision and depth perception. Within this field, trace a line from the horizon to yourself, and back out. Invite both eyes to see at the point of your attention. Let your eyes lead your head, so the head nods on the top joint of the neck, and be aware that your highest point is your crown.*
- *From mind in the brain, observe whether you are straining or holding the in-breath, and invite this not to happen. Let your out-breath be a little longer, rest there even, and find your springy in-breath that widens your ribs. Allow this to travel down your body.*
- *Be aware that your heels are at the bottom of you, hip-width apart, your crown is at the top of you, your ribs are expanding at the side of you, your back is expanding, you are a three-dimensional form, with volume, standing in three-dimensional space.*

Don't worry if your experience of some of these is still rudimentary, or you cannot find them all at once. Just keep gently having a go.

- *Keeping all this in play as best you can, have another go at your single leg balance. Has your score improved?*
- *To keep your sense of perception going with your eyes shut, explore the difference between closing your eyes, or instead gently lowering your eyelids till they meet.*

(I learned this last point from Peter Grunwald at his annual Eyebody retreat, Wales, 2017.)

My own sense is that when I close my eyes, I close myself down, losing any sense of the world. I might also slump physically. But when I lower my eyelids, the world and I stay present and fully expanded.

- *Now bring in the biomechanics of Chapter 7, done together in exploration 7.21: iliac spines back, sitting bones towards the back of the knees, pubococcygeals engaged, elbows forward and outward so the upper back widens and lifts forward and up off the lumbar, top of sternum lifting up from the sitting bones, hands rotating back. Think the directions without responding then give yourself a 1-2-3. Sustain this while you allow your natural breathing to wash out excess tension, then try your balance again.*

Balancing on one leg, or on a wobble board, wakes up the body schema. Sandra Blakeslee defines our body schema as our felt experience of our bodies. It is composed of the network of body maps in the brain, along with the interaction of touch, vision, proprioception, balance, and hearing (see also Cacciatore et

# Single leg balance

al. 2020). The body schema even includes the space around the body. Many trainers and health professionals are now using wobble boards with very overweight people who have often lost contact with their core (often due to trauma) and have extremely poor self-awareness (Blakeslee and Blakeslee 2008: 32, 45). As the body schema wakes up, contracted muscles relax, lengthening muscles come back into play, and curve patterns equalize, improving our balance and relationship with gravity. When the body feels physically safe again, it can come out of emergency mode, cortisol levels drop, enabling weight loss.

## Lesson 2 The vestibular organs and the three directions of space

Balance is not purely postural, the nervous system plays a crucial role. For us, perceptual information from sight, vestibular system and other senses is needed to stand; even a slight loss of consciousness immediately affects our balance.

Balance involves a continuous dynamic interplay of vestibular information along with proprioceptive, visual, auditory, and other sensory information, which continually update our sensorimotor maps in the brain and brainstem to maintain our uprightness. We do not *hold* a balance, but *maintain* it, moment by moment.

> Postural control has two main functional goals: orientation of the actively aligned trunk and head with gravity, our support surfaces and surroundings, and maintaining equilibrium in our center of body mass when balance is disturbed by any movement (Horak 2006). It used to be thought that this was done through reflexes. It is now known to involve complex feedback and feedforward pathways in which feedforward pathways stabilize us before a movement is initiated and then integrate dynamically with feedback pathways once we are in movement. It also involves the coordination of all the joints simultaneously, to modulate them in multiple planes. This involves neural cross-talk, which increases as balance is challenged (Bojanek et al. 2020).

### *Vestibular system directions*

Thanks to Missy Vineyard for introducing me to the vestibular system (VS), and the exploration below (Vineyard 2007, ch. 18).

The vestibular organs (VSO) are known popularly as the balance organs. They were not discovered till 1830s, as they are deep within the temporal bone for protection. They are the oldest sense organ in vertebrates and are the first sensory system to develop in the fetus. The key sense for any animal is to know which way is up! Any other sense can be lost, and a fairly normal life maintained. But when the VSO are knocked out, for example by illness, a person is helpless, with no orientation in space and no idea which way is up. When the VSO are working well we are completely unaware of them; they work below the level of consciousness.

The VSO are two organs in one. The semicircular canals respond to rotations, while the otolith organs sense accelerations – including that of gravity. This much you can read in any scientific tome. But much less mentioned is that their sensory input is crucial for our spatial awareness: both internally and also externally – the perception of the space around one's body (see Chapter 18).

*Use them or lose them!* Alexander work, in common with running, swimming, cycling, and many daily activities, generally only uses the forward and back movement plane. Tilting and turning are often under-represented in our movement vocabulary. We need, in whatever way, to play with rolling, spinning, twisting, rocking, swaying, balancing, etc., along with coordinating our eyes within these movements, so that we activate our VSO and brain-maps as we exercise all our whole-body spiral and curve patterns. Without this we lose stability and spatial navigational ability as we age. This is becoming recognized as a huge problem: "The overall prevalence of vestibular dysfunction in adults aged over 40 in the USA is 35.4%" (Arshad and Seemungal 2016).

Notice that if you are balancing on one leg and begin to wobble, touching something even with

# CHAPTER eight

one finger can help to stabilize you. You have added another layer of spatial information which helps the body orient. Walking sticks and walking aids are designed to be used with this light touch, and should only be used to lean on as a last resort.

If we find single leg balance with eyes closed difficult, we may be substituting visual verticals for VSO information. Likewise, when we wobble, we are probably being drawn down into *feeling* the muscles to help them, which also pulls us away from vestibular and orientation systems. Tensing the body against the wobble then impedes the subtle body adjustments which are needed continually to stay upright.

### Exploration 8.3  *Waking up our vestibular organs*

We can encourage the optimal use of the VSO for balance by tuning into the three coordinates of space: up/down, right/left, and front/back.

As you find these lines in this exploration, watch for any sense that the line feels blocked. If so, invite it to extend through and beyond the block. Likewise, if you notice that a line is not running true to its direction, but veering off to one side/twisting, etc., then gently invite or project it into the pure direction.

- *Stand upright in physical alignment. Visualize that you are standing on a vertical imaginary line, a coordinate, much longer than you, that aligns with your axis. Don't feel it, or try to see it. Know it goes far above your head, far down below your feet.*
- *Become aware of the front/back line, going from your nose forwards to the wall, and beyond, far beyond where you are. And from the occiput back behind you a long way.*
- *Become aware of the side/side lines, each going many miles each way.*
- *When you sense all these are running smoothly, in the right planes, without blocks, then project all three lines together. Do you feel expanded? Is that familiar or unfamiliar? If this feels unfamiliar, keep projecting the outwards lines till your VSO resets. (I felt quite weird, and then "seasick" for a while, the first time I did this, but it passed, and has not happened since.)*
- *Explore your balance again. How is it now? And with the eyes closed? When you wobble, notice whether you brace, feel into the body, or simply panic and stop focusing anywhere. Instead, continue projecting your spatial directions, and see what happens.*

## Lesson 3 Finding our secure base – the ball of the foot and the sesamoid bones

Goldie would ask me to lift the big toe, then, keeping it lifted, to swivel on the heel to take the foot out to 45 degrees or so, and then in again to parallel. It felt nice, but I had no idea why she did it.

How do we balance on our feet? The key came from AT teacher Bob Britton in a great workshop called "Move like a Dinosaur" (Dublin 2013), which inspired me to explore functional anatomy.

The sesamoids are two little bones under the ball of the big toe (Fig. 8.1B). Sesamoids are floating bones; others include the hyoid and kneecap. Feel the ball of your big toe. The most prominent point is the outer sesamoid. The inner one is not so easily felt. Rub the balls of your feet to wake them up.

Why are they there? "The function of sesamoid bones is to reduce friction between the tendon and other rigid structures, producing a more efficient gliding mechanism between adjacent tissues" (Longo et al. 2013). The standard understanding of weight distribution on the feet is that we balance on a broad triangle: ball of the big toe, ball of little toe, heel. If this was so, our feet would have no dynamic movement. Bob gave us a more interesting picture: the weight triangle is heel, outer sesamoid, inner sesamoid. Much of the weight of the body goes through this point as we walk. I presume that the sesamoids, with the web of fascia around them, also form a weight-dispersing area – a protective cushion for the underlying bones. The outer toes function like stabilizers on a bicycle, to balance us over rough ground.

# Single leg balance

For optimal balance and movement, we need to understand the functional anatomy of the feet. The bones of the feet divide neatly into the bones of the medial arch and those of the lateral arch (Fig. 8.1B) (Myers 2014: 149). The big toe bones are hugely bigger and stronger than the other four. (Fig. 8.1A and B). In Figure 8.1C, trace the path of the weight distribution from the body coming down into the ankle bone, from which weight goes *back* into the heel bone, and *forwards* down the instep into the ball of the big toe, under which are the sesamoids. Between each of these bones are broad, flat surfaces for the transfer of weight. There is also some transfer of weight into the second and third toes (Fig. 8.1B). The outside of the foot transfers weight from the heel forward into the outer toes, but it is clear from their size that this is for short-term weight balancing only (see Fig. 8.1D).

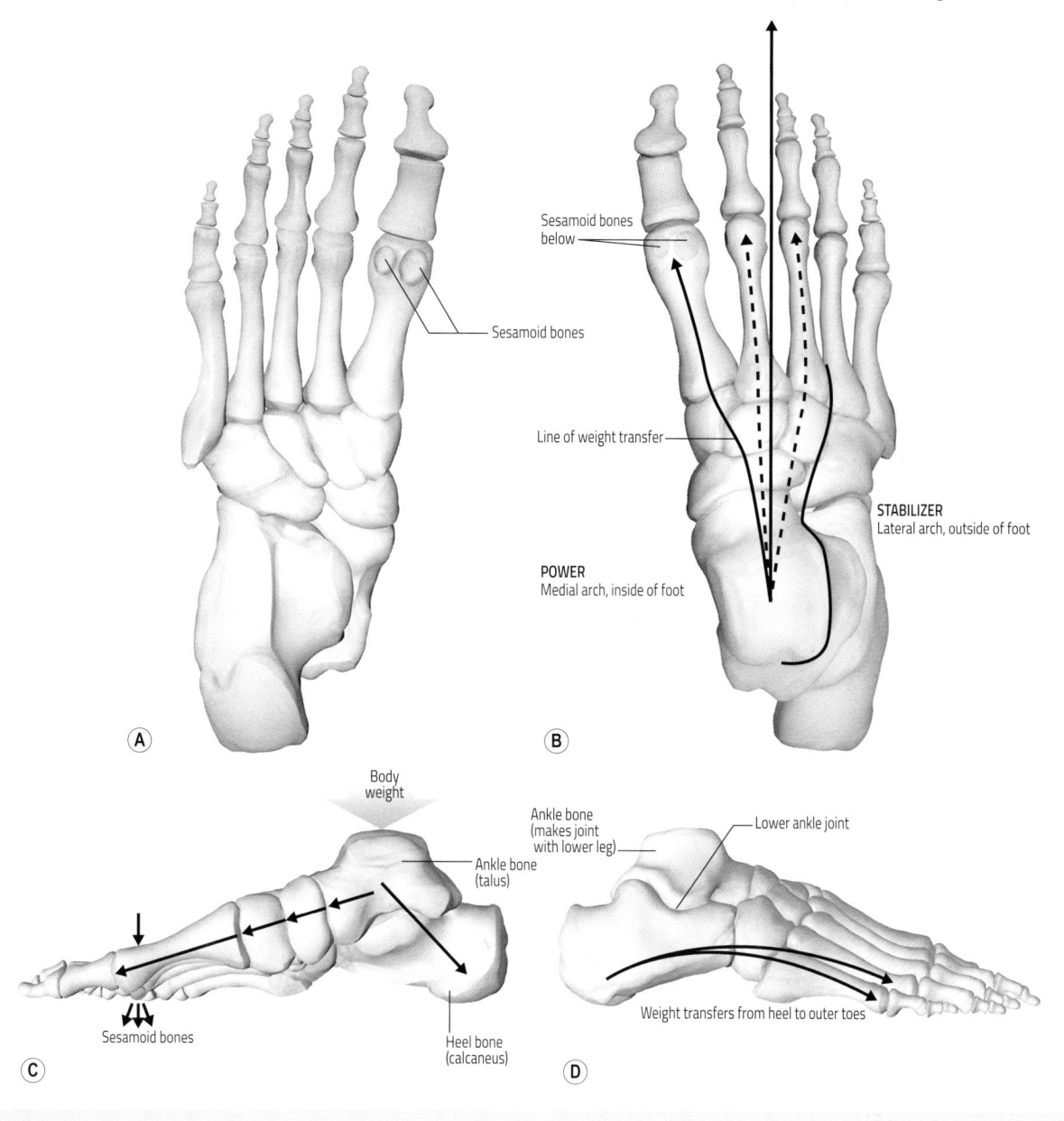

**Figure 8.1A–D**
Anatomy of feet: (A) from below; (B) from above; (C) from medial side; (D) from lateral side

# CHAPTER eight

*Exploration 8.4  Exploring the ball of the foot*

**Video link for exploration 8.4**

- *Is the weight through the big toe ball?* Put one foot forwards and the other back. Keeping the front knee straight, press up from the back foot as if you were walking (Fig. 8.2A). In the back foot, notice whether the power is in the ball of the big toe, through the sesamoids. If not, you are probably sickling your ankle outwards, to bring the weight onto the outside of the foot (Fig. 8.2B).
- *Use a mirror at floor level if needed, to bring your foot up straight over the ball of the big toe.*
- How fully are you using the big toe joint? This *joint is so crucial, so little considered, and often under-used thanks to stiff-soled shoes. All shoes should bend!!!*
- *It is worth taking time to ensure you are getting a clean bend at the big toe joint, with the weight over the big toe joint.*
- *Bring your feet parallel and bounce a little, be aware that the power driving you up off the ground is in the big toe joint.*
- *Activating the big toe joint also activates the core muscles of the body. Go onto your toes, staying on the balls of the big toes (or do this as a slow bounce) and you might notice that the adductor muscles up the inside of the thighs have come into play, lifting the arch of the pelvis (see Fig. 8.11).*
- *Now, connecting from your pelvic floor, down your inside legs through to your big toe balls, try your single leg balance again. Do you notice the adductors working to stabilize you? These are huge muscles which are often not fully engaged (see Fig. 10.9).*

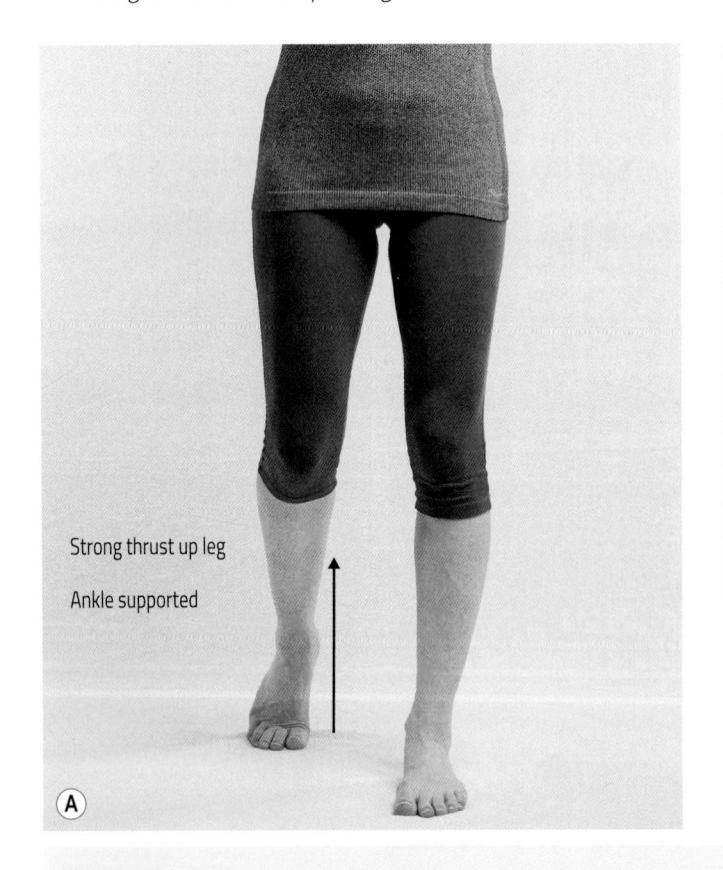

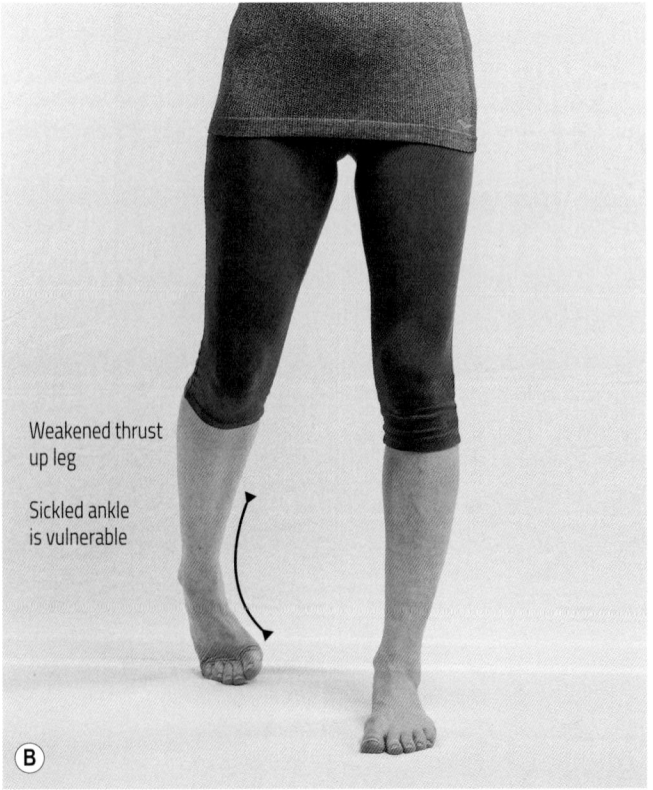

Strong thrust up leg

Ankle supported

(A)

Weakened thrust up leg

Sickled ankle is vulnerable

(B)

**Figures 8.2**
Walking. Weight through (A) the ball of the big toe; (B) the outside of the foot

# Single leg balance

## Lesson 4 Finding our secure base – the hip stabilizers

The hip joints are the key to successful movement, as anyone knows who has undergone a hip replacement. Of course, if we learned to use the hips better in the first place, maybe there would be fewer replacements needed. So many people stand and walk with the weight collapsed into the hip joints, which then calls up compensatory patterns to move. This, I realized, was a key part of what Goldie was after when she asked me to step to the side without displacement in any plane. She would talk about the torso being a rectangle – with level shoulders above level hips, connected by vertical sides, all facing forward – never distorting.

### Exploration 8.5  *The torso as a rectangle*

- *Test this by watching yourself in a mirror as you stand on one leg. How much do you displace sideways onto the supporting leg? Does the supporting hip, or the torso above, sag down or otherwise compensate? Does your torso stop being rectangular (Fig. 8.3A–C)?*

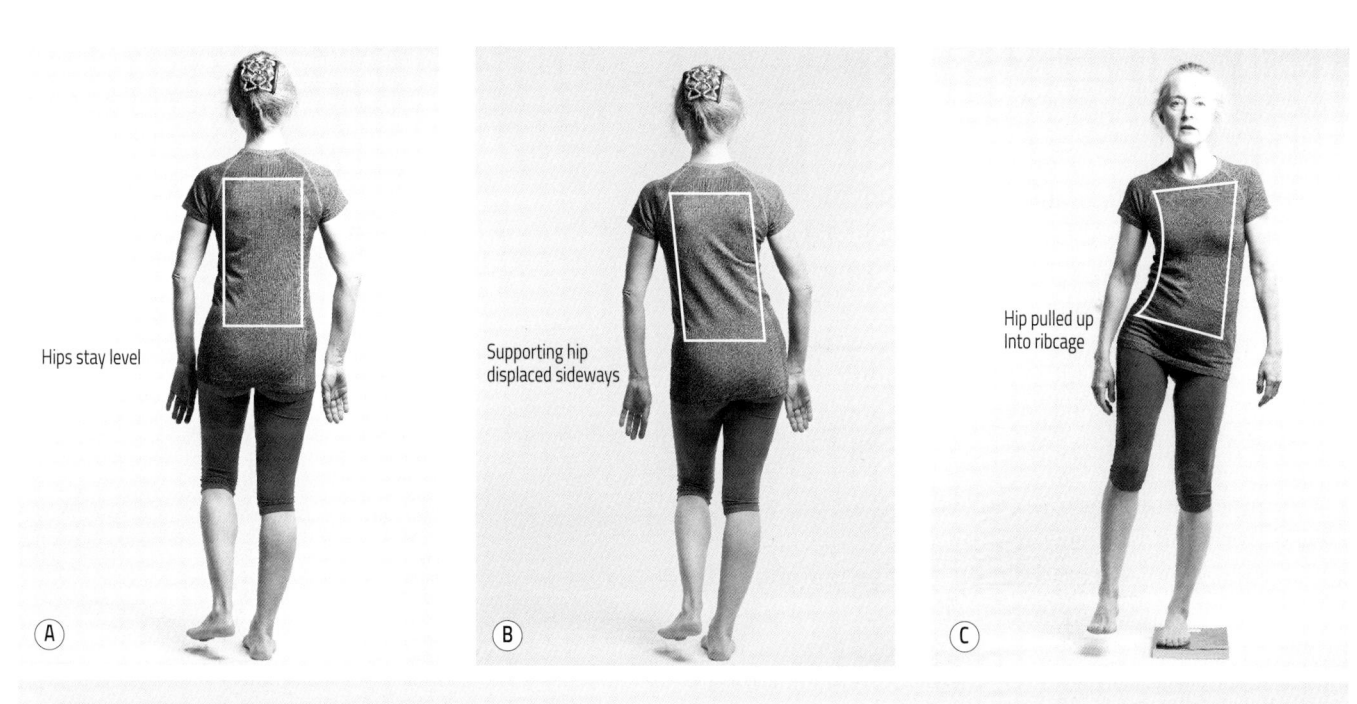

**Figures 8.3A–C**
The rectangle of the torso. (A) Lifting a leg maintaining square hips and torso. (B) Lifting a leg with sideways displacement. (C) Lifting the other leg from lower torso

# CHAPTER eight

We need to find the key stabilizers of the hip joints. There are very many small but powerful muscles around the hip joints, connecting between the top of the leg bones and various points of the pelvic girdle, that act together to maintain the integrity and stability of the hip girdle. Of these, a major group for stability while standing or walking are the muscles of the lateral line (Fig. 8.4): the gluteus maximus, medius, and minimus, the tensor fasciae latae and the IT band.

> I call this group the hip laterals. The gluteus medius and minimus and the IT band are usually called the abductors, as when not standing, they act to lift the leg away from the body. Since while walking they work differently, working in the stance leg to prevent the other hip from collapsing inwards Myers 2014: 121), I have renamed them the hip laterals to reflect their more crucial role of lateral stability.

The tensor fasciae latae muscle and the gluteus maximus (the body's biggest muscle) connect strongly with the IT band, which is a huge band of fascia strong as steel, running down from iliac crest to the top of the tibia. When the two muscles contract, the IT band is tightened, adding huge stability across hip joint and thigh for safe movement, keeping the pelvic girdle and leg at right angles to one another.

The hip lateral group is evolved to take the whole weight of the body when we shift the weight onto one leg, so that complete torso stability can be maintained (Bowman 2017: 184). At least, that is what is supposed to happen. But the tensor fasciae latae is chronically shortened by excessive sitting, while gluteus maximus is over-lengthened, weakening the smaller muscles also and destabilizing the hips. This is even more of a problem than we might assume, as the hips are the primary joint through which we feel secure, whether standing or sitting.

Retired osteopath Everard Peters solved his walking problems by practicing single leg balance. He

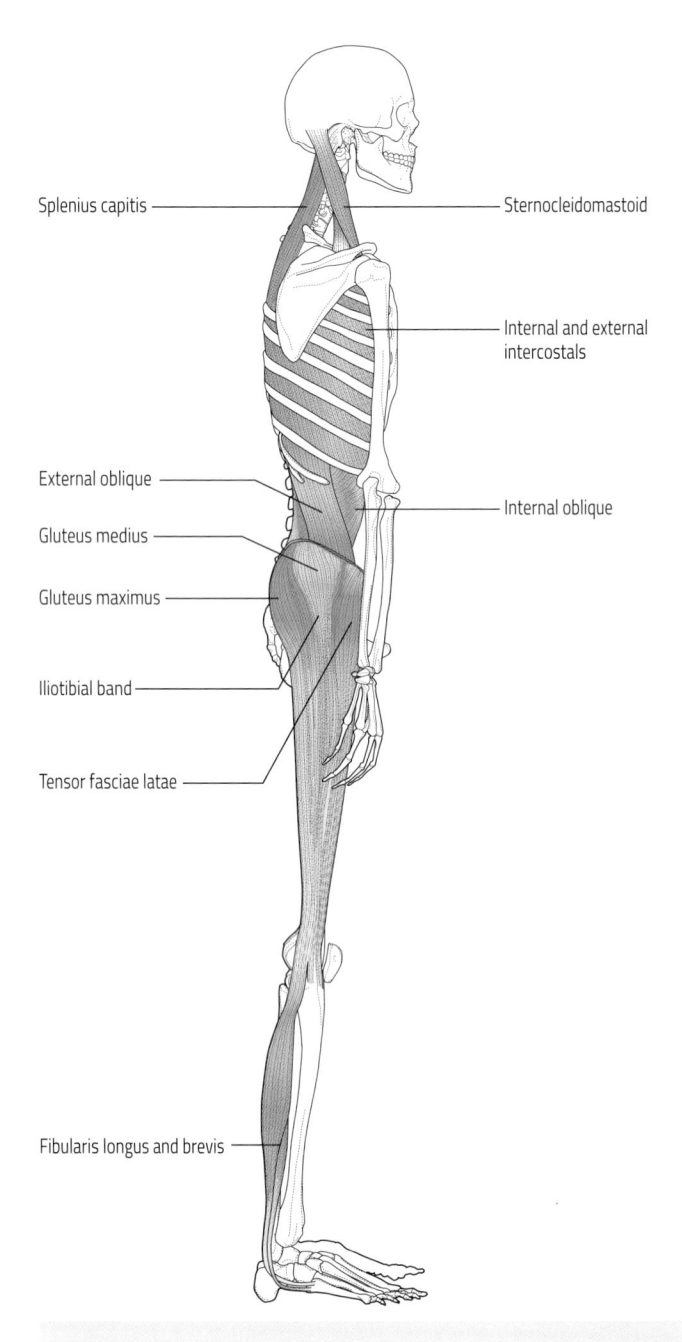

**Figure 8.4**
The lateral line includes the "hip laterals" that support the weight in the hips

# Single leg balance

observed: "The primacy of accurate weight-bearing through the hip joint is of central importance for the organisation not just of walking, but also of the body as a whole. It functions as the primary joint of postural security, so that finding a precise balance through it has enormous potential not just re-organising the functioning of the hip joint itself, but also the whole way that the body balances itself with regards to its weight-bearing point of contact with the earth" (unpublished work).

### Exploration 8.6 Pelvic lifts

- *Stand without shoes, with one foot on the floor and the other on a book large enough for your whole foot, about 3/4 inch (2 cm) thick. Have your feet hip-width apart so your legs are vertical. Keep your feet pointing forwards with your big toe balls engaged and both knees straight throughout all these explorations.*

- *Raise the floor-level foot off the ground without bending the knee. How do you do this? Do you lean to the side? Or shift your weight completely across (Fig. 8.3B)? Do you pull up the hip on the lifting leg side, by tightening your side or lower back into the ribcage (Fig. 8.3C)? Or can you lift the foot, keeping the leg straight, without any distortion (Fig. 8.3A)?*

The first three of these moves act to distort the torso and do not engage the key muscles. How can we move without distortion?

To understand the action of the hip laterals, see them like a bench with the legs inset – if someone sits on the very end of the bench, it tilts down and tips up the other end. This is how hip lifts work, except that instead of *pushing* the end of the bench down, it is *pulled* down. The gluteus medius (Fig. 8.5) runs from the top of the iliac crest, down to the greater trochanter (the knobbly bit at the outside top of the thigh bone) and when it contracts, acts to *pull* the pelvic girdle into a tilt. This tilts the other side of the pelvic girdle up, drawing up the other leg.

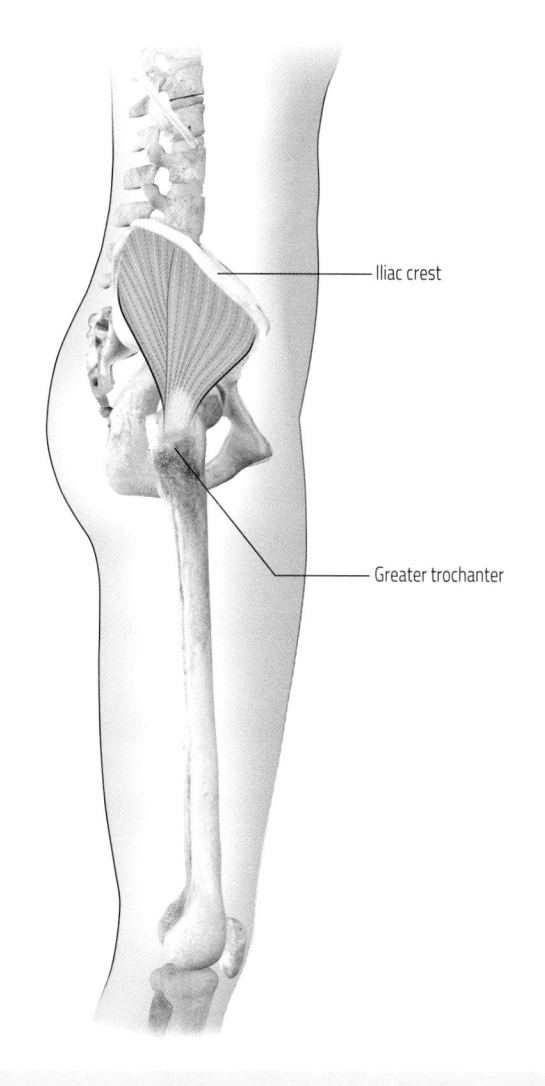

**Figure 8.5**
Gluteus medius

# CHAPTER eight

### Exploration 8.7  Finding your gluteus medius and other hip stabilizers

Video link for exploration 8.7

- To get your hip lateral group working, invite the gluteus medius to pull down from the iliac crest of the supporting hip. (It can help to put the heel of your hand on the iliac crest – your palm will be on the gluteus medius – and push down gently to give your body a cue.) (Figs 8.6A, B.) The upper part of the gluteus maximus will engage with this move.

- Avoid pushing your hips forward and swaying back in your upper body by keeping iliac spines back, hamstrings and pubococcygeals engaged and upper body toned. This keeps the pelvis vertical and balances the pulls of tensor fasciae latae and gluteus maximus. The IT band is only fully engaged when these muscles that tighten it are in balance.

- Keep breathing throughout the torso, especially into (or from) from the pelvic floor.

It may take a few minutes to find the muscles involved, and until then you might notice yourself wobbling or compensating with other movements of ankles, arms, pelvis, knee bends, or torso tilts.

#### The link to the ball of the big toe

Notice that if you simply push down the outside of the hip and down to the outside of the foot, you will need to lean outwards on the supporting leg.

- To prevent this, think of the big toe ball pressing down on the inside of the leg, as the hip pushes down on the outside.

- You might notice your adductors now coming into play, so that both sides of the leg are stabilized. Encourage the adductors by pushing down on the top of the inside of the leg with your opposite fingers (or a stick; Fig. 8.6C).

### Exploration 8.8  The muscle spirals of the legs

Notice that though the downward movement initiates in the outside of the hip and upper leg, it terminates in the big toe ball. This is because of the spiral arrangement of muscles in the legs, which connects these two crucial places via the IT band and its tensioning muscles from outside hip to outside knee, and the tibialis anterior from outside knee to the inside of the heel (Figs 3.24 and 3.25).

- Do a hip lift with your supporting foot turned out, and then with it turned in, so that the big toe is slightly inside the line of the heel. In which is it easier to engage the whole of the hip laterals?

- Observe that the hip laterals are part of the external torque chain and will twist the leg out, while the adductors through to the big toe balls are part of the internal torque chain and will twist the leg inwards, and these must balance each other. Notice that with the foot turned in, there is a much clearer linkage of force from the big toe ball into the side and back of the hip. The two sides of the leg are working together to power the movement. (More on foot placement in lesson 6.)

# Single leg balance

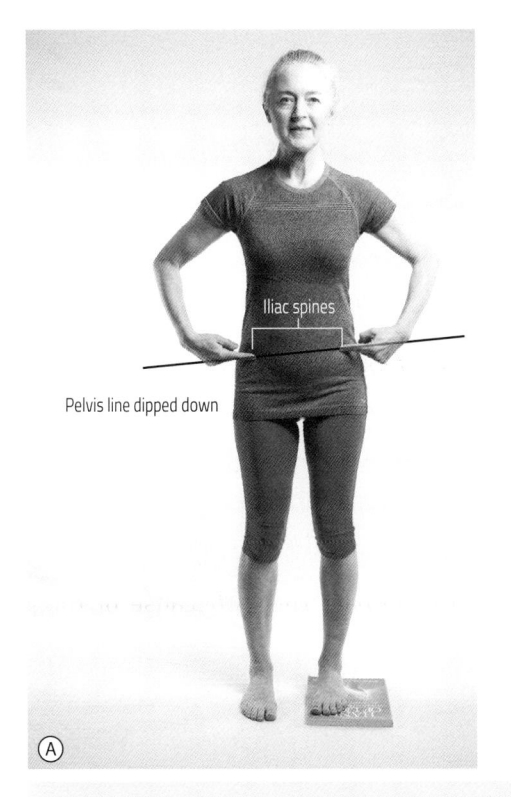

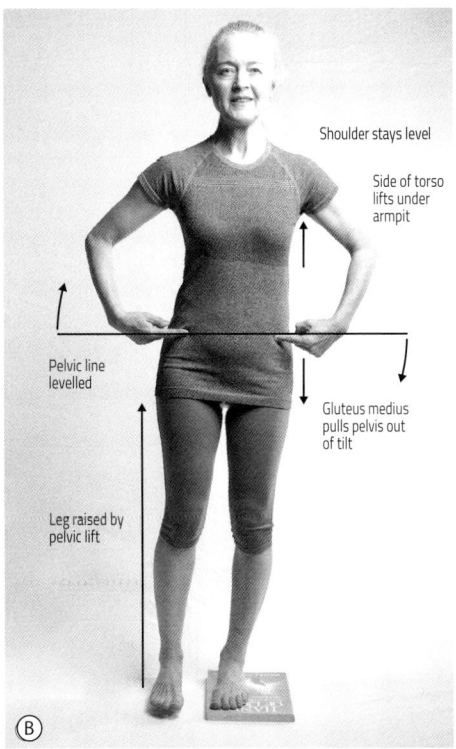

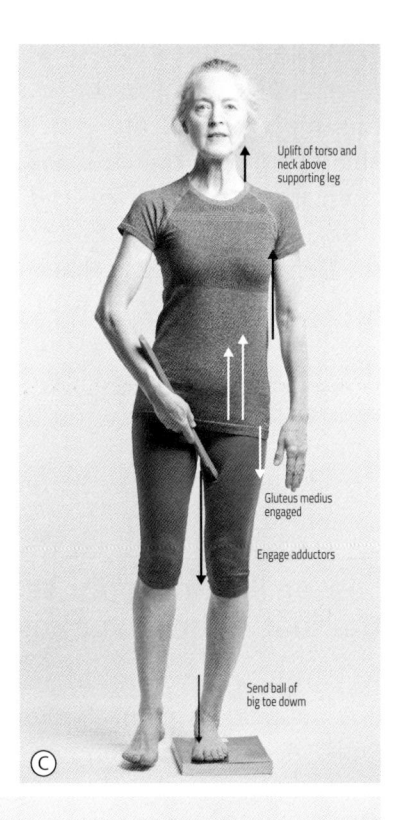

**Figure 8.6**
Pelvic lifts. (A) Standing with one foot on a book tilts the pelvis.
(B) Contracting the gluteus medius tilts the pelvis back to level and lifts the other leg. (C) Engaging ball of big toe and adductors with pelvic lift

### Exploration 8.9  *Support up into the torso*

- Do this move again and notice the response of the torso above the supporting leg when you send the hip, big toe ball and inside leg down.
- You may notice that the supporting side of the body lifts up off the hip joints, right up under the armpit. (But having noticed this, don't help it along! Just let it happen.) The shoulders are not involved. This all further stabilizes the torso, as the oblique muscles of the spiral lines, and the intercostals of the lateral lines, all are engaged. The sternocleidomastoids are part of both these lines, and these engage to lengthen the side of the neck.
- When you engage the adductors, it also brings in the muscles at the front of the body on the supporting side, particularly the rectus abdominis (Figs 8.6B and 8.6C).

# CHAPTER eight

I love this move. These small "abductor" muscles (that I dub the hip laterals), along with IT band and the upper part of the gluteus maximus have to be able to support the entire weight of the torso apart from the supporting leg, and to do it repeatedly, step after step, taking all of our weight. Moreover, when they engage, it seems that almost all of the body's muscles engage with them – lateral, spiral, core, front and back lines all come swinging into play on the supporting side. So leave a book lying round on your floor, preferably for a month or two, and keep working it. When you have mastered this with a shallow book, try a deeper one, or a yoga block. You can only get stronger.

## Lesson 5 Finding our secure base – tilting the foot – the lower ankle joint

As bipeds, we pivot on our ankle joints, and for many it is the weakest point. For good balance, these little joints need to be strong and flexible across many planes. Functionally, the ankle is two joints in one. The true ankle joint allows the sole of your foot to hinge down and up again. This is the movement we need to walk.

### Exploration 8.10   Finding our ankle joints

- *Put your finger and thumb on the bony bumps either side of your ankle – the lateral and medial ankle bones – and flex your foot up and down. You can feel the ankle bone (talus) hinging between them.*

But the foot needs also to be able to tilt sideways to accommodate rough and uneven surfaces. The joint that allows this is really several joints functioning as one, and they are between the heel, ankle bone, and the middle foot bones (Fig. 8.1D). Because we stand and walk mostly on flat surfaces, for many people these have stiffened up with lack of use.

- *Place your feet flat on the floor. Taking one foot at a time, can you tilt your foot inwards, by pulling the instep towards the other foot, so that the little toe and outside of the heel lift off the floor? Can you do this while holding your knee still (Fig. 8.7)?*

- *Tilt it outward then in again a few times to waken up the joint, emphasizing the inward movement, until you can experience a clear movement. Leave your toes relaxed as you do this; they may want to lift or curl. Can you now slide a finger under the outside of the foot from front to back? This may take several sessions.*

## Lesson 6 Placement of the feet – untwisting the leg spirals

That feet should turn out was a social norm, part of "noble posture" (Fig. 8.8), perfectly placed for lunging with a sword, or curtsying. To raise the chest tightens and arches the lower back, pushes the pelvis forward and rotates the feet out: it is part of an over-pronounced secondary curve. Even though Alexander and Delsarte were against a pronounced curve, I wonder if they could have challenged the foot placement: it was so culturally accepted.

Many movement instructors advise pointing the big toes straight forward. But anyone who has been skiing may remember the inward placement of ski boots on the skis, which brings the ankle joint into correct alignment, without which it would shear at high speeds. I was first introduced to this by Jeando Masoero, from whom I learned exploration 8.12. It is also recommended by Katie Bowman (2017: 96, 112). Bowman gives similar advice on rebalancing the accompanying leg muscle imbalances.

This fits with our exploration (in muscle spirals of the legs, above), that the external torque and internal torque chains of the hips and legs only balance in this placement, providing full support and power to the torso. This becomes even clearer when we progress to walking uphill (see Chapter 11, lesson 3).

# Single leg balance

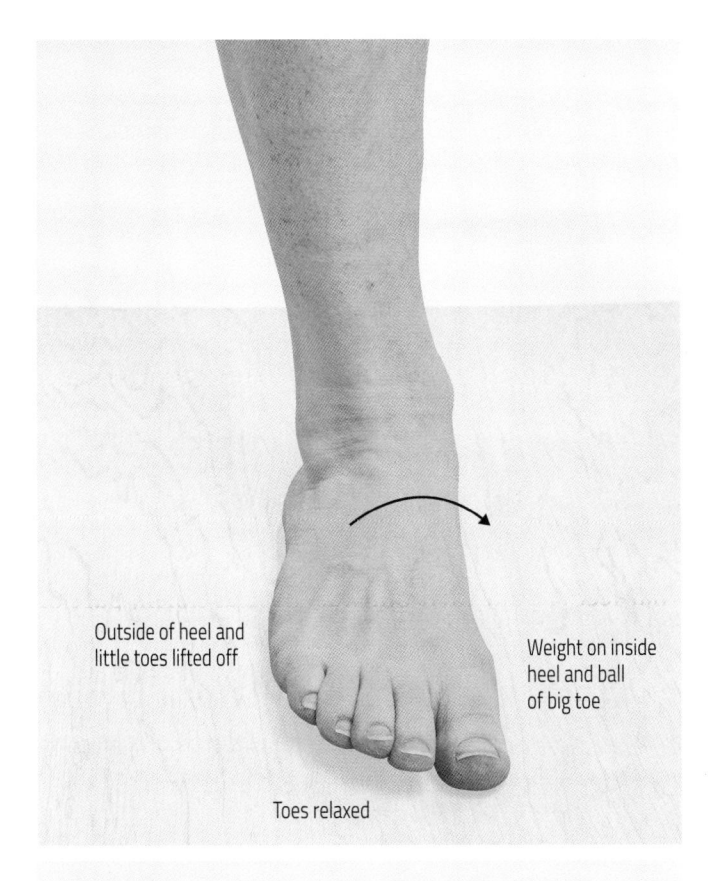

**Figures 8.7**
Instep pulled to midline

Outside of heel and little toes lifted off

Weight on inside heel and ball of big toe

Toes relaxed

### *Exploration 8.11  Foot placement affects the deep hip rotators*

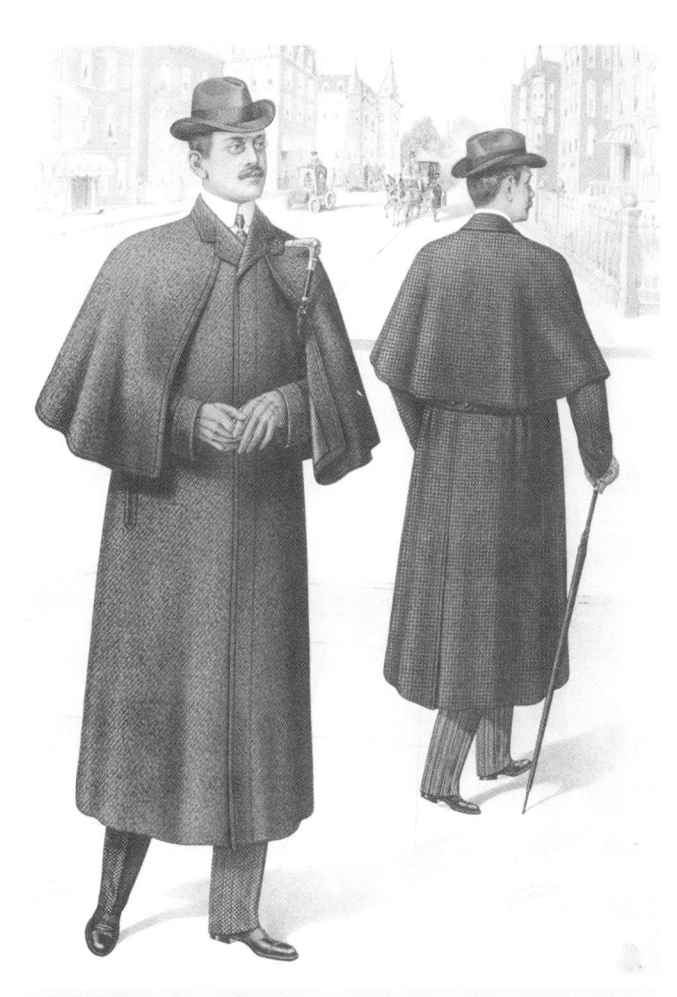

**Figures 8.8**
Magazine fashion shot, New York, 1903

These six little muscles run laterally from the lower pelvis and sacrum to the greater trochanter of the femur, and act to rotate the thighs outward. They are also important stabilizers of the pelvic girdle, linking to the adductors and core muscles.

- *Play with turning your feet slightly in, and notice it opening and stretching all the deep hip rotator muscles under the gluteus maximus. Then turn the feet out again, and notice the area tightens (Fig. 8.10C).*

The deep hip rotators are also core stabilizers of the pelvis. All except one (obdurator externus) act as powerful extensors of the hip joint, maintaining our torso vertically above the hips and opposing the flexors – psoas, iliacus, adductors, tensor fasciae latae and rectus femoris. Roll slowly up from a forward bend to feel these deep muscles under your gluteus maximus working with the hamstrings to straighten and stabilize the pelvis. They make fascial links to the pelvic floor and adductors. In particular, the obdurator internus inserts on the inside of the sitting bones and pubic bone, making extensive fascial connection with the pelvic floor. When we engaged the pubococcygeals to anteriorly rotate and stabilize the pelvis (exploration 7.16) I suspect it is this muscle doing the work – but it is much harder to visualize!

# CHAPTER eight

### Exploration 8.12   Untwisting the leg spirals

But there is more to it than simply turning the feet in. Gravity is precise and our response to it is equally precise, for better or worse. Realigning one part of the body will show up any restrictions and long-term tensions that were concealed by the misalignment.

- *Align your feet: turn your feet inward, so that the outer lines between the heel and 5th metatarsal – the bump one third of the way up the outside of the foot – are parallel (Fig. 8.9).*

- *Does this now throw you onto the outside of the foot? If so, it is revealing tight muscles on the inside ankle that draw up the foot, and underactive muscles on the outside of the ankle (Fig. 8.10A).*

- *Pull the instep of each foot towards the midline, as in exploration 8.10), and see if the outside of the foot will lift off – this will be harder in this pattern (Fig. 8.10B). Keep breathing! Does this then drag your knees together? Notice that this pulls you out of the lateral muscles of the hips and might also tilt your pelvis forward again.*

We have now brought the inside leg muscles (internal torque muscles) into play and need to balance them with the external torque muscles (hip laterals).

- *Counter-rotating the top of the thigh outward to realign the knees. Maintain the inward-instep pull – send your big toe balls and the inside of the heels down. Keep this going as you counter-rotate the top of the thigh outward. To do this, think your iliac spines coming back and up off the outside of the knee, while the pubococcygeals pull forwards. This engages your hip laterals again. It may feel very tight, as we are applying counter-twists to old patterns (Fig. 8.10C). Keep breathing!*

- *To lift the arch of the foot: take these pulls very slowly and gently, to engage a stretch up the inside of the leg from below the instep. You may discover that this lifts the arch of the foot, and counters flat feet.*

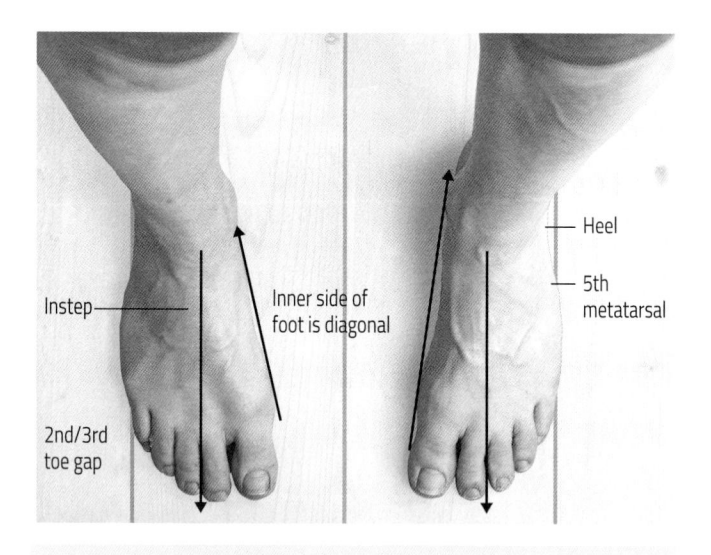

**Figure 8.9**
Feet aligned with heels to fifth metatarsals parallel

**Video link for exploration 8.12, part 1**

Now the risk is that the feet may twist outwards again. If you walk, or come onto tiptoes, do the feet revert to their old alignment? We need a directional pull that will stabilize the new angle of the foot, whether stationary or in movement. This next move can take a while to find, but is immensely stabilizing for the ankle.

- *"Screwing the ankle": while standing, put your left foot on a chair, aligning it as in Figure 8.9, and take hold of your ankle bones from behind with left hand finger and thumb. Notice that the inside bone is slightly forward of the outer one. Pull it back and up, and notice that it pulls the heel away from the big toe on a diagonal, and the instep is lifted up.*

- *Can you now do this from the ankle itself?*

**Video link for exploration 8.12, part 2**

# Single leg balance

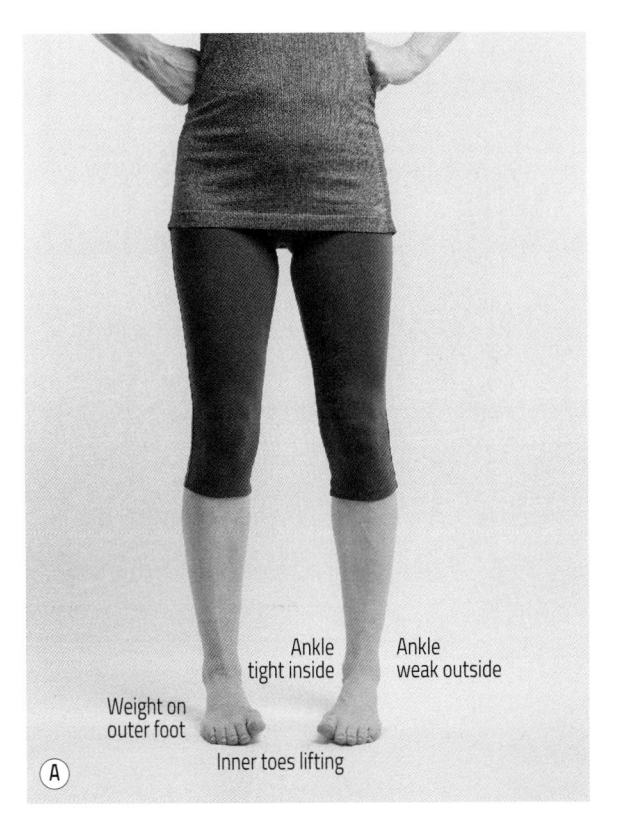

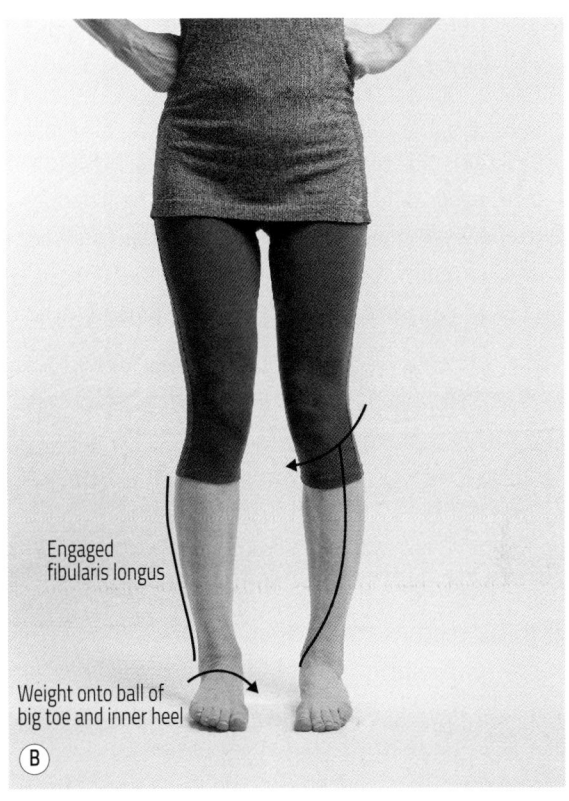

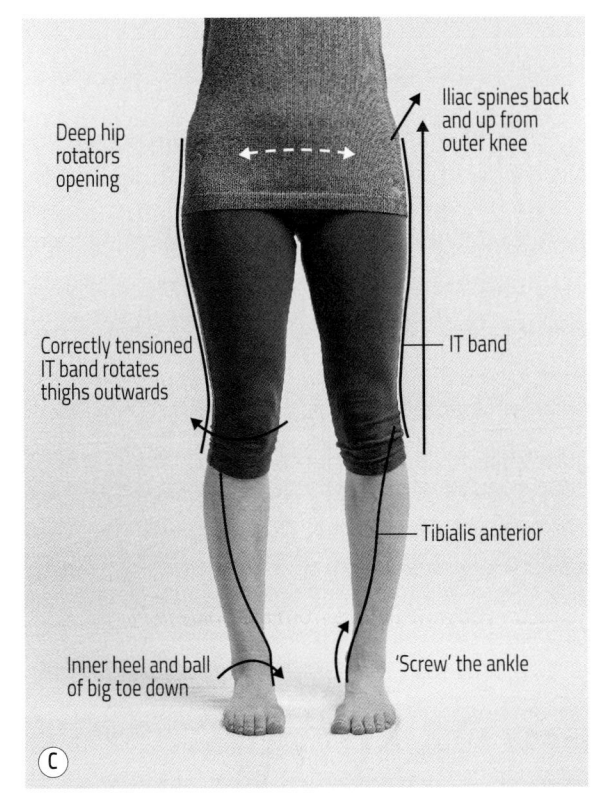

**A**
- Weight on outer foot
- Ankle tight inside
- Ankle weak outside
- Inner toes lifting

**B**
- Engaged fibularis longus
- Weight onto ball of big toe and inner heel

**C**
- Deep hip rotators opening
- Correctly tensioned IT band rotates thighs outwards
- Iliac spines back and up from outer knee
- IT band
- Tibialis anterior
- Inner heel and ball of big toe down
- 'Screw' the ankle

**Figure 8.10**
Rebalancing the leg spirals. (A) Aligning the feet often throws the weight onto the outside. (B) Bringing insteps to midline can drag the knees in. (C) Counter-rotating the thighs to balance the leg spirals. Right leg: directions to use; left leg: muscle responses

# CHAPTER eight

These are strong moves, and probably will feel initially as if your leg is being twisted in two opposite directions at once – which it is, undoing the contra-twists that your legs have endured for years.

- *While standing, focus your heels down – you may notice you settle back on your heels. Then change your focus to the inner ankle bone. You may notice a better balance of weight through the foot, and a lift up the leg and torso.*
- *Keep focus on "screwing" the medial ankle back and up as you walk or come onto tiptoe – does it now maintain the foot alignment? What else happens?*

## Anatomy of all this

Several things are happening together.

- Pulling the insteps towards each other is waking up the fibularis longus (and also fibularis brevis), the muscle of the lower lateral line which runs down the outside of the leg and crosses under the foot to insert on the base of the first metatarsal (Fig. 8.4 and Fig. 3.25). This is underworking in most people – seen when ankles easily twist and collapse outwards on rough ground, or wobble on high heels.
- The counter-rotation of the thigh is brought about through the external torque of the hip laterals group muscles. As the gluteus maximus wakes up and engages, it lengthens the tensor fasciae latae again. This correctly torsions the IT band which then acts to pull the knee outward. They are aided by the sartorius muscle – which goes from the inside of the knee to the iliac crest. It pulls the knees away from each other, such as when we sit cross-legged on the floor. (*Sartorius* is Latin for "tailor" – a profession who always sat cross-legged.)

**AT info:** Another of Alexander's puzzling instructions was "knees forward and away." This move is "knees away," i.e. away from the midline of the body.

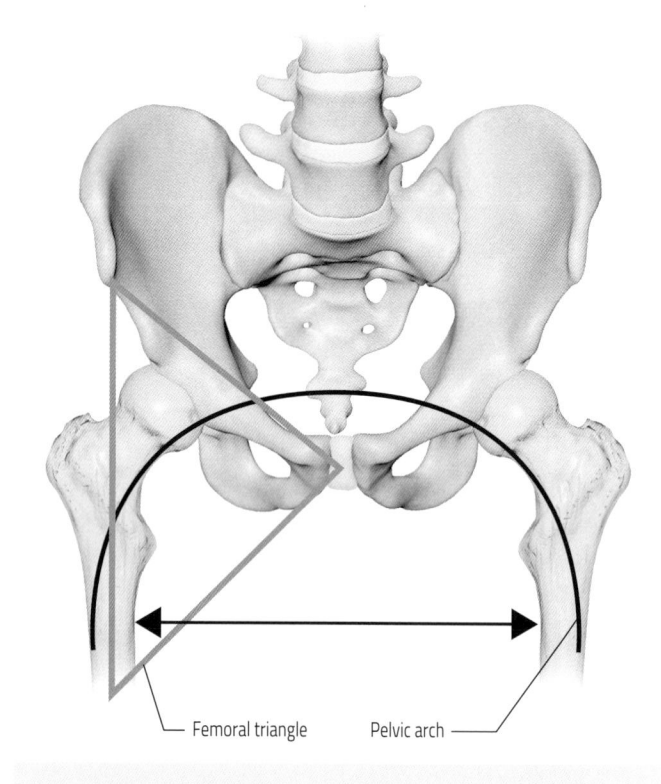

**Figure 8.11**
The pelvic arch and femoral triangle

- The fibularis longus, on the outside of the lower leg, and tibialis anterior, running up the front to the outside shin, are in balance together and are in fascial continuity under the heel – forming a sling around the foot (see Fig. 3.25, spiral line back view). When one is slack, the other is often tight, tilting the foot inwards or outwards. When we bring the knee out we are stretching this muscle on the inside of the heel and lower leg, and so lifting the arch of the foot.

IT band injuries are common in sports, and the solution is often seen as rolling or stretching it. The real cause is not the IT band itself but the imbalance of many muscles around the hips and legs (Ferber et al. 2010) and indeed the whole-body. There is serious rehabilitative potential with this work.

# Single leg balance

## Lesson 7 Widening the hips with the breath – opening the femoral triangle

The pelvis is commonly conceived as an arch, transmitting weight from spine to legs (Dimon 2011: 54). While many people are aware of fallen foot arches, less comment is made on what I call fallen pelvic arches, when the muscles of the pelvic region are not holding balanced tone to support the skeletal arch and the legs collapse towards each other. When the thighs are drawn together, the incorrect alignment of the hip joint and thigh bone creates misplaced pressures all through the leg regions. It also constricts the femoral triangle (Fig. 8.11) through which all the big blood and lymph vessels, along with nerves, pass to the legs. This has to be a recipe for poor pelvic and leg health. The lowest "corners" of the belly are often places of congestion – contributing to the development of appendicitis, constipation, etc. We need to widen the pelvic arch that is so crucial for both our support system and health.

To widen the pelvic arch from the inside, we will work with the breath.

For most people, the belly wall pushes forward on the in-breath. This is because, with a tight lumbar spine, the rectus abdominis is overstretched and cannot maintain tone. All this narrows the pelvis. We need to use the transversus abdominis to create widening, which will open out the tight lumbar region and allow the rectus abdominis naturally back into play.

### Exploration 8.13   Widening the pelvic arch with the breath

- Stand with legs and feet aligned. Or explore this in child's pose (see Fig. 14.4A), which can be easier.
- Find your spatial awareness. Allow your natural breathing as in Chapter 6; rest at the bottom of the out-breath so that the in-breath becomes a springy response that moves down the body, until you are aware of the lumbar spine then the pelvic girdle widening. Notice the deep hip rotators under the bum muscles widening a little.
- Be aware that you can pull your iliac spines back as you breathe out, to send the out-breath back and up. Now play with keeping your iliac spines pulled back as you breathe in – enlisting the power of the transversus abdominis to widen the belly. Keep them back as you continue to breathe, so the widening continues and deepens. Discover that the in-breath can now widen the belly muscles, rather than push them forward.

Now you are supporting your internal organs in the correct location, rather than letting them bulge forward over the front of the pelvic girdle. You can now take your awareness into the soft tissues of the pelvic bowl, wider and deeper.

- Place your hands either side of the pubic bone, and be aware of the soft tissue here widening too, then take this awareness out to the sides of the lower belly right into the corners.
- Be aware of the pelvic floor descending on the in-breath. Then find your sitting bones (maybe feel them with your hand), be aware of them moving apart on the in-breath. Let this widen to include the hip joints as the deep hip rotators engage, then through the hip joints into the thigh bones – out to the trochanters. From there you might pick it up going down into the thighs, and even to the lower legs and feet (Fig. 8.12).
- Keep breathing and engaging the deep hip rotators as you try your single leg balance again, bringing in your hip laterals, etc. Does this help to maintain the pelvic arch and displace less as you transfer the weight onto one leg?

## Summary

### Exploration 8.14   The five moves for aligning the feet while standing

1   Stand with heels under hips, with free knees.

2   Turn your toes so the outside line of heels to 5th metatarsals are parallel (see Fig. 8.9).

# CHAPTER eight

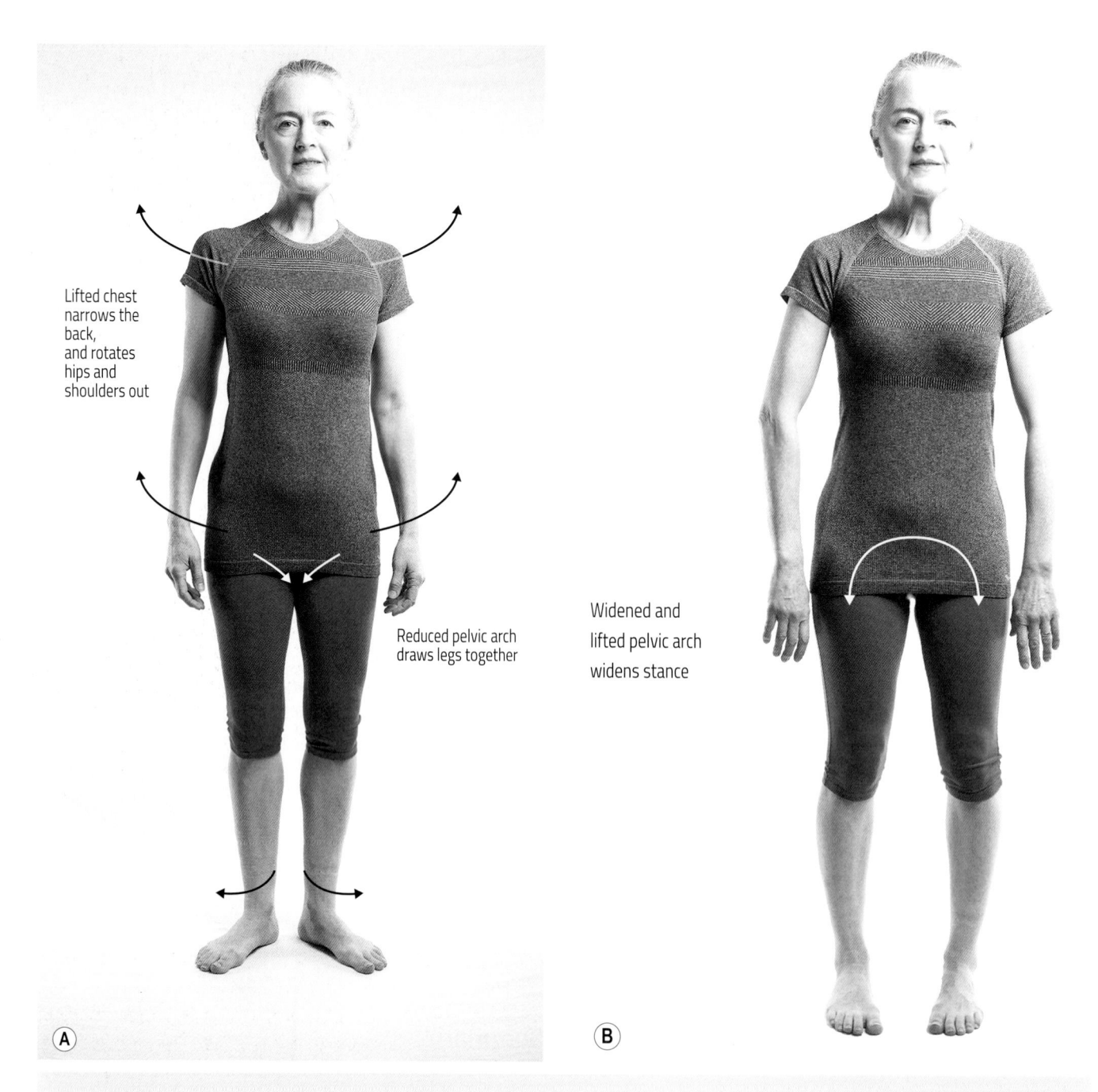

Lifted chest narrows the back, and rotates hips and shoulders out

Reduced pelvic arch draws legs together

Widened and lifted pelvic arch widens stance

(A)

(B)

**Figure 8.12**
Summary of changes to new body geometry. (A) External rotation patterns of standard (noble) posture. (B) New body alignment

# Single leg balance

3  *Pull the insteps to the midline, so the weight is now on the big toe balls and the inside of the heels (Fig. 8.10B).*

4  *"Screw the ankle" by taking the inner ankle bone back and up to pull the heel back on the diagonal and lift the instep.*

5  *Maintain this as you gently counter-rotate the thighs: send your lateral hip stabilizers down, bring the iliac spines back and up off the outsides of the knees and pubococcygeals forwards (Fig. 8.10C).*

(To do this sitting, see exploration 10.2.)

Caution: these moves can cause short-term discomfort – and long-term benefit

Standing habitually with the feet rotated out causes the shinbone to rotate outwards, which then pulls the kneecap slightly out of its groove (Bowman 2017: 179). Since this happens gradually, the tissues have adjusted gradually and we unaware of it. When we realign the feet, and with them the shinbone, the muscles, ligaments, and tendons around the knee joint realign, changing the forces within the joint. This can cause soreness for a few days and is ok – just take it gently until it passes. Sometimes other joints can also be sore for a short while as the forces change for the better within the leg system. This is no different to the soreness or pain that can result from the first few days of wearing corrective insoles or adjusting to barefoot shoes, as the balance of muscles changes. I suggest that people who have stood for years in a strong turn-out (including dancers), and those who have had prior foot problems, may need to take these realignments in stages.

It was a few years ago that I first did these corrective moves which felt so weird and briefly made my knees hurt. I took the pulls very gently for a few days, and my knees soon recovered. To my amazement, after only two weeks, I placed my feet in the new alignment and it felt so good! Over time, it has brought much more ease and greater strength to my feet and legs, and also for many of my pupils and colleagues, some of whom also had initial short-term discomfort.

This alignment seems to be old wisdom in the Eastern traditions, as several people have told me that they have learned it from their Tai Chi or yoga teacher. If you are disbelieving, I invite you to try it for yourself and see what happens.

9

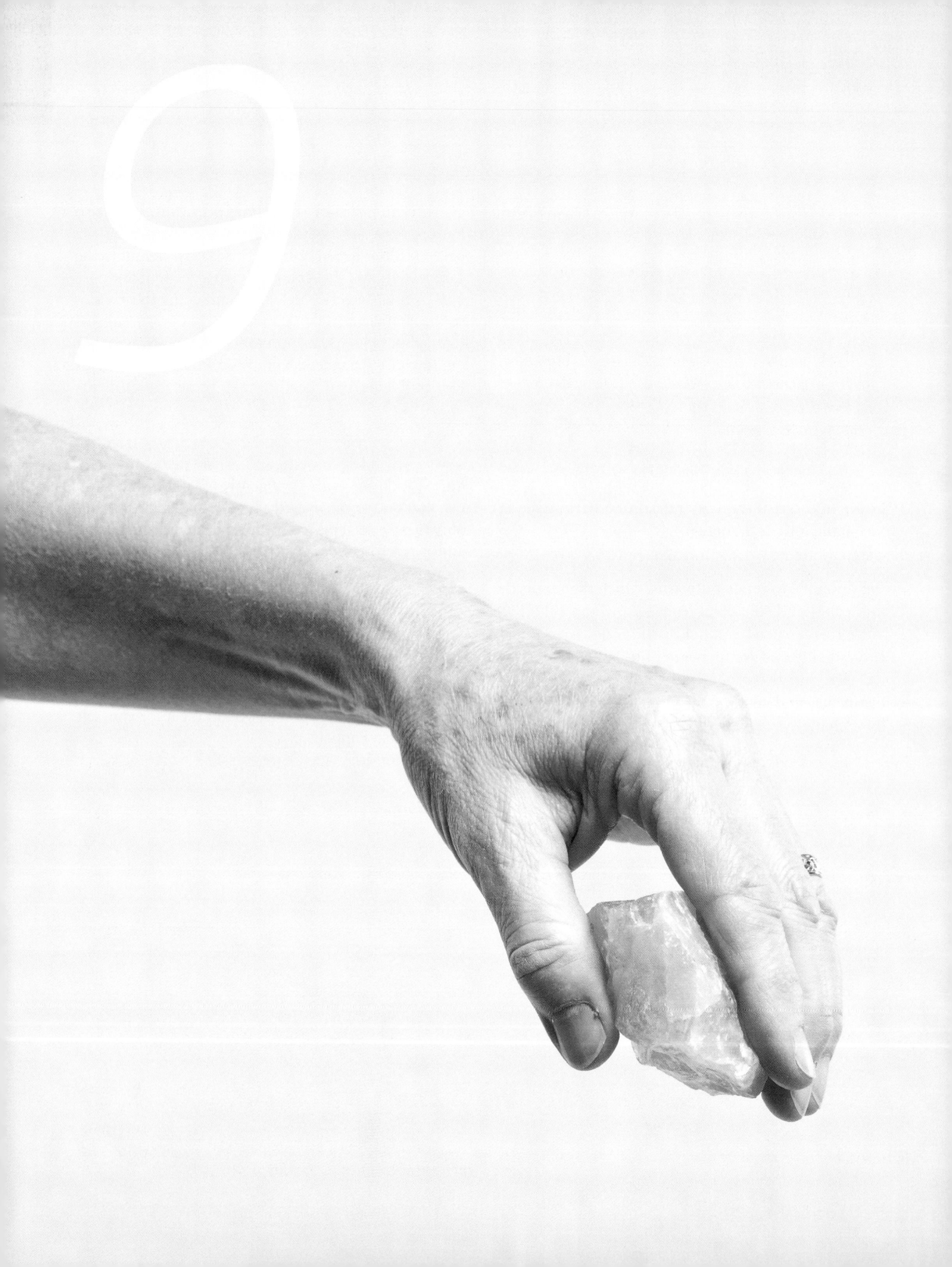

# Spatial relationships and use of the upper body and arms

## Coming into relationship with our world

Integrated movement involves expanding our space. With calm presence (parasympathetic dominant), we self-engage, becoming more aware of interoception, proprioception, and embodiment, and the fullness of space within the body. From this embodied place, we find the awareness of space around us, within which the hands are active in daily tasks. We need to expand the physical body to restore our lengthening antagonistic muscle relationships so that the full range of muscles is at our disposal. With the imbalance of primary and secondary curves, and the nervous system imbalance that goes with this, many of our muscles are working sub-optimally. Here we will explore the functional anatomy of the upper body in relation to spatial awareness. Then in Chapter 12 we will do the stronger active stretches of Initial Alexander technique for the upper body.

I began playing the violin when I was eight. Four of us stood in a line and tried to copy what the boring teacher showed us. The result was indifferent playing, and not very enjoyable. At fourteen, I was allocated a new teacher. The first lesson was an eye-opener when she took the violins from me and my fellow learner and made us bounce up and down on the spot, simultaneously swinging our arms. I was intrigued, though the other girl soon left.

Over the next year my playing was transformed with real teaching, as she guided me through supporting the violin and moving my arms with no reactive tightening. The new movements I learned felt natural to my body balance, although were often strange initially, such as the way she brought my fingers to the strings. Instead of closing in with the front of the arm, I felt I was pouring the fingers on from above by lengthening up the back of the arm, hand, and fingers, and over onto the strings. The necessary pressure was then funneled from my back and my new, amazing vibrato worked from the whole arm. I was now in relationship with my violin, and my whole-body was the sound-board.

Unfortunately, I never thought to apply any of this to the rest of my tense life, and once I left school, I left the violin behind too. I did not think of it again until, a few years into teaching, I had my first string-player pupil. Suddenly I realized this learning fitted completely with AT and particularly with Miss Goldie's teaching.

This is the route we will take here with arms: discovering how lifting the arms is not the heavy or straining activity most people conceive, but that the arms can happily balance in many positions, providing there is support from the torso. We can then move them without contracting into the joints, maintaining length at all times, and finding integrated strength in this. We will discover how optimal use of the arms involves conscious presence and spatial relationships with the objects we touch or grasp, the whole-body and mind involved in even the simplest hand movement. We are working against the cultural imperative of our fast lane societies to "grab and go."

We are always exploring our dynamically balanced structure of lengthening antagonistic relationships, within which the arms and shoulders are self-supporting. This is because all the muscles adjust to hold each position moment by moment, in dynamic oppositions between fingers, elbows, back of the armpits, etc. While the weight of the shoulder girdle and arms is being transmitted down through the vertebral column, no additional misaligned loading is being sent through onto the structures below – ribcage, lumbar spine, etc. – which are therefore free to maintain their own balanced self-support and self-organization.

Although the directions given for the use of the arms can be precise, I am not delineating the "right way" to move the arm or the "best posture" for it. As humans, we are uniquely capable of an incredible diversity of arm movements, and defining the right way to move would limit this. Our intention is always to reconnect the brain links to muscles and joints, so that all muscles are brought back into embodied play in a flow of dynamic balance. Then when we move, the nervous system has the full choice of muscles with which to optimize a potential movement, rather than being restricted to a few overworked muscles that are often not the ones fit for purpose.

# CHAPTER nine

Thanks to Ted Dimon's excellent books *Anatomy of the Moving Body* (2001), and *The Body in Motion* (2011) for so clearly explaining the functional anatomy of the upper body from an AT perspective.

### Exploration 9.1  Observing your current use

- Do some common movements, such as pick up a cup, open a door, type, pull on socks, grasp a phone, and observe the relative tensions in your arms and chest. You will need careful attention as habitual use can feel comfortable.
- Do your shoulders lift or contract as you move?
- Does the angle of your breastbone drop or lift?
- Are you comfortable using your arms above shoulder height, such as lifting plates from a higher shelf? Do your arms feel heavy or light when you lift them?

## Lesson 1  The supportive torso

### The arms and shoulders as a self-supporting integrated system

While the pelvic girdle is a solid construction, firmly joined to the sacrum, the shoulder girdle is a much lighter structure floating on top of the ribcage. It is attached to the breastbone only by the slender collar bone – the clavicle – with no bony attachments whatsoever to ribs or spine. When the shoulder girdle is balanced in this way on a self-supporting torso, the arms can float up seemingly without effort, and stay up all day – as is needed for violinists, painters, or AT teachers using hands-on work. But if the torso slumps, the shoulders fall forwards, rounding and tightening inwards, whereupon the arms become extremely heavy to lift and their movement becomes restricted.

The most superficial layer of muscles of the back are the trapezius and latissimus dorsi, which between them widen the back and take it slightly upward (see Fig. 3.6). Both Alexander and Goldie called the latissimus dorsi the "lifter muscles" (Alexander 1987: 115). Along with the deeper layers of the back, these support the torso in what Goldie called the rectangle of the back (Fig. 8.3A).

### Exploration 9.2  The weight of the arms

- Sit in a good old slump. Curl your upper back forward, let your shoulders hunch, collapse your mid-back backwards, and let your lower back and hips fall behind the sitting bones. Your neck will constrict with backwards tilted head as you look forward. Notice that the shoulders are now in front of the body and pulling down on it.
- If you try to lift your arms in this position (imagine playing a violin or try holding up a book), they will feel immensely heavy and won't hold up for long. They are lifting against the downward pressure of the shoulders and will have limited movement.
- To come out of the slump: let your head roll forward on the top of the neck, let it follow the crown upward and allow your whole spine to extend upwards. As it lengthens, notice that the body can once again breathe into the back at the floating ribs, the shoulder blades, and maybe the lumbar spine too, as the body widens as it expands.
- Let your visual arc track down and up, your head and aligned torso can follow to pivot at the hips forward and back – this will help to integrate the back. Can you now sit upright comfortably?
- Try lifting the arms again, are they lighter, and can you float them up to shoulder level with little effort? Can you take them fully up?

In an integrated system of dynamic balance, support is always two-way – the torso needs tone to support the shoulders and arms, while tone in the shoulders and arms is part of support for the torso.

### Exploration 9.3  There is no switching off

- Lift your arm above your head then release the tone to drop it down by your side, as we mostly do. Do you notice a loss of tone in the torso also? Repeat this, possibly with

# Spatial relationships and use of the upper body and arms

*a mirror, and notice that the whole system loses tone when the arm is released in this way.*

- *Lift one heel and put it slowly down again, thinking an up-thought from Achilles tendon, up the legs, the sacrum, the back and to the crown (see explorations 3.11 and 3.12). Alternate your heels, until your whole system is streaming up.*

- *Become aware of the distance between mind in the brain (eyes seeing forward) and the fingertips by your side. Maintaining the up-streaming thoughts, let your fingers describe a huge arc that takes the arm above your head. Now let them trace the same arc down again, maintaining the up-streaming of the body. You might notice the sensation in the arm is now no different whether it is moving upward or downward.*

- *When the arm returns to your side, do not switch it off again!*

- *Do the same for the other arm and observe whether you can maintain tone in the first arm as you do it.*

Notice all the areas in life where we drop the arms after the action is done. For instance, brushing hair, finishing a text, opening a cupboard. For AT teachers/therapists, what happens when you remove hands from your pupil/client? Does the hand switch off and drop when the action is done? Can you lower the hand instead of dropping?

Notice that sustaining tone also requires a sustaining of attention, of presence, while normally we switch off at this point. It takes a while to retrain your nervous system and consciousness to maintain tone in the arms and hands.

## Lesson 2    The shoulders and upper arms – opening the deep back arm line

There are complex chains of muscles in the arms allowing an immense range of movements. Thomas Myers found four arm lines: a superficial line and a deep line for both the front and the back of the arms (Figs 9.1 and 9.2).

We will discover that mostly, we overuse the first three and underuse the crucial fourth – the deep back arm line (DBAL). Only when this is engaged can all four come into balance. The DBAL links the upper spine, through the rhomboids, to the muscles around the scapula that form the rotator cuff – the joint which gives the full mobility to the upper arm. This links, via the back of the armpit, to the triceps – the extensor muscle of the upper arm – and through to the hypothenar muscles of the little finger. The rhomboids also link at the scapula to the serratus anterior and into the spiral line (see Fig. 3.25) so are crucial for support of the whole torso. We will discover that only when the DBAL is engaged do we have the full strength of the body available to the arms.

### Exploration 9.4    Finding the arm lines

- *Using Figures 9.1 and 9.2, track the different muscles that engage if you hold the arm straight out sideways at shoulder level (from Myers 2014: 154).*

- *With the palm facing forward and stretching along the fingers you activate the SFAL, while stretching the thumb upwards activates the DFAL. With the palm facing down, stretching along the back of the hand activates the SBAL, while with the little finger leading the DBAL is activated.*

Myers emphasizes that these lines are not always as neat as they look (2014: 153). Because of the huge mobility of human arms, the lines can link and double up for stability, strength, and flexibility.

### Exploration 9.5    The movement possibilities of each part of the arm

Shoulders and arms move in many planes, but each joint has a specific role, which can be surprising.

- *Play with each of these in turn and discover how mobile you are (or not) at each joint.*

The shoulder girdle is composed of two bones: the scapula (shoulder blade) at the back and clavicle (collarbone) at the front; these hinge together at the top

# CHAPTER nine

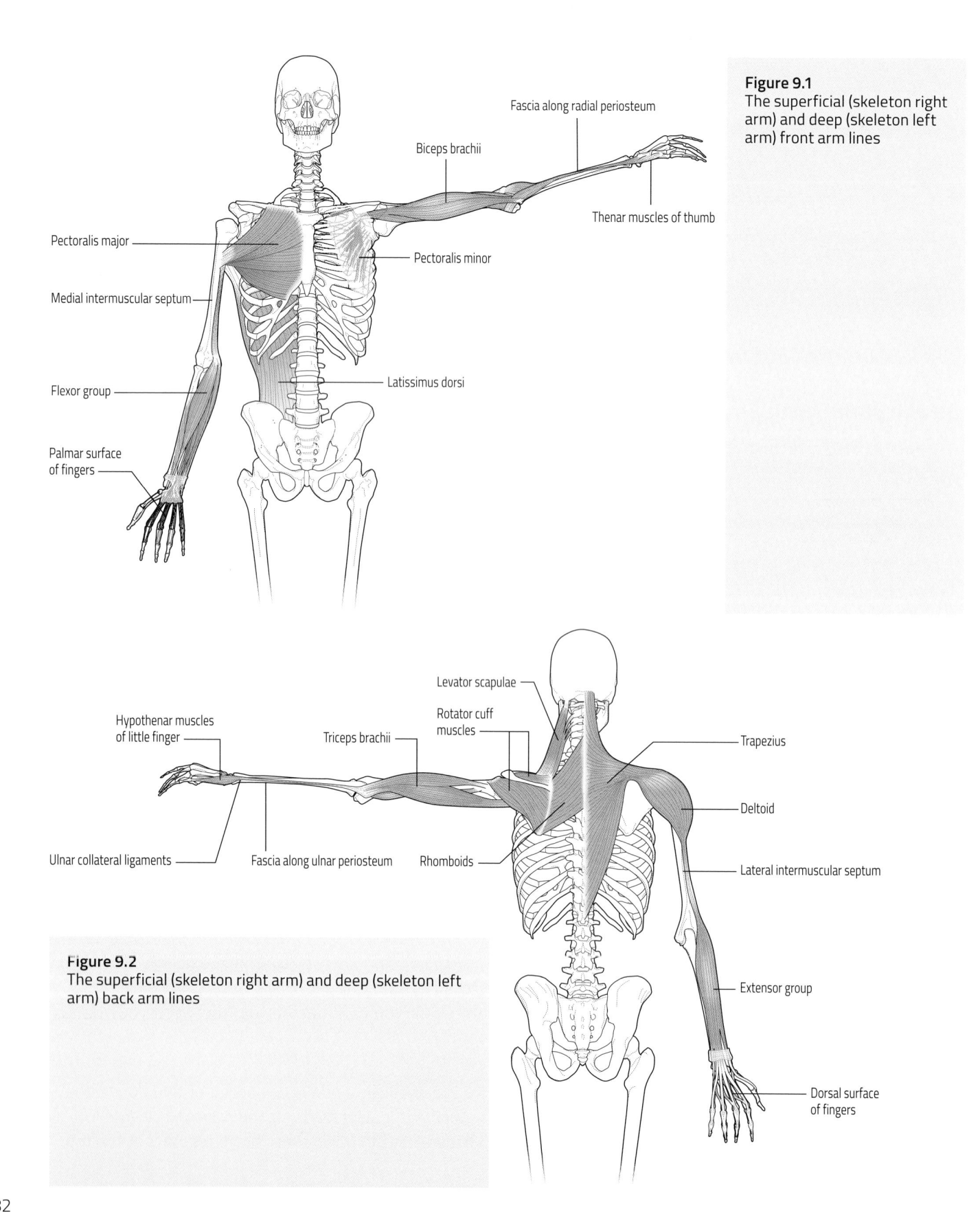

**Figure 9.1**
The superficial (skeleton right arm) and deep (skeleton left arm) front arm lines

**Figure 9.2**
The superficial (skeleton right arm) and deep (skeleton left arm) back arm lines

# Spatial relationships and use of the upper body and arms

of the shoulder. The only skeletal attachment is at the sternoclavicular joint, where the clavicles meet the top of the sternum. There is no bony connection to either the spine or the ribcage. This means the shoulder girdle floats on top of the ribcage and is extremely flexible: for manipulation, grasping, throwing, hanging, pushing, grappling; all the incredible range of movements possible to human arms because we are bipedal. The torso and breathing need not be involved, destabilized or restricted by our arm and shoulder movements.

The shoulder girdle itself can move in three planes: up and down; forward and back; in and out.

- *Play with these one arm at a time, while holding your clavicle and then scapula to experience the incredible mobility of this. (If there is little mobility, keep working these movements.)*

In this, the clavicle acts as a yardarm around its pivot point to allow the shoulder girdle a huge range of motion, while the scapula has a huge sculpted surface for the attachment of the many muscles that create and power the arm movements while stabilizing the shoulder girdle with the back.

The upper arm has one bone, the humerus, which meets the scapula at the glenoid socket, a shallow ball and socket joint, allowing an incredible range of movement. It is held in the joint by the rotator cuff muscles.

- *From this shoulder joint, the whole arm can lift forward to shoulder height, or backward to a lowish angle. This gives the swing of walking. The arm can lift to the side and pull back into the side of the body. The upper arm can rotate through about 180 degrees, taking the elbow out to the side or in toward the body.*

The lower arm has two bones, ulna and radius, which make very two very different connections:

The elbow is a hinge joint, between the humerus and ulna bones, moving the lower arm towards or away from the upper arm.

The wrist is a complex joint, between the radius of the lower arm and the carpal bones of the hand. The turning action of the hand (pronating – turning palm down – and supinating – turning palm up) happens from the elbow joint. In this, the ulna bone, on the little finger side of the arm, stays still, while the radius bone leading down to the thumb rotates around it.

- *Hold one elbow in the palm of your other hand and rotate your hand to see this.*

At the wrist, the hand can bend forward and back (flexion and extension of the wrist), and can move sideways, towards and away from the body (adduction and abduction, also called ulnar deviation).

The hand itself comprises 27 bones – 8 carpals making the wrist, 5 metacarpals in the palm culminating in the knuckles, 2 digits in the thumb and 3 in each finger. It has a whole range of movements in several planes of palm, fingers, separately or together, and opposable thumb. The fingers start at the knuckles, on which they can flex, extend, and move sideways (abduction and adduction). The thumb also has a knuckle on which it flexes, extends, abducts, and adducts, but it starts deeper down at the wrist – two carpal bones are also part of the thumb. This enables the whole thumb pad to move right across to the little finger to make the opposable thumb.

## Lesson 3   How safe do you feel? Opening up the chest and armpits

The shoulder joints and upper chest are highly reactive areas; they indicate how fearful or relaxed we are at a deep level. When we tighten the front of the shoulders to pull the arms across the body, tightening the elbows and possibly wrists as well, we are making a highly defensive "shy" gesture, often seen in stroke victims or the mentally ill. Contrast this with a dog, relaxed on her back. Her legs swing so freely in the joints that you can take her paw between your hands and throw the leg from one hand to the other with no resistance (until the dog gets fed up!). You can do the same with a relaxed small child, but rarely with an adult or even an older child. This is a state of safety it is wonderful to return to.

# CHAPTER nine

When we squeeze the arms into the side of the body, we are particularly tightening the big pectoral muscle – pectoralis major – at the front of the chest, along with pectoralis minor underneath it (Fig. 9.1). Both pectoralis major and latissimus dorsi twist into tendons that attach onto the underside of the humerus bone, and these tendons form the back and front of the armpit.

### Exploration 9.6  Freeing the armpit – the starting point for a free arm

- *Discover how tight you are in the armpit: bring your left hand to your right armpit, your palm on the side of the chest with thumb pointing up and fingers curling round under the armpit. Breathe normally – is there sideways movement under your fingers? Try the other side, is one side freer than the other?*

We need to open the pectoral muscles (and surrounding muscles) to release movement back into the side ribs. Do one arm at a time, initially keeping your opposite hand under the armpit to monitor what is happening.

- *Stand in balance with your hand by your side. Look out with spatial awareness; be aware how far away the tip of your elbow is.*
- *Imagine a string coming from the tip of your elbow. Then imagine it being drawn out to the side and up, the tip of your elbow following like a puppet arm, with the hand hanging passively down. Let the tip of the elbow rotate slightly forward with this so that the shoulder blade opens. You are lengthening the tendons of the pectoralis major and latissimus dorsi. Notice stretching in the muscles of the upper arm. If your shoulders lift, this will not happen (Fig. 9.3).*
- *Lower the "string" back down again (don't drop it!). Are your ribs now moving more under your hand?*
- *Take the hand further round towards your back. Can you feel the back of the ribcage expanding and latissimus dorsi widening?*
- *Repeat with the other elbow.*

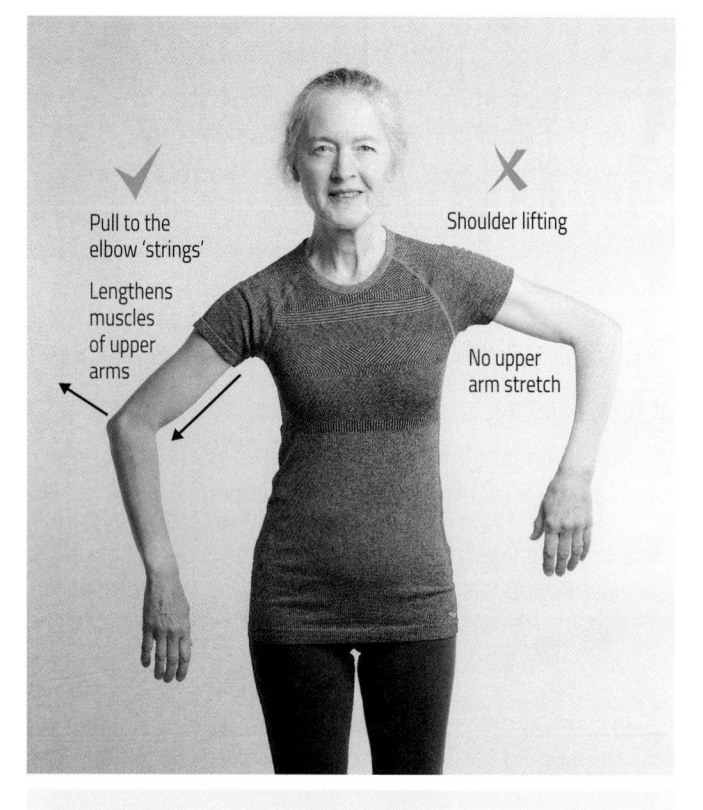

**Figure 9.3**
Pull to the elbow "string"

The pectoralis minor lies under the pectoralis major, running from the 3rd to 5th ribs and attaching onto a small spine (the coracoid process) on the inside surface of the scapula. It acts to stabilize the scapula by drawing it forwards and downwards. However, if it is tight, it pins the scapula to the ribs, restricting movement even further.

In polite society you keep your elbows in, for instance when eating or sitting on a bus. I can remember being told this as a child. This pushes us into overuse of the front arm-lines while disabling the back and access to our real strength. This can also be looked at psychologically, as an instruction not to access our full size. Women especially are encouraged to keep themselves small and weak by this constriction of the side of the body.

# Spatial relationships and use of the upper body and arms

### Exploration 9.7 Freeing the pectoralis minor to open the shoulders, and activate the deep back arm line (DBAL)

**Stage 1:** tension pins the scapula

- *Squeeze your arms into the side of the body in a defensive gesture; notice you cannot move your shoulder blades – they are pinned tight to the front of the chest.*
- *Explore how you would lift the arm while maintaining this tension – notice that the rotator cuff is effectively disabled so that the upper arm does not rotate at the shoulder; instead you must lift the shoulder and arch the chest to create a limited and strenuous upward movement (Fig. 9.4).*
- *Keeping everything pinned, force an in-breath, and notice that because the shoulder blade cannot move, the chest arches instead – you may feel the pull of the pectoralis minor on the 3rd, 4th and 5th ribs lifting the chest.*

**Stage 2:** finding the DBAL as we lift one arm

- *Free off your arms again with a pull to your elbow strings. Notice that your upper arm will now rotate at the shoulder joint.*
- *Place your hand under the side of the armpit again, the thumb pointing up over ribs 3–5. Send the fingers of the free arm away in a huge arc; let your hand follow so the arm comes up in front of you. With your thumb, monitor when the ribs begin to lift even slightly, and stop at that point. Let the breath open the armpit – at both front and back; you may notice the front ribs dropping gently as the pec minor opens again (feeling flat-chested is ok!). The sternum will drop with this; it may feel hollow chested. The back also readjusts at each stage to hang down (Fig. 9.5).*
- *When the ribs move freely again, rotate the lower arm so that the little finger now leads the movement upwards. If or when you notice the chest arching again, stop and repeat the previous instruction. At each further lift of the arm, notice that the back could be pulled up, but instead can readjust itself to hang down.*

If the top of the shoulder becomes involved, the front arm lines have taken over and the arm will be drawn in towards the neck.

- *Watch for the top of the shoulder lifting, drawing the arm toward the neck. Stop and let your elbow string draw the underside of the arm long, so that the movement comes once again out of the back of the armpit, and the deep back arm line.*
- *You may notice that when the arm lifts higher now, the movement has a different quality. Once the scapula is unpinned it is free to rotate and the whole DBAL comes into play under the trapezius, from little finger, to triceps, to rotator cuff, to rhomboids, and onto the thoracic spine. The arm lengthens up out of the side of the back.*

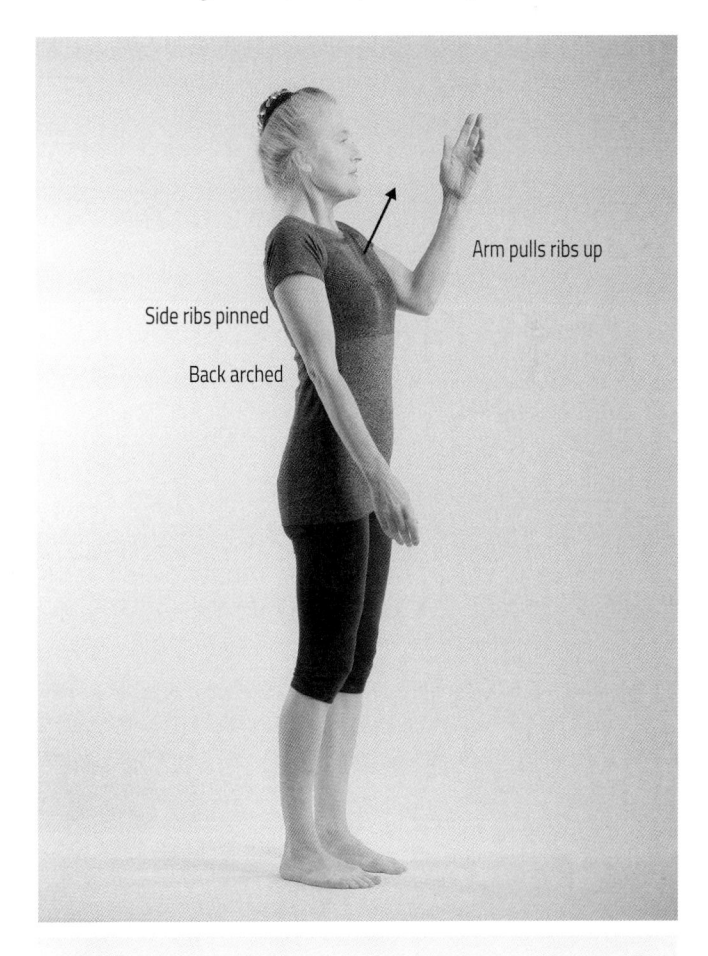

**Figure 9.4**
A tight pectoralis minor pins the scapula and disables the rotator cuff. To lift the arm, the chest must lift instead

# CHAPTER nine

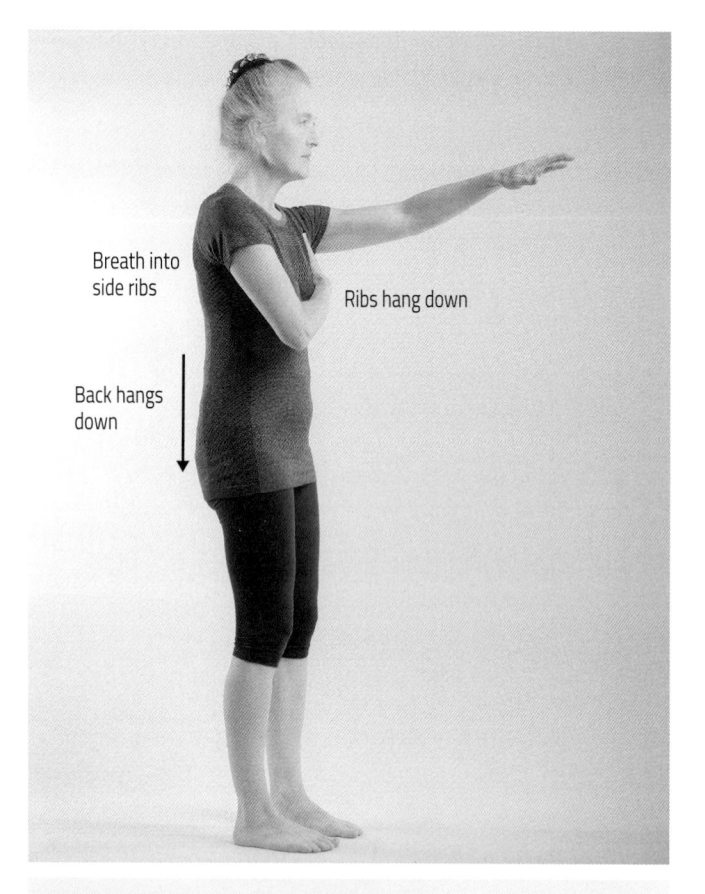

**Figure 9.5**
With a free pectoralis minor the scapula is mobile and the arm can lift without distorting the torso

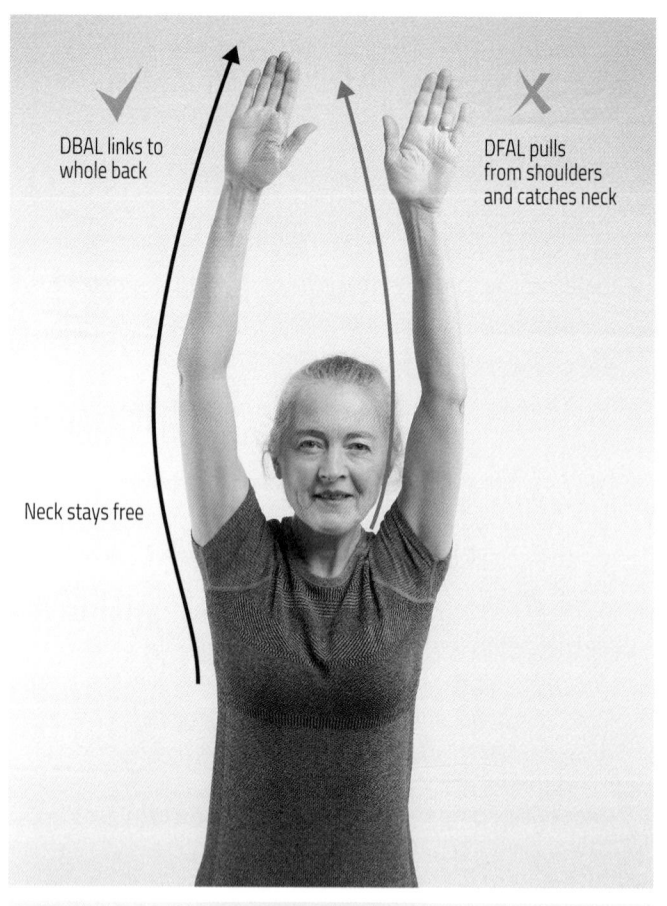

**Figure 9.6**
Little finger leading arm engages deep back arm line (DBAL); thumb leading engages deep front arm line (DFAL)

- *Play with alternating the little finger leading to rotate the arm inward, then the elbow leading, rotating the arm out. Notice the different qualities of these, and how they work together to tease more lengthening out of the back (Fig. 9.6).*

**Video link for exploration 9.7**

By focusing on extension in the tip of the elbow and little finger, we are opening the DBAL with all these moves, connecting into the back. We reduce the overuse of the front arm line flexors, and by not using the top of the shoulders we are stopping the trapezius and deltoids from dominating the movement. Instead, one is aware of the movement coming from under the shoulders, as the muscles around the scapula are employed, rather than those above it. This brings a beautiful sense of fluidity and dance into the arms.

## Lesson 4  Opening the forearm flexors

The overuse of the flexor system particularly affects the lower arm. The elbow joint is often very reactive, over-tightening the lower arm in towards the upper, and the pectorals join in with this, tightening the whole system into the shoulders.

# Spatial relationships and use of the upper body and arms

### Exploration 9.8   Letting the hands hang down freely

- *Are you comfortable letting your arms hang by your sides? Or do your hands feel like spare parts when they hang freely? Notice if, as you walk around, you keep your elbows bent like the queen carrying a handbag, your arms folded, or hands clasped or thrust into pockets – anything other than hanging freely.*

These are deeply rooted habits in many people, that I suspect stem from deeper tensions in the nervous system and lack of embodiment.

- *With spatial awareness, invite your elbows to open and arms to drop, then find a connecting link – maybe of "liquid light" (exploration 4.8) – through from your head, trickling down the neck and out to the shoulders, through the upper arm to the elbows, down the lower arm to the wrists, through the hand to your knuckles and fingertips. Can you now let your arms hang freely?*

### The opposition between fingers and elbow

The grip and extension of the hand is worked by extrinsic muscles whose muscle bulk is on the forearm, with tendons that connect into the hand. When the flexors on the underside of the arm are overused, these tendons become tight. This can become a serious problem in repetitive, precise tasks such as writing and computing or playing an instrument, leading to repetitive strain injury and carpal tunnel syndrome. The solution is to balance the flexors with the extensors.

Alexander called the move we need "a pull to the elbow." In fact, there are three pulls.

1. We have already found the "elbow string," taking the tip of the elbow away from the back of the armpit, opening the tendons of the pectoral muscles and latissimus dorsi, and widening the upper body. It also lengthens the triceps muscle along the back of the upper arm and encourages the upper part of the deep back arm line to open, right back to the spine.
2. The second pull is between the elbow and the fingertips, especially along the extensor line from the top of the lower arm to the little finger.
3. The third pull, to the wrist (ulnar deviation), will be considered below.

We need to activate these three opposing pulls together to maintain length in the whole arm, and then maintain them in all activities to access strength and precision in arms and hands.

### Exploration 9.9   The opposition between fingers and elbow, opening the forearm flexors

- *Make a pull to the elbow "string" as in exploration 9.6.*
- *While keeping a gentle opposing pull to the tip of the elbow, send your fingertips forward (focus the back of the hand to activate the SBAL), to send the hand out in front of you. Draw the elbow back again, letting the fingers gently oppose the movement. Play with the opposition created by these two directions, each resisting the other, lengthening the lower arm (Fig. 9.7).*
- *Play with sending the arm in different directions (in the air, across the body, etc.) led by pulls from the backs of the fingers and elbows. Can you also bring the rotation of the forearm in while doing this?*
- *Keep the elbows rotating forward in all these pulls (and the iliac spines thinking back) to prevent the upper body leaning back. This will keep opening the shoulder blades and the deep back arm line.*

**Video link for exploration 9.9**

Notice that when you activate these opposing directions from spatial awareness, the upper arm swings

# CHAPTER nine

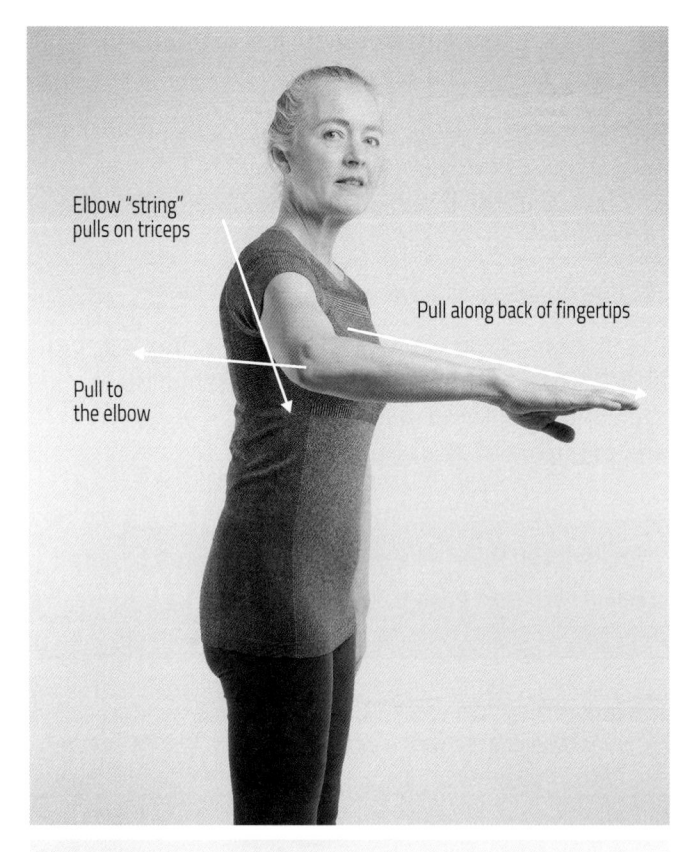

**Figure 9.7**
Opposition between elbow and fingers to balance extensors and flexors of forearm

(Labels on figure: Elbow "string" pulls on triceps; Pull along back of fingertips; Pull to the elbow)

easily in the shoulder joint, without tightening the pectorals. You are opening out all the arm flexors (the front arm line muscles) and bringing the extensors (the back arm line muscles) into play. Keep the little finger active to keep the DBAL in play.

It also maintains the sense of space between us and our hands. Normally, we constrict this by pulling forward mentally into what we are doing.

Ulnar deviation allows us to access the front arm lines in balance with the back arm lines. Once one can keep these oppositions going it is possible to access both lines together in stronger moves, such as kneading bread, or in press-ups or pull-ups.

### Exploration 9.10  Ulnar deviation for opening all the arm lines together

- *Stretch your hands down by your sides, palms facing back.*
- *Tilt your hand sideways and outwards on your wrist so that the inside of the wrist and thumb now stretch down while the little fingers point out diagonally. Notice that the inside of the arm – the flexor line – is now being stretched from armpit to thumb, giving an opposition between the inside wrist and the front of the armpit.*

This is ulnar deviation, and in this position one can stretch the thumb forward, while the little finger and elbow stretch out and down, and so stretch all the arm lines together (Fig. 9.8).

## Lesson 5  Gripping without grabbing – balancing flexors and extensors as we grip

As we reach our hands towards an object, our brains are already organizing the shape of the hand that will be required and the tensions that we expect to employ. (This is "affordance"; see Blakeslee and Blakeslee 2008: 106–8). Since our habit is to use too much tension in the flexor muscles, I notice these predictive mechanisms are often out of sync with what is really needed.

### Exploration 9.11  Balancing flexors and extensors as we grip

- *Reach towards the sides of a mug or glass. Watch your hand already molding to the shape and size needed. Notice whether as you touch, your palm and fingers immediately tighten to grip (Fig. 9.9).*
- *Return your hand by your side. Bring in awareness of the space between yourself and the glass or mug and the spatial relationship of your hand to your body.*
- *Reach towards the mug again, leading with the fingertips, staying back in the back of the armpit. Let the fingertips*

# Spatial relationships and use of the upper body and arms

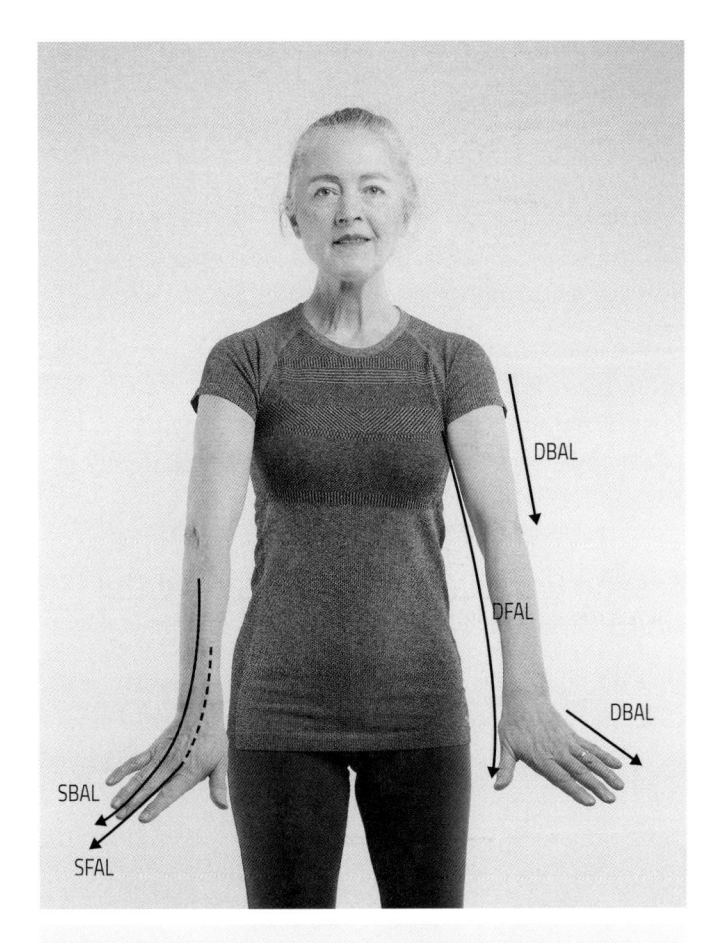

**Figure 9.8**
Using ulnar deviation to find all the arm lines together

again. Play with this in different planes and be aware of your arm joints opening and closing without tightening or straining, as if the mug is flying.

- Play with this with a full mug, engaging only sufficiently to take the weight. If the DBAL stays involved, the weight of the mug is held from your back muscles. Keep the oppositions and spatial awareness alive and take a drink. Do your head, neck, and mouth need to move as much as usual?

## The rotation of the lower arm and hand

I think the movements we use to pick objects up can tell us how we relate to our world. When we are in a hurry, we tend to snatch. The flexors overwork, shortening the arm, gripping at the elbow, grasping the object from above then holding it away rather than turning it towards us. The sense of space is constricted and there is no sense of relationship with what we encounter. This is the movement of our "grab and go" culture.

When instead we use the rotation of the hand from the lower arm, the fingers often close more gently

brush across the object without any attempt to grip it. Be aware of the delicacy of the sensation in this. Bring your hand away and back, to let go of the desire to grip.

- Let the fingertips lead in again to brush the mug sides, then invite the back of the fingers to fold around, instead of the front of the hand gripping it. Notice that this gives you enough purchase to lift and manipulate it (Fig. 9.10).

- Notice whether your hand wants to tighten in as you continue to hold it, and say no to this. Continue to maintain the spatial relationships between you and the mug.

- Send your fingertips away from you to take it further away and then use your elbow "string" to bring it back

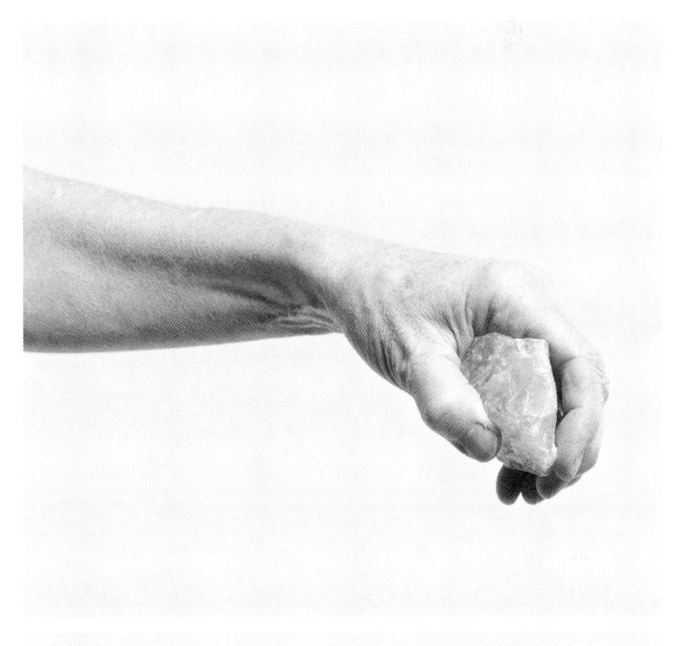

**Figure 9.9**
Grabbing an object, flexors of hand overworking

# CHAPTER nine

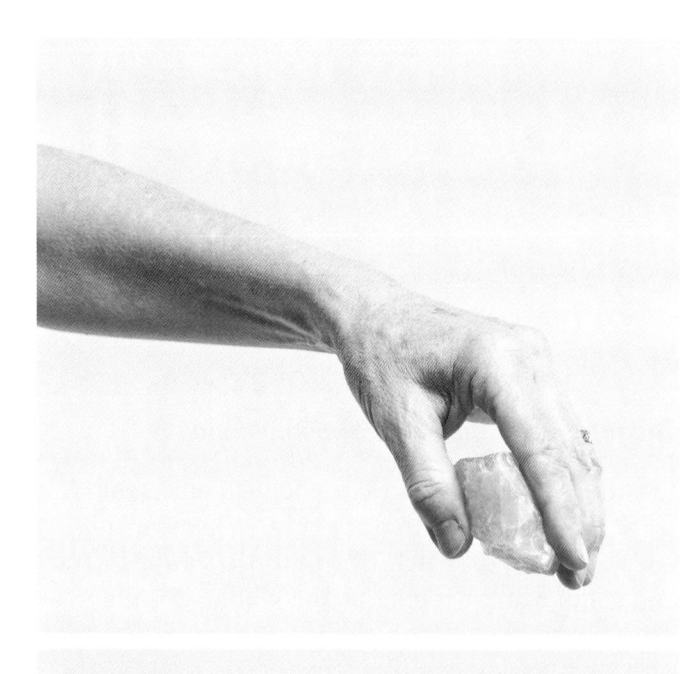

**Figure 9.10**
Hand folding round an object, extensors active, flexors in balance

- *First, pick it up as if you are in a great hurry. Does the elbow tighten sharply? Do you snatch? Is there any sense of space, gentleness, or relationship in the movement?*
- *Now take your time, let the hand fold around the object, and use the rotation of the lower arm so that your hand scoops it towards you. What is the sense of space, gentleness or relationship now (Figs 9.11 and 9.12)?*

We are encouraged to be gentle with ourselves, but often do not know how to get there without feeling false. If we learn to use this simple rotating movement of the lower arm and hand in everyday life, we bring a gentler relationship to our lives.

## Lesson 6  Delicate movements of the hand

Within the hand are three groups of intrinsic muscles: those for working the thumb and little finger in different planes, and those of the hand, called

round the object, there is a possibility of caress in it as the finger pads awaken to sensitivity. The fingers can play on the object as the hand comes alive. The rotation turns the object towards us, so that we come into relationship with it.

The two movements involve a different engagement of shoulder muscles: the snatch from above involves the deltoids and the trapezius muscles across the top of the shoulders, so that we hunch our shoulders a little. In contrast, the scoop leaves the deltoids and trapezius muscles more neutral. Instead, the torso lifts from the base, employing the latissimus dorsi and all the trunk muscles of the lateral and spiral line, along with the upward and opening movement of the arm.

### Exploration 9.12  The rotation of the lower arm

- *Find an item that requires your whole hand (rather than finger and thumb), such as a ball or mobile phone.*

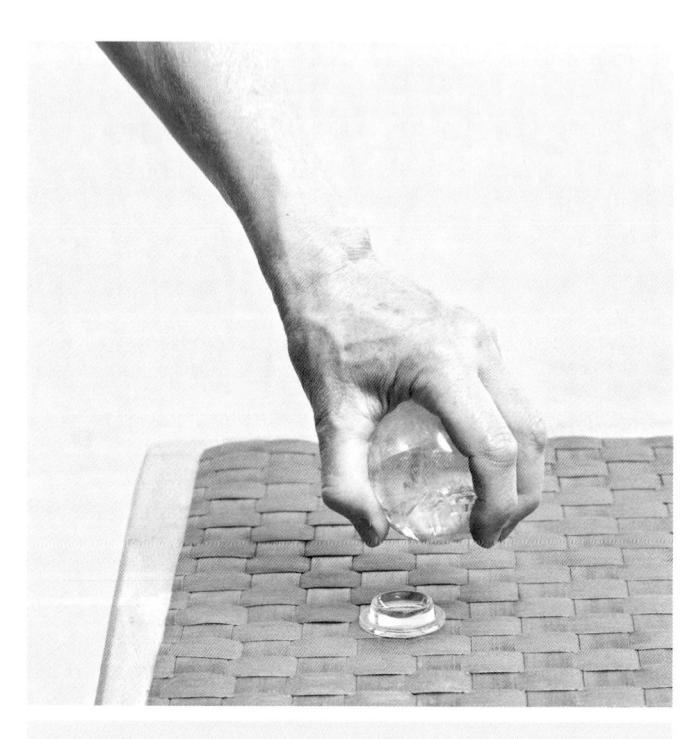

**Figure 9.11**
Snatching an object from above

# Spatial relationships and use of the upper body and arms

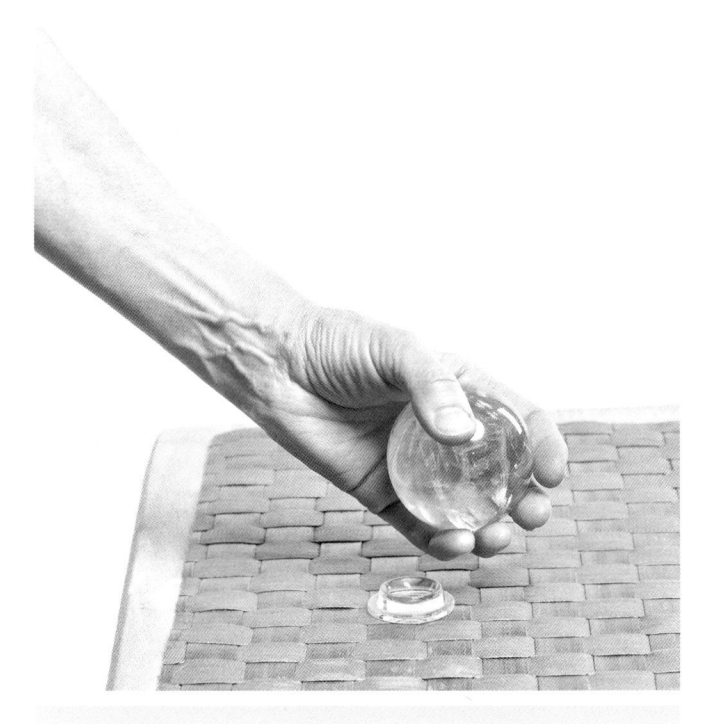

**Figure 9.12**
Using rotation of the lower arm to scoop an object towards oneself

I once took some piano lessons with a very gifted pianist, who asked me to turn my hand into a dead spider by putting it limply upside down on the keyboard. The fingers curling upwards did indeed look like a dead spider – fortunately I am not arachnophobic. Then he asked me to rotate my lower arm so that the hand was turned passively over – becoming a live spider. The fingers were now correctly placed to run all over the keys, with strength, and without interference from the arm. He told me that sometimes, when playing some complex piece of music, he would look down at his hands rampaging up and down the keyboard and wonder whose they were! This total aliveness of the hands, along with a sense of separation, is what we need at all times, and particularly for keyboard use.

### Exploration 9.14    Finding fluidity and strength in the hand, coming from the back

Do all these explorations from full spatial awareness (see Fig. 4.1). Your whole-body is expanding in all planes. This gives a unity from which we can expand into action.

Crawling the fingers:

- Use spatial awareness and oppositions of back of armpit, elbows, and fingertips to bring your fingers to a desk.
- Let your fingertips land like a spider, with the fingertips touching, the lower part of the fingers curled but the knuckles and wrists straight, on a level with the elbow (Fig. 9.13).
- Let the fingers crawl forward gently, pulling the arm behind them. There is friction under the fingertips as the knuckles pull forwards. This results in strong, rolling, conscious movement. You are using the extensors of the hand. If the flexors dominate, the hand will scuttle.
- Crawl the fingers in different directions, playing with the oppositions between knuckles, elbow tips, and inside wrists – the elbow might pull them backwards or sideways, the inside wrist might pull them across the body. Does the ribcage stay open and breathing? Notice that all

the interossei and lumbricales. This latter group act to bend the fingers at the knuckles but straighten the digits, as when we make the hand into a beak (Fig. 9.10).

### Exploration 9.13    The quality of touch

- Contract your arm, pulling it in at shoulders and elbows. Pick up a small object – a pencil or rubber maybe – and play with it between your fingers. Notice the quality of this.
- Put the object down again and open out into extension by using your elbow string and pull to the fingertips. Using opposing directions with spatial awareness, allow your fingers to reach then fold around the object, but keeping the fingers themselves somewhat straight, bending mostly from the knuckles. Play with it there and notice the quality of touch.

# CHAPTER nine

*the joints of the arm can open and close without tension, led by the fingers (Fig. 9.13).*

Snaking the hand in all planes through the air:

- *Let the fingers lead up into the air in the same way, so that the whole arm follows behind. Take your fingers on a snaking journey in all directions and notice all the arm joints opening and closing as needed, the body staying in expansion, balanced, steady and breathing. The arms can play around the torso without response from it.*

- *Without any preformed idea or preparation in the fingers, let them make contact with a light switch and turn it on, open a drawer, etc.*

### Exploration 9.15  Delicacy and strength in the hand for typing, light switches, and cupboards

Typing:

- *Play with typing on a keyboard (or piano), keeping the oppositions between fingertips, elbows and the back of the armpits (and also between inside wrist and front of the armpits if you can manage that many thoughts).*

- *Think of your elbow strings and little fingers to float your arms away from each other over the keys, and inside wrists to float them back in again. Notice that all the strength needed for the task can be provided through these opening lines; you do not need to tighten anything (Fig. 9.14).*

## Lesson 7    Spatial relationships in the arms in everyday life

### Exploration 9.16    Everyday movements

You can explore many movements using these oppositional pulls. Horizontal plane movements, whether circling (e.g. stirring a saucepan) or straight (e.g. cutting bread). Lateral movements of the arm across the body include bowing a stringed instrument, passing the salt, ironing (if you can remember what that is …) or opening

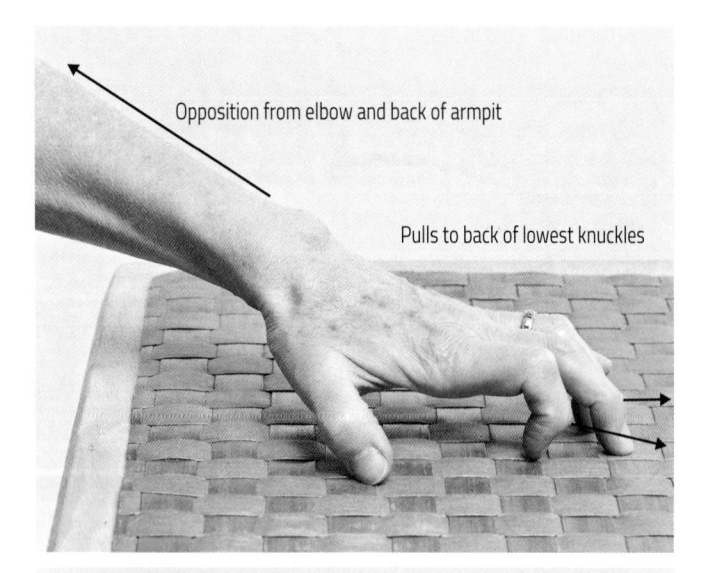

**Figure 9.13**
Playing with oppositions in the back arm lines to find strength in the hand

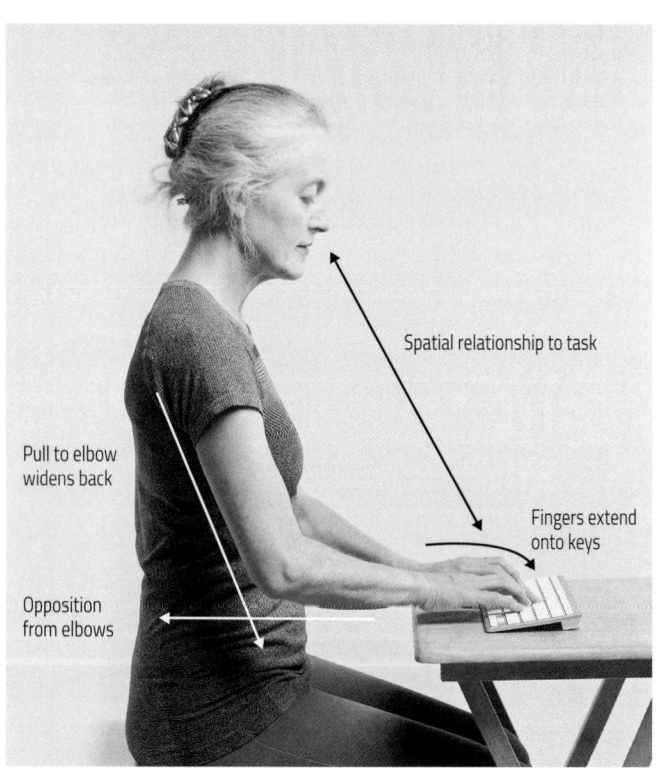

**Figure 9.14**
Typing while maintaining oppositions

# Spatial relationships and use of the upper body and arms

a sliding door or curtains. Vertical movements include painting a wall, pulling down a blind, lifting something off a shelf, wiping down the shower. Combing long hair is a similar action, though in trickier planes. Then there are precise movements, such as writing, sewing, or cutting your nails.

- *Always start by finding your balanced stance, with spatial awareness. I suggest you explore all these movements on their own before you try it with spoon, brush, door handle, etc. Then allow the backs of the fingers to fold around the object, if needed pouring strength from the back and down the back of the arm to hold it more firmly.*

### The connections of the arms to the back

Figure 9.15 is one of Thomas Myers's functional lines that come into play during activity. He comments that the latissimus dorsi and pectoralis major are in effect the trunk extensions of the arm lines through their insertion on the humerus bone. They offer a counter-balancing link from one arm to the gluteus maximus and vastus lateralis (the outer quadriceps) of the opposite leg, then spiraling down the tibialis anterior to the medial arch, in actions such as walking, lunging, or throwing a ball. Since movement is always changing, they are moments of connection in a sweep of forces (Myers 2014: 177). However, I see them as more integral than that. When we utilize the arms and torso as described here, we have ongoing widening of back and chest that keeps the latissimus dorsi and pectoralis major in extension and linked into the toned arms, along with a deeper stabilizing connection through the thoracolumbar fascia. Then they can underpin and strengthen the arm movements possible at any moment.

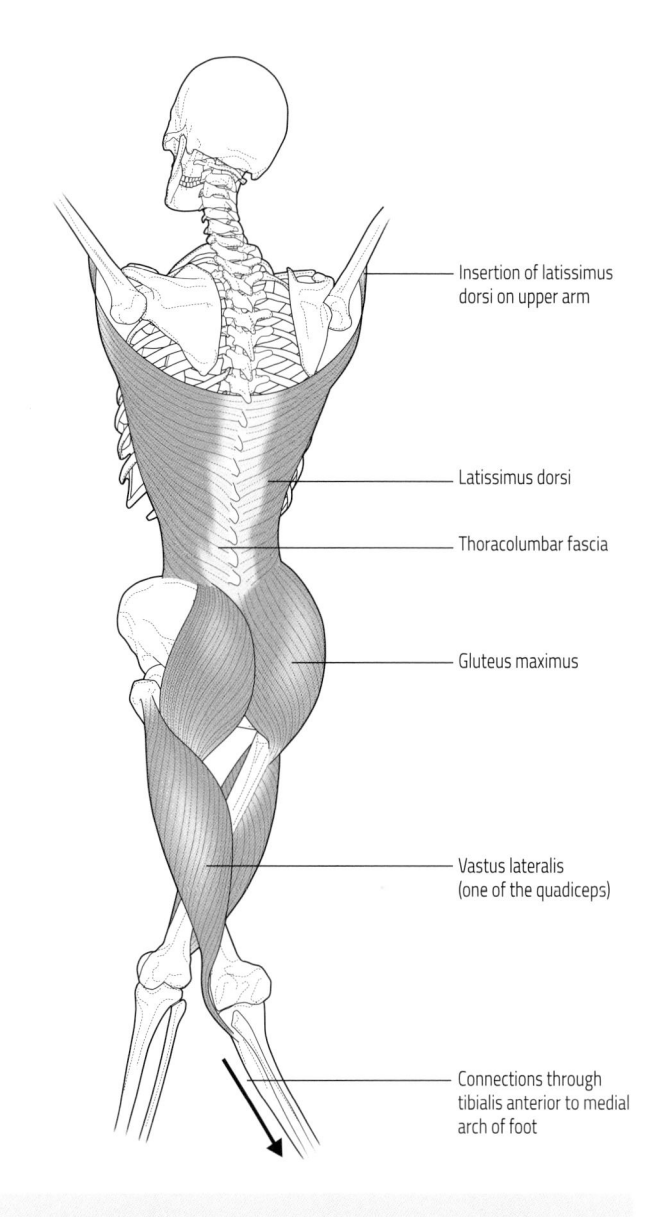

**Figure 9.15**
The functional line

### Exploration 9.17 Giving a massage or kneading bread

- Play with an action that requires pressure from both hands together, such as massaging, or kneading bread. Notice that when the elbows fall in, one is pressing from above and the flexors of the arms take the strain of the action. Then rotate the elbows out and the hands in; notice the whole balance of the movement changes as the extensors come into play and the arms are underpinned by the latissimus dorsi, the supporting muscles of the torso, and the big muscles of the gluteus maximus and legs. A push into the hands now comes right from the back, legs, and feet (Figs 9.16 and 9.17).

# CHAPTER nine

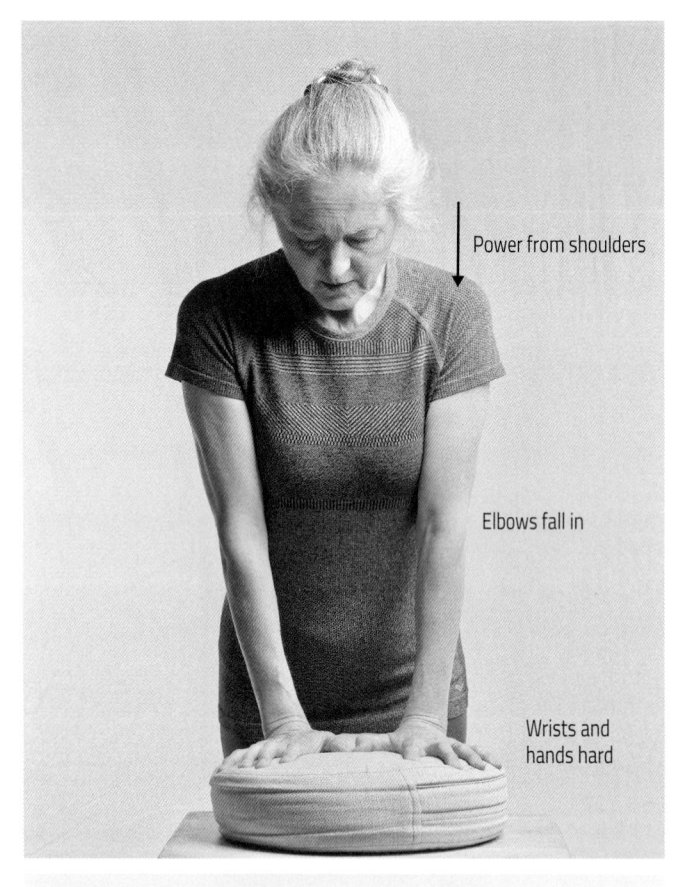

**Figure 9.16**
Narrowing to press down

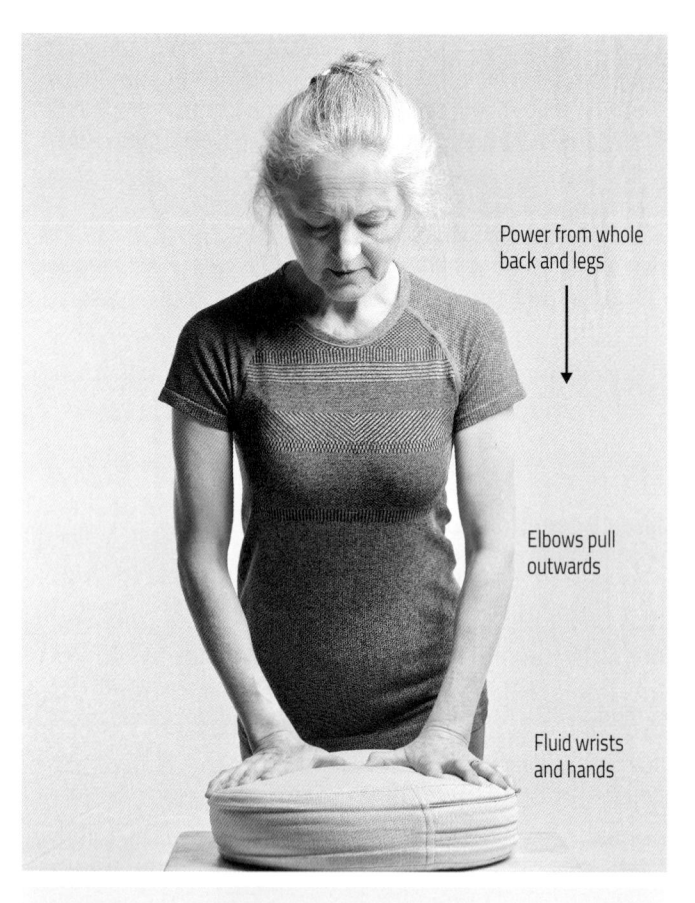

*Labels: Power from shoulders; Elbows fall in; Wrists and hands hard*

**Figure 9.17**
Widening to press down

*Labels: Power from whole back and legs; Elbows pull outwards; Fluid wrists and hands*

## Gesturing as we speak

Gestures are an integral component of communicating; people blind from birth still gesture as they speak (McNeill 2012: 13). But many of us use harsh movements as we gesture, and our hard-won alignment and quietness is lost the moment we open our mouths.

### Exploration 9.18  Playing with gestures

- *Observe your gestures as you speak (or video yourself in conversation). Observe your hands, shoulders, face, and whole-body.*

- *Are your gestures choppy? Are they large and expansive, or tiny, confined within a narrow radius? Do you ever prevent or freeze your gestures? Do your fingers and toes "talk" even when you are still?*

- *Now invite yourself not to make any gesture at all as you speak. Hands are the easiest place to start as we can directly see what they are doing.*

- *This is a useful middle stage, where we let go of habitual patterns of movement that are probably mainly serving to reinforce our tensions and pull us off balance. This initially can feel very boring but will slowly bring a different and much more enjoyable quality.*

- *Once you can leave everything alone as you speak, invite the gestures back in as you talk. Let the hand gestures come from below, maybe rising up off your lap, involving rotation of the hand, rather than from the shoulders and down-slashing movements. Let the backs of the hands and arms be involved, let them flow and swirl. Let the upper body expand and breathe as you talk (Fig. 9.18).*

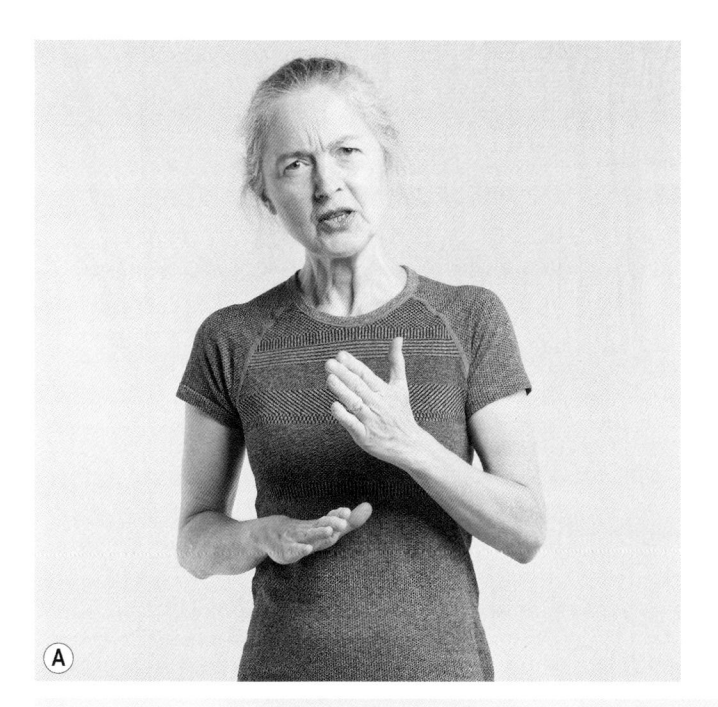

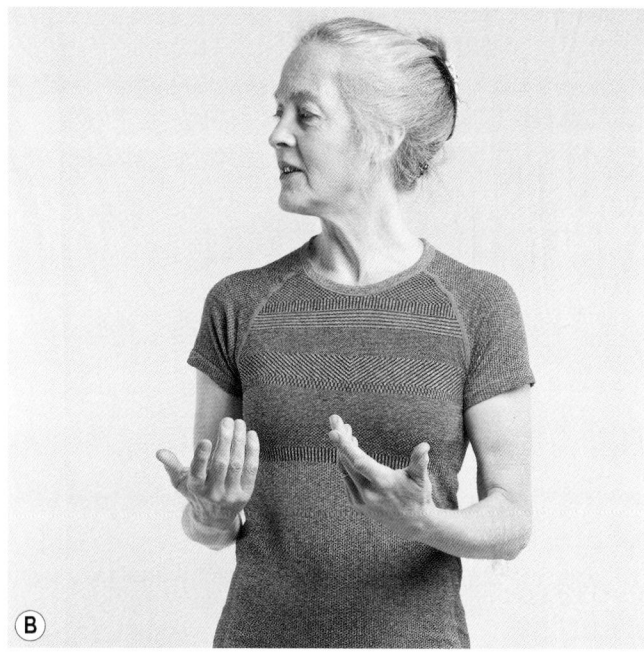

# Spatial relationships and use of the upper body and arms

**Figure 9.18**
Gestures while speaking. **(A)** Harsh downward gestures. **(B)** Gentle upward gestures

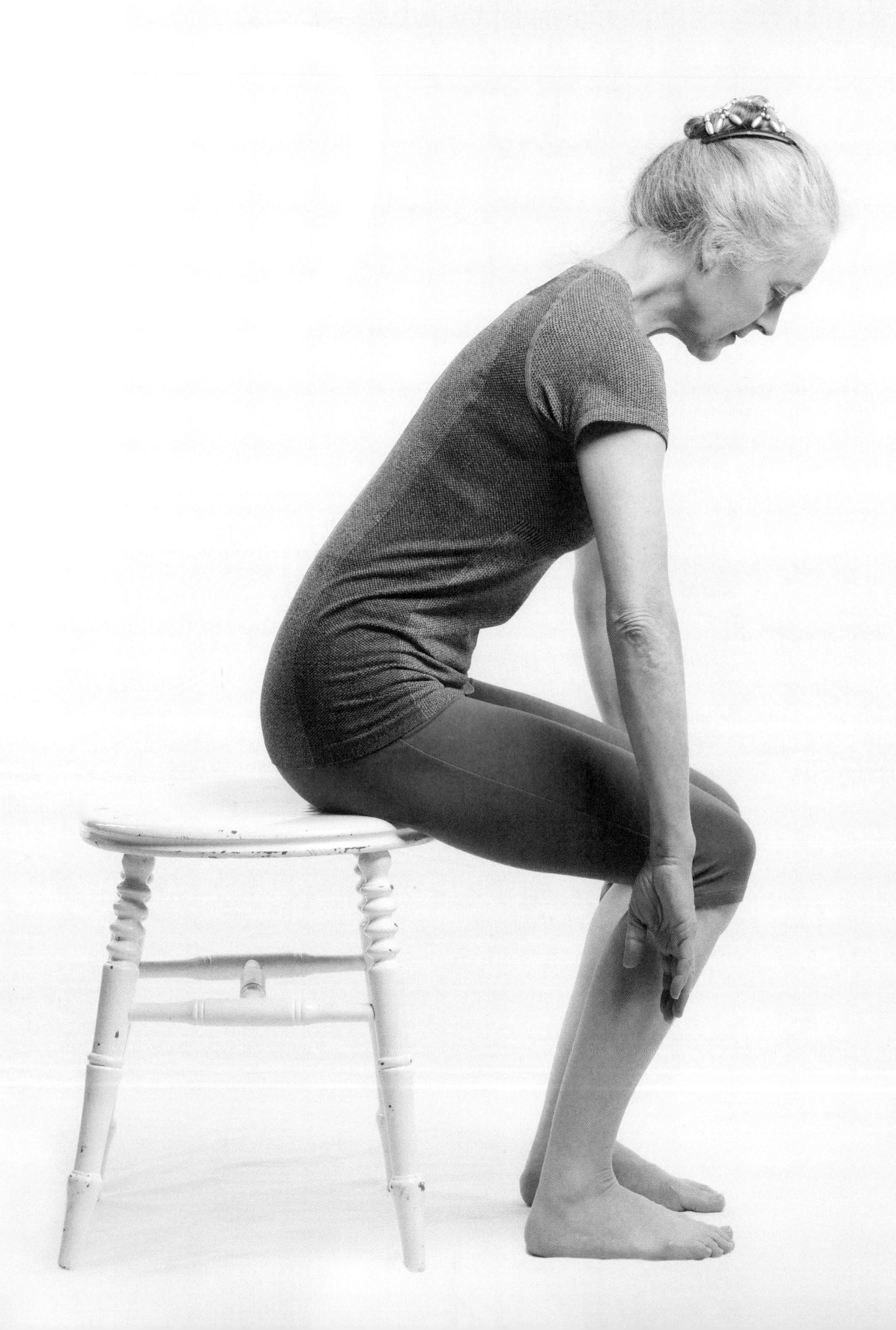

# Toned sitting – integrating the core muscles

## Introduction – why work at sitting and standing?

To move lightly and easily between sitting and standing is an Alexander ideal which is often poorly understood. What are we really trying to achieve, and why do we work quite so hard at it? Why is it so difficult? I consider the core of human movement to be the folding squat, which small children do so effortlessly, though most Westernized adults have long lost this ability. Even those who can squat are often aware of tensions and rarely find its pure, easy form as dynamic modulation of postural tone. To sit on a chair is to perform half a squat. But as we saw in Chapter 3, most people perform all sorts of distortions to bring about this apparently simple movement.

Successful bending requires that the whole system is acting in expansion, rather than collapsing into itself. Particularly, the whole area of the lower body needs to be expanded rather than collapsing into the legs. Since many people are not present in their lower bodies, they have no idea of the extent of the problem. Indeed, I have very rarely seen anyone with full integration through from torso to legs. This chapter seeks to give a full road map of the process.

> **AT info:** As Alexander technique teachers, we have been committed to non-doing. But this requires that someone else makes the strong changes for us. If our teachers do their work well, the changes integrate so fast that there is little or no sensation in the muscles, so that we have as recipients little sense of how the change was brought about. Beautiful though this is, it is unhelpful if later we lose touch with what happened, as we have no road map to recreate it.

Researcher and AT teacher Tim Cacciatore researches how people sit and stand. He has demonstrated (Cacciatore et al. 2014) that trained AT teachers can perform a sit to stand movement (STS) in a smooth sustained manner, shifting weight gradually onto their feet. However, healthy but untrained adults (the control group) cannot do this; they speed up as they approach lifting off from the seat and are unable to change this pattern at will. To perform a smooth STS movement requires:

- moving the mass of the body over the feet while
- using our extensors in legs and back to prevent postural collapse against gravity as we stand.

So we need our extensor muscles, in particular, engaged and always ready to adapt. Flexion (hinging at the hips) happens as gravity pulls the torso into a forward tilt, weighting the feet. In this, the extensor musculature adapts both to allow and to control the forward tilt, from which to stand us up.

Cacciatore observed that the control group could not flex forward sufficiently over their feet while simultaneously weighting the legs/feet. This difficulty could result from stiffer hips and knees, or torsos which hinder the forward movement, or from insufficient adaptivity of postural tone to continuously match the changing forces on the body during weight shift, which is necessary for a slow, smooth movement. They avoided the problem by swinging forward to take off at speed from further back in the chair.

We will look at increasing both springy muscle tone and mobility of the legs in lessons 1 and 2. In lesson 3 we will look in more detail at flexing forward – hinging at the hips, ready to find the full adaptive, springy tone of the torso in Chapter 13.

### *Flexibility versus mobility*

People assume that to stand or sit, one needs flexible hips, knees and ankles, and strong legs (and back). In general, it is thought that flexibility must be addressed separately from strength: for instance, you can watch runners stretching their calves before running, then repeating the stretches after the run has tightened them again. But flexibility work is passive stretching which can leave joints vulnerable. StrongFit coach and physical therapist Dr Sara Solomon runs an online splits program in which

# CHAPTER ten

she distinguishes *flexibility* (the amount you can passively move a joint) and *mobility* (the range of motion that a joint can achieve actively). "The nervous system is always alert for instability in a joint and responds by 'splinting' the joint by tightening various muscles around it. This results in a tight joint, but the answer is not passive stretching. By learning how to engage your proximal stabilizers, you can minimize distal chaos. This frees the joint, giving its full natural mobility" (personal correspondence, August 2019). In other words, when we engage our core hip stabilizers, the outer muscles no longer need to protect the joint stability and can lengthen and engage appropriately.

So going into a squat or sitting requires full *mobility* in the hips, knees, and ankles. The more we can use and stabilize the core muscles, staying with quiet attentiveness, the more mobility we will have in the joints. This works strength, freedom of the joints, and stretchy responsive muscle tone together.

Miss Goldie taught me about the integration of this region as no other teacher could, because she lived it completely herself. What was she doing that was so different? I have been helped in my understanding of this by Masoero's work on the Initial Alexander technique; and by Philip Shepherd's work on Radical Wholeness, through which I learned fully to inhabit the lower body through into the legs. The difference in stability, not just of the physical body but also on my sense of being, was worth the work. The functional anatomy of this can be explained by the head to toes connections of core muscles in the deep front line and the front to back connectivity of the thoracolumbar fascia.

### Are these moves "doing" or "non-doing"?

When we start this unfamiliar work, we will probably be working quite physically opening out tensions. During this, I notice the brain is re-connecting to the re-awakened muscles, so that we can use integrated programs for change. We want to do these from brain/embodied intelligence so they become completely non-doing. With time, you may find these movements happening by themselves, demonstrating that they are the natural alignment of the body, in harmony with relaxed and fully alive states of being. Remember FACTISPAL (see Chapter 7).

## Lesson 1   Keeping the legs switched on while sitting, even at a desk

### Introduction – how are you currently sitting?

The writer Aldous Huxley was a keen pupil of F. M. Alexander's in the 1930s. Despite the technique then being almost entirely chairwork, Huxley saw its full potential and excitedly shared it with the Indian guru Krishnamurti. The guru didn't get it. He responded drily that there is more to life than getting in and out of a chair.

But in modern life, for many people, is there more to life? As we discussed in Chapter 2, sitting, the curse of the computer age, is the new smoking – and chain smoking at that. Many people are aware they collapse their torsos into a slump as they sit. What is more surprising to discover is that we lose much of our support for the torso by collapsing the legs and feet. This is so endemic we mostly do not know what full leg and foot tone looks like.

> Alexander stated the ideal that one could sit at a desk and yet be exercising. "If ... he had learned to use his muscles consciously ... In his most sedentary occupations he could have been using and exercising his muscular system without resort to any violent contortions, waving of the arms or kicking of the legs ... he should have used his muscular mechanism in such a way that its uses could have been applied to the simplest acts, such as sitting on a stool in writing at a desk ... the whole physical machinery would have been coordinated and adapted to his way of life" (Alexander 2011: 92).

# Toned sitting – integrating the core muscles

### Exploration 10.1    How do you sit on a chair?

- Observe yourself sitting on your chair. Are you slumped, behind your sitting bones, or braced upright, with slight forward tilt of the pelvis?
- Now observe your legs. Are they drawn in towards you, crossed, or pulled under you? Does that help maintain your upright position by bracing the lower body? Let them move to flat on the floor and observe what changes in your torso.
- Are they now "relaxed" – with feet flat and weighing on the floor? Goldie observed that such legs are often heavy and lifeless, even though they offer some support to the torso.
- Now bounce your legs up and down for a minute, finding their springiness. Bring them back to stillness, but without letting the tone go (as in stopping without stopping, exploration 6.15), or bracing the back or belly. What do you notice?

Goldie reminded me repeatedly to keep my legs alive. This next exploration switches the legs on much more fully, and through this wakes up the whole torso. Initially it will be unfamiliar to hold this much tone while sitting still, so build it up gently. Then you can use it during desk work, with a 1-2-3 to restore flagging tone, say every half an hour. Alexander's ideal is possible – we can get fit while sitting still.

In exploration 8.12 we explored the placement of the feet and untwisting the leg spirals while standing. Here we explore this while sitting. You will need a mirror at ground level.

### Exploration 10.2    Aligning the feet and legs while sitting

**Stage 1:** bring your legs and feet into the alignment they would have when standing

- Sit on the edge of your chair so thighs don't touch the chair – it is easier to maintain an upright spine when the pelvis is able to move freely. (Try sitting back and notice the difference.)
- Align your thighs parallel to each other (look down at your thighs to check).
- Bring the lower leg vertical, with heels hip-width apart (look in the mirror).
- Align the outside of your feet parallel (Fig. 8.9), by lifting and swiveling the big toe. You can now see your big toes between your knees. There is now a diagonal between your big toes and your inside heels (Fig. 10.1; compare Fig. 3.9).

**Stage 2:** the three pulls to rebalance the foot

Your legs and feet are now parallel as when standing, but may feel twisted or imbalanced.

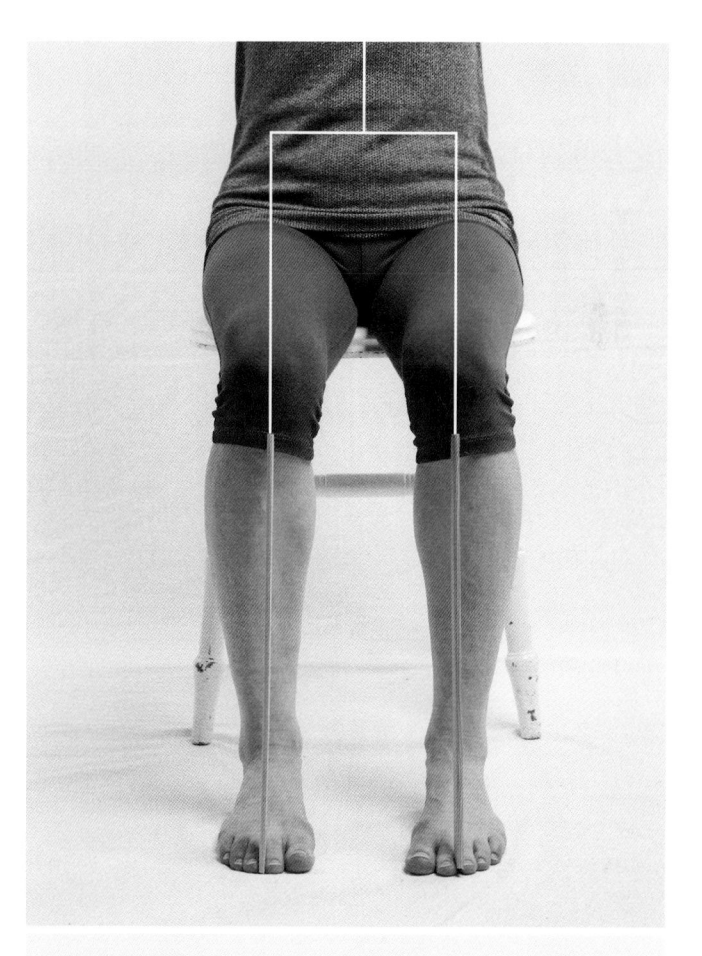

**Figure 10.1**
Support from feet and legs while sitting

# CHAPTER ten

We use the three pulls of Chapter 8 to rebalance the muscle patterns: play with them to start with until you loosen up the ankle joints, and your foot understands them.

- *Pull the instep of each foot towards the midline, until the outside foot will lift off. Keep the inside heel pushed firmly down.*

- *"Screw the ankle" by pulling the inner ankle bone away and up from the big toe back on the diagonal. Can you feel your calves working (Fig. 10.2A).*

- *This can pull the knee in too. With the inside heel and ball of the big toe pushed firmly down, use your hand to pull the knee away from the instep (i.e. outwards). Do this very gently until you feel a resistance under the instep as tibialis anterior is stretched (Fig. 10.2B). This can feel like hard work!*

- *Keep watching your toes — have they turned out? Keep them aligned with the big toes inside the line of the heels (see Fig. 8.9).*

- *Once you have the sense of this inside leg stretch, keep screwing the ankle while you rotate the thighs outwards, by bringing iliac spines up and back, up away from the outside of the lower knee. Take the pubococcygeals forwards and ribs back so you do not arch the lower back (Fig. 10.3).*

Your legs and feet are now switched on! Do this whenever you sit, initially in short bursts of a few seconds each.

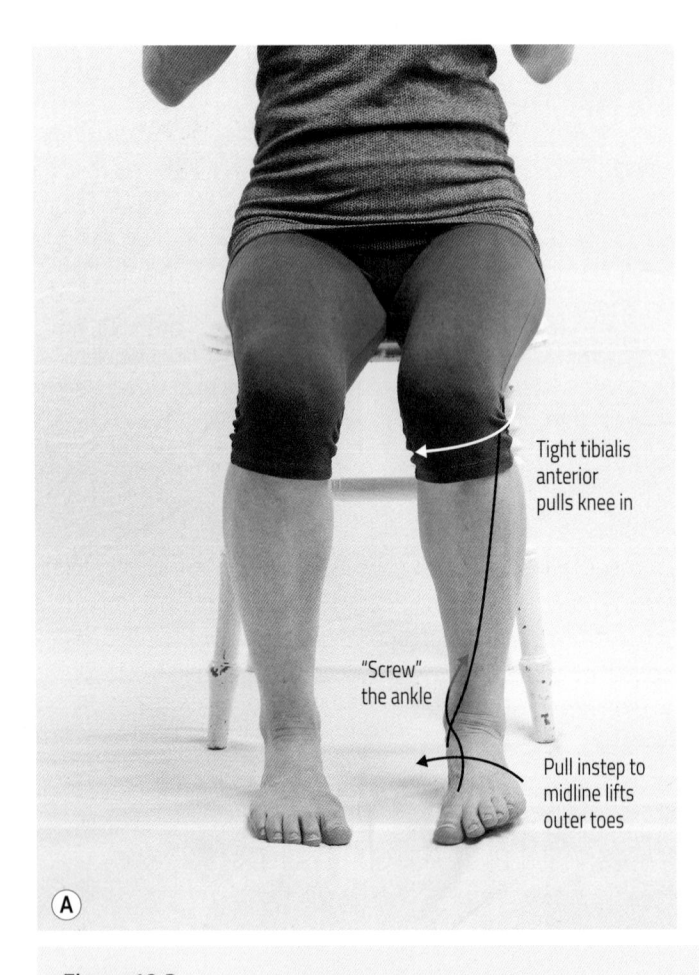

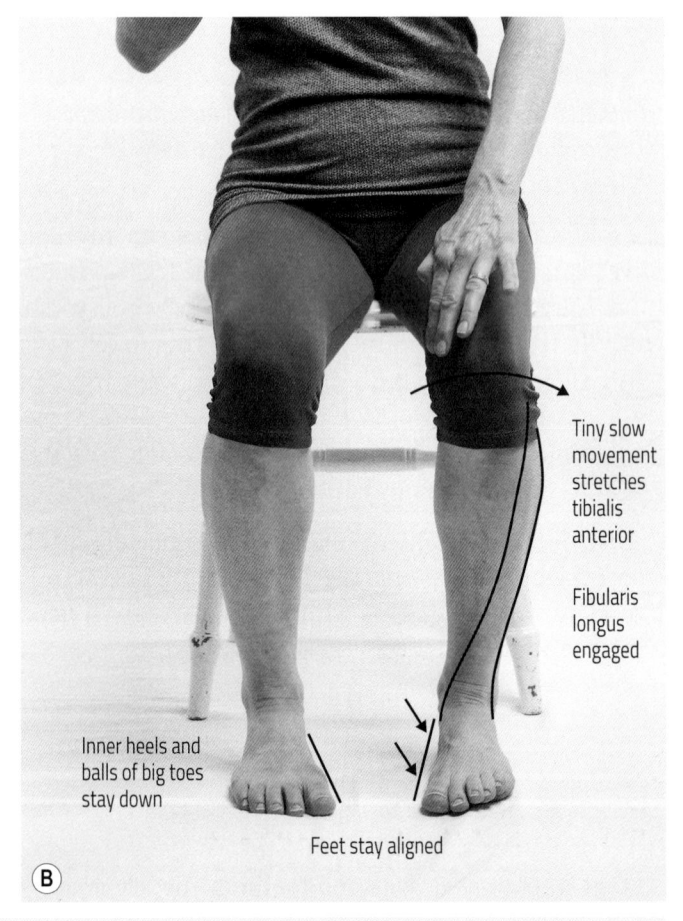

**Figure 10.2**
**(A)** Pulling instep to midline engages fibularis longus. **(B)** Counter-rotating the thigh stretches tibialis anterior

# Toned sitting – integrating the core muscles

*Exploration 10.3  Integrating the directions for legs and feet*

- While sitting in a balanced position, think your directions precisely, from embodied intelligence and spatial awareness. Initially, do one foot at a time. Video yourself or use a mirror – remember that sensory perception of new movements is notoriously unreliable. Directions are a map into the unknown, and it may initially be uncomfortable.

  *I send the big toe balls and inside heels to the floor (1).*

  *I pull the inner ankle bone back and up on the diagonal (2).*

  *I pull the iliac spines up and back, up away from the outside lower knee (3).*

  *I pull the ribs back and the pubococcygeals forward (4).*

- Move to a count of 1-2-3 (Fig. 10.4).
- Check all the details of your alignment now; did you manage all the movements? Keep having a go until your nervous system has integrated these moves. Check for unnecessary tension (see exploration 7.7).
- Once you have these three moves working together, add in directions for the upper torso (see exploration 7.10).

This reintegration will take time! Keep giving your nervous system another chance to sort it out. You are getting somewhere when you notice different movements or qualities afterwards.

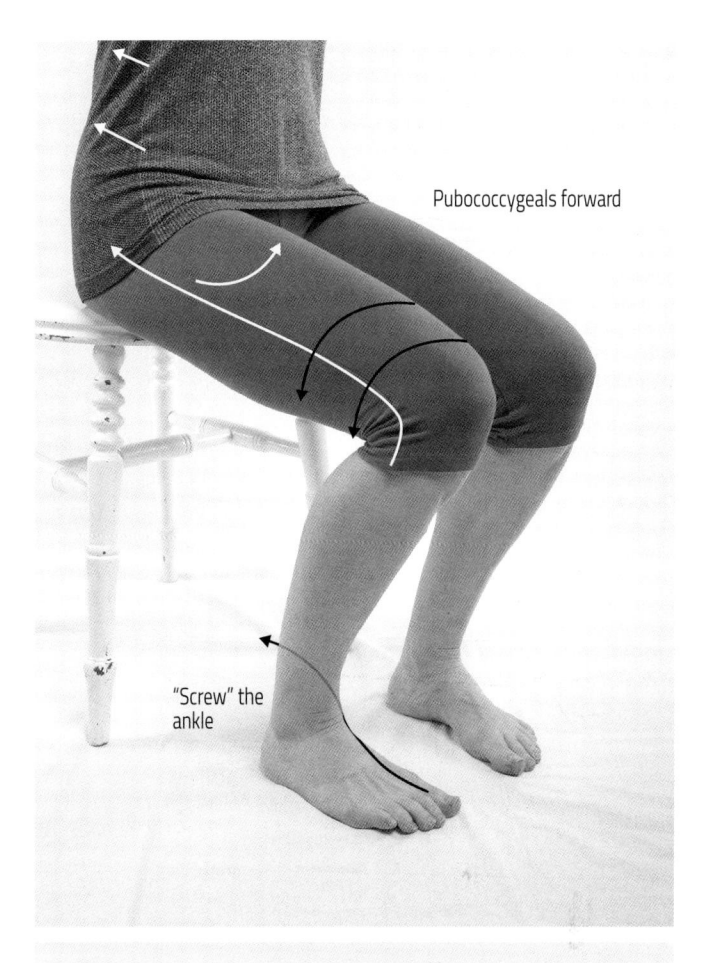

**Figure 10.3**
Counter-rotating the thighs

I explored thinking these pulls to the feet in a swimming pool, where one has no resistance to work against. The flipper stroke of my feet for crawl, which had always been weak, suddenly powered in, and I shot across the pool!

## Lesson 2  Sit to stand using the new alignment of the legs and feet

As people age, they often push more heavily on their legs to stand, applying force in increasingly inappropriate ways. By the time they are elderly, their legs seem too weak, and they haul themselves around with their arms using hand-rails, walking frames etc. If muscles are wasting with age, why do they not waste equally? Muscles mostly weaken with lack of use. When we use these new alignments to stand and sit, we can observe how usually we do not fully engage the leg muscles in everyday actions. Poor alignment with gravity, poor core muscle patterns, insufficient use, and lack of embodied consciousness are all factors. I speculate that this is partly why legs weaken disproportionately with age.

# CHAPTER ten

### Exploration 10.4   To stand utilizing the full engagement of the legs

We are going to take this in four stages, repeating the directions each time to keep all muscles engaged throughout.

**Stage 1:** engage legs and torso

- *Sit on the edge of your chair, with legs and feet aligned.*
- *Draw your feet back towards the chair to make standing easier.*
- *To engage the core muscles and the inner torque chain, we emphasize the weight through the inside of the knee, the inside heel, and the big toe balls, de-emphasizing the outside of the foot.*

   *I send big toe balls and inside heels to the floor (1).*

   *I pull the inner ankle bone back and up on the diagonal (2).*

   *I pull the iliac spines up and back, up away from the outside lower knee (3).*

   *I pull the ribs back and the pubococcygeals forward (4).*

   *I pull the top of the sternum up away from the sitting bones (5).*

   *I pull my elbows forward and outwards opening the deep back arm line (not pictured).*

- *Think the directions with spatial awareness while inhibiting any response, then give yourself a 1-2-3 (Fig. 10.4).*

**Stage 2:** tilting forwards

- *Give yourself another 1-2-3, as you incline forwards, keeping legs, feet, and iliac spines engaged as the weight comes onto them.*
- *Do not jump, push, or lift your shoulders! Don't be impatient!*
- *Let the arms hang vertically, as you tilt, and stop when your extended fingers point to an inch (3 cm) beyond your instep, and the top of your sternum is over your instep. Keep front and back of upper body supported by widening through the arm lines.*

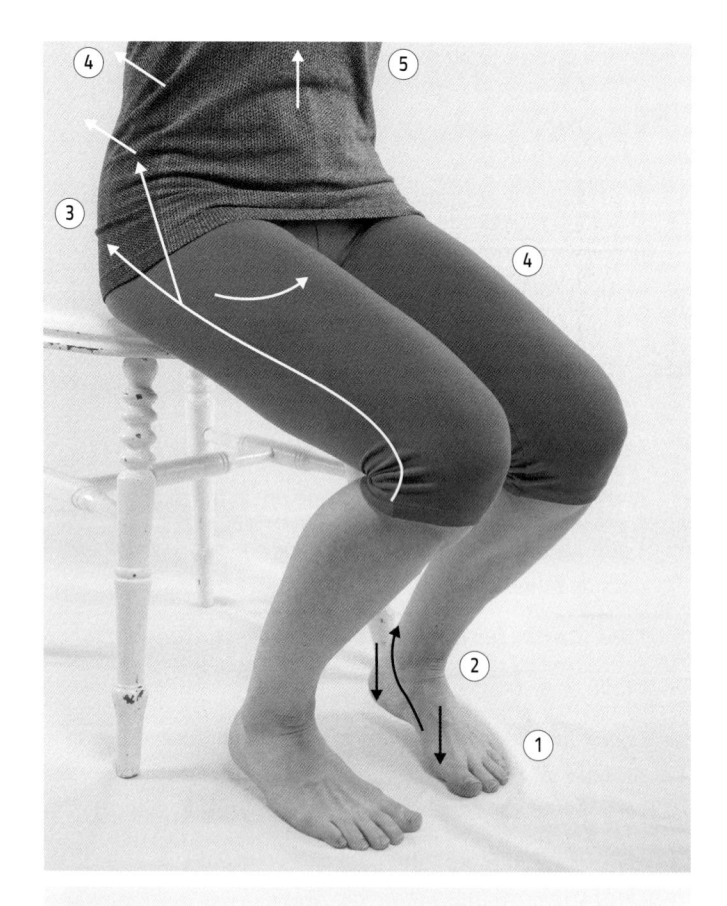

**Figure 10.4**
Integrated pulls to engage feet and legs (see text for directions)

**Stage 3:** engaging friction and downforce with the whole foot

- *Push your heels forwards towards your toes, but do not let them slide. Notice that the forward impulse is translated into a strong downforce. This provides friction and downforce that will send the body back and up.*

**Stage 4:** to stand

- *Repeat the directions, then as you count 1-2-3, push your heels towards your toes, engage the legs strongly and you may stand easily! We have activated all the major support lines – superficial back and front lines, lateral, spiral, and deep front lines (see lesson 3) by fully engaging the feet and legs (Fig. 10.5).*

**Stage 5:** to sit again

# Toned sitting – integrating the core muscles

## Lesson 3   The anatomy of integration, finding our core muscles, and active hip folding

### *The integrating psoas muscles*

The lumbar spine transmits most of the body weight but has no obvious supporting structure around it. There have been many theories over the years of how best to protect it (Bowman 2017: 144). In the 1980s: press your back flat on the floor (particularly with sit-ups and ab-crunches). This force-loaded the back and caused injuries. In the 1990s: keep a curve in the lumbar spine. The ensuing shortening and narrowing of the lumbar region forced other muscles to overwork to compensate. In the 2000s: the transversus abdominis was employed, with the instruction "pull the navel back to the spine and hold it there." This is preferable, but simplistic. "The belly supports the back" was a concept many of my pupils had been told by physios. It made no sense to me – surely there were back muscles that supported the back?

Alongside this, researchers were investigating the real functions of the mysterious psoas muscle group. The psoas major is the deepest muscle in the body and is *the only muscle that links the spine and legs* – running from the inside thigh to the sides of the lumbar spine. The iliacus runs from the inside thigh to the inside of the iliac crest. (The psoas minor is weak or absent.) Together, they are called the iliopsoas (Fig. 10.6). They were known to be hip flexors, but were they also spinal rotators? or lateral flexors? This thinking is too specific. I understand them as the fluid, supporting, integrating core, involved in *all* the movements of the lower body, transmitting and integrating the movement between the torso and legs, in cooperation with all the surrounding muscles.

Look again at Figure 6.6 for the front to back connectivity of the lumbar region. The psoas major muscles nestle on the front of the lumbar spine, while the erector spinae and deeper multifidi surround it at the back (Fig. 10.6). Together they support the lumbar spine – *but only if the back is lengthening and widening.* Then they are also aided by the balanced tone of the quad-

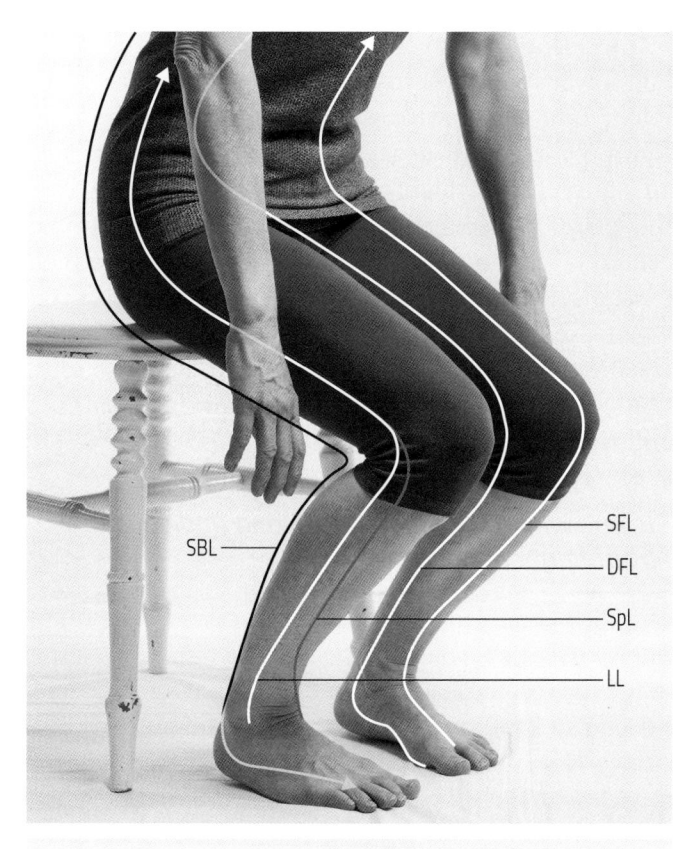

**Figure 10.5**
Integrating pulls of feet and legs engage all muscle trains to stand. Spiral (SpL), lateral (LL), superficial front (SFL), superficial back (SBL), and deep front (DFL) lines

- *Engage everything again to return to the chair: prepare, then repeat your 1-2-3 as you move.*

### How strong are your legs?

Watch yourself in a mirror. Can you come to standing or sitting without the knees moving toward or away from each other? You may need to engage the pelvic area, legs, inside ankles and feet repeatedly till the legs stay stable during the movement. *When the right balance of muscles engages, strength arrives by itself.* We will need these strong, fully engaged legs for stronger walking and movement patterns in later chapters.

Sit and stand in this way each day at the beginning of desk work, or before a meal. Once we are involved in the task, we often forget our use again. So work towards refreshing this with a 1-2-3 each time you take a break.

# CHAPTER ten

Erector spinae

Psoas major

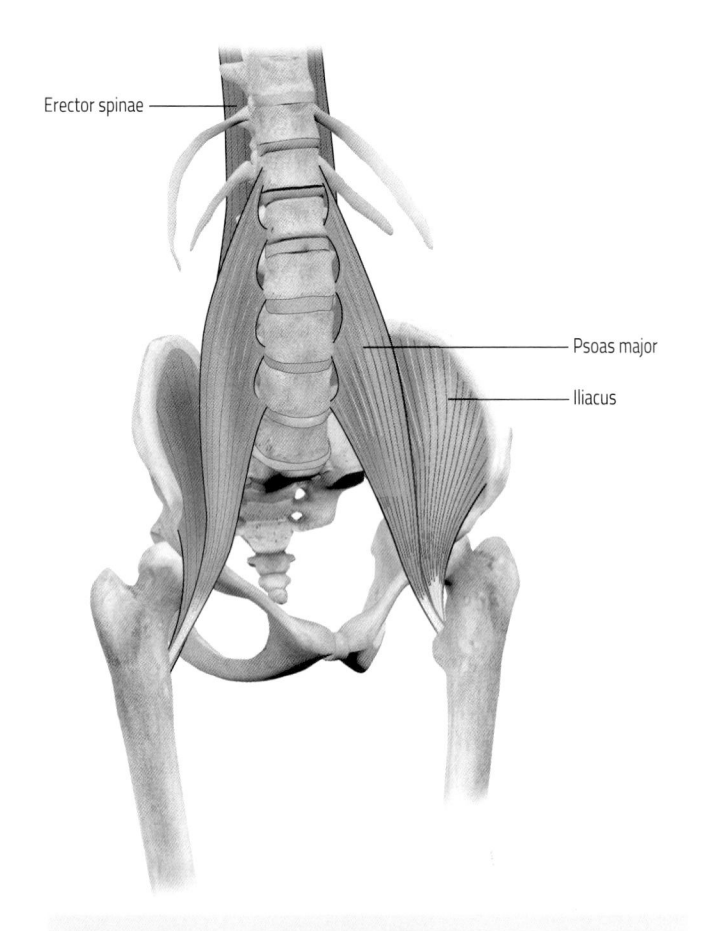

Iliacus

**Figure 10.6**
Balance of erector spinae and psoas to support the lumbar spine

The psoas are also crucial for integrating the upper and lower torso, where the upper parts of the psoas major interweave with the roots of the diaphragm. Many people "fall apart" here in a slump, or "fix" an apparently straight spine by constriction across this zone. The solar plexus, an important emotional center, is here, along with the adrenal glands, which explains why we quickly clamp this area up again when stressed. When we open and calm this zone by freeing the floating ribs to breathe, we begin to integrate the upper and lower body, linking breathing and walking (Myers 2014: 198).

## Playing with the belly muscles, and finding your natural flat stomach

The instruction to "hold one's tummy in" was one I knew well as a teenager, especially in dance classes; it made me feel tense and rather sick. Like most people, I used my upper rectus abdominis – the muscles that run vertically from pubic bone to ribs. These are flexor muscles, on the superficial front line (Fig. 3.22). When engaged directly, they pull the ribs down toward the pubic bone, and so shorten and narrow the stature.

### Exploration 10.5    Exploring the belly muscle problem

- *"Pull your tummy in" – notice how the front of the body caves slightly and narrows, and the pelvis tucks under. Can you now breathe freely (Fig. 10.7)?*
- *Let your belly muscles go, so that your belly hangs forward. Does this tilt the top of your pelvis forward? Fig. 7.17A)*

ratus lumborum, the latissimus dorsi, and all the belly muscles which come naturally into play around them.

But mostly, the balance of these deep muscles has been disrupted by years of sitting. With the hips in constant flexion, the psoas (and quads) shorten to this new length (see Fig. 2.1). When we stand, these shortened muscles pull the pelvis into a tilt. This contracts the erector spinae, arching the lumbar spine, tightening the quads into the hips. The rectus abdominis is now over-lengthened, and the belly spills forward. Without knowledge of how to use a quiet nervous system to lengthen all these deep, over-contracted muscles, no wonder the belly muscles were frequently invoked to help.

The general advice in Alexander circles is to leave one's tummy alone. This was certainly a relief to me on starting AT lessons, so I let my belly protrude and told myself this was how women really are. Then on moving to London I found a new teacher, who put her hand on my belly and announced: "Nice little pot we have here! We can soon do something about that!" Within a few months she had taken an inch off my

# Toned sitting – integrating the core muscles

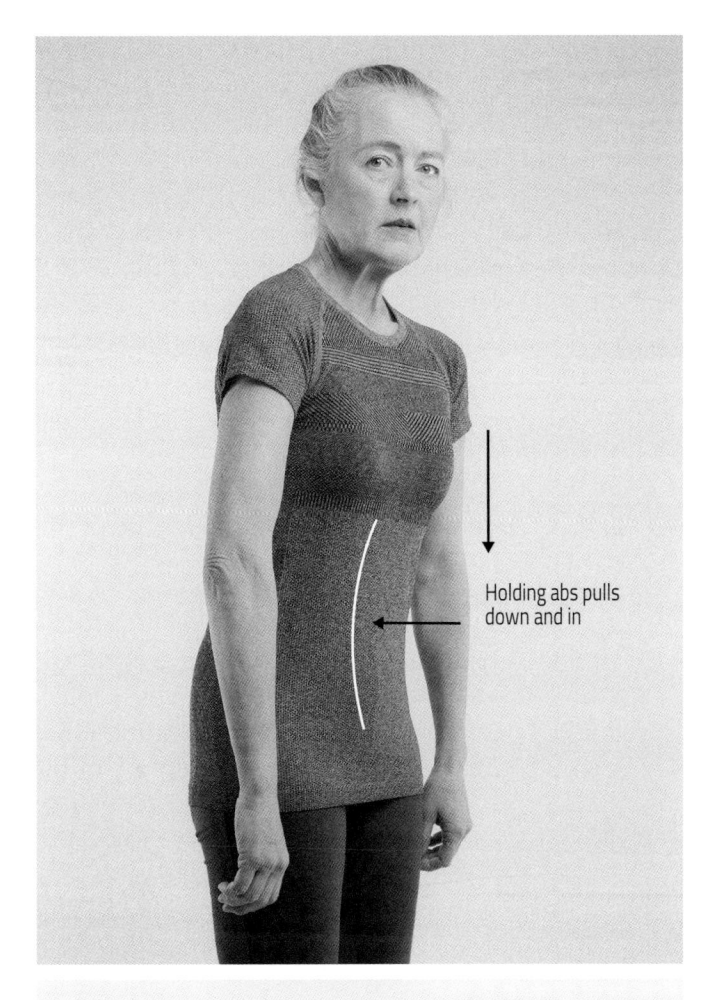

**Figure 10.7**
Holding the belly in with rectus abdominis (abs)

*Holding abs pulls down and in*

> Alexander describes the beneficial organ positioning and massage brought about by positions of mechanical advantage such as leaning back in a chair (2011: 157–9, 228). Thomas Myers also discusses the relationship between organ position and the "myofascial superstructure" of the body, with the need for free movement between them for optimal health, giving us "spatial medicine" (2014: 30). This free movement can only happen when the body is in physical balance.

In Chapter 8, lesson 6 we explored widening across the hips with the breath, rather than letting the belly fall forward. This encourages more tone in the belly muscles, though without ever gripping them. Methods that encourage the tight holding of core muscles miss the fact that muscles need to be responsive to changing circumstances. Toned belly muscles can engage responsively to the load placed on them, while tightened ones are locked and flaccid ones are unresponsive (Bowman 2017: 145).

Of the four layers of belly muscles, external oblique, internal oblique, rectus abdominis, and transversus abdominis, the last is the deepest layer– except at the very lowest part. About halfway between the navel and pubic bone, the rectus abdominis dives through pockets in the transversus abdominis to become the deepest muscle (Fig. 10.8). When we can bring awareness and aliveness to these deepest muscles, the base of the body really engages and many actions we are exploring in this book become much easier. We began to explore this with breathing (exploration 6.13), and now we will take this further.

### Finding the core muscles of the deep front line

The deep front line of the body is complex (Fig. 10.9), and encompasses many areas. Rather than trying to understand it intellectually, we will use breathing to discover it from the inside. Myers comments that it is better envisaged as a series of volumes (2014: 145). These can be spaces, such as the pelvic floor, abdominal or chest cavity, or groups of muscles that

waist measurement and left me much flatter, which was wonderful, but as usual I had no idea how she did it. Now I do!

There are girdles sold for women – flat tubes of rubber, which encircle the lower body to hold the belly in. The transversus abdominis (Figs 10.8 and 7.15), along with the external and internal oblique muscles, forms just such a girdle, already installed in our bodies. We only need to learn to use it. When engaged, these muscles bring the abdominal organs back into better relationships within the body, allowing them to work much more efficiently (Fig. 7.17B). This is evidenced by frequent improvements to pupils' constipation and gut problems, period pains, and menstrual problems, etc.

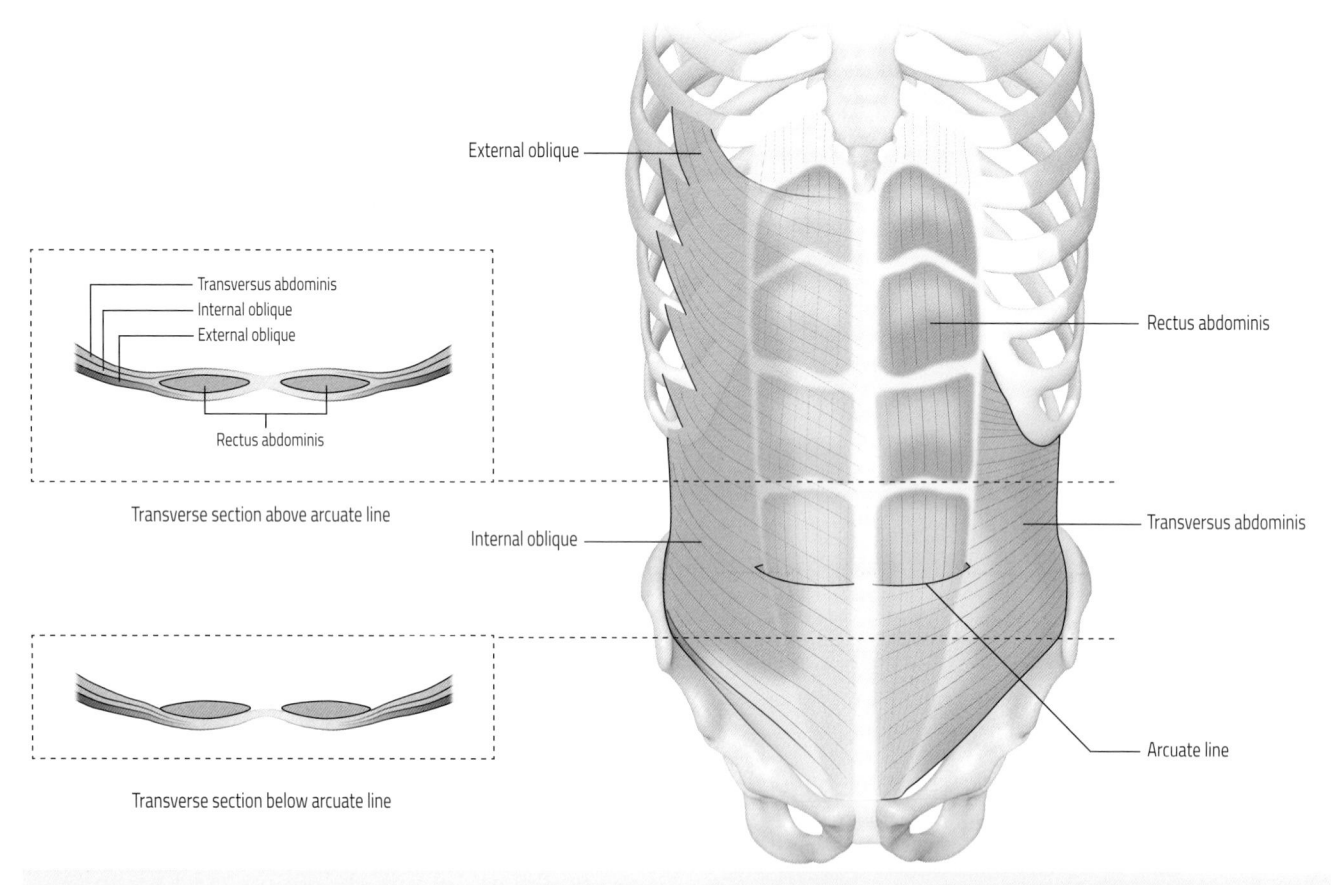

# CHAPTER ten

**Figure 10.8**
The four layers of belly muscles. The rectus abdominis dives below the transversus abdominis at the "arcuate line"

form three-dimensional arrangements, such as the adductors, psoas, or infrahyoids. We will use six stages; I suggest you take them a bit at a time until your embodied intelligence comprehends the whole picture.

### Exploration 10.6  Finding the core muscles of the deep front line through breathing

**Stage 1:** preparation

- *Lie in semi-supine and let go of over-involvement with the breath. We can only find core muscles from quiet awareness.*
- *See the ceiling with spatial awareness, being aware of the breath flowing in and out. On the out-breath, the belly falls towards the back, and the in-breath takes care of itself. How little can you do? Disengage from tensions and over-involvement by keeping mind in the brain (Chapter 4, lesson 4). You may notice the out-breath becoming much longer.*

**Stage 2:** the connection between the back and the legs

Finding the back wall of the abdomen – the psoas and quadratus lumborum (see Fig. 6.3).

- *Take the consciousness deeper within the belly. On the out-breath the organs fall back towards the spine, and up along it. On the in-breath, they move down and wide into the pelvic floor.*

# Toned sitting – integrating the core muscles

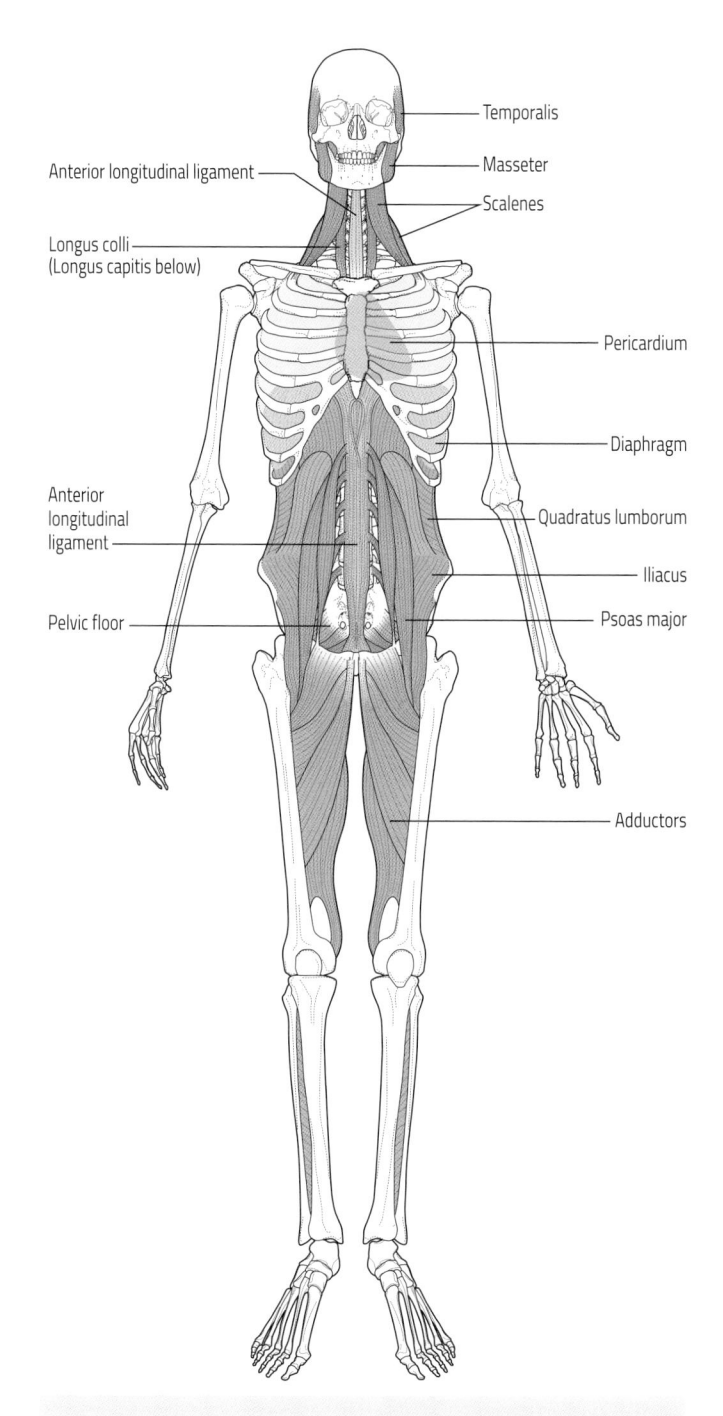

**Figure 10.9**
Deep front line, front view

- We are inviting the psoas muscles to lengthen, and with them, the erector spinae. Notice the lower back flattening and widening on the floor.

  The adductors make fascial links to the psoas.

- The out-breath moves the torso up and off the legs, allowing the legs to lengthen away. Notice the thighs lengthening upward as the psoas lengthens. The inner line of the legs – the big adductor muscles – are also lengthening and working, sending weight down into the balls of the big toes.

- Let your consciousness fall back with the out-breath, till you are aware of the inside of the iliac crest. You may be aware of the iliacus lengthening from inside the iliac crest to inside thigh. Above the iliac crest, the quadratus lumborum muscles angle back in towards the spine. Can you feel them widening on the in-breath?

  The pelvic floor – the bottom of the abdominal cavity – makes numerous fascial connections to adductors and psoas.

- Be aware of the pelvic floor moving down and wide on the in-breath, up on the out-breath. It holds tone throughout its range.

  The diaphragm forms the top of the abdominal cavity, and its roots intermingle with the top of the psoas major and the quadratus lumborum.

- The movement of the diaphragm is in parallel to the pelvic floor.

**Stage 3:** finding the very deepest belly muscles

There are fascial links from psoas, to pelvic floor, to pubic bone, to lowest part of the rectus abdominis, and up this to the ribs at the solar plexus.

- Gently engage your pubococcygeals, running from coccyx to pubic bone. This will slightly tilt the base of your pelvis forward so that the lumbar spine lengthens still further.

- Be aware of the pubococcygeals on the pubic bone now linking to the very lowest part of the rectus abdominis and toning this lowest part of the belly.

# CHAPTER ten

- *As these deepest belly muscles engage, the superficial front line lengthens. Then the superficial back line can also open, so that the neck lengthens upward.*

**Stage 4:** widening the whole torso on the in-breath

- *Notice the sitting bones widening on the base of the pelvic floor. Let this widen the groins and femoral triangle (see Fig. 8.11).*
- *Notice the deep hip rotators widening across the back of the hips.*
- *Notice the back of the pelvic floor widening. This includes the piriformis muscle (which when tight, causes sciatica). Be aware of the lumbar spine widening – the thoracolumbar fascia, quadratus lumborum, and latissimus dorsi.*

Widening from the belly muscles.

- *Keep pulling the iliac spines back and wide on the in-breath, so that the belly cannot puff forward (as in exploration 8.13). This further widens the lower back.*
- *Put your hands cross-wise on your hips, your forearms mirror the line of the obliques. Invite the in-breath to come fully into the sides and back of the abdomen rather than puffing up the front. This widens the mid-back. Here you might notice the inferior posterior serratus muscles pulling the lower ribs wide as the diaphragm descends.*

The whole volume of the abdominal cavity.

- *The whole abdominal cavity is being opened into a wider and straighter stretchy tube. Be aware how much easier movement now is for the wave of displacement that flows like a plunger down from diaphragm to pelvic floor and up again. This ensures the organs are moved and massaged as intended, without being displaced forward or compressed in inappropriate planes.*

**Stage 5:** the volume of the chest

From the diaphragm, there is connection into the pericardial sac around the heart, the pleural sacs around the lungs, and the fascia around the esophagus (gullet) and trachea (windpipe). At the top of the chest, there are fascial connections into the deep front arm lines – perhaps giving the healing link between heart and palms of hands. The transversus thoracis (see exploration 12.9) widens the front of the chest from the inside.

- *Be aware of all these opening with the breath. Can you be present in these deeper layers, rather than caught in superficial ones? Can your breath now flow into the back of the neck, rather than catching in the front?*

**Stage 6:** linking the deepest belly muscles up the body to the neck and head

All the deeper muscles of the front of the neck – the throat (the pharynx), and the infrahyoid group running between the back of the top of the sternum, the larynx, hyoid bone, and jaw – are part of the deep front line (see Chapter 14, lesson 1). They make a fascial link to the psoas along the anterior longitudinal ligament, which runs up the front of the spine.

- *When the breath sinks back in the body, the deep front line engages, and the front of the body lengthens upwards right from its deepest point. Observe that this frees the throat and deep neck muscles, rolling the head gently forward.*

The deepest muscles of the neck are longus colli and capitis on the front of the neck spine, and the tiny rectus capitis anterior, deep flexors that pull the head forward on the neck.

- *As the head rolls forward gently, you may notice these engaging.*

The big jaw muscles make fascial links to the infrahyoids.

- *As all this happens, does your jaw release?*

## *Maintaining tone as we hinge the legs on the back*

The only table turn Goldie ever gave me was to demonstrate the connection of the legs to the back. First, she brought them over my body to connect them up into the back, then she kept that connection as she brought them down again so the feet rested again on the table, with knees up. It was such a clear sensation and brought about such change in the relationship of my back and legs. I now realize she was showing how

# Toned sitting – integrating the core muscles

to maintain tone in the psoas and lowest belly muscles – the bottom third of the rectus abdominis and the transversus abdominis over it.

### Exploration 10.7  Active hip folding – maintaining tone as we hinge the legs on the back

These moves are mostly done for us in an Alexander table turn. I first learned them as an active process with breath with my Viniyoga teacher.

- Staying in semi-supine, bring your knees up over your body. Engage all these deep muscles on the out-breath, drawing everything up and back along the spine. The psoas and iliacus flexing (not the quads) will draw the thighs towards the chest, and the belly moving back will make room for them. I call this active folding of the hips.
- Keep the surface of the belly soft, falling back to the spine from the pubic bone, bringing the lowest part of the rectus abdominis into play. The pubococcygeals come forward and up in opposition to the psoas.
- Keep the iliac spines back, do not let the belly push the legs away from you on the in-breath. Instead, use the in-breath to widen further into the back of the pelvis and sitting bones while you maintain this tone in the deep muscles (Fig. 10.10).

**Video link for explorations 10.7 and 10.8**

Play with this quietly for a while, giving the nervous system time to sort out and build new links, until something really connects in your back and legs. Then attempt taking the legs down without arching the back.

### Exploration 10.8  Maintaining active hip folding as we lower the legs

- On the out-breath, begin to lower the legs away from you (one at a time initially) back into semi-supine. If you do this without holding tone in the deep muscles, the weight of the legs will pull the lumbar spine into an arch. Play with this to observe it.
- Instead, maintain the tone, as if the thighs are still drawing in toward the chest even as they are moving away. Then the back will continue to lengthen and widen against the floor as the legs are lowered slowly. Stop when you can no longer maintain the connection and the back begins to arch, then draw the legs towards you again to repeat the action.

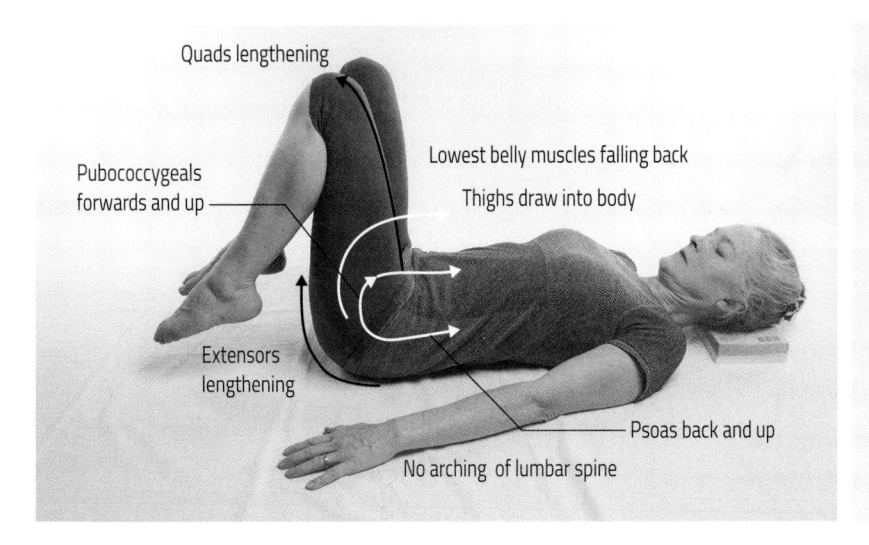

**Figure 10.10**
Active folding of hips

# CHAPTER ten

Initially you may not be able to go very far before the back arches; stay within your limits of connection. Do this regularly, to strengthen this vital connection for flexing forward to rise from a chair without strain, squatting and many other movements.

- *Play with cycling the legs in the air while keeping the connection on all parts of the breath.*

## Lesson 4    Finding the anatomy of integration by inclining back on a chair

This procedure is the best way I know to open out the lumbar arch with its over-contracted quads and psoas group. This engages the erector spinae and core muscles of the belly, and balances the hip flexors and the muscles around the hips.

Then sitting can be supported from deep in the body. Do it a few times, until your brain/body intelligence can sort the task out and integrate it. Then the psoas and erector spinae can come into a deep dynamic dance to support the lengthening lumbar spine, aided by the belly muscles and thoracolumbar fascia.

### Exploration 10.9    Inclining back on a chair

**Stage 1:** finding the balanced torso

- *Lead with your vision to sit on a firm stool, low table, or sideways on a chair. Sit upright with legs and feet supporting the torso (Fig. 10.1).*
- *For each of the following set of directions, think them first, then move over a count of 3. Maintain the tone after each, rather than "relaxing."*

  **Bring your feet and leg spirals awake (Figs 10.2 and 10.3, Fig. 10.11 group 1).**

  **Pull your iliac spines back, sitting bones to the back of the knees and pubococcygeals forward (Fig. 10.11 group 2).**

  **Rotate the elbows forward and outward, bring the wrists back, and pull the top of the sternum up, to widen the upper torso (Fig. 10.11 group 3).**

All this will open the back, so that the vertical from sacrum to T8 is straighter.

Help this along:

**Pull T8 (between the shoulder blade tips) up away from the heels (Fig 10.11 pull 4).**

- *Do not let go of the upright sitting stance you are now in. Take a moment to breathe in this position, being aware of the widening on in- and out-breath, across the back of the back. Be aware of the breath in the pelvic region, with the iliac crests, the sitting bones, and pelvic floor widening also.*

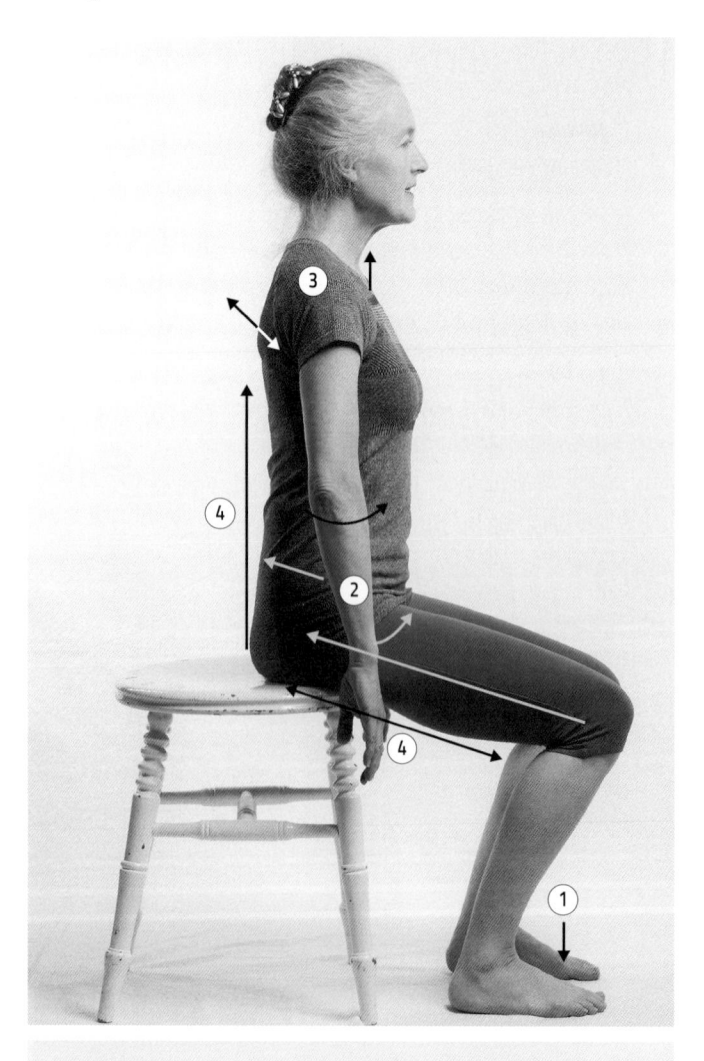

**Figure 10.11**
Directions for active sitting (see exploration 10.9)

# Toned sitting – integrating the core muscles

**Stage 2:** inclining yourself back

- *Pull the iliac spines back in space and pubococcygeals forward; your whole torso will tilt back away from your knees. The ribs must come back too; if not, the back arches. You may feel curved forward (think of curving back along a universal banana) (Fig. 10.12 group 1).*

- *Deeper in, you may be aware of the iliacus and psoas working, back and up, helping to open and support the lumbar spine. Keep awareness of widening throughout the back and pelvic floor (Fig. 10.12 group 2).*

- *Keep breathing so that nothing grips.*

**Use a finger check:** put your finger on your iliac spine, and thumb on lower rib. If you come back with ribs and iliac spines, the thumb will lead back behind the finger, and the distance between them will not change. You may notice the side of the body lengthening up, legs lengthening down. If you roll your pelvis, your thumb and finger will move closer together. If the finger moves less than the thumb, you are arching, and you will be gripping the body.

You can also hold a stick against your back to see that sacrum to T8 stays straight.

### Troubleshooting

*You are hanging on for grim death in the stomach area.* If your upper back gets ahead of the lower back, you will fall backwards, unless your stomach area is gripping to hold you. Trust that you can bring iliac spines and ribs back.

*Your feet are lifting up.* The quads, used to holding tight, need to lengthen away to allow your back and core muscles to work. If they hang on, your feet will lift. Put your feet down, send your knees away from you, and trust to your back and core.

Help this by spatial awareness of the lowest areas of the torso – pubococcygeals pulling forward and lowest part of rectus abdominis coming back and up.

You may be aware of the lower back, back of the pelvic floor, and sitting bones widening and supporting you.

Can you breathe in your lower body in this position?

When we come into balanced muscle tone in this position, we are not aware of what is holding us there. This is a state of dynamic balance – core, middle and outer muscles all working appropriately throughout, even in a position that is apparently anti-gravity.

At first you may only be able to go a small way, but with time, improved body geometry and trust in yourself, you can go surprisingly far back.

**Stage 3:** to come back to upright

- *Keep thinking all these directions, the iliac spines back and pubococcygeals forward, as you bring yourself back up to vertical.*

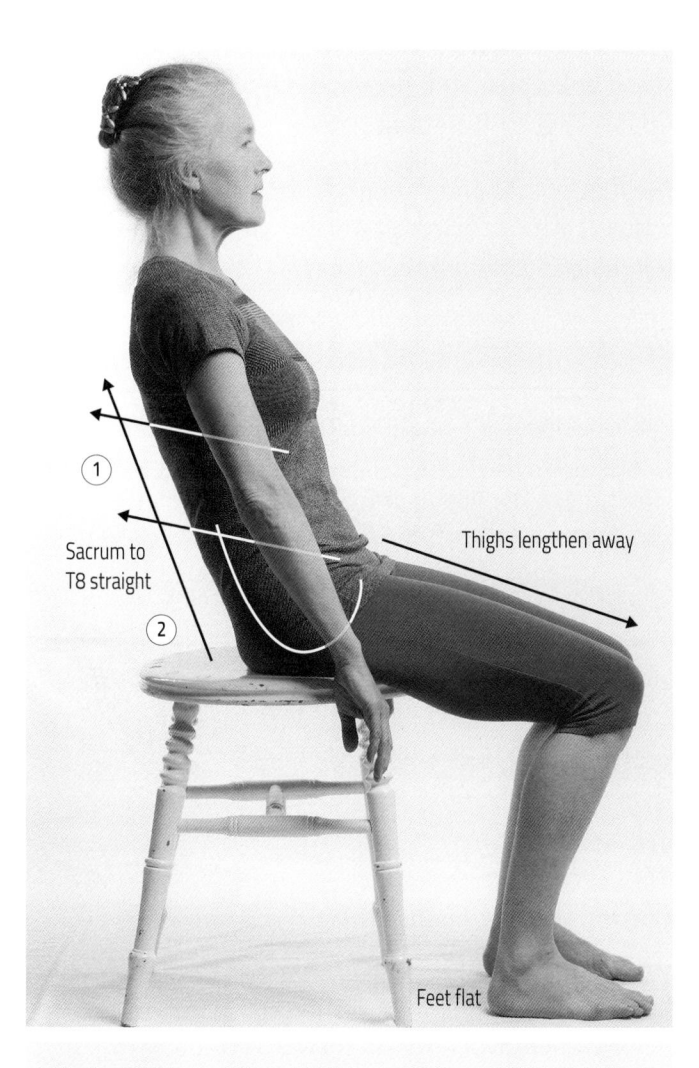

**Figure 10.12**
Inclining back in a chair

# CHAPTER ten

- (If you find this difficult, get another person to pull forward on your knees as you bring yourself back to vertical; this stops you pulling the front of your pelvis down into your quads.)

- If possible, keep conscious of the volume of the body, with connection to the back of the abdomen, pelvic floor, and legs. It will help to think of seeing from the back of the head.

- You may be aware of using the transversus abdominis muscle which runs like a seat belt between your iliac spines. It is working to keep the hips free, so you do not pull the pelvis down into the quads. Instead, you are using the psoas and iliacus deep inside for pure hip flexion – that you probably cannot feel.

Video link for exploration 10.9

**AT info:** Leaning back in a chair is such a useful teaching procedure, but not all training schools teach it. Goldie often took me back in the chair. While it had been a regular move in my training, we were instructed to give our weight over to the teacher, so they could swing us freely in the hip joints. We kept the spine lengthening but were to let go of the legs. Goldie's approach was completely different. I was forbidden to give her my weight, but had to stay self-supporting, without gripping, which initially seemed impossible. She would prod me over and over in hips and ribs (or as I now realize, iliac spines and costal arch ribs) as she took me back millimeter by millimeter. Eventually I got it, but did not understand how it worked. Once I was angled back, she would often wander off to look at her clock or answer the phone, and I was to hold there without fixing or gripping in my belly till she returned.

It used to take me quite a few lessons before I could bring somebody back in the chair and then remove my hands, as Goldie had done many times with me, showing that the deep muscles of their back and abdomen were now working. Now, with anatomical understanding, I can teach them to do this for themselves very quickly.

While modern AT seeks to get the torso working in one piece, this is the end result sought, not the "means whereby" to bring it about. In his first book (2011: 42, 167 and many other passages), Alexander writes repeatedly of how poor use displaces parts of the body (narrowed collapsed chest, hollowed back, protruding abdomen, etc.) and the need to restore displaced parts to their proper positions. We need to change the relationship of the pelvis and lumbar regions, thorax and ribcage relative to each other. Only then will the spine integrate and move in one piece, while still integrating with the legs. Notice that pupils can only stay self-sustaining and swing easily in the hips when the iliac spines and ribs come back as described here, without which their hips are locked by the quads into the upright position.

Alexander's cigar box procedure (2011: 158) refers to this position as a position of mechanical advantage. It demonstrates the self-supporting organization of the body, that the human frame can balance comfortably in positions (at least for a certain amount of time) that would be impossible if the body was simply gravity-stacked. Marjory Barlow told me that once, Alexander's brother A. R. took her back into this position and left her there for fifteen minutes while he walked off on some errand. She was shaking by the time he came back, but she was able to maintain the position!

## Playing with pendular arms

When not actively engaged, the arms are evolved to hang vertically below the shoulders. But what happens to them when we tilt forwards or backwards?

# Toned sitting – integrating the core muscles

### Exploration 10.10   Find your pendular arms

- *Play with tilting yourself backwards and to upright, then tilting forwards and back to upright, thinking back with your iliac spines and ribs throughout.*

- *What happens to your arms?*

  *Do they swing freely in the shoulder joint as you tilt, maintaining their vertical position, as would a pendulum?*

  *Do they hold stiffly at an angle and not move at all?*

  *Or do they stay fixed then catch up to vertical?*

  *Or go in the counter-direction as a balancer?*

- *Take your movement very slowly, being aware that the torso is actively engaged in the task but that the shoulders are uninvolved – see if you can disengage the arms.*

- *If you find this very difficult, you might stand and play with moving your torso around, tipping forwards and back, swiveling, marching, and see if you can allow the arms to swing freely while the torso stays supported. It can help to pretend you are very drunk ... I'm not usually in favor of letting everything go, but sometimes it has its place.*

### Exploration 10.11   Tilting forward on the chair to stand

To tilt forward, we mostly let the lumbar spine fall forward somewhat, so that we become heavy in the legs, which must then work harder to stand us up (see Fig. 3.1C and B). To prevent this, we need to keep working the lumbar spine back and up using all the directions above. (This is "back back" in AT speak.)

- *Follow all the instructions above for tilting back, but this time tilt forward. Remember your pendular arms.*

- *Keep your legs and feet aligned and engaged.*

- *Once your top of sternum is over your feet, keep thinking back, wide and up in the iliac spines, and in the ribs, and of the psoas coming back and up, helping to open and support the lumbar spine. Keep awareness of widening throughout the back and pelvic floor.*

- *You may find yourself rising smoothly out of the chair, pulled up by the upwardly lengthening torso, the legs lengthening underneath you.*

- *Once your bottom lifts off, don't let the legs take over and push, but keep thinking back and up all the way to standing fully upright (Fig. 10.13)!*

**Video link for exploration 10.11**

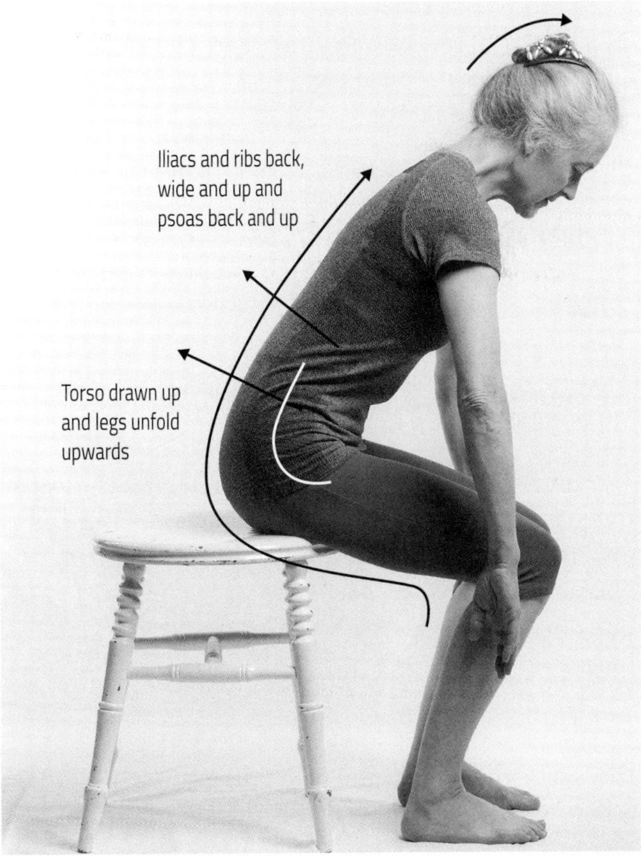

**Figure 10.13**
Directions to tilt forward to stand

Iliacs and ribs back, wide and up and psoas back and up

Torso drawn up and legs unfold upwards

Once you have explored each of these stages, integrate each stage by speaking the relevant directions first and engaging them with a 1-2-3, and then move as you repeat 1-2-3 while maintaining the engagement, as in exploration 7.19. In lesson 2, we engaged the leg spirals strongly to move from sit to stand; in this lesson we powered the movement from the back. Now let's join these up, using the deep front line linkage from big toe balls, past the inner ankle, up the inside of the calf, through the adductors to the psoas (see Fig. 11.6).

### Exploration 10.12  Linking the psoas with the leg spirals

- Sit upright, and "screw the ankles," pulling the inside ankle bone up and back off the big toe balls. Notice that the pull will travel up to the adductors, into the psoas major; let it draw you forward into a tilt.
- Notice that this may pull your knees together. So find a pull into the iliacus (Fig. 10.6), which comes up the inside of the iliac crest, fanning from the anterior iliac spine at the front, to the posterior iliac spine at the back. Focus on these points, either side of the sacrum (Fig. 7.15) and notice this helps to counter-rotate the thighs again.
- Take this into tilting forward to stand as above, to bring all the muscles into play together.

I observe that focusing here also activates the upper gluteus maximus (see below) along with the spiral and superficial back lines, integrating and lifting the whole torso.

### Undoing primary curve patterns, and the importance of the bum muscles.

The vertical sacrum and pelvis is uniquely human. When we first stood on two legs as hominids, it was not only our brains that enlarged beyond all other primates – so did our gluteus maximus, with a new segment originating on the back of the iliac crest and posterior iliac spines, and inserting on the IT band and vastus lateralis (Stern 1972). Other animals only have the lower portion of the gluteus maximus linking sacrum and femur. This new, superior portion is a key part of the hip laterals, stabilizing us as we walk, while the inferior portion does the major thrust (see Chapter 11) (McAndrew et al. 2006).

As already stated, all the explorations work for both primary and secondary curve patterns, though one can adjust the emphasis for individual patterns of use. Here is a case history that used pelvic lifts (exploration 8.7) alongside the work of this chapter, and taught me a lot about undoing primary curve patterns.

Ultan was in his late eighties and slumped, his head fully sunk onto his chest. We worked on lengthening his sternum upwards, and soon he could look forward and join in conversation at meals. But he still needed his hands to push himself up – his torso would not support itself, and months of classic Alexander work hardly began to awaken the muscles.

His arms did all the work to move him – hauling himself slowly out of a chair, or propelling himself on sticks, his legs seemed as weak as his torso. The breakthrough came when we did pelvic lifts on a book – lots of them. Over some months, the hip laterals and lateral line slowly woke up. We then added tilting back in the chair and forward again, awakening his thoracolumbar fascia and belly muscles, supporting first the lumbar and then the thoracic spine. His legs began to connect with his back and sit to stand became much faster. He discovered the toe push. Shortly before his ninetieth birthday, he found he could uncurl himself to fully upright by using his torso muscles alone. Sadly he never could maintain this fully while taking a step and so couldn't walk upright without a frame. But by using the back leg thrust (Chapter 11), while staying back in iliac spines and looking forward to keep everything working, he could use a much lighter hold on the frame. We could then take long walks round the nursing home gardens including rough ground and moderate inclines – impossible before – all to the amazement of his family and nursing home staff! Covid 19 has now stopped his lessons, and he has maintained all this since for himself.

11

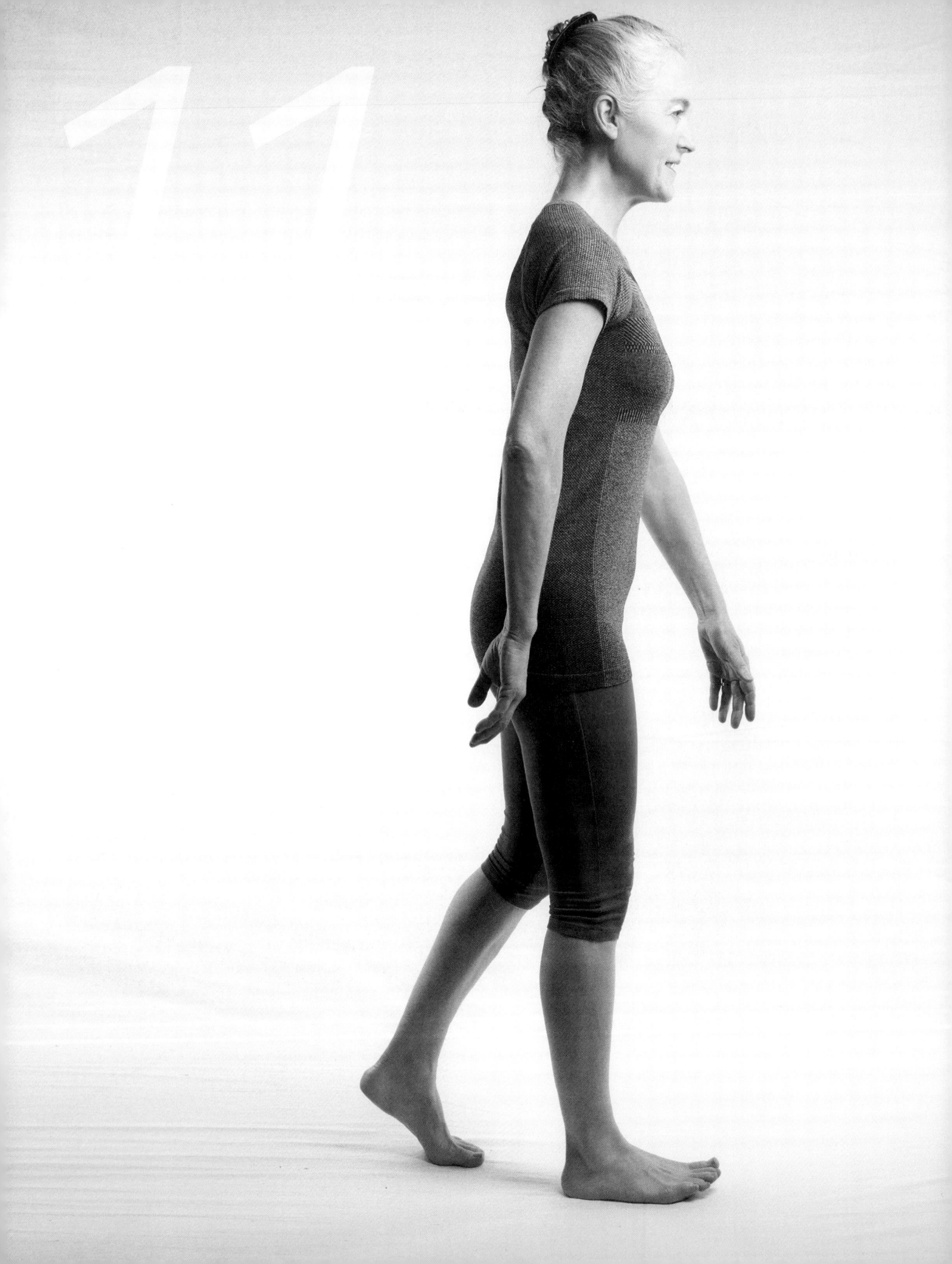

# Walking as you've never walked before  11

## The standard model of walking

In 2009 the book *Born to Run* (McDougall 2009) was published and soon became a best-seller. It told the story of finding the Tarahumara tribe of Mexico who do ultra-running (50–100 miles or more at a time) for fun, barefoot. Barefoot running was already known to use a different biomechanical balance from the style of running promoted by the big shoe companies, who were selling increasingly cushioned heeled shoes to enable a longer front stride and heel strike (Fig. 11.1). *Born to Run* exposed the fallacy of this marketing, which far from preventing foot problems, was in direct proportion to them. It also backed up the findings of AT teachers (such as Malcolm Balk 2006) who were exploring barefoot running – that the torso should always be over the leading foot, while the driving foot is behind the body (Fig. 11.2).

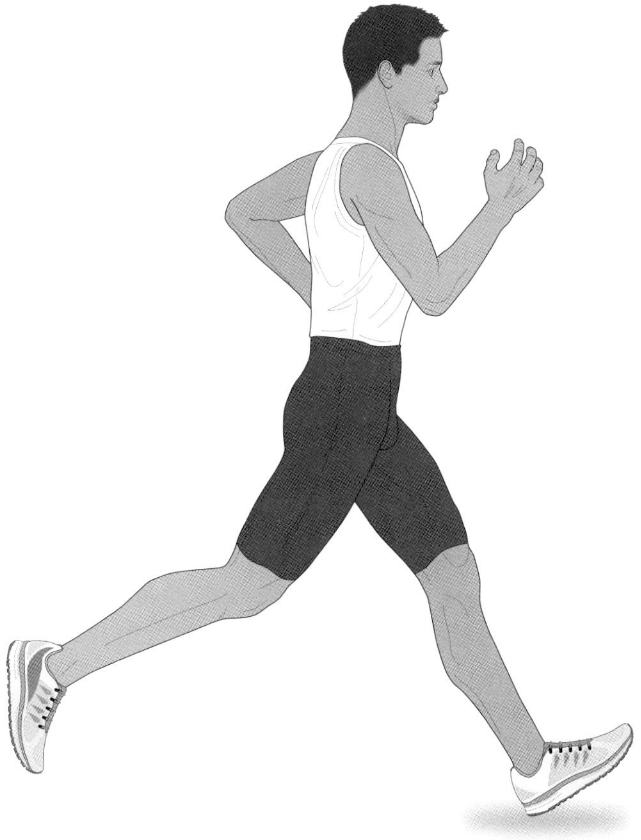

However, up till now, there has been little application of the same analysis to walking. Katy Bowman (2017: 169) points out that the imbalance in thigh muscles caused by too long sitting is key: for a powerful toe push, the driving leg must be squarely behind the body. But in most people the hamstrings and gluteus maximus are now too lax to pull the leg back behind the body, while the quads and psoas no longer have sufficient length to allow this. Then a wide variety of compensatory patterns must be developed to find the power needed to move.

The majority of people walk as a controlled fall, with the movement driven by the front leg and arm, using the quads and the biceps. The swinging leg is kicked out in front of the body, the knee fully straightening, and with the foot (and often toes also) pulled upwards. Then the heel lands – with an audible heel strike – and the rest of the foot flops to the floor as we let our weight fall onto it. We then swing what is now the back leg forward and kick it out in turn. We often help this by marching with the arms, for added forward swing.

**Figure 11.1**
Standard running – leg ahead of body with heel strike

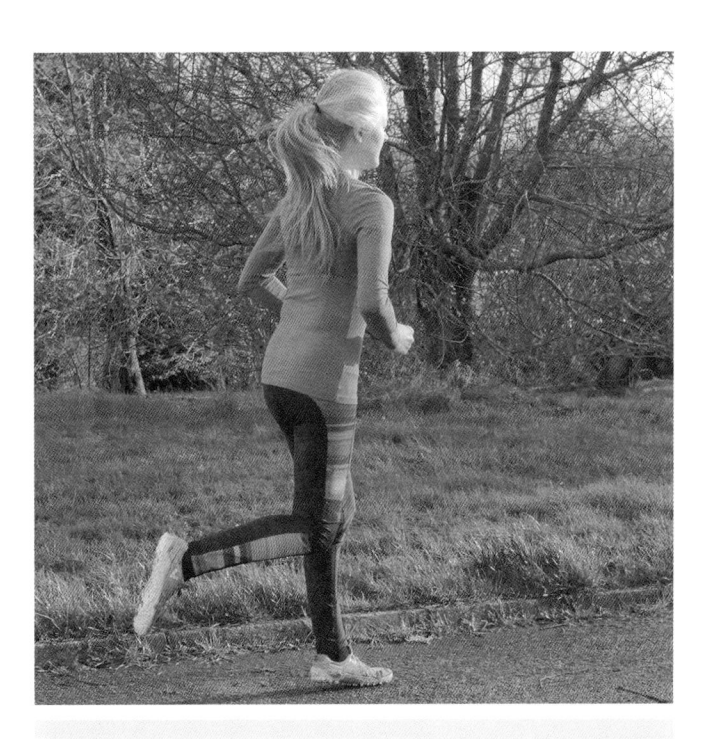

**Figure 11.2**
Landing toes first, with instep under top of sternum

# CHAPTER eleven

Meanwhile, the torso is often inclined backwards in the upper body, with the head tightened back on the neck, and a lumbar curve. The lumbar curve can also cause the legs to rotate outward slightly so that the toes point outward. Just as in the standard running model, the whole movement happens in front of the body, and acts to drive the body backwards even as we are moving forwards. Each step then drives the body weight down into the ground, so that the footfall is clearly audible. This walking is hard work! Walking over shifting surfaces such as sand, pebbles, or rough ground generally is then even harder work. No wonder we like tarmac (Fig. 11.3).

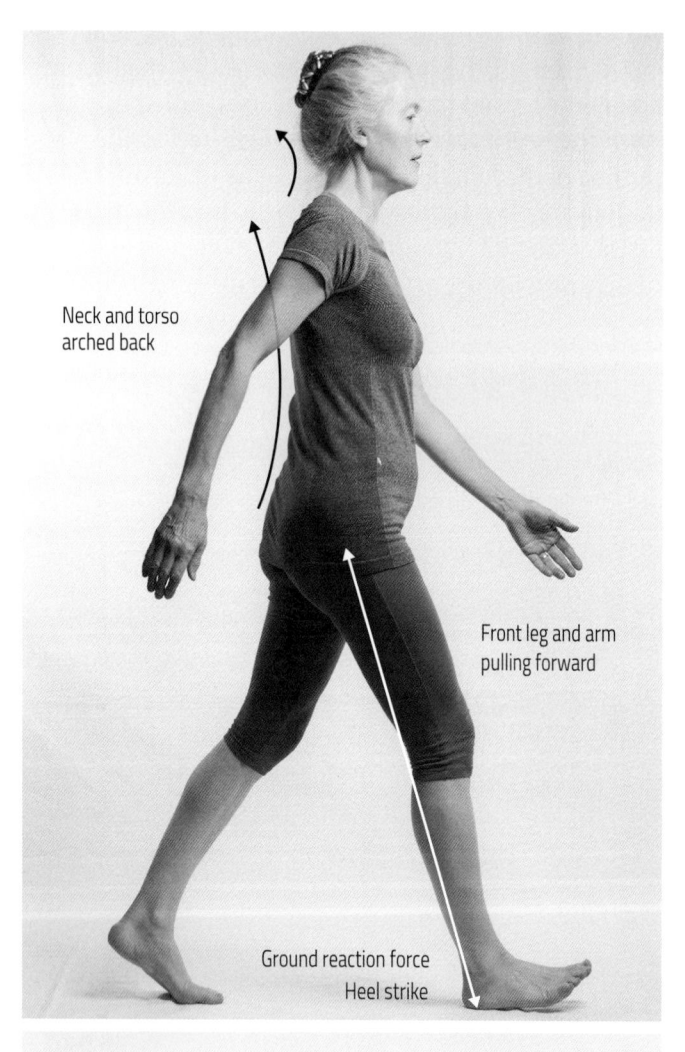

**Figure 11.3**
Standard walking, driven by front leg with heel strike

### Exploration 11.1  How do you walk?

- *Ask someone to video you side-on, walking purposefully. Does your leading foot extend in front of the body? Does your torso stay rectangular, or distort in some way: shoulders swinging, hips swinging, chest and back arching or collapsing, arms rowing or not moving at all, head poking forward ... Observe it carefully.*

This sort of walking is heavy and effortful, because the ground reaction force both forces the heel into the ground (heel strike) and also sends the force of movement backwards (see Fig. 11.3). We want to find an easy but powerful walk that is light and springy, that moves over the ground rather than into it, and in which all the forces generated serve to take us forward. Such a walk can also zoom us up hills, and glide us over rough ground or shifting pebbles.

We will look at the mechanism of walking in four aspects: stability, mobility, coordination, and torque.

## Lesson 1  Stability enables mobility

When, because of misalignment, there is instability in the hip joint, the nervous system will co-contract the joint by tightening all the big muscles around it. This draws the head of the femur up into the hip socket, giving tight hips. In Chapter 8, we worked on re-awakening stability in hips, legs, and feet. When the stabilizers work, the big muscles can release, bringing full mobility back to the joints.

In walking, there is always a stance leg, taking the weight of the body with straight knee, and a swing leg, traveling forward. With painful knee problems such as arthritis, people use excessive co-contraction of the knee joint for stability as they step onto it. Research has shown that AT lessons reduce such co-contraction (and also reduced the pain) (Preece et al. 2017). (Does co-contraction cause arthritis, or does arthritis cause the co-contraction? We do not know.)

Our first task is to stabilize the stance leg, so the swing leg can be much less involved, rather than driving the movement.

# Walking as you've never walked before

### Exploration 11.2   Strong supporting (stance) leg, and freely swinging thighs

- Stand with the feet parallel and hip-width apart. Find the up-line up the back of the legs and body through to the crown. Find your natural breathing, lengthening and widening throughout on the in-breath, to self-support the torso from the inside with active psoas and core.

- Keep this going, and shift the weight slightly onto your left leg, sending the hip laterals down so that the torso springs up from this hip, yet keeping the weight over the inside of the heel and the big toe ball, with the inside ankle coming up and back. This is now your stance leg.

- Gently use your right hand to push the back of your right thigh forwards, pivoting on the ball of the right foot. The thigh should swing easily in the hip joint forwards and backwards, without any displacing of the pelvis in any direction. Explore this also on the other leg (Fig. 11.4).

We are finding a balanced use of the extensors and flexors of the legs. The result seems effortless as each knee slides forward from under the hips (this is Alexander's instruction "knees forward"). With the hips stabilized, the swing leg can both pivot and stabilize through hip and ankle. Does adding the thought to bring the inner ankle up and back help further to stabilize the ankle and release the knee forward?

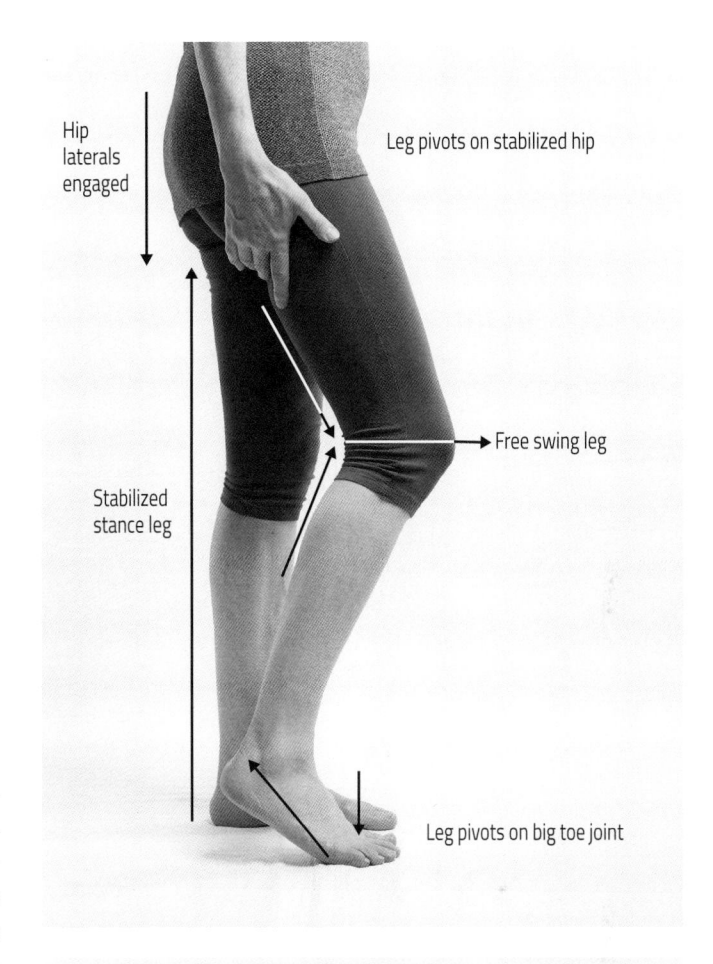

**Figure 11.4**
Freeing the thigh in the hip by stabilizing the stance leg

### Exploration 11.3   Taking your first steps

- Take a step forward on your left leg, and stabilize on it (as above) with the front knee straight. This is now the stance leg – the right (back) foot will come onto the ball. Gently push this back thigh forwards, and notice that the knee can swing forwards under the body, and back over the big toe ball, with no displacement of the torso (Fig. 11.5A).

- Once you have the stability, let the right knee swing forwards (as if pushed from behind) and this time carry through (Fig. 11.5B). Do not fully straighten the knee, so that the traveling foot lands on the flat of the heel, only slightly beyond the toes of the left foot. You will need to use very small steps for a while, until your quads and psoas lengthen. The ball of the foot lands a fraction of a second afterwards and the weight of the whole-body can rock forwards, pivoting on the ankle, until it is directly above the right foot. The right leg is now the stance leg.

- As the right foot lands, the heel of the back foot will lift and send that knee forwards from behind, and that action rocks the torso forwards to transfer the weight (Fig. 11.5C).

**Video link for exploration 11.3**

# CHAPTER eleven

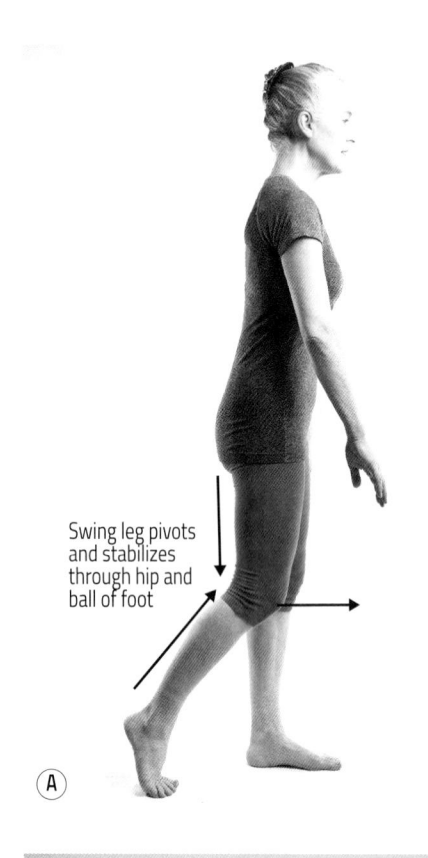

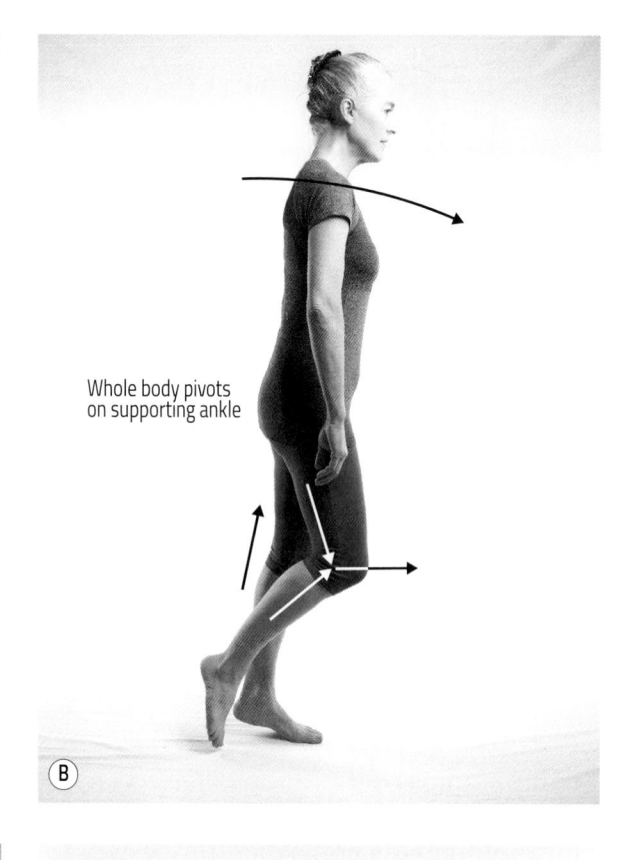

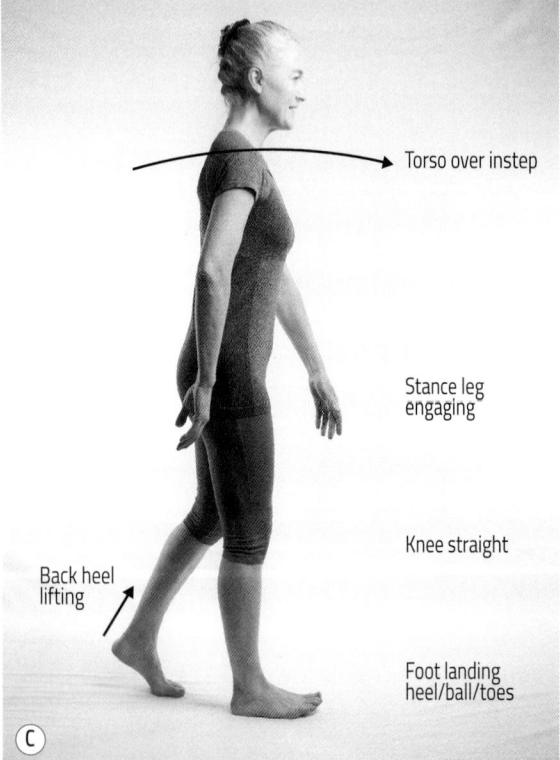

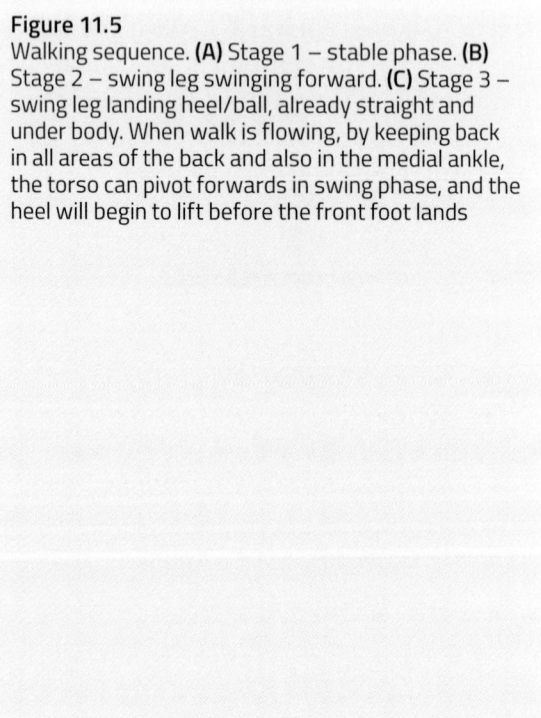

*Labels in figure:*

**(A)** Swing leg pivots and stabilizes through hip and ball of foot

**(B)** Whole body pivots on supporting ankle

**(C)** Torso over instep; Stance leg engaging; Knee straight; Foot landing heel/ball/toes; Back heel lifting

**Figure 11.5**
Walking sequence. **(A)** Stage 1 – stable phase. **(B)** Stage 2 – swing leg swinging forward. **(C)** Stage 3 – swing leg landing heel/ball, already straight and under body. When walk is flowing, by keeping back in all areas of the back and also in the medial ankle, the torso can pivot forwards in swing phase, and the heel will begin to lift before the front foot lands

# Walking as you've never walked before

This is very different from most adults walking, it flows quietly over the ground. The whole direction of the movement is forwards, at no point does the torso weight fall backwards. The walk is powered from behind the body, at no point is the foot in front of the body weight.

Figure 11.6 shows how the toe push powers the walk through the deep front line: through the medial arch, to the inner ankle coming up and back, to the calf muscles, adductors and to the psoas.

### Exploration 11.4  The angle of the lower leg should not move forward past vertical

This strange idea makes more sense when we discover that the action of the lower leg is often dependent on the angle of the back or neck.

- Tip your upper back backwards as far as you dare and try walking. The front foot will kick out way out in front of you. Taken to extremes, this becomes like a sketch from Monty Python's "Ministry of Silly Walks."
- Stretch your head and neck out in front of you like a chicken, to notice also that the foot must reach in front.
- Now tilt your whole-body forward in a straight line from ankles to head until you lose balance and begin to fall forward. Your thighs must swing forward while your feet catch up under you as you continue to tilt, making a toddler-like run. Notice that the lower leg only extends to vertical, at which point the foot lands to take your weight. The steps are small as each foot lands just in front of the other one.
- Once you have the feel of this action of the lower leg, slow to a walk again, but invite the same action of the legs and short stride. It can help to think of the back leg being lazy. The back heel then lifts before the front foot lands.

### Exploration 11.5  Breathing and walking

If you get boggled with biomechanical detail, come back to letting the natural walk emerge, led by the eyes and the goal of movement. Use natural breathing to help this. The roots of the diaphragm interlink with the psoas, which link to the adductor muscles of the inner thighs and so to the knees. Any movement is freer when begun with a softening at the knees, in conjunction with the breath, gently unifying the whole-body (see exploration 3.14).

To begin, take only one step per breath cycle, keeping the steps small. Keep looking forwards.

- Find the natural breath to the base of the torso, inviting it to widen across the pelvic floor into the hip joints. Notice when the in-breath connects, maybe loosening your hips. The out-breath comes back and up along the lumbar spine, activating the psoas and lengthening the quads, maybe softening the knees.
- As the next out-breath happens, let the back leg swing forward and land, as an emergent movement. Let the in-breath happen, and wait for the next out-breath to let the other foot step forward.

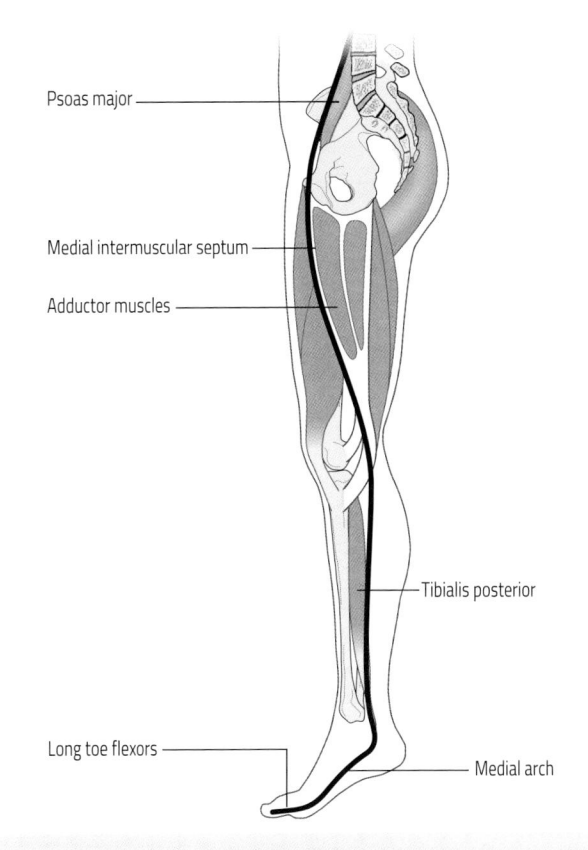

**Figure 11.6**
The deep front line in the leg

# CHAPTER eleven

### Exploration 11.6 Engaging the core muscles of the torso

Many people push forward in the lower spine as they walk. To bring the pelvis vertical and stabilize the lower spine, we need to engage the lower belly muscles, hamstrings, and pubococcygeals. Then the psoas muscles stay lengthened and active, smoothly swinging the thigh forward, while the lumbar spine stays back, lengthened and widened. (This is "back stays back" in Alexander-speak.) This brings wonderful stability to the pelvis and lower body, and incredible freedom to the legs.

Notice that the lower you can engage the belly muscles, the easier it is to breathe fully while maintaining tone. This also takes more pressure off the front of the body, allowing greater freedom of movement.

1  Preparation

- *Stand in alignment, and find the natural breath as in exploration 11.5. This engages your psoas.*
- *Give instructions from spatial awareness and brain/whole-body intelligence, while inhibiting any movement. Keep the knees straight throughout:*

   **I send my heels down and send an up line up my legs to sacrum and then T8.**

   **I pull the sitting bones to the back of the knees, and the pubococcygeals gently forward.**

   **I send the iliac spines back in space.**

   **I pull the tips of the elbows forwards and outwards to open the deep back arm line.**

- *Move over a count of 1-2-3 to engage these altogether.*
- *Keeping the iliac spines back throughout the breath cycle (as in exploration 8.13) helps you maintain dynamic tone rather than tension.*

2  Emergent walking

- *Give another 1-2-3 as you walk forward on the outbreath, led by your eyes and knees.*
- *Once this is working for you, can you now walk throughout the breath cycle, maintaining this stability and mobility in the hip and knee joints?*

### Video link for exploration 11.6

### Exploration 11.7 Walking backward

When walking backward, we have to open the lumbar spine and stabilize the pelvis to avoid falling.

- *Use the instructions of exploration 11.6 to walk backward, while looking forward with spatial awareness (Fig. 11.7).*
- *Stop and walk forward again. Does your lower body push forward? If so, go between walking backward and*

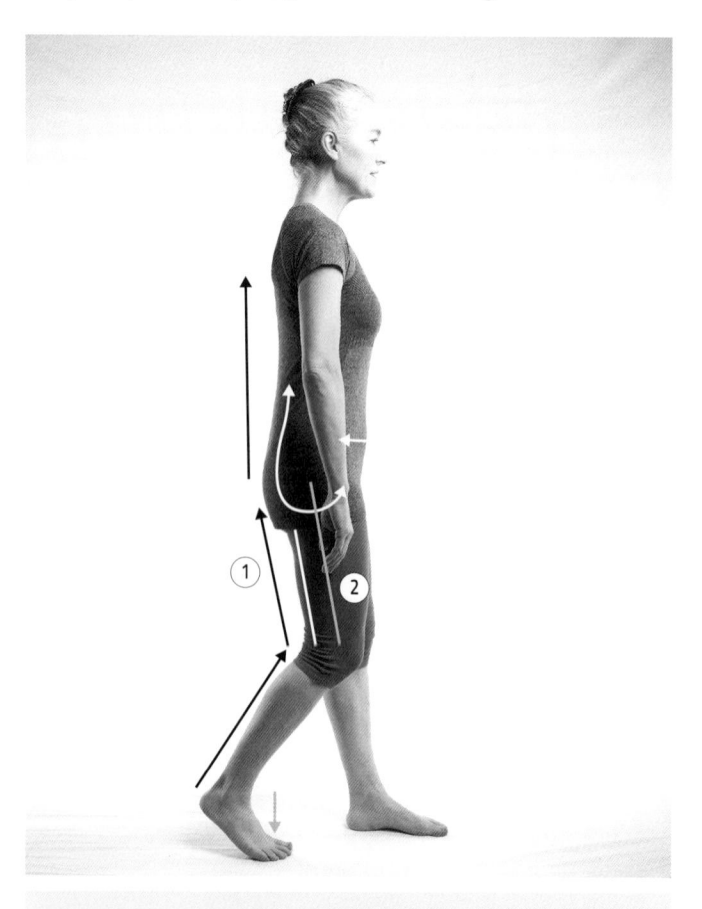

**Figure 11.7**
Walking backwards: 1: psoas, pubococcygeals, hamstrings and iliacs all take the back back and up. 2; the hip laterals and ball of big toe stabilize the movement as you step back

# Walking as you've never walked before

*forward until you can walk forward while staying back in your back.*

I use this a lot when out walking – taking a few steps backwards to find my back coming back, then going forward again without losing this. It feels mad, but no one ever stares. I probably look like I've forgotten something.

## Lesson 2   Stability enables coordination – finding fully active feet

A flat uniform surface gives no challenge to the foot, so that we switch off signals from it. Stepping-stones, where we need precise placement of the feet, can encourage them to wake up. You can create some stepping-stones by laying a wide circle of books on your floor.

As a child in rainy North Wales, our country walks would often cross marshes. I learned to stabilize on the supporting leg, often with bent knee, while the swing leg looked for the next secure foothold – a clump of grass or stone. Then I always tested it before transferring my weight, in case it sank me into the bog. This is what we are doing here – though with no risk of wet feet.

### Exploration 11.8   Waking up the soles of the feet

**Video link for exploration 11.8**

- *In bare or stocking feet, tread your "stepping-stones" book path, using your stabilized, emergent walking.*

I find most people can do this without a problem. If you have balance problems, please use your judgment or a helper to stay safe. If the books slip a bit then you will need to pay attention!

- *Explore doing this with bent legs, keeping the weight over the inside heels and the big toe balls, with hip laterals engaged, iliacs back, and pubococcygeals forward. The bent stance leg (and maybe angled torso also) will give even more stability, so you can pause, mid-step, to choose the next book, and test before committing weight to it. Can you wave the free leg around in the air, or step over an imaginary or real obstacle? Can you sense your system waking up?*

Weight transfer is tricky, as mostly people swing across from the hip or the foot. Instead,

- *send your inside thigh and back of knee forward and away over the big toe balls, opening out the adductors and the pelvic arch. Then the weight seems to pour itself across (Fig. 11.8). Play back and forth between two books to find a slow, smooth weight transfer.*

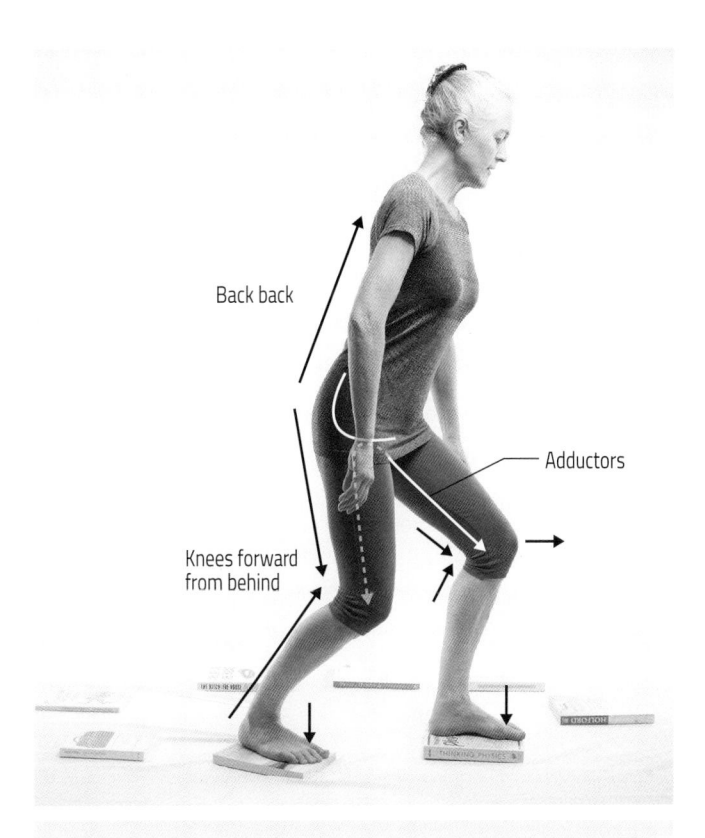

**Figure 11.8**
Weight transfer between books

# CHAPTER eleven

- *Once your system is awake, can you now tread your path with straight legs?*

Our feet are evolved to flex in several planes over a rough surface, but often they have stiffened up and have forgotten this.

- *If you feel confident, test your stability and foot flexibility by landing only partly on the books, supporting your weight with different parts of your feet. Keep those lateral stabilizers and big toe balls working!*

- *Challenge yourself by walking backwards, feeling with the ball of the foot for the book behind you. Keep seeing forward with spatial awareness, breathing, and stabilizing. You will be even more aware of weight transfer over the foot as you step back.*

- *Step off the books onto the floor. Notice whether the soles of your feet instantly switch off again. Step back on the books again to reawaken them. Step off again, choosing to keep them awake. How long can you maintain them awake?*

### Exploration 11.9  Walking in shoes

**Five essential criteria** for your everyday shoes. Please bin any shoes that don't meet these criteria.

1   A flexible sole – so that the ball of the big toe can work fully.

2   A big enough toe-box so the toes, especially the big toe, have some room to spread and maintain their forward direction – it can be very hard to find women's shoes particularly that do not cramp the big toes inward.

3   Shoes need to stay on your foot – without you looking after them.

4   The ankle needs to be able to flex – this is especially an issue in boots.

5   Heels – as low as possible.

- *Now step back into your shoes, inviting your consciousness to flow through the shoe to the ground, as if the shoe were not there.*

- *As you walk, do not look after the shoe with the foot. So often the foot is more involved with the shoe than the ground. If the shoe slips a bit, let it! See if you can bring back full awareness of the ground through the shoe.*

- *Try your "stepping-stones" again, then see if you can find this aliveness of the feet in shoes on flat surfaces. There are 200,000 nerve endings in each foot – let's use them.*

### Exploration 11.10  Rough ground versus tarmac

We live on floorboards, pavements, and tarmac, all smooth surfaces with no challenge to the feet. Rough ground wakes up the outside of the foot, which operates like trainer wheels on a child's bicycle, actively engaging when the weight tips onto them. But this is about more than feet. Balancing through constantly varying angles activates myriad different muscle groupings with every step. We need to walk on rough ground regularly to activate our feet and our whole bodies. Where I live now in Ireland I am blessed with a large garden with rough paths and paddocks, and can take pupils on little hikes to wake up their feet, legs, and whole-body maneuvering.

- *Find rough ground to challenge your feet and whole-body. Most towns have areas with decorative cobble stone paving or rough grassy areas. Maybe you have access to a stony beach, or a wood where you can step off the path. Notice that walking sometimes in slight "monkey" helps to bring everything alive, especially if you step on or over, duck under and weave around real or imaginary obstacles. Then notice that when you get back to the flat tarmac your feet (and body) will again switch off, unless you choose not to let them.*

I have become passionate about feet and legs. Penfield's homunculus shows that the sensory area of the brain devoted to the foot is almost as large as that for the hand. With switched-off feet, how much of this are we using?

# Walking as you've never walked before

## Lesson 3  Stability and mobility enable torque – finding the power in your walk

Our walking explorations so far have been gentle and meditative, perfect for a seaside stroll. But mostly we need to move with more dynamism than this, to get jobs done, climb a steep hill or stairs.

Torque, a combination of twist and thrust, is the driving force for human movement. A twisting force has more power than a straight-on force – this is why tornadoes are more dangerous than high winds. The physics of biomechanical torque is complex but simply put, torque is how much a contractile force can rotate a lever (a bone) about its fulcrum (a joint). Most muscles are on an angle, and so their activity creates twist across the joint, which then moves the bone. While traditional biomechanics analyzes one joint at a time, we will look at torque chains and whole-body spirals. But first, let us examine how torque evolved for land animals.

### The evolution of human movement – the spinal engine theory

The general perception is that the legs locomote us, and the body is carried along, more or less passively. Alexander countered this with his theory of primary control: that movement is organized through the head-neck-back relationship: the head leads forward movement. This is more obvious in animals, where the head does lead the body. But is this the force that powers movement? Alexander never addressed this. By looking from an evolutionary perspective, a different picture emerges. In the introduction to Chapter 6, I described evolution of vertebrate movement, and how the axial locomotion of fish and then reptiles was overlaid in mammals with flexion–extension. The power in the back end that had driven the fish forward through the water was conserved, with powerful hind limbs and stabilized head with sense organs.

When lateral bending in the lumbar spine is combined with flexion–extension, it creates a twisting force. Gracovetsky points out that this happened in evolution, from which he argued that all mammalian movement is powered from the small of the back (his spinal engine theory). Think of the cheetah running. Flexion brings the legs underneath, while extension stretches them out for the stride. But as cheetahs run faster, you see a rotational movement around the central axis as the pelvis rotates. Watch videos of great runners to see this contralateral twist – the reach of the legs extended by the pelvic rotation, the spinal twist opposed by the contralateral arms before it can reach the head.

Others disagree with Gracovetsky, as do I. The torque chains that power movement include the back muscles, but the real power is in the buttocks and thighs, not the lumbar spine. However, I think he is right that the spine is deeply involved, twisting and stabilizing in balance with the overall spirals of movement.

The conventional idea of the spine was as a compressive rod, stabilizing everything, around which the bigger muscles move. But spines – these curving towers of complex multi-jointed bones – are held in expansion within a complex balance of opposing forces, allowing the potential for small movements in many planes. Since all contractile elements are in myofascial connection, the spine cannot stabilize in isolation from larger movements, but must take up its own curve in balance with the curves of movement. Since, with integrated movement, the torso is primary to the limbs, it is logical that if a twisting motion is to flow through the body for running or other big movements, it must originate in the spine to stabilize the core for the bigger movements to follow. According to Gracovetsky (1988), this rotation originates in the small muscles closest to the spine, and ripples outward to the big muscles of the spine, hips, and legs.

The nerves innervating the buttocks, hip muscles, and legs emerge from the spinal cord at the lower lumbar vertebrae and sacrum. They do not go directly to their destinations but first interconnect like railway points in the sacral plexus. One can speculate that this is for exchange of information in

# CHAPTER eleven

which all the shifting layers of movement and stability for this region can be coordinated. In Tai Chi, both the twist that powers movement and the stability of it are initiated in this lower lumbar/sacral region (Ong 2017).

### Exploration 11.11  Play with a mock frisbee throw (backhand)

- Let your whole-body spiral with the movements, both to prepare and throw. Notice the twist is imbalanced if it happens only from the upper body and arm (Fig. 11.9), or from the knees. But when it happens from the waist and hips, spiraling down into the knees then up out of them, there is tremendous stability, power and flow in the movement (Fig. 11.10).

We need to be free to rotate the pelvis or not, according to the level of power required. In Alexander work, as one comes out of dominant secondary curves into balanced use, visible pelvic rotation while walking markedly decreases, along with other unwanted pelvic and spinal displacements, as the pelvis is no longer tangled with the tight lumbar region. But to stop it entirely is a mistake. Just as the shoulder moves to give us a longer reach with the arm, so pelvic rotation gives us a longer active stride length when we need that extra oomph. Legs provide a bulk of muscle which amplifies the movement, and they too are in double spirals. If all these spirals are in balance, they prevent undue twisting at the pelvic level. By their length, they vastly increase the reach of the movement generated. But such big movement is energetically costly – it is only for when the power is needed.

### The upper limbs and stability of the head

For us, walking is still a four-legged exercise, in which the arms help direct, coordinate, and balance locomotion. The counter-twist of the upper body balances out the rotation of the pelvis and lower body, so that by the time it reaches the head there is no twist remaining, and the head stays stable.

The forward swing of the arms points the direction, while the backward thrust helps drive the movement forward, particularly when running. At an Art of Running workshop (August 2016), Malcolm Balk pointed out that paralympic runners without legs

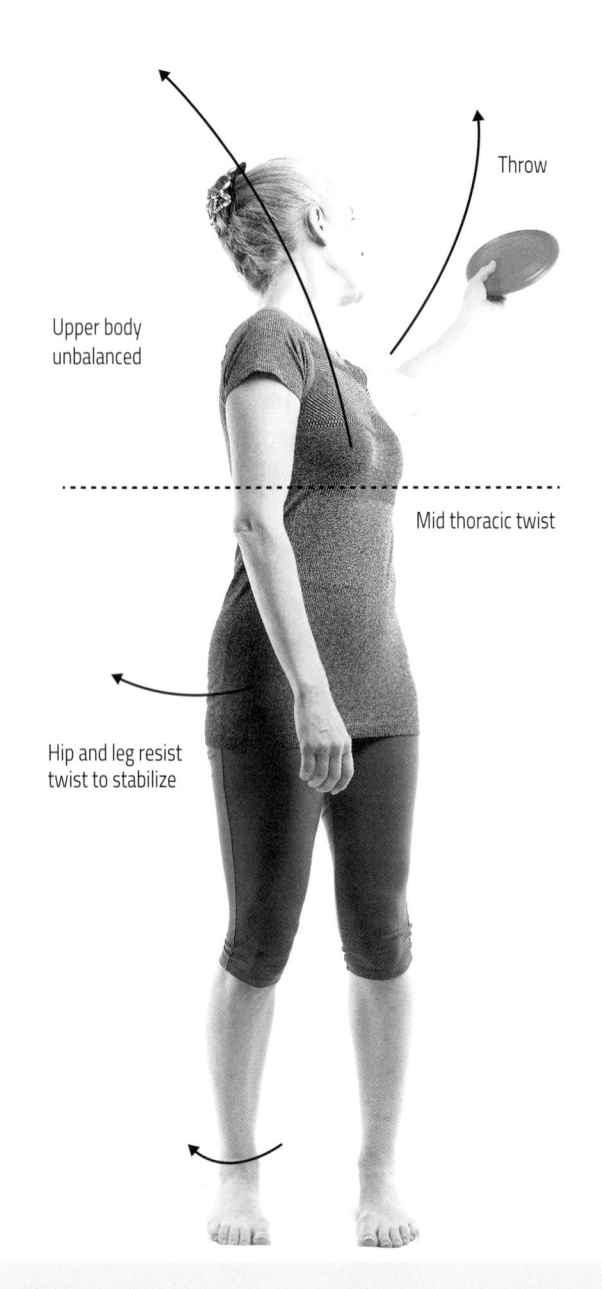

**Figure 11.9**
Twist from upper body. Lower body must resist while upper body is imbalanced by arm movement

# Walking as you've never walked before

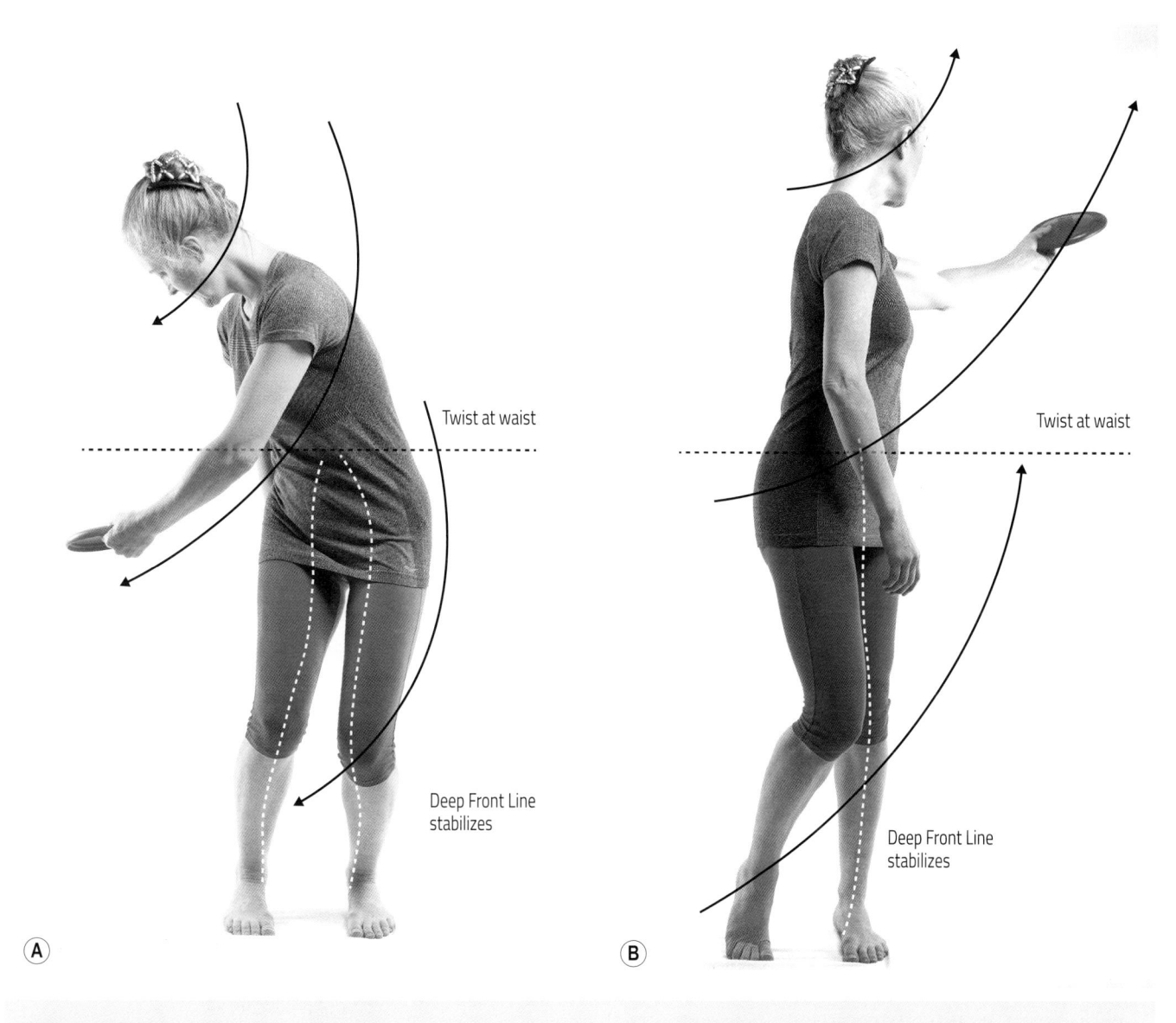

**Figure 11.10A, B**
Twist at waist. Movement stabilized through lumbar region and core muscles and powered through big muscles of legs and buttocks, connecting through thoracolumbar fascia, latissimus dorsi and obliques to arms

have won gold medals, but runners without arms have a much harder time.

## Stability of the feet

Just as the head must be unaffected by rotational movements of the torso, so the feet must also be stable, under constantly varying conditions, so that they can always transmit power reliably to the ground and bounce off it again. The structure of the human foot provides beautifully for this stability, with its small muscles and tendons making three arches, which evenly distribute and store energy throughout its structure. This allows for rapid initial stabilizing

# CHAPTER eleven

on ground contact – stretching the arches, which then becomes a spring-like release of the stored energy in the swing phase. Friction between foot and ground is also crucial, utilizing shearing forces between skin and underlying tissues that increase the power generated at the toe push. The force from the feet also connects back up to the torso. The toe push coincides with firing of the extensor muscles – the hamstrings and gluteus maximus – which then connect up through the extensor line of the body (the superficial back line) and to the ribs and latissimus dorsi – the lifter muscles.

### Exploration 11.12  Waking up the instep by coming onto tiptoes

- *Stand with aligned torso and head, feet, and legs. Be aware of the vestibular directions: the vertical line from heels to crown and beyond, and your front /back and side lines also. See forward; allow your natural breathing.*

- *Keep back in your iliac spines and ribs so you do not rock forward, and forward and wide with the shoulder blades so the upper body does not tip backwards. Hold the back of a chair lightly if needed for balance.*

- *Pull your left inner ankle back and up, so that the arch is activated and the heel lifts, and the foot comes onto the ball, onto "tiptoe." The activation of the inner ankle will prevent your ankle from sickling – the weight stays through the big toe balls.*

- *Now bring that one down again, and as you do so, activate the right inner ankle/arch/heel lift.*

- *Alternate your feet, being aware of the insteps working.*

  *Keep the iliac spines back and up from the outside of the knee so that the IT band stabilizes the knees from falling inward. Keep pubococcygeals pulling forward to prevent the pelvis tipping forward.*

  *Is the upward-moving instep weight-bearing? Or is the stance leg taking all the weight? For this move, both feet take equal weight, so that one heel is moving up as the other*

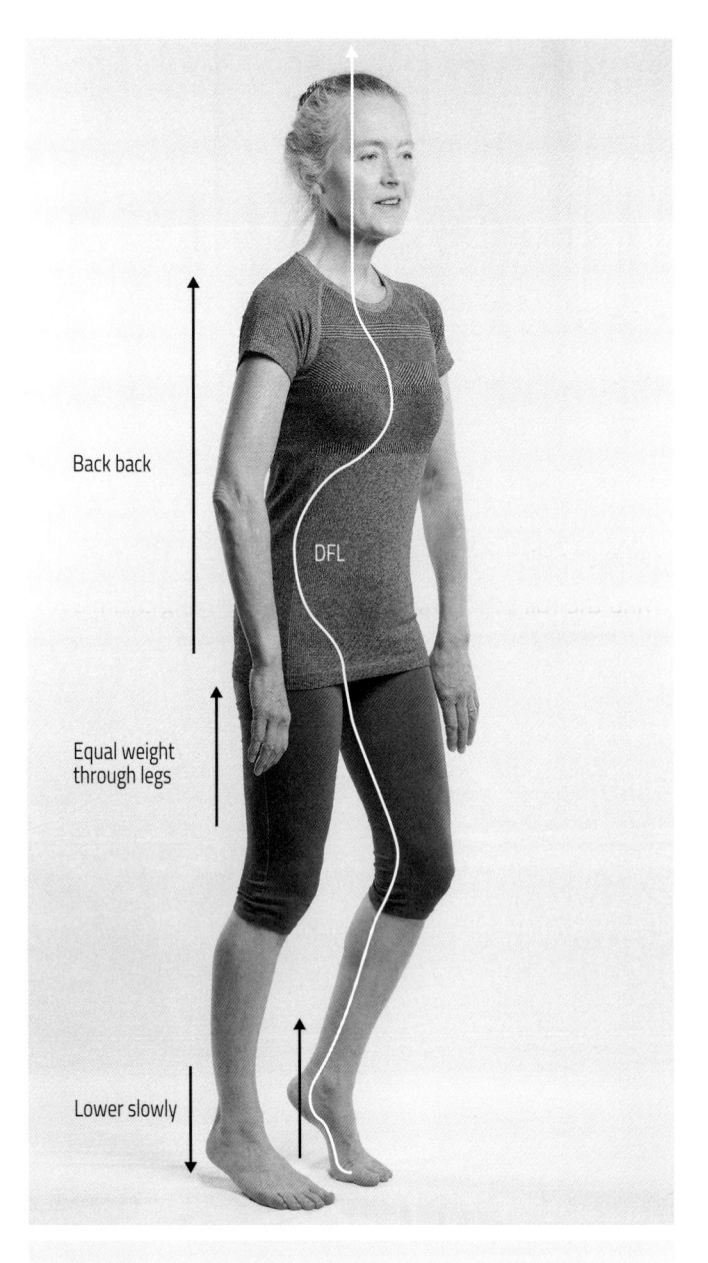

**Figure 11.11**
Waking up the insteps

moves down, and the upward moving instep is powering the movement, through the deep front line up to the crown (Figs 10.9, 11.6, 11.11).

- *Find your balanced walk again, noticing that the heel of the back foot pushing up powers the ball of the foot to drive you forwards (see Fig. 11.12).*

# Walking as you've never walked before

*Exploration 11.13  Finding the power of the stride*

Video link for exploration 11.13

So far, we have focused on the legs as the prime movers, keeping the pelvis uninvolved, to find a free walk with short stride and not so much power. This was needed to let go of unwanted pelvic movements and compensatory patterns, so common in Westernized populations. The pelvic rotation needs unencumbered freedom to move around the vertical. Now we need to find the full stride and power again, keeping this freedom by maintaining the balance between internal and external torque.

It is easiest to find this on a hill. Any small slope will work, such as a wheelchair ramp into a shop or grassy bank in a park.

- *In exploration 8.7 we found pelvic lifts on a book. Now find this while standing level. Your hip laterals pull down; the weight stays on the big toe ball and inside heel, working the adductors; which tilts the other hip gently up and lifts the foot off. When the torso on the stance side extends upwards with this, you know you have engaged the right muscles.*

Now continue this action as you walk forward.

- *The hip laterals (external torque muscles) are now pushing down and backwards to thrust you forward,*
- *while the inner ankle of the back foot pulling back and up powers the instep and ball of the foot (internal torque) to drive you forward.*

This counterbalance of torques both keeps the foot straight and increases the power generated.

These two movements are working in opposition to power the leg, one pushing down, one pulling up. The link between these is the spiral line (Fig. 11.12).

Spiral line – IT band, tibialis anterior

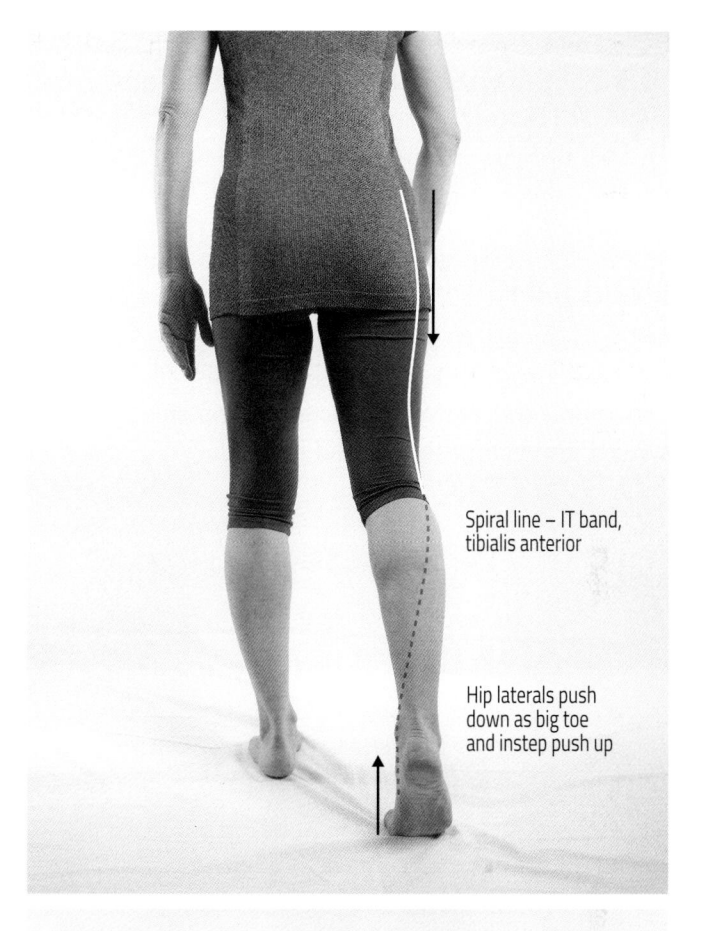

Hip laterals push down as big toe and instep push up

**Figure 11.12**
Balanced leg spirals maintained while walking

Notice that as you increase the power in these two movements, the stride lengthens. The quads (front of thigh) are now extending, while the hamstrings (back thigh) are contracting.

- *Notice that you need to keep your feet aligned so the second and third toes point forward, then all the leg muscles and gluteal muscles come into play. Then the stance leg can support for longer as you rock forward on the ankle, allowing the longer stride.*

The pelvis rotates slightly backwards with the hip lateral thrust (the spinal engine). But the pelvis and spine does not twist outwards. This is because it is opposed by the screwing of the ankle back and up, keeping the inside heel directing outward, so the ball of

## CHAPTER eleven

the foot thrusts inwards along the inside of the leg to the adductors and the psoas, along the deep front line (Fig. 11.13).

- *Play with allowing the foot and pelvis to rotate out, notice that the stride is still long but power is lost (Fig. 11.14).*

### Note about arms

While walking slowly, the arms can hang vertically with very little movement. Once we power the walk, the arms come into play. In the usual stance, the arms hang with slightly bent elbows, and palms facing the side of the body. This means that when we walk, the lower arm swings further forward than the upper arm (Fig. 11.3).

With the new balanced alignments, with elbows rotated forward, the arms hang vertically and the palms face back. Now the elbow does not bend during walking, instead the whole arm swings from the shoulder joint. This feels seriously weird to start with (Fig. 11.15)! Notice that just as with the legs, the power from the arm now comes from the back swing, while the front arm swings freely to counterbalance and point the way.

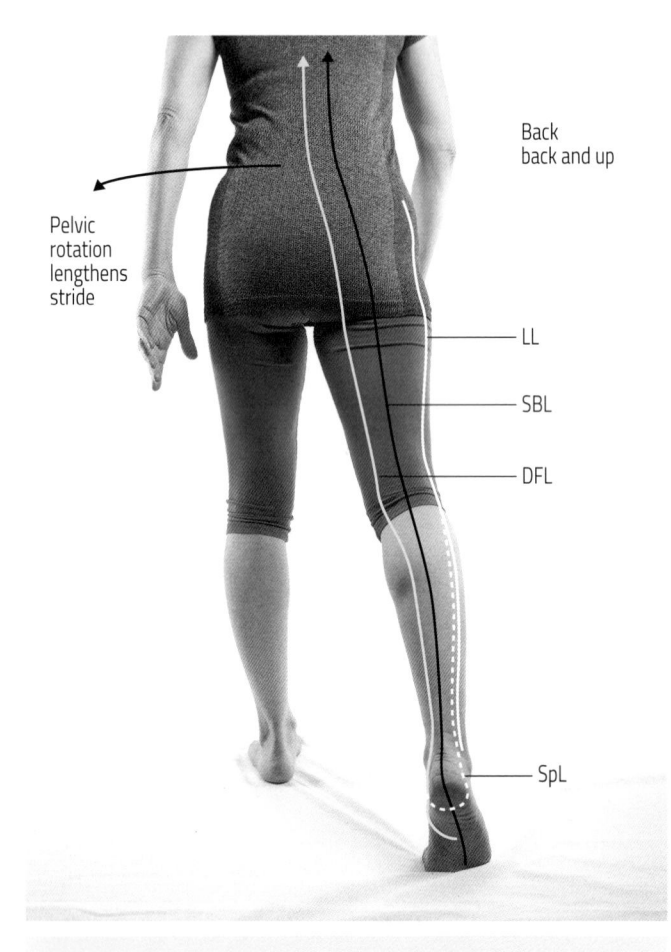

**Figure 11.13**
Powering the walk with balanced leg spirals/torque chains rotates the pelvis and lengthens the stride. Spiral (SpL), lateral (LL), superficial front (not shown), superficial back (SBL), and deep front line (DFL) all engaged together

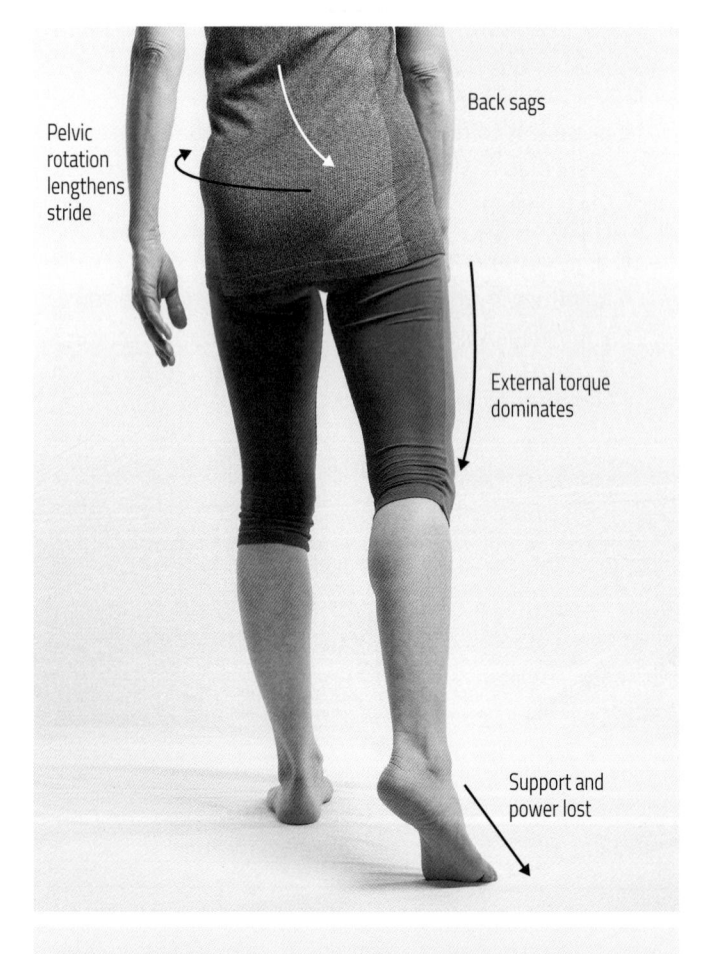

**Figure 11.14**
Allowing hip and foot to twist, secondary curve winning

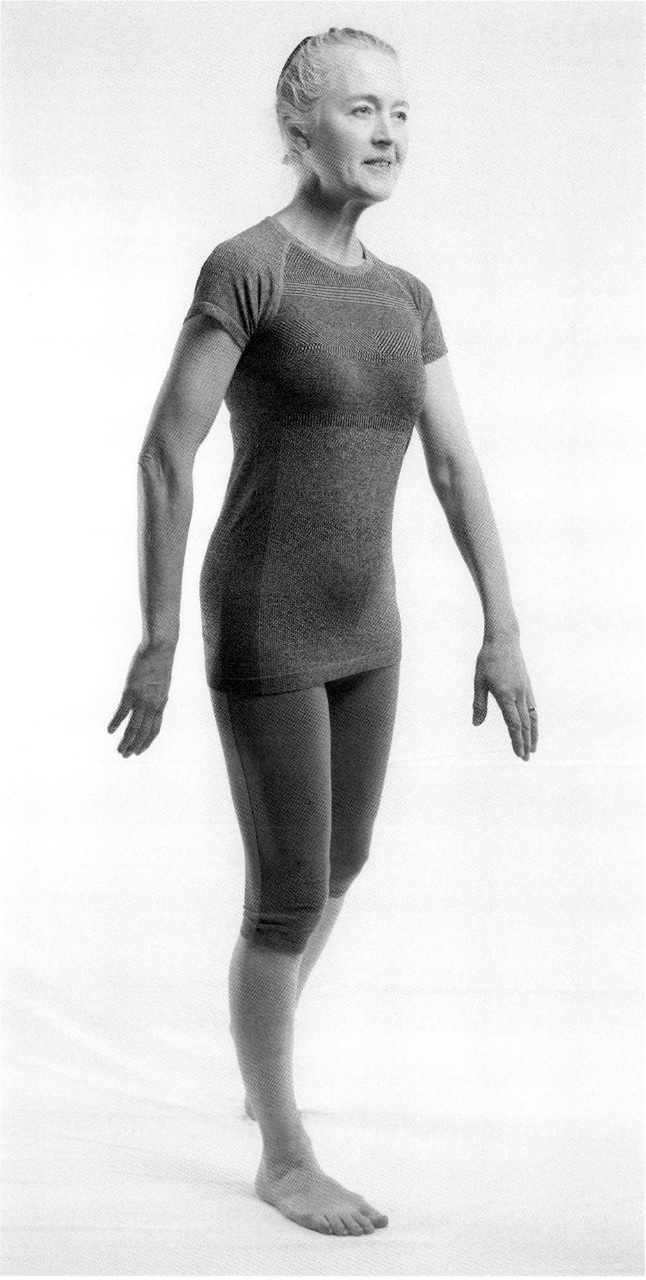

# Walking as you've never walked before

**Figure 11.15**
Arm swing with balanced walking

### Exploration 11.14  Climbing a hill

Finding a hill – even a wheelchair ramp – will help you understand what is happening here, and it is amazing how easy this action makes even the steepest hills.

- The head stays level – spot ahead with your eyes, and let what you see draw you forward.

- Notice that you do not need to lean into the hill, instead your torso is driven upward by the pelvic lift, through the lateral lines. These extend along your sternocleidomastoid muscles (between top of sternum and back of ear) extending the side of your head, taking your head forward and up.

- Keep taking your iliac spines and ribs back, breathing into the upper back, widening the deep back arm line. This will give your lungs and heart more space, and the rib expansion will widen the latissimus dorsi (the lifter muscles), sending your upper body forward and up.

- On the in-breath, widen into your pelvic floor and down into the hips, helping the hip lateral thrust; on the out-breath come back and up along the deep front line, to continue to take you up as you breathe out, and lengthen the legs.

- Use the contralateral movement of the arms to stabilize and help power you up. Notice that it is the arm swinging back, activating the latissimus dorsi (though without lifting the shoulders), that brings power to the walk – ensure the shoulder stays level (Fig. 11.16).

### Exploration 11.15  Coming down a hill

This is usually harder because there is more risk of falling, and gravity drives the body weight down into the knees. Thinking back and up in all its forms helps both

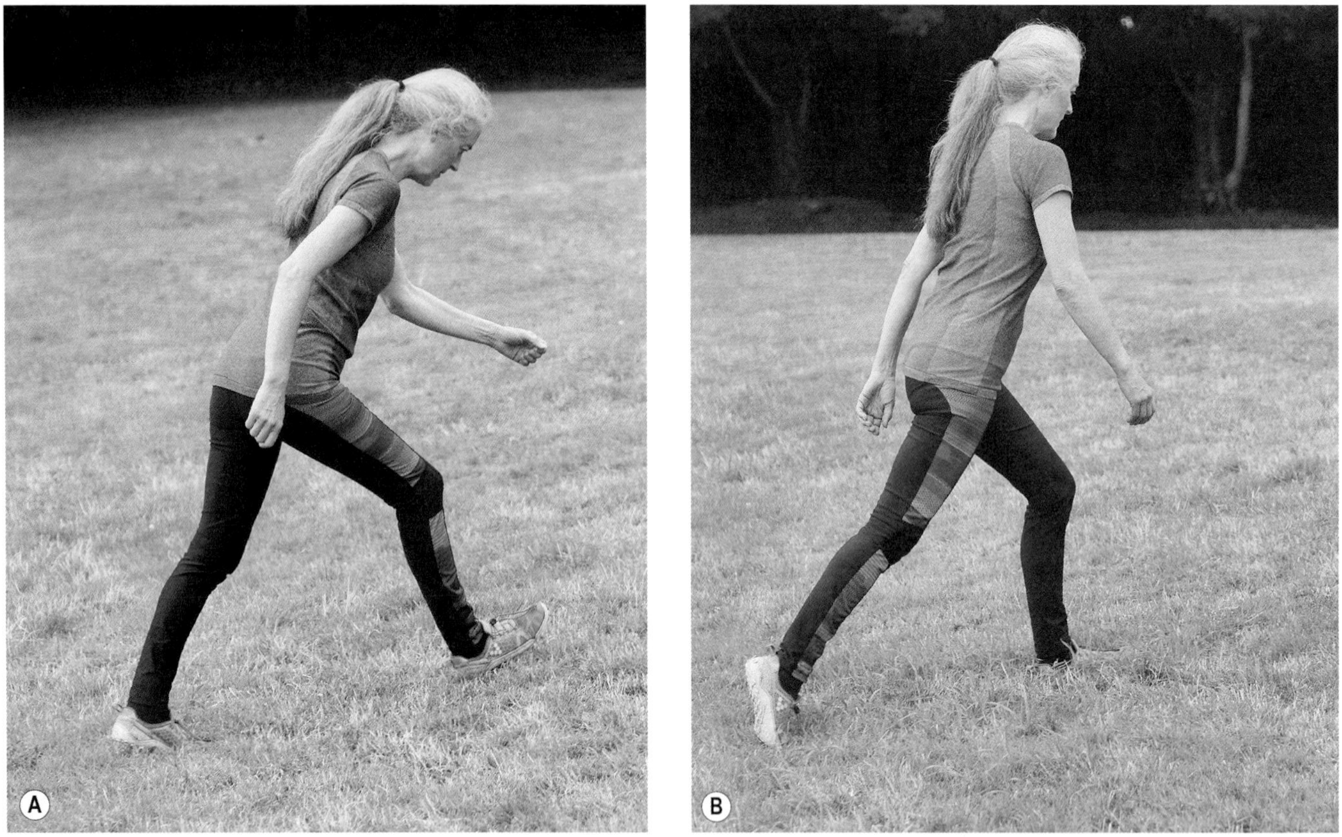

# CHAPTER eleven

**Figure 11.16**
Walking uphill. **(A)** Imbalanced torque chains are pulling against the directions of movement. **(B)** Balanced torque chains work together to take the body up the hill

of these by prioritizing the extensor system, and takes pressure off the front of the body.

- *Avoid falling by keeping the iliac spines back, to lean back from the hips not the upper back.*
- *Think up from the heels to sacrum to T8 as each foot touches down, and let the spring in the movement bounce you up. Do not plod!*
- *Stay with the back of the legs and let the knee joints open from behind.*
- *Play with all our other stabilizing methods also (Fig. 11.17).*

### Learning to walk naturally again

I love barefoot shoes. But initially, when walking distances on hard surfaces – such as interminable airport corridors – I felt I wanted that small heel of the standard "flat" shoe. Then I discovered hip stabilizers and soon after, began walking fully barefoot every morning, and my feet began to contact the ground in a new and positive way.

Then I took another trip. In the long corridor, I thought of my hip stabilizers driving the back foot, opposed along the length of the leg by this new contact with the ground, and suddenly everything I teach happened by itself. The feet turned in and the weight came onto the big toe balls, the knees rotated out and went forward over the second and third toes, the foot came strong, the back widened and came back, the shoulders broadened and came forward, the torso lifted off the legs. The movement was easy and powerful and for the first time my barefoot boots were completely

# Walking as you've never walked before

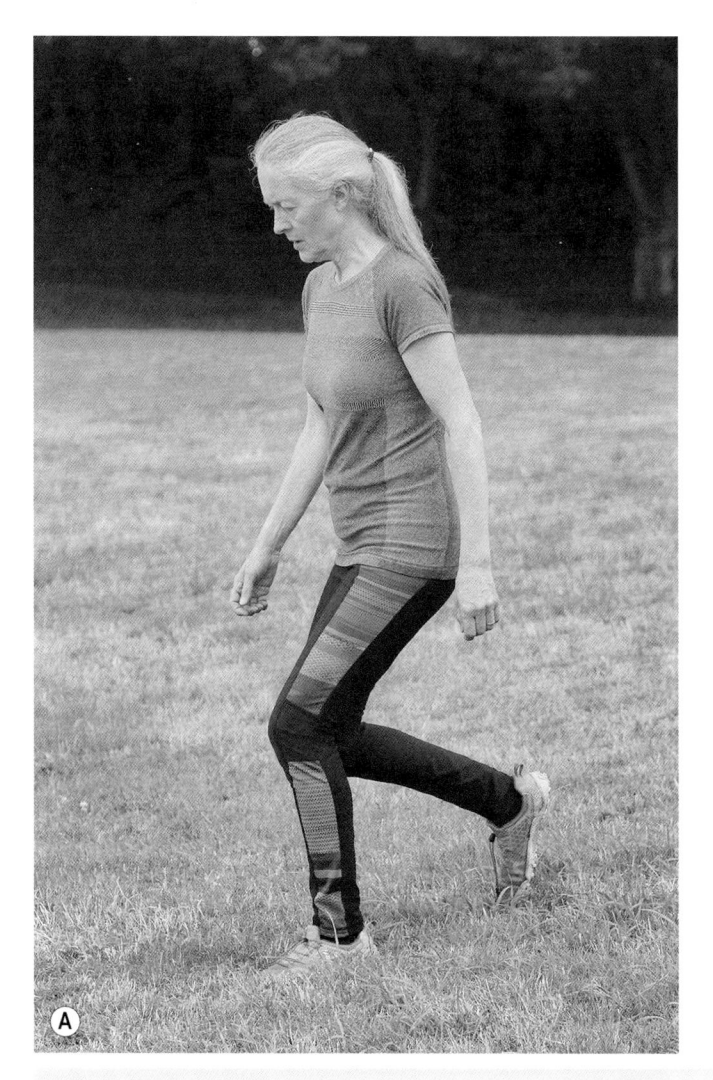

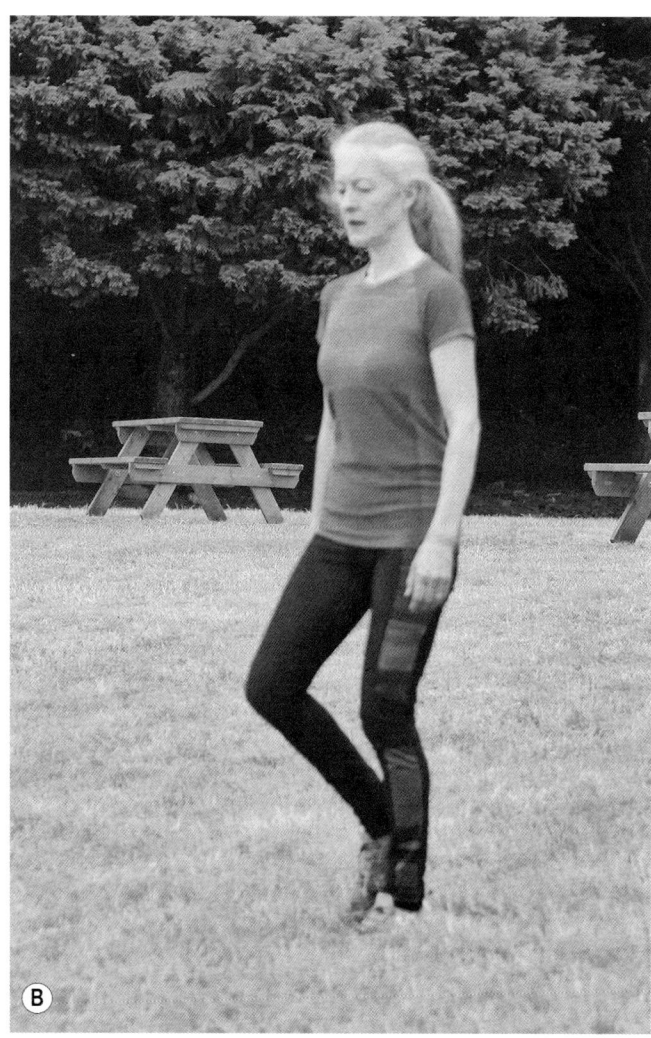

**Figure 11.17**
Walking downhill. **(A)** Extensor system weak, elastic energy lost, body weight dropping into knees; risk of falling. **(B)** Extensor system working back and up for safety; elastic rebound keeps body light

comfortable. I was easy in my body and the surroundings together, as the biomechanics of movement morphed into action by themselves. Truly a game changer!

Your walk may currently feel self-conscious and awkward as you struggle to keep all the various directions happening together. Keep alternating with letting it happen from spatial awareness and embodied intelligence, including awareness of the ground under your switched-on feet. We are aiming for the complexity of movement to be managed by self-organizing pathways, probably in the lower brain and spinal cord, to which the cortical brain can send modulating messages as needed. More on the coordination of walking in Chapter 16.

## Brief introduction to natural running

As you walk faster, you can either distort your body (as competition walkers do), or break into a run. This gait change happens quite naturally if we let it, with

# CHAPTER eleven

the foot still landing below the top of sternum. (The argument is on-going whether we should land on front of foot or whole foot.) As we land, the back foot comes up behind, from which position it will naturally cycle forward to stretch in front of the body in the flight phase. The faster you run, the higher the heel will come, resulting in a longer stride. However, at landing, because the torso is not pulled back, the instep is always under the top of sternum (see Fig. 11.2). Some runners lean forward, and some run more upright; whichever we do, we need to keep directions going to stop the back either sagging forwards or arching back.

Running arms, like walking arms, swing forward and back from the shoulder joint. But in running, the elbow bends into a right angle, with the palm facing the body, so that the pull back of the upper arm helps to power us forward. Many runners let their arms flop around, and lose out on this.

The shoulders and pelvis need to be unrestricted and free to move as needed in all three planes, while maintaining stability through the torso. At a lower speed, the arms are relaxed at waist height; as we speed into a sprint the hands arc between hip and nipple.

There are excellent courses run by various AT teachers on natural running for those who want to know more.

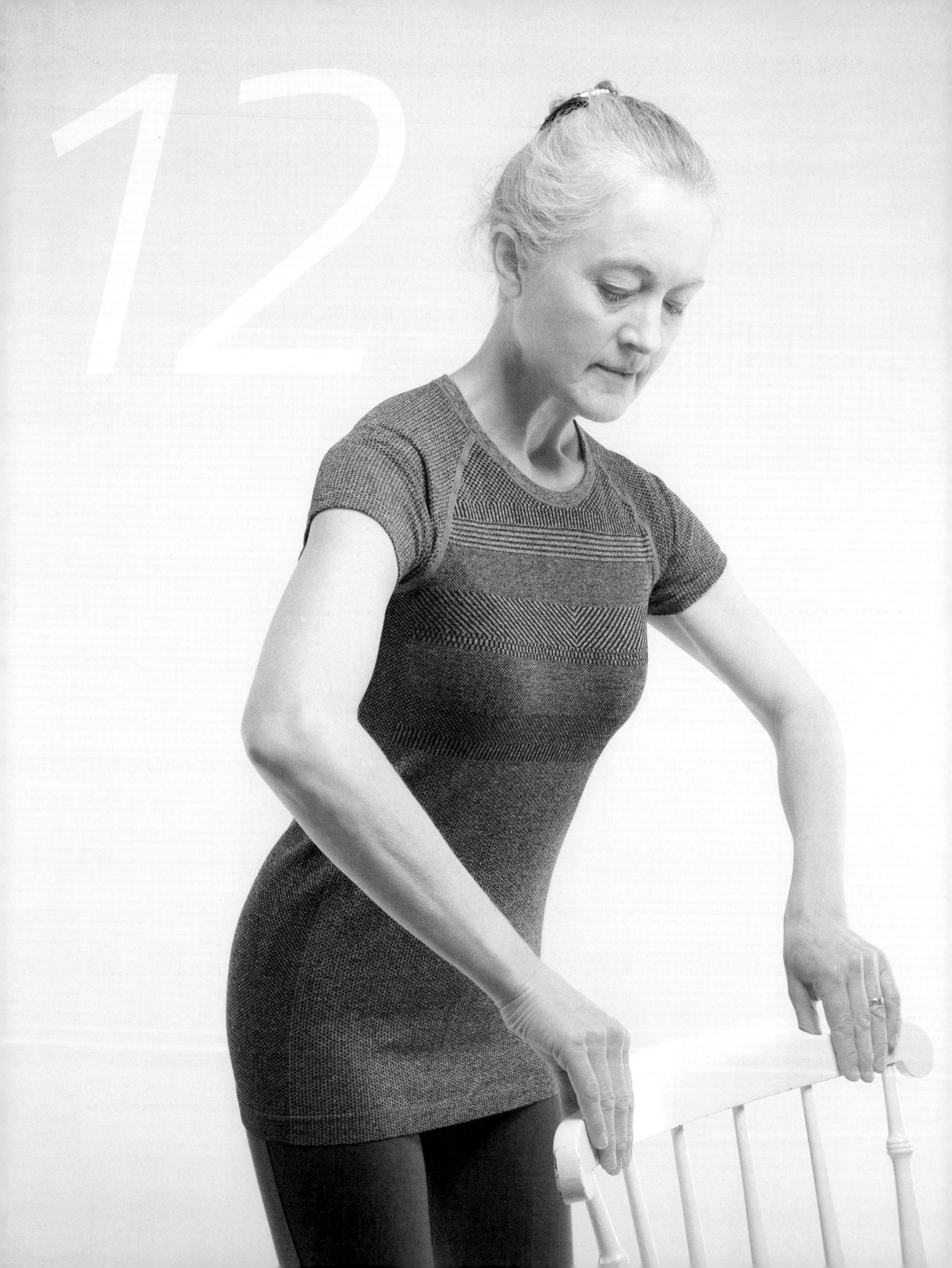

12

# Alexander's biomechanics for expansion of the upper body

## Introduction

I was a slender quick-footed child, but with little upper body strength. There was neither power nor aim when I threw snowballs – I once missed a boy in my class from one meter away! So embarrassing. I always tried too hard, putting too much effort into everything – my poor arms would often shake uncontrollably after strong activity. In my Alexander lessons and training it was a relief to learn to do less in every activity, and to leave my arms and hands quiet. I learned to let my arm hang heavy in the hands of my teachers, to be lengthened and released out of the shoulders. I learned to leave the hands alone, almost limp, as I brought them softly up onto a pupil, so that my back could communicate through them.

Soft hands and non-doing hands have become a hallmark of modern Alexander training and work. But the first-generation teachers used their hands quite differently, with immense strength, though they were often not that sensitive to where the fingers landed – they could be sticking in your throat or even up your nose. They were spiky and clear and powered from their backs. I wondered how they generated that power without forcing it; after all, wasn't that why we needed such soft hands? Wasn't this what Alexander had taught? But if people attempted to tell Miss Goldie – as I did once – that her hands were too rough on my neck or throat, her counter was that it was your neck or throat that was fighting her hands, and you should use your technique to stop it!

My understanding of every part of me changed with her lessons, and hands and arms were no exception. Her emphasis was not on release and softness, but on integration, aliveness, and connection – to my back and body, and to the world. This wasn't about a nice floaty feel, it was tangible – there was so much more sensation in my fingers when I touched things, and there was a gentleness in it I had never had. Paradoxically, there was also much greater power for throwing or lifting and much more accuracy of aim. Despite the increased strength, my arms were more non-doing than before, coming from a quiet connectivity with the rest of me that was both gentle and strong. As with my legs, I struggled to understand this from the learning she had given me, and while over the years I came to understand much, there were many missing pieces.

Again, Jeando Masoero and his understanding of Alexander's initial technique has completed this for me and allowed me to access the full strength of my hands, arms, and upper body after I lost it with years of illness; thanks to him for nearly all the explorations in this chapter. Just as we found how little we use the full tone of the legs, so most people also do not access the full tone in expansion of the upper body.

## Active, integrative stretching versus passive, single muscle stretching

Most of us use our bodies like a machine: alternating between pushing them into action with the big limb muscles, mostly flexors, and passively disengaging them when not in use. In neither is there much engagement of those extensors which would integrate the limbs with the muscles of the torso.

We have already explored bringing all the muscle groups for legs and arms into play, letting them unfold into action, and then *not* switching them off again. In this chapter, we will use Masoero's Initial Alexander technique (Initial AT) explorations for actively opening the deep tensions we carry in arms and torso (see box). These can bring even more fluidity, strength and coordination, but they will be unfamiliar, and can initially be difficult. However, perseverance will produce change over time. We are up against our proprioceptive databanks in the brain – those guardians of our current habits – which will tell us repeatedly that these moves are wrong. It won't help that the stretches may hurt. But have a go, then afterward, notice what has changed in your springiness and freedom of movement. I sometimes still resist the hard work and discomfort of these stretches, but now, knowing the benefits they bring, I can welcome it. It will take time and repetition to work through these explorations. If needed, do feel free to intersperse them with explorations of the next chapters or Part 3.

# CHAPTER twelve

This is very different to the standard approach to stretching. Consider the standard triceps stretch (Fig. 12.1). This is a passive stretch, where the muscle is put into a position it could not easily hold actively. Muscle trains do not work when the angle of connection is acute (Myers 2014: 67), just as a trailer cannot be pulled when it has jack-knifed. After passive stretching, no attention is usually given to maintaining its length in the ensuing activity, which will inevitably tighten it up again.

In contrast, the active pulls we do here are linking up muscle trains for real life movement patterns that we can then utilize and maintain the lengthening.

**Important:** *once you have the basics for each of the explorations, add in the procedures in Chapter 7 for removing unnecessary tension (exploration 7.7) and playing with temporal relationships (exploration 7.25).*

> Masoero describes the Initial AT as the "the means whereby any student can self-experiment with conscious guidance and control to self-regulate his/her own use" (Masoero in conversation, October 2019, Ennis, Ireland). He added: "It's not just a matter of defining instructions: it's a matter of defining how you are going to do the movements all together." This chapter uses the sequences I learned from him to access and re-activate the upper body, opening out deep tensions. This also familiarizes the learner with the body geometry and pulls involved. In Chapter 13, lesson 6, I give the method as I understand it for using these methods as experiments in constructive guidance and control as Alexander wanted.

## Lesson 1  Finding the supportive torso

To lengthen the arms, the shoulder girdle must be supported correctly on the torso, for which the parts of the torso must be aligned together and with gravity. We discovered in Chapter 7 that often, an "upright torso" is in a reverse curve. You could describe this as a D shape (Fig. 12.2).

Initial AT, drawing on biomechanics as well as Alexander's books, teaches a different body geometry. This is flatter at the front with ribs draping down and sternum vertical; straighter at the back from sacrum to T8, from which point the head springs forward and up (Fig. 12.3). That this is what Alexander was teaching is clear in the picture of the first training course (Fig. 7.21). He called this forward slope of the very top of the torso the "hump"; Bowman (2017: 227) calls this connectivity of upper thoracic and cervical spine "ramping the head" – a much more acceptable name to modern ears.

To undo the D shape, we need to reverse these deep tension patterns (Fig. 12.4). This is more easily done in three stages:

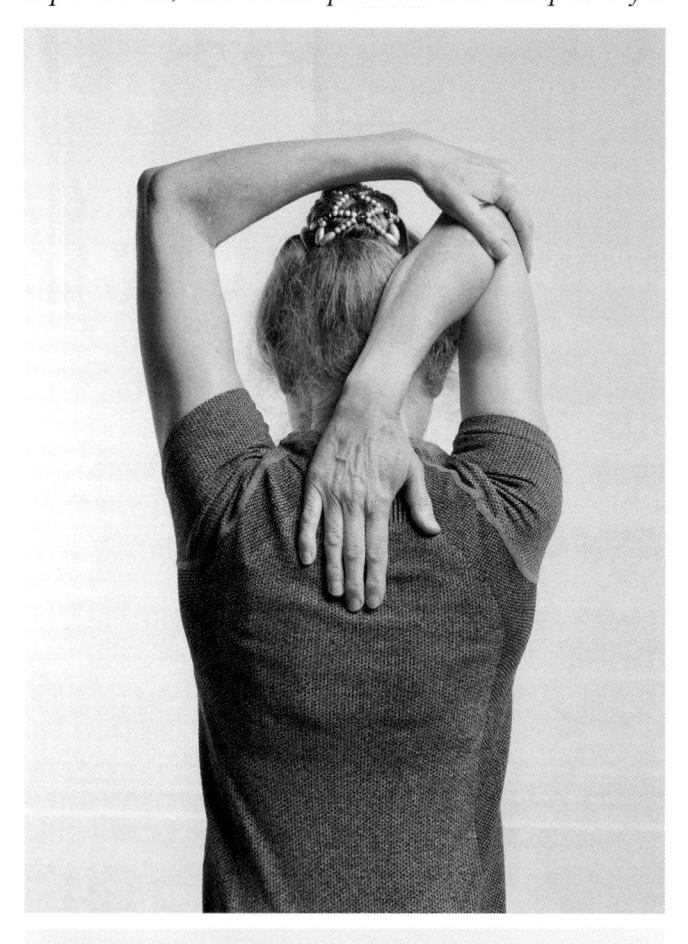

**Figure 12.1**
Standard triceps stretch

# Alexander's biomechanics for expansion of the upper body

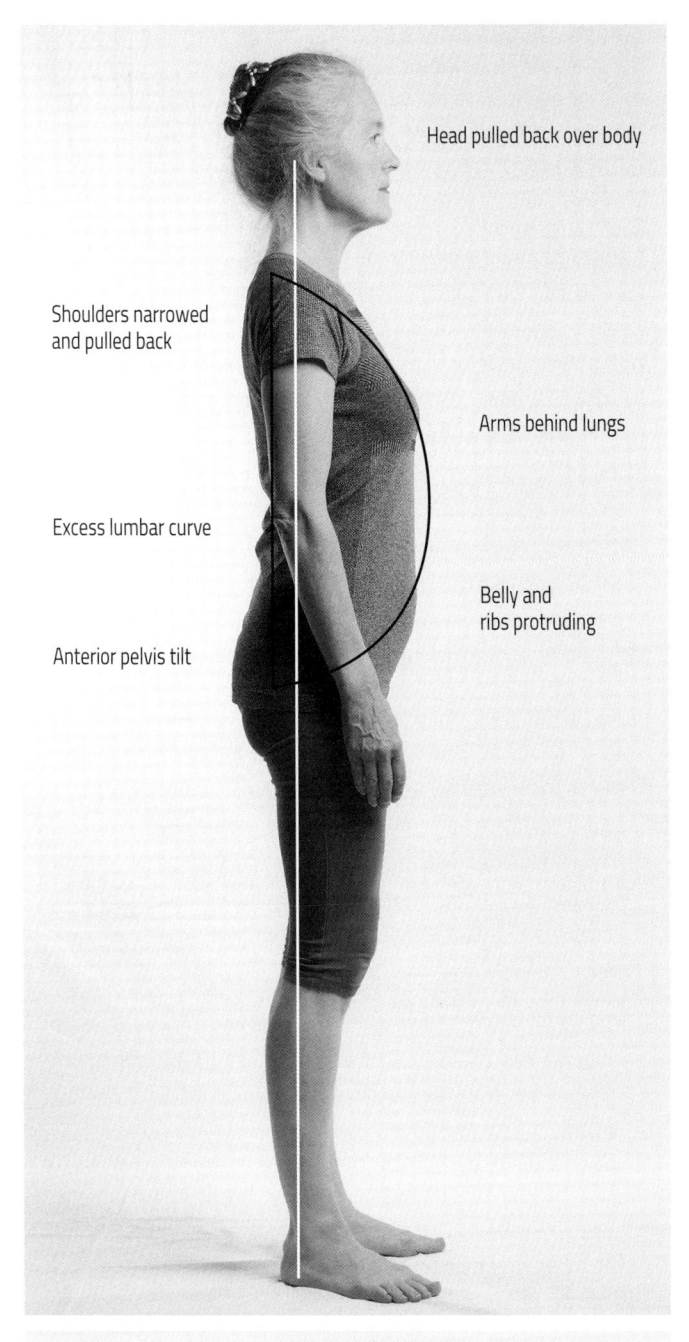

**Figure 12.2**
Standard "correct" posture describes a D-shape

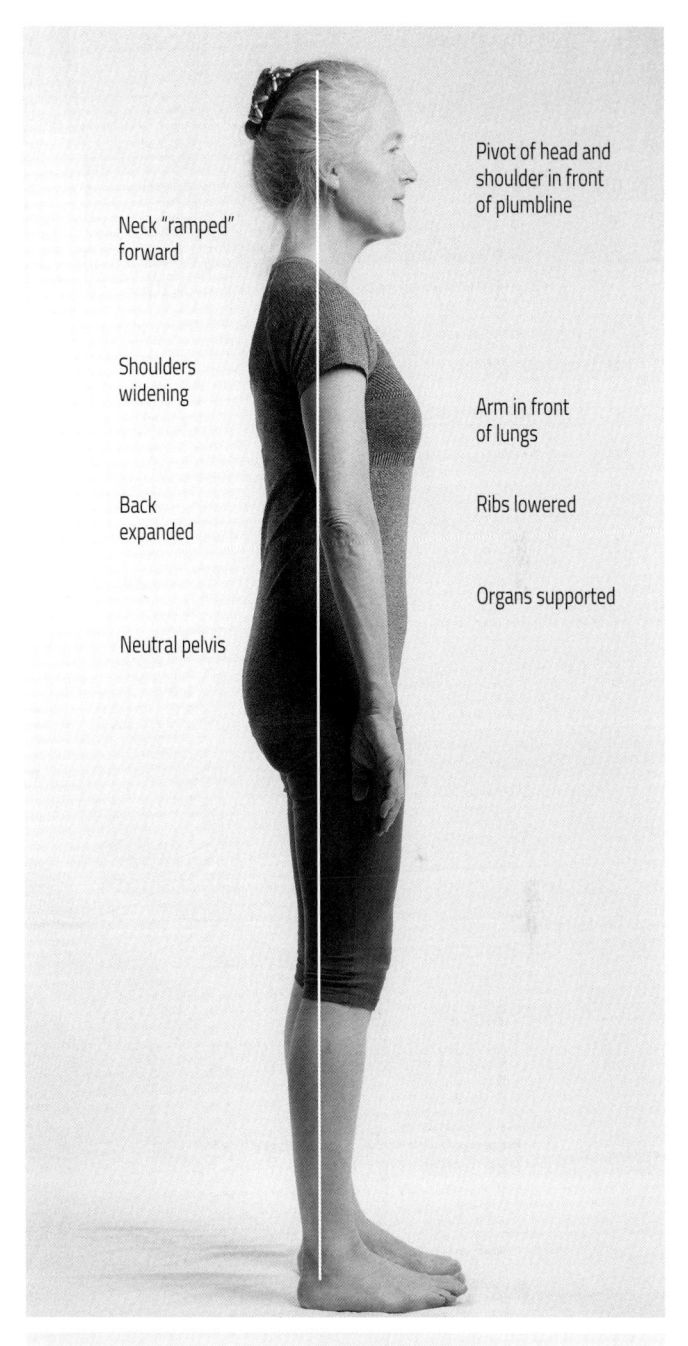

Labels: Head pulled back over body; Shoulders narrowed and pulled back; Arms behind lungs; Excess lumbar curve; Belly and ribs protruding; Anterior pelvis tilt

**Figure 12.3**
New body geometry is straight up and down

Labels: Pivot of head and shoulder in front of plumbline; Neck "ramped" forward; Shoulders widening; Arm in front of lungs; Ribs lowered; Back expanded; Organs supported; Neutral pelvis

1. The ribs need to come back and up in space, and
2. T8 (between the lower tips of the shoulder blades) needs to come back and up from the sacrum and heels.

These two moves are part of one process, which is to lift the upper body up off the lower body, and open out the arch in the lumbar spine. It also widens the back.

# CHAPTER twelve

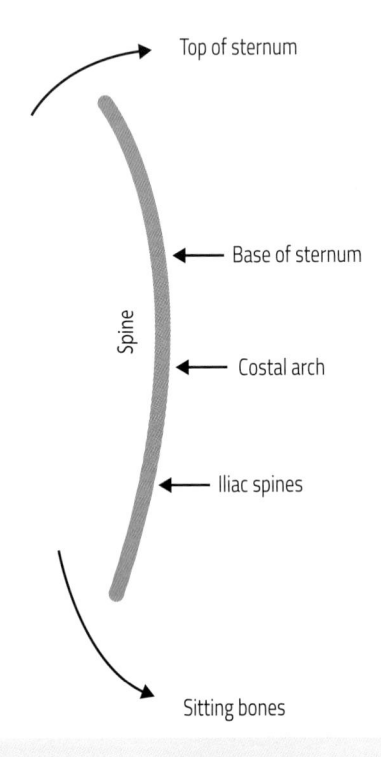

**Figure 12.4**
Directions needed to reverse the D-shape

*(Diagram labels: Top of sternum, Base of sternum, Costal arch, Iliac spines, Sitting bones, Spine)*

3  The top of sternum needs to lift forward. This brings the line from the 8th to the 1st thoracic vertebra *forward*, to allow the head to go forward and up.

*These are unfamiliar pulls which may take time to sort out.*

### Taking the ribs back and up

Just as pulling the iliac spines back flattens and widens the lower back through the action of the transverse abdominals, so pulling the ribs back flattens and widens the middle back through the action of the external obliques (see Fig. 3.24).

### Exploration 12.1  Using the wall

The wall was used on the first training course and is still used by many teachers to open out the lumbar spine, but the body geometry was never clarified verbally by Alexander. That he was using the body geometry described here is recounted by Robert Best, who took lessons with him from 1929 on: "When F. M. was staying with us I gave a demonstration [of using the wall] in the bedroom. Of course he corrected it and showed how the hump should be coming away from the wall and the hollow of the back *going towards* it" (Best, sometime in the 1930s, cited in Murray 2015: 169).

In explorations 10.6 and 10.7 (active hip flexing) we found the core muscles of the deep front line, then maintained the tone as we hinged the legs on the back. This is the same work, done against a wall. You are going into the unknown, so work from spatial awareness and embodied intelligence, thinking the directions first then, if possible, doing them all together with a 1-2-3. By staying out of the way, we allow the body to self-organize; to check our perceptions we need to use video.

- *Stand flat against a wall, heels 3–4 inches (8–10 cm) from the wall, and sacrum the lower tips of the shoulder blades (with T8 between) touching the wall. Probably, your mid-back will not be touching. What does it take to flatten this against the wall? You could push your front ribs down, folding in your middle, but this would round your spine, drop your chest, and T8 would come away from the wall.*

- *Instead (1) invite the back to widen on the in-breath, especially at the costal arch level. The ribs drape down and move back, from where they widen and lift back and up. You are widening your external obliques and latissimus dorsi – the lifter muscles. Rotating your elbows forward and outward to open the deep back arm line will also help.*

  *Then (2), on the out-breath, bring your breath up and back along the lumbar spine, out of the legs, and engage your pubococcygeals to open out the lumbar spine.*

- *Lastly (3), bring the pelvis more vertical by thinking iliac spines and the lowest belly muscles back, pubococcygeals forward, and hamstrings engaged. Keep taking the ribs back and up (Fig. 12.5).*

There is real work going on here, to pull out deep old tensions – you are putting yourself on the rack! Some

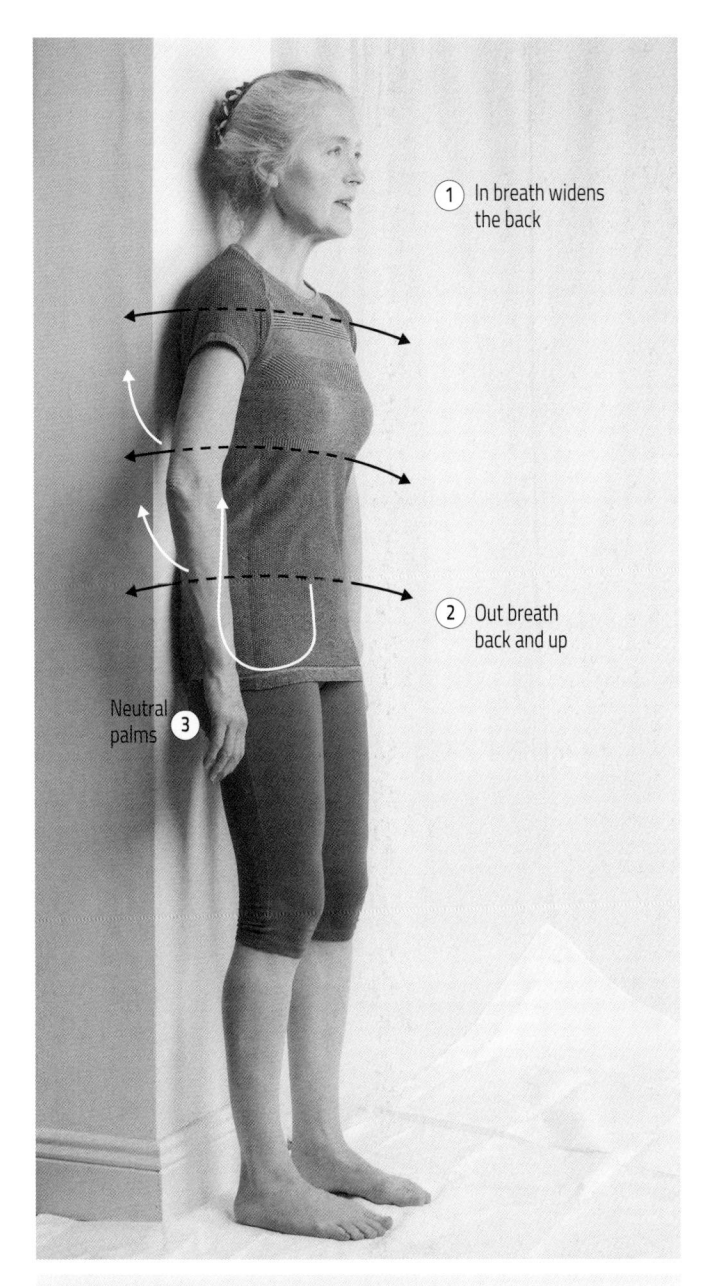

# Alexander's biomechanics for expansion of the upper body

**Figure 12.5**
Lengthening and widening against a wall

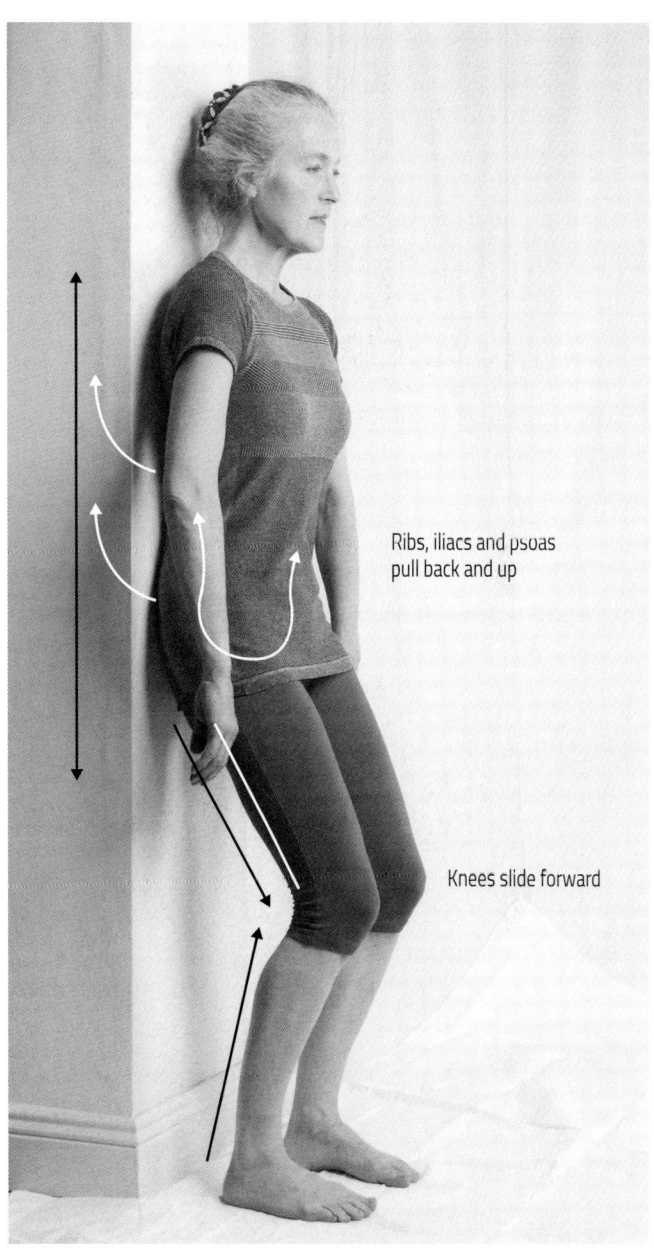

- ① In breath widens the back
- ② Out breath back and up
- ③ Neutral palms

**Figure 12.6**
Sliding down and up a wall

- Ribs, iliacs and psoas pull back and up
- Knees slide forward

people will by now be flat against the wall, and others will not. To help, do the full wall procedure:

- *While keeping all this going, let your knees slide forward from behind, so your back slides down the wall, opposed by the ribs and out-breath pulling back and up. Do not go too far down (Fig. 12.6).*

- *Breathe in, widening everything.*

- *On the next out-breath, pull the ribs, iliac spines, and psoas back and up the wall. The legs will lengthen by themselves – they do not need to push.*

# CHAPTER twelve

- *Will your back now stay flatter and wider against the wall? Play around till you can find this; give it time. If you have deep spine tensions it may take several attempts to see a difference.*

You will now feel as if you are in a reverse curve (like a bracket shape). This is faulty sensory perception, as the wall proves your back is now straight, in an I shape. Since this will feel so very wrong I suggest you do not worry about shape, but think of it as muscle activation work. Trust your embodied intelligence to self-organize, and you may notice afterwards that you are moving differently.

Can you now find this opening and widening of the back while freestanding? Check it with your long stick against your back.

Video link for exploration 12.1

### Bringing the line sacrum to T8 to vertical

#### Exploration 12.2    Sacrum to T8

- *While standing, play with bringing T8 strongly up and back from the heels and sacrum. This will bring the ribs back and up, lift the upper body forward and open the lumbar spine.*

### Taking the top of sternum forward in space

For most people, the sternum is angled forward at the base and back at the top. Another whammy for our cultural body image is that the sternum line should be approaching vertical, but you will not see this in anatomical drawings (Figs 12.7 and 12.8).

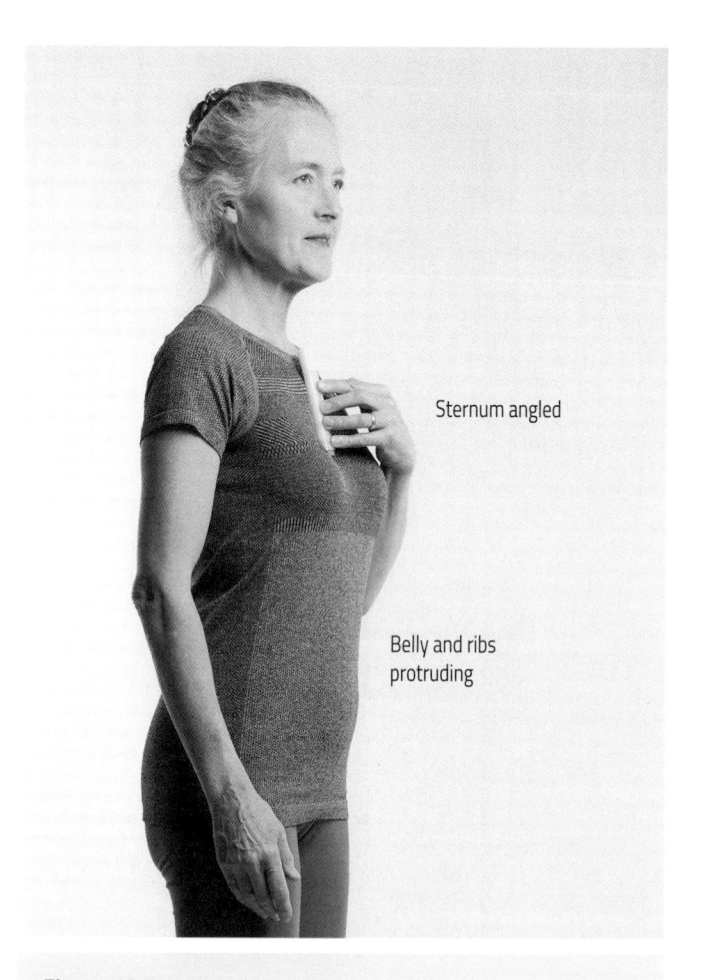

**Figure 12.7**
D-shape posture angles the sternum

#### Exploration 12.3    Anatomy play – the sternum line

- *Find the line of your sternum, by putting a pencil along it vertically.*
- *Bring T8 back and up from the heels and sacrum as above. Notice that as the ribs come back and up, the base of the sternum is pulled back with the ribs, bringing it more vertical.*
- *You may now feel hollow chested and hunched – that is ok!*

To bring the head forward and up, we need to pull the top of sternum forward in space, to take the 1st vertebra forward of the 8th vertebra.

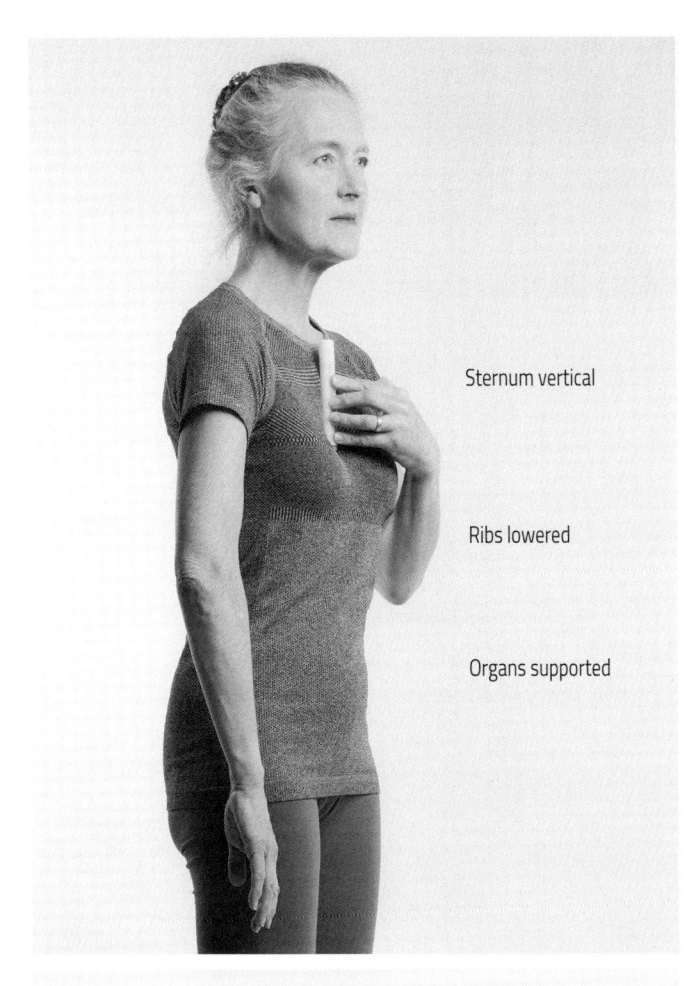

# Alexander's biomechanics for expansion of the upper body

**Figure 12.8**
New body geometry has vertical sternum

- Sternum vertical
- Ribs lowered
- Organs supported

back, with a corresponding force to take the top of sternum forward.

This difference can be defined in engineering terms:

*Kinematics* – the study of describing movement (with displacement, velocity, etc.). It looks at movement with shape and alignment.

*Kinetics* – the *forces* acting on your torso that cause motion (torque, gravity, friction, etc.) which can feel like over-engagement of the muscles and tension.

To consider a cyclist – kinematics would study the changing relationships of our thighs, lower legs and feet articulating at hips, knees and ankles, interacting with the circular movement of the pedals, to produce seemingly effortless movement forward on the bike. Kinetics would look at the real forces being applied through the legs to produce this movement, and the oppositional forces needed from the cyclist's seat, torso, and arms to prevent twisting as force is applied through each leg.

To change his back, without the help of a teacher, Alexander had to find and use these forces. Many teachers do this for their pupils with strong, directional pulls. With Initial AT, we can learn to do this for ourselves.

If you simply try to pull your top of sternum forward, you will probably curl and hunch yourself, maybe also pulling your chin down, as T8 moves forward too. These are unwanted movements; we need to be able to isolate the movements we need. For this we need oppositions: when the ribs come back and up, T8 stays back, from which T1 can move forward.

## Kinematics versus kinetics

We do need to apply real forces on the torso, matching the force used to take the iliac spines and ribs

### Exploration 12.4  Finding an opposing force from the top of the sternum - anatomy play

- *Stand upright, and using the flat of your hand, push back on the top of your own sternum. If you do nothing in response, you will bend backwards with the upper body.*

- *To stay upright, you need to resist the push with the top of your sternum. Notice that you also need to take your iliac spines back, or you will bend forward instead. Watch that you have not involved your shoulders or neck; it may take a few goes to isolate the opposition to the top of sternum alone. Keep breathing.*

# CHAPTER twelve

- *As you take your iliac spines back, can you now find this push forward without using your hand?*

This is easier to play with another person, applying the pushes to each other. You may be surprised just how much resisting power we can generate here. There are important muscle links here that we are not using fully.

## Making an integrative change

Now we will use all the moves in Figure 12.4 to open out the D shape.

### Exploration 12.5  Stacking the torso for balanced shoulders – opening out the curve in the torso

Give directions from spatial awareness and embodied intelligence, while not responding to them, then count 1-2-3 as you make all the movements together (refer to Fig. 12.9).

*Align your legs and feet. Send the heels down.*

I pull T8 up away from the heels (1a), which brings the base of the sternum back (1b).

I pull the ribs back and up in space (2).

I pull the top of the sternum up and forward – and stay looking forward (3).

To stabilize these moves,

I pull the iliac spines back in space (4).

I pull the sitting bones towards the back of the knees, and gently engage the pubococcygeals forwards (5).

You may now feel bowed forward, which is probably faulty sensory perception. Check with your sticks whether your ribs and top of sternum are now nearer the unity line (see Fig. 7.3), and whether your sternum line is more vertical. (Fig. 12.9).

**Video link for exploration 12.5**

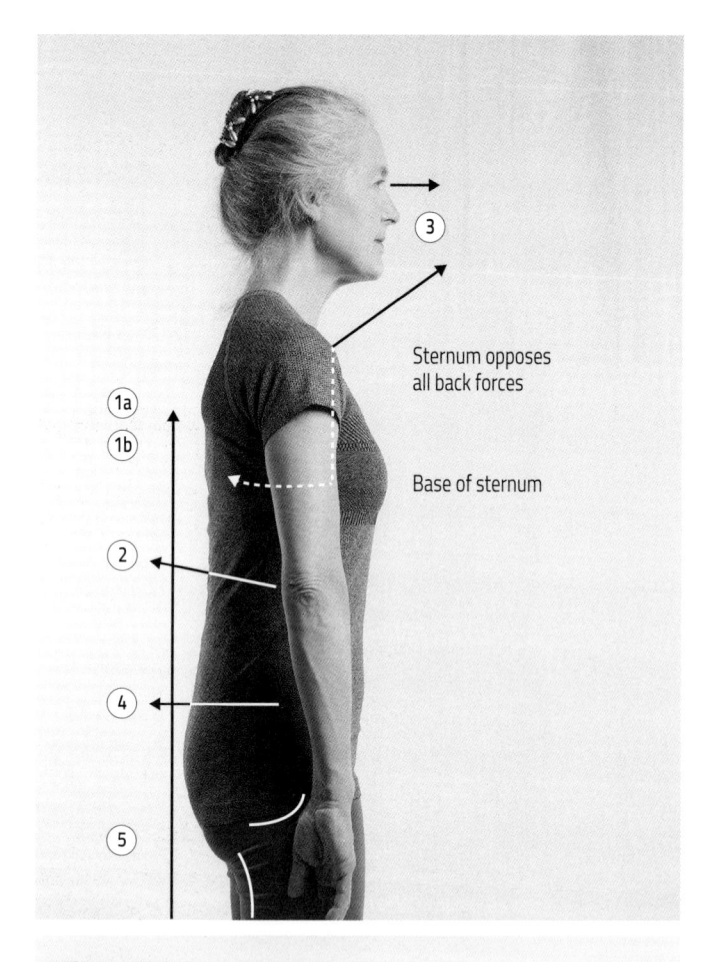

**Figure 12.9**
Pulling the upper vertebrae T8 to T1 forward

## Lesson 2   Shoulders and clavicles

Having supported the shoulder girdle securely on the torso, we can address the geometry within it: the relative positions of the shoulder blades and clavicles.

### Exploration 12.6   The shoulder shrug

The shoulder shrug is a temporary game only to understand the body geometry of shoulders, at the back and the front. At the back, the shoulder blades are often held too close together, by over-tight rhomboids. Instead they need to lie on the sides of the back. This hugely widens the back, frees the breathing, and activates the deep back arm line (DBAL). When, at the front, the clavi-

# Alexander's biomechanics for expansion of the upper body

cles also widen, it makes space for the neck to lengthen up between the shoulder blades.

### Anatomy play

Initially, play with this with one arm at a time; you can use your other hand to direct the clavicle out sideways.

#### Stage 1 (Fig. 12.10A)

- *Find the lower tips of your shoulder blade (scapula) and T8 between them.*

*Pull your scapula tips (and so T8) right up away from your heels.*

*Send the iliac spines back in space.*

*Keep looking forwards.*

Your shoulders will hunch up and forwards to your ears, bringing your top of sternum forwards. Taking the iliac spines back stabilizes this move. Try this while holding your little stick to notice whether your sternum line changes angle.

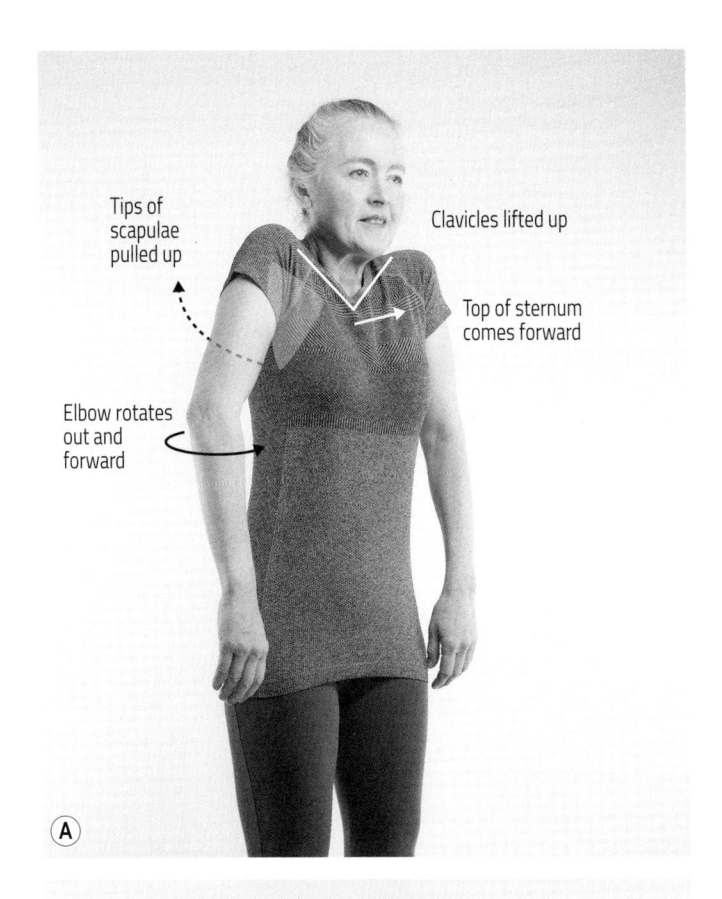

**Figure 12.10**
Shoulder shrug. **(A)** Stage 1, lifting the scapulae up and forwards. **(B)** Stage 2, pouring the shoulders down and widening

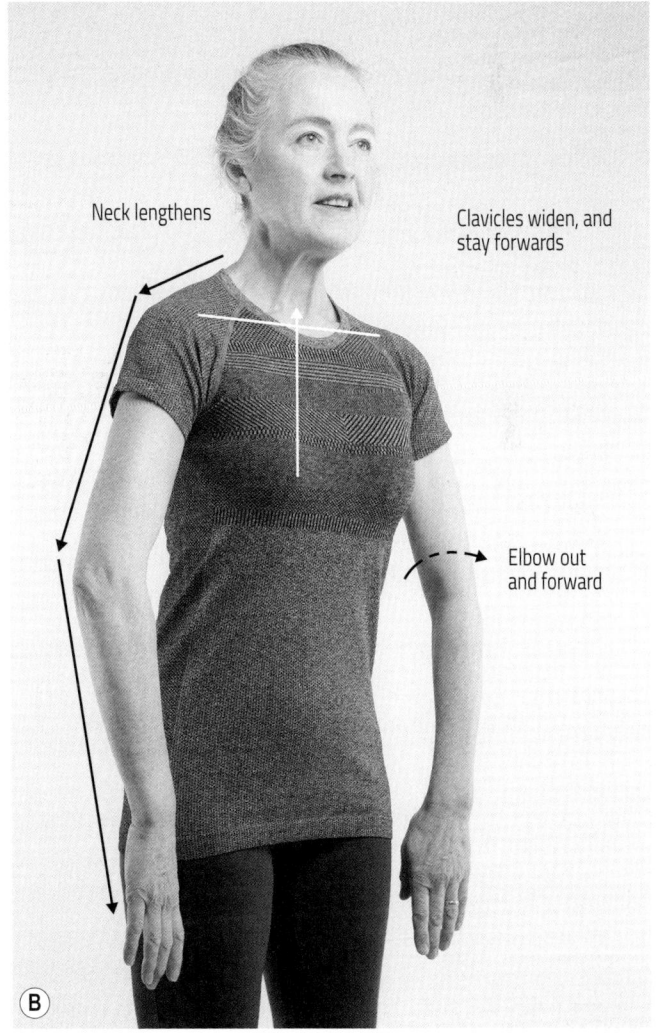

# CHAPTER twelve

**Stage 2 (Fig. 12.10B)**

*I send my elbow tips and little fingers down, to pour the shoulders downwards.* (Do not let the shoulders fall back, keep them forwards.)

*I widen my clavicles away from my top of sternum, following the sideways pull of the elbow and little finger.*

*I leave the neck alone, I keep looking forwards.*

- *If your chin and gaze want to drop, add an opposing thought that the neck does not go down with the shoulders - mentally find the space between them. (Wobbling it and then thinking it to stay free will help.)*

- *Use the directions given to do this as an integrated change for each stage in turn.*

*You may feel hunched forward but is your back more open? Is your front wider?*

## The fall of the shoulder and the clavicle line

### Exploration 12.7    The fall of the shoulder and line of the clavicle

- *Using a mirror, put a small stick along the topmost line of your shoulder, from the side of your neck to top of the arm. Is it horizontal, or does it slope downward from neck to shoulder?*

We want the fall of the shoulder to be angled downward. If the shoulders are raised, the muscles between shoulders and neck are tight. These need to lengthen to let the head be free on the neck.

- *Put a pencil along your clavicle. How does it slope: horizontal, upwards, or downwards (Figs 12.11 and 12.12)?*

While most people's clavicles are angled up and back, ideally, the clavicles are level, and even slope slightly downwards from sternum to shoulder. Notice that pushing them further down is counterproductive. But we can change the slope of a line by working from

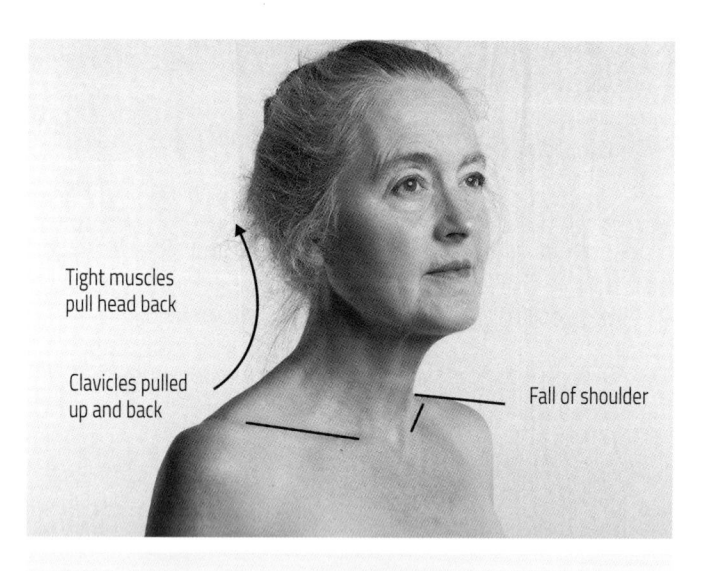

**Figure 12.11**
Clavicles pulling up and back, neck tight

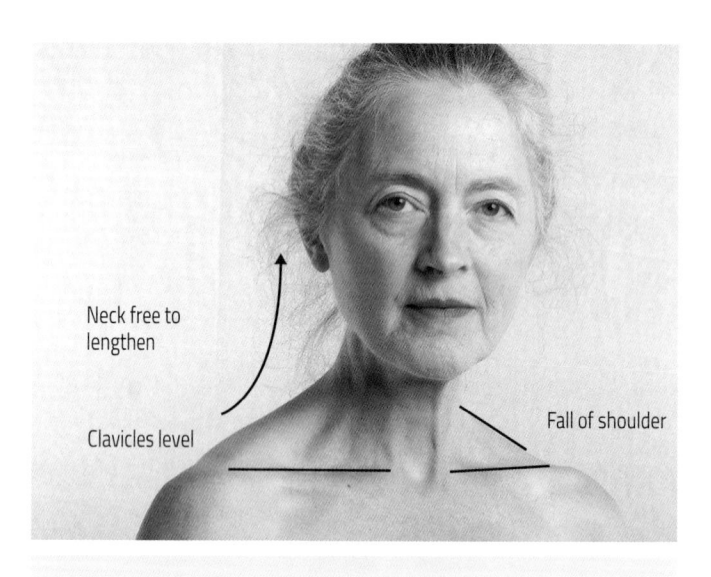

**Figure 12.12**
Level clavicles lengthen the neck muscles

both ends. We took the shoulders out and down in the shoulder shrug. Now we need also to take the top of sternum up.

# Alexander's biomechanics for expansion of the upper body

### Exploration 12.8   Find the diagonal – top of sternum to tip of elbow

Initially, do one arm at a time, but always give the pulls to both iliac spines or the torso will twist.

Explore these two stages separately. Then think the directions, and move on a count of 1-2-3.

> I pull my iliac spines up and away from the outside of the knee, and my ribs back and up.
>
> I pull my top of sternum forward and up, away from iliac spines and ribs.
>
> I pull the tips of my elbows down, away and forward from my top of sternum,
>
> and my top of sternum up away from the tips of my elbows.

Check your shoulder and clavicle lines. Have they altered? See that as the fall of the shoulder and the clavicles go down, the top of sternum is taken higher. (Fig. 12.12).

The tops of the lungs project above the level of the first rib. If the clavicles are angled back and up, they cross over the 1st rib, which impairs breathing into the top of the lungs. All these procedures that bring the top of sternum, the clavicles, and the arms forwards are disentangling these so that the shoulder girdle, ribcage, and lungs can function as intended (Figs 12.13 and 12.14).

## Lesson 3   Opening, widening, and deepening the chest

When invited to expand the chest, most people lift and arch into a secondary curve, narrowing the back.

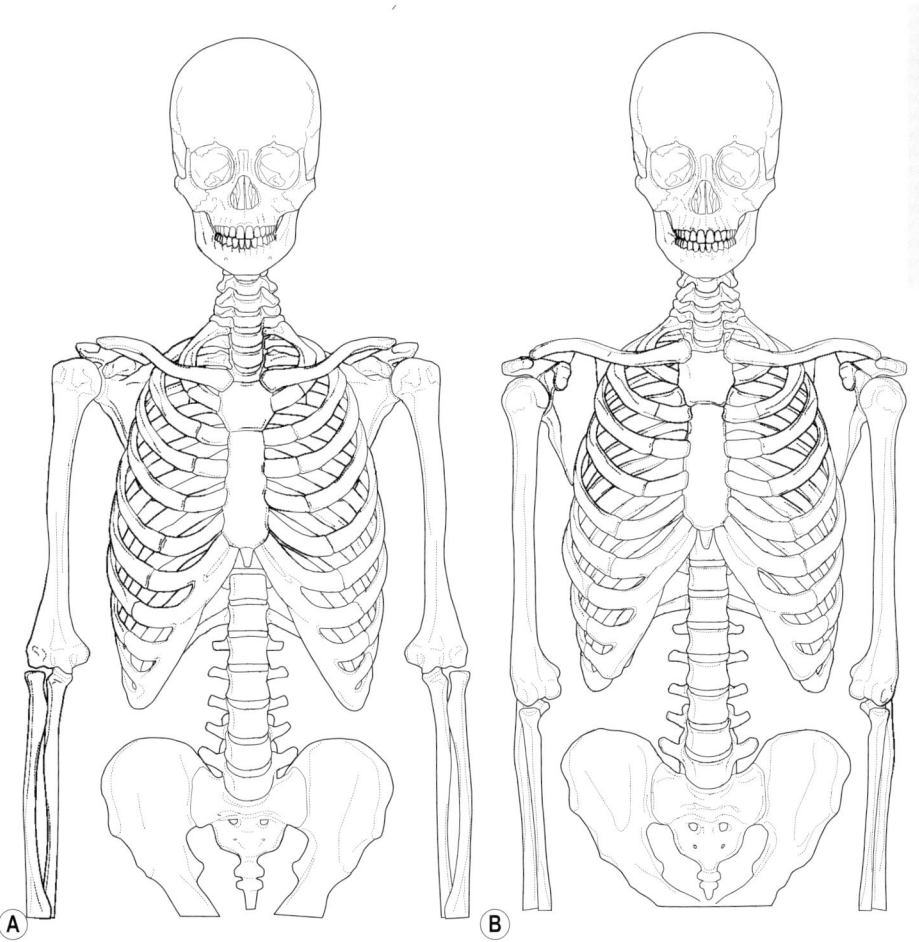

**Figure 12.13**
Ribcage model front view. **(A)** Shoulders pulled back angles clavicles up and back, tangling with first ribs, taking arms behind ribcage. **(B)** Shoulders widening and coming forward brings the clavicles lower, untangling them from first ribs, bringing arms forward

# CHAPTER twelve

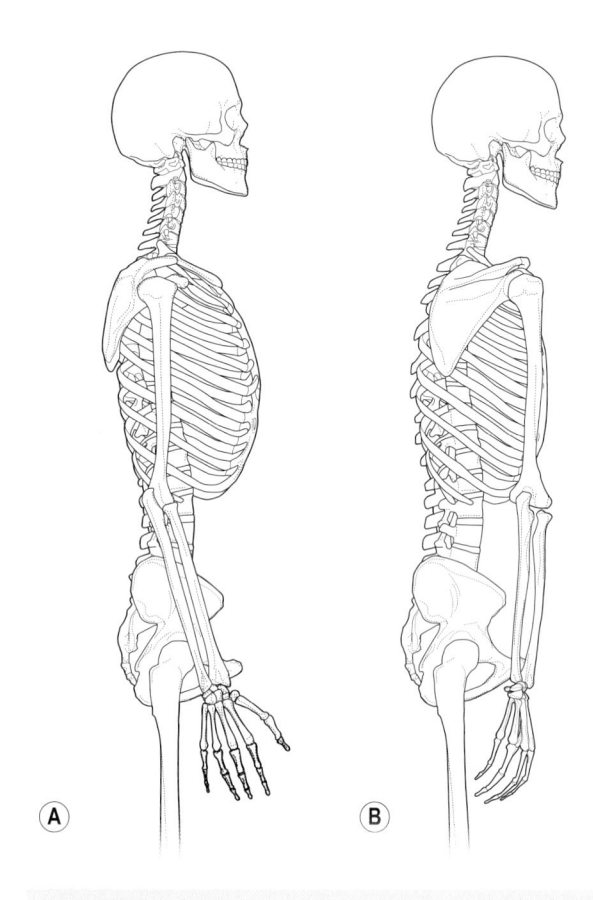

**Figure 12.14**
Ribcage model side view. **(A)** Shoulders back brings T8–T1 vertical, lifting base of sternum and costal arch, compressing top of lungs. **(B)** Shoulders forward and widening "ramps" T8–T1 and neck, so that top of sternum lifts forward and up. It brings base of sternum back and allows top of lungs to expand

We will explore opening the chest while keeping the back expanded also.

With the shoulder shrug, we discovered how to widen across the upper part of the arms by taking the clavicles away from each other. In explorations 9.6 and 9.7 we discovered breathing into the armpits to open the side of the ribs. Now we need the ribcage itself to widen across the front. All the ribs attach to the sternum by elastic cartilage, allowing some flexibility. But through poor breathing patterns the chest often becomes very rigid, and the cartilage can even ossify, showing up on chest X-rays. Be patient with yourself, it may take a while to reawaken movement here.

### Exploration 12.9  Fanning the ribs

The transversus thoracis is a muscle on the *inside* wall of the front of the chest. It goes from the *back* of the sternum, and fans out and up across the inside of the ribcage (Fig. 12.15). It acts to contract the ribcage to help us exhale sharply or cough.

- *To find it, try coughing – can you feel the center of the chest hollow and contract in?*

Initially your ribcage may drop as you do this, so play around until you find a lateral movement.

Now experience the reverse – that on the in-breath the middle of the ribcage fans out. This is the action in expansion of the transversus thoracis muscle.

- *To feel it in action, put fingers and thumb of one hand either side of the lower part of the sternum.*

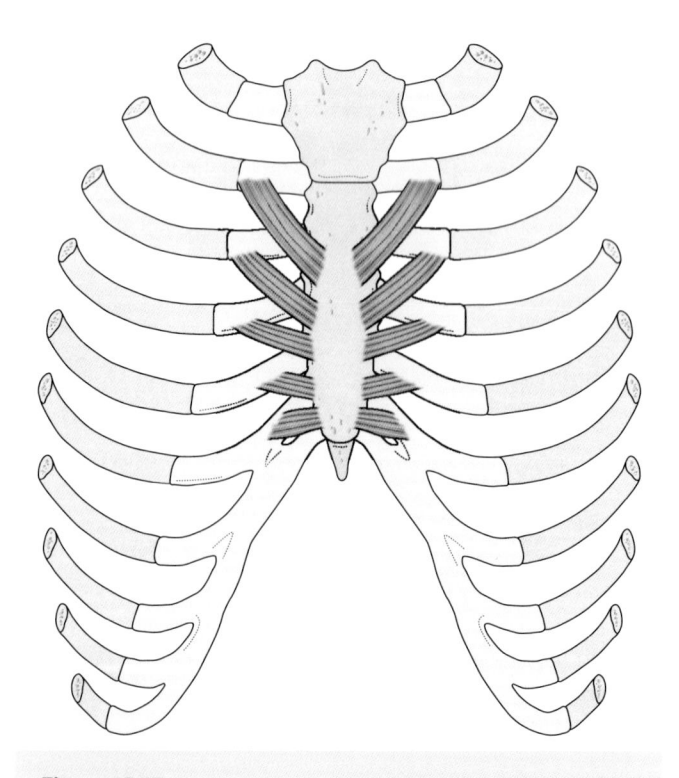

**Figure 12.15**
Transversus thoracis

# Alexander's biomechanics for expansion of the upper body

*Now push back as if you want T8 (between the lower tips of the shoulder blades) to move back,*

*but continue to bring your clavicles and elbows forwards while widening.*

*Breathe in and feel your fingers widening apart as you breathe.*

With this muscle we can widen the chest when we lengthen the back.

The transversus thoracis is fanning out the front of the ribcage.

Discover that the ligaments between the sternum and ribs are elastic! But notice this is much less when the sternum is tilted.

- *Notice whether your sternum now moves more vertically up and down with the breath, rather than tilting from the base.*

## Exploration 12.10  To create a firm chest

This widening needs to be maintained on all parts of the breath, so the chest is always supported and firm. (This also supports the breasts!) Alexander writes that vocalizing requires: "a firm but not 'fixed' position of the upper chest during vocalisation" (Alexander 2015: 45).

- *Touch either side of the base of sternum again, pushing back gently; breathe in and be aware of the ribs widening apart.*
- *Then, on the out-breath do not allow the ribcage to move back in; the fingers stay expanded.*
- *This is like a parachute coming down from the sky; the parachute stays inflated by the air pressure inside it. The ribs descend slowly when all the muscles used for the in-breath continue to work eccentrically on the out-breath.*
- *You may be wondering how to breathe out! We need to allow the lifting of the diaphragm to exhale, which also gives internal upward support to the torso.*

This creates a firm expanded chest, but not a rigid one, as it is always in responsive movement at the front, back and sides. By not letting the ribs fall back in, your top of sternum will go much higher than before because you are no longer pulling it down on every out-breath.

---

Serratus posterior inferior (Fig. 3.5) works similarly to transversus thoracis. Feel it by putting hands on your lower ribs either side of the spine, make a sharp exhale and notice the narrowing that results. Breathe in and notice it widening the centre of the back. Now maintain the expansion on the out-breath.

---

## Exploration 12.11  Expanding the triangle between T8 and the front of the shoulders (FSh)

The front of the shoulder (FSh) is the top of the humerus bone of the arm. The clavicle hinges with the acromion of the scapula just above this. We want to take the clavicle ends wider still, to free tight muscles in the neck (especially the trapezius, scalenes, and levator scapulae) and bring the top of sternum forwards.

- *Imagine lines between T8 and front of shoulders (FSh) (Fig. 12.17A).*

It will make a broad triangle, with T8 at the back and FSh wider and higher at the front. We need to expand this triangle (Fig. 12.16).

*I pull the iliac spines and ribs back (1).*

*I pull the FSh forwards and away from T8, and I pull T8 back from the FSh (2).*

*I pull the tips of the elbows down, forwards, and outwards, away from the top of sternum (3), (and top of sternum away from tips of elbows) (this stops FSh going higher).*

The front of each shoulder is widened forwards and away from the spine; this is making the top of the serratus anterior work. This was the goal of the shoulder shrug; here it is more precise.

- *Play with this first, then do it as an integrated move.*
- *Count 1-2-3 as you activate the movements together.*

# CHAPTER twelve

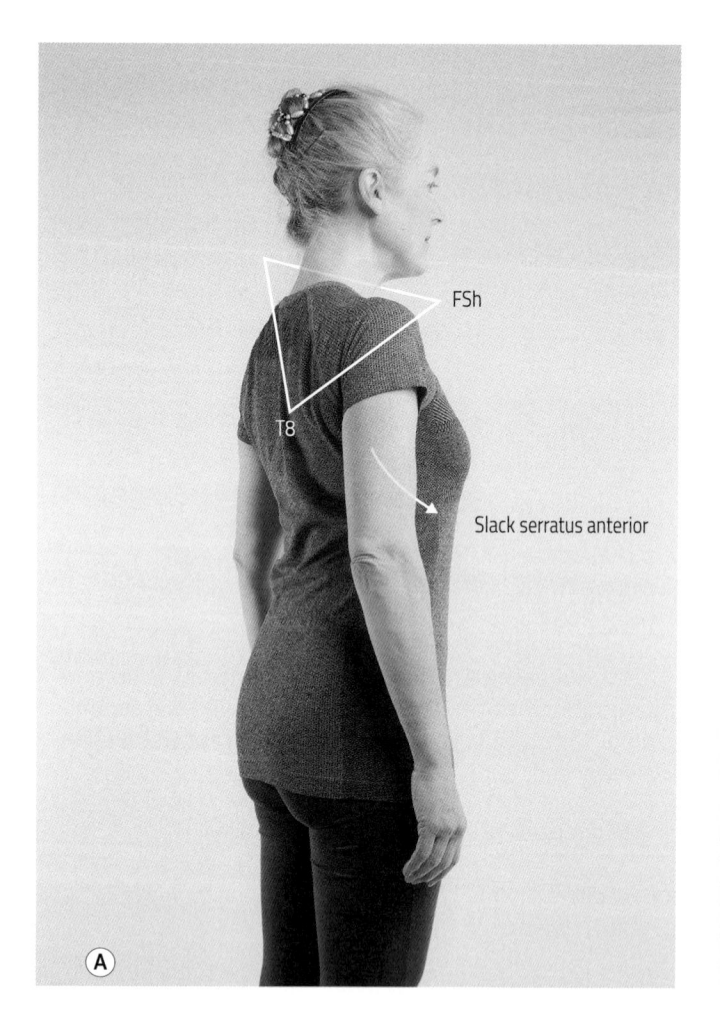

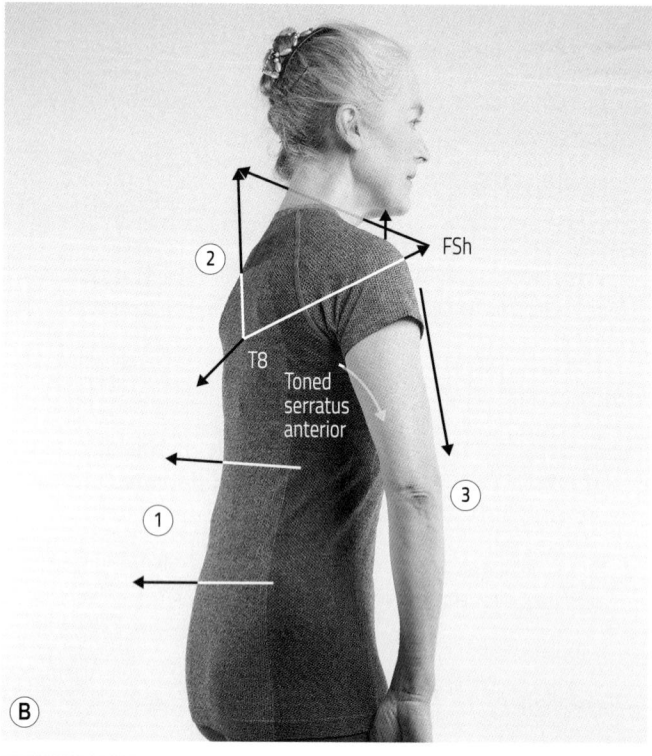

**Figure 12.16**
Expanding the triangle between T8 and front of shoulder (FSh). **(A)** Before; **(B)** directions for change

### Exploration 12.12  Widening and deepening the top of the chest

If the FSh are where we widen the front, the rib at the back of the armpit (RBAP, the 4th or 5th rib, depending on your current body geometry) is another significant point where we widen the back backward. If we pull the FSh points away from RBAP, we both widen and deepen the top of the chest. This brings much more tone to this area, by working all the arm lines together.

- Find RBAP. Send elbow away and down, and put your hand under the opposite armpit (as in exploration 9.6), and feel with your finger for the rib at the back.

*I pull the FSh away from RBAP, and RBAP away from FSh (Fig. 12.17B).*

### Exploration 12.13  Lifting and widening the back

If we think to take the RBAP away from the sacrum, we create another triangle, this time a vertical one. We can both lengthen and widen this triangle at the top to lift and tone the upper body.

*I pull RBAP up and away from the sacrum (see Fig. 7.9 dotted lines).*

**Video link for explorations 12.11 to 12.13**

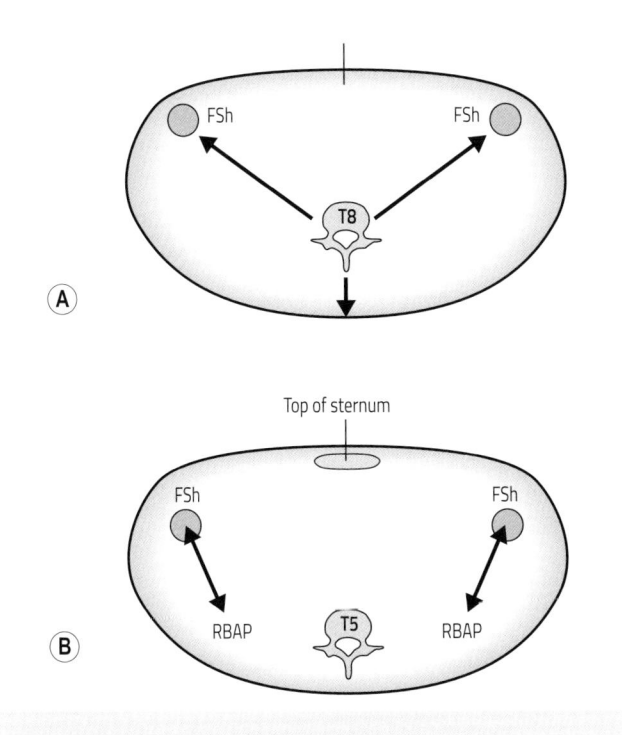

# Alexander's biomechanics for expansion of the upper body

**Figure 12.17**
Widening and deepening the top of the chest. (A) Front of shoulders (FSh) away from T8. (B) Front of shoulders away from ribs at the back of the armpits (RBAP)

### Exploration 12.14  Breathing into the front and back of the chest together

When we breathe to widen the back, we risk narrowing the front, while breathing into the front risks narrowing the back. When we breathe into both together, we are opening both front and back deep arm lines (DBAL and DFAL, Figs 9.1 and 9.2). For this, we need anatomical clarity.

At the back, we are widening the DBAL, from rhomboids to rotator cuff muscles to the back of the upper arm and the top of the triceps. But at the front, we are widening the DFAL from pectoralis minor to the front of the armpit only (Fig. 12.18), because when the arm is down, the angle from shoulder to biceps is so acute that the line of pull is broken.

- With spatial awareness, allow the breath to widen front and back of chest together, and into the back of the arms.
- Raise the arms to the sides; observe that the in-breath can now connect into the front of the arms.

## Lesson 4  Straightening the arms from both ends

### Exploration 12.15  Observation of arms

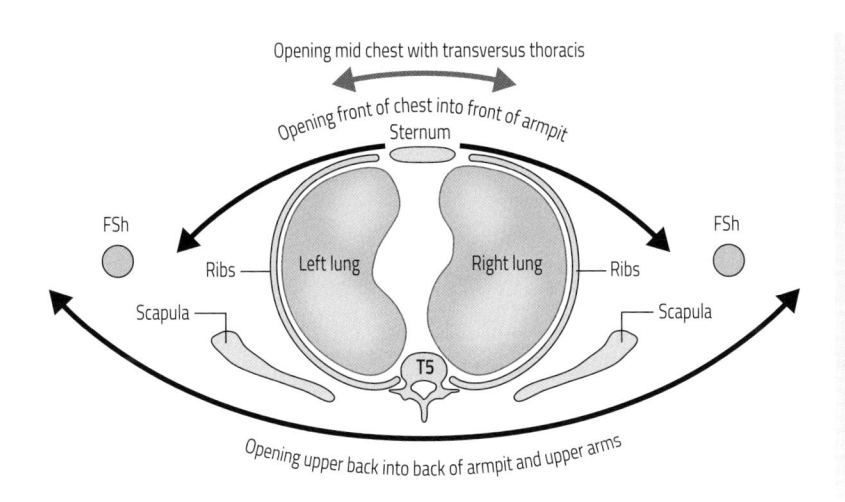

**Figure 12.18**
Expanding front and back of chest together with the breath (FSh, front of shoulder)

# CHAPTER twelve

We all have a habit of over-flexing the arms, under-working the extensors. Usually the elbows are bent and falling behind, while the wrist hangs forward of the upper arm. Then people cross the arms or put their hands in their pockets, etc., because to let them hang freely is uncomfortable. Since most people stand in a D shape, with the ribs pushed forward, the upper arm hangs behind the ribcage (see Fig.12.2).

- *Check your starting point with a side-on selfie – are both of these still true for you?*

Imagine the slanting line between your wrist and the ribs at the back of the armpit (RBAP). This line will be shorter when your arm is flexed. We need to extend this line. Both ends are movable: we can take the RBAP up and out from the sacrum, or we can take the wrist down from the RBAP.

### Exploration 12.16    Extending the ribs at the back of the armpit (RBAP) up away from the wrist

Align your legs and feet. Explore these directions in two stages initially, then put them together (Fig. 12.19). Play with each direction to check you understand it. Then, using spatial awareness and embodied intelligence, think or speak them aloud without responding, then move over a count of 1-2-3:

**Stage 1:** to open the lumbar spine and lift the upper body forward

*I pull the sitting bones towards the knees and the pubo-coccygeals forwards (1).*

- *I pull the iliac spines and the ribs back (2).*
- *I pull RBAP up and away from the sacrum (3) (exploration 12.13 above).*

**Stage 2:** to open the upper body

This involves expanding another triangle, of top of sternum forwards and away from RBAP (find this yourself on Fig. 12.17B). Do not let the chin drop as this will take the top of sternum down. (Play with wobbling the neck.)

*I pull the FSh away from RBAP, and RBAP away from FSh (4) (bringing the shoulders forward and widening; exploration 12.12).*

*I pull the top of sternum forward and up from the RBAP (5) (opposing the backward movement of RBAP and iliac spines).*

*I breathe to fan the ribs out from the base of the sternum (6) (using the transversus thoracis – exploration 12.9).*

- *Is your top of sternum now closer to the unity line? (Use your stick to check; see Fig. 7.3.)*
- *Has this move lengthened and straightened your arm?*
- *Is your arm now in front of your ribcage (Fig. 12.19)?*

Video link for exploration 12.16

### Exploration 12.17    Extending the hand down away from RBAP

This needs your arm to be in front of the ribcage, otherwise it will pull you into an arch. We started this in exploration 9.10, working all the arm lines together in ulnar deviation. Explore one arm at a time, playing with each instruction, and notice their different effects, then put it all together. (See Fig. 12.20 for numbering.)

*I pull the RBAP up away from the sacrum and away from each other (1).*

*I pull the tip of little finger away from RBAP, down and out from the body (2).*

*I pull the side of the wrist away from RBAP, down and in towards the body (3).*

*I pull the tip of the elbow away from RBAP, down and out from the body (4).*

*I direct my top of sternum away from RBAP, forwards and up (5).*

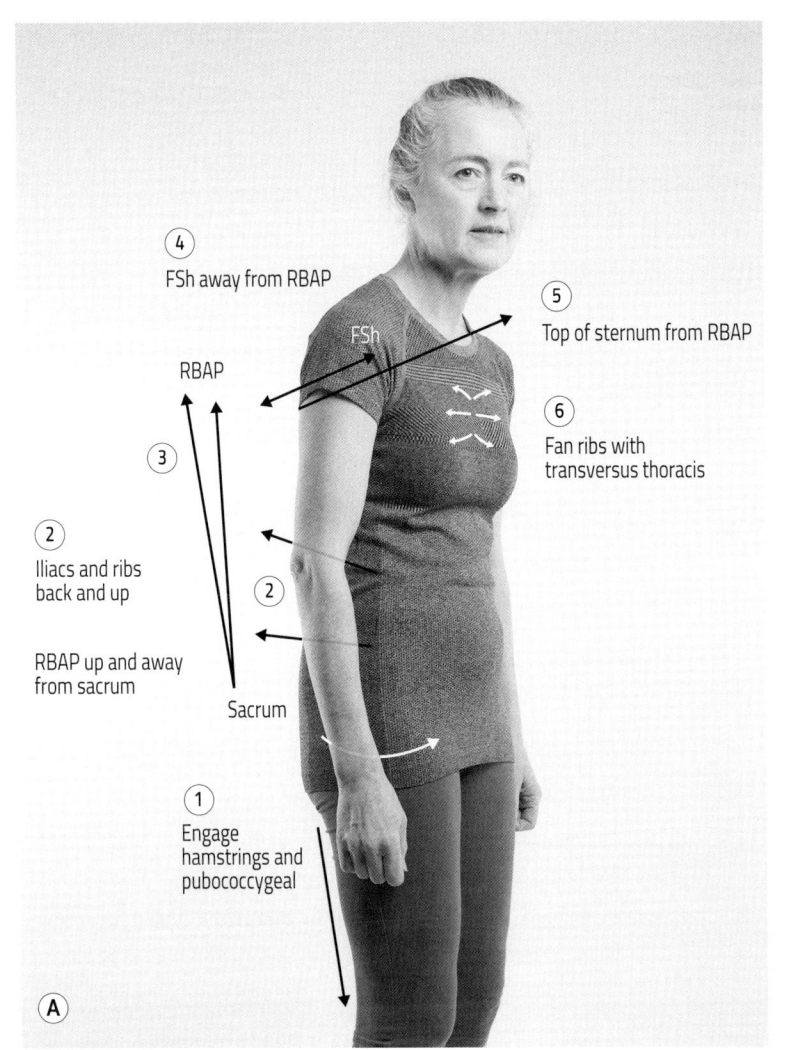

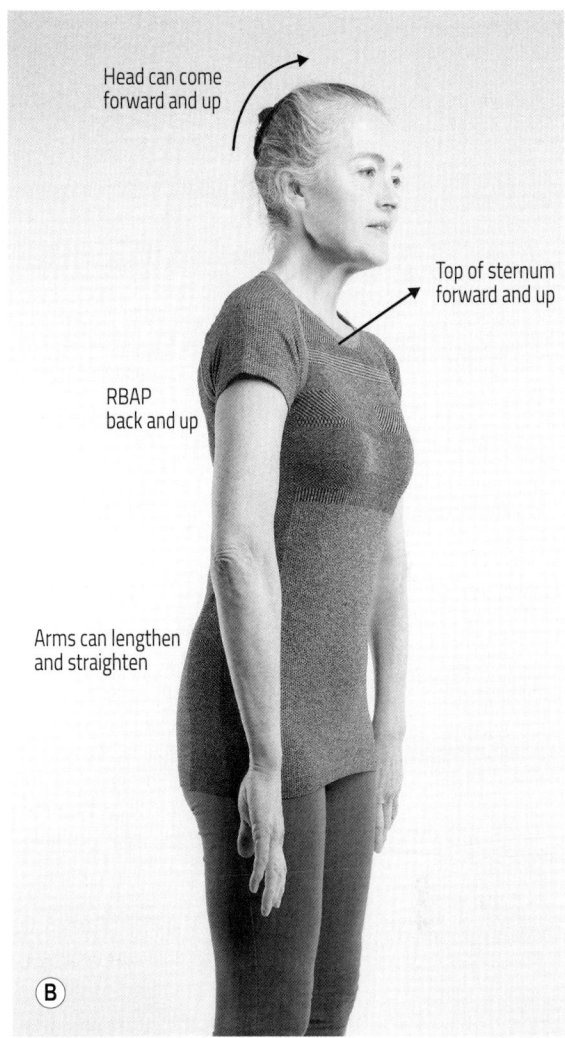

# Alexander's biomechanics for expansion of the upper body

**Figure 12.19**
Opening and lifting the upper torso back lengthens the arms. (A) Directions needed. (B) The new body geometry

Check what has happened:

- *Are your arms now in front of your ribs?*
- *Has your chin pulled down or is your head moving forwards and up?*
- *Are your arms straighter (Fig. 12.20)?*

When all the arm lines are lengthening, with the arms hanging vertically down and free to move (pendular arms, exploration 10.10), it shows that we are truly supported by our legs and torso, rather than using our shoulders for support.

## Integrating these in life activities

Expanding the triangle between RBAP and sacrum is a useful move that supports the whole torso back, widening and upright, while taking the top of sternum forwards and up from RBAP brings T1 forwards. Now our arms are free to lengthen into movement forward from the RBAP: using the three pulls, the elbows are supported away from the body while the hands are alive and strong to work. By lengthening all the muscles of the back and arms we have woken up their tone and springy strength. If we add

# CHAPTER twelve

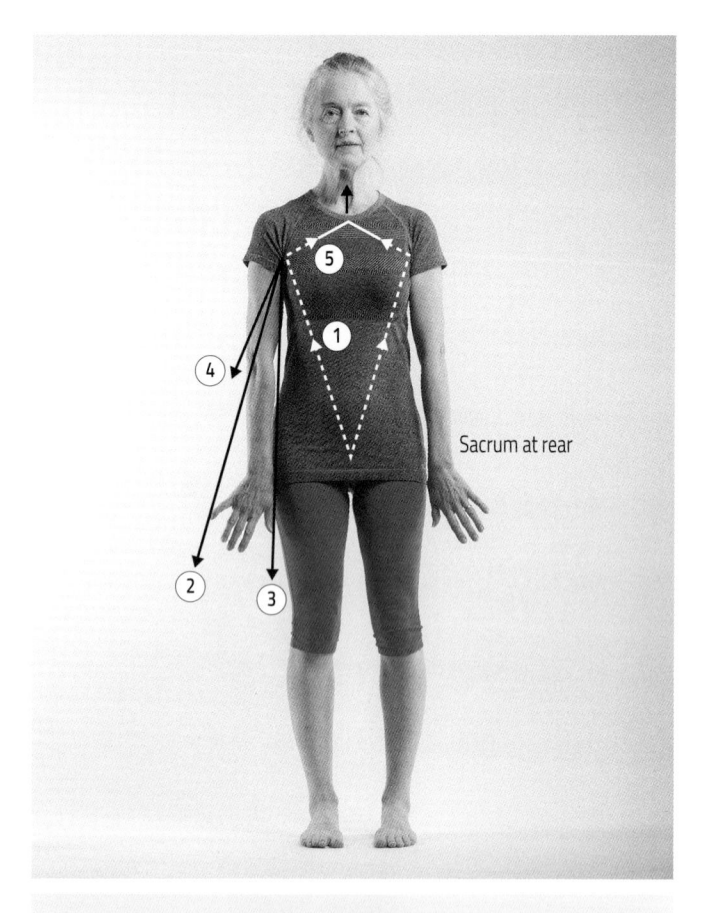

**Figure 12.20**
Lengthening the arms from ribs at back of armpit (RBAP)

the thought to breathe with transversus thoracis – fanning the front of the ribs – it will bring gentleness to this. Think these directions as you work on a computer, turn a tap, etc., as in exploration 9.16.

## Lesson 5  Opening the top of the ribcage – the reverse whispered Ah

I always start natural breathing work in the lower body and back, because without this grounding, the body is unsupported. Now we need to open the very top of the lungs. The lungs extend much further up than most people realize, going higher than the clavicles. When the top of the ribcage is arched back, the 1st rib tangles with the clavicles and the intra-thoracic capacity of the top of the lung is compromised. We have worked in stages towards opening this:

- bringing iliac spines and ribs back opens the lumbar curve and lengthens the torso
- widening the shoulder-blades so the front of the shoulders and clavicles can drop down, untangling from the neck
- then moving the top of sternum forwards so the neck can lengthen forward and up from T1, untangling the top of the ribcage.
- To help this along, we will use the pneumatic power of the lungs.

### Exploration 12.18  Channeling the breath into the top of the lungs

This exploration is a device to give the breath nowhere to go but upwards into the top of the lungs.

- *To open and support the torso, repeat the directions of exploration 12.16.*
- *You are now fanning the ribs with transversus thoracis, expanding the ribcage. Gently refuse to release this expansion on the out-breath so that the diaphragm must work instead (as in exploration 12.10).*
- *Pull the iliac spines back and wide to work the transversus abdominis, and refuse consent for them to release again, to prevent the belly from expanding on the in-breath.*
- *Be aware of the whole internal torso moving down and wide into the pelvic floor on the in-breath, connecting into the legs, and up under the diaphragm on the out-breath.*

It is not only the lower belly that bulges out with the breath; the upper part of the rectus abdominis often does also, so that the stomach area bulges forward. To prevent this, we need more tone in the external oblique muscles.

1  *Cross your arms in front of you and place the fingertips of each hand on the opposite iliac spine. Now the in-breath cannot bulge forward and so expands the upper back, driving it up further into the top of the lungs.*

# Alexander's biomechanics for expansion of the upper body

   2   *Draw the pelvic floor up and back. This is a temporary device.*

   *The breath now has nowhere to go but back and up into the upper chest. The tops of the lungs are free to expand, the top of the sternum lifts forwards.*

   *Once you have found this, release the pelvic floor (but not the belly muscles) and allow the whole internal lengthening and widening movement of the breath.*

   3   *For an even stronger move, actively stop the costal arch moving wider on the in-breath, or collapsing together on the out-breath, and notice the opening of the upper back that follows.*

Breathing work needs to begin by expanding the floating ribs, as so many people fix across this zone. However, Alexander comments (along with an amusing observation) that many people show an "undue lateral expansion of the lower ribs. This excessive expansion gives an undue width to the lower part of the chest, and there are thousands of young girls who present quite a matronly appearance in consequence … adequate *contraction* is equally important … the expiratory movement [often] calls for more attention than the inspiratory" (2011: 254).

The reverse whispered Ah was discovered by AT teacher Alex Murray after a lifetime of breathing exploration (2015: 166). He notes that in AT training, teachers are encouraged not to lift the chest, but to breathe from the floating ribs, and to breathe only through the nose. Sometimes good things happen when one does the opposite! This method makes the Ah sound as we draw the breath into the very top of the lungs, it is an activation to get the upper lungs working. It reinstates "full chest breathing" – the first name Alexander gave to his own work in 1900.

### Exploration 12.19   Reverse whispered Ah with hands on a wall

This is Masoero's development of reverse whispered Ah. If you find this too hard, do one arm at a time to start with.

It will feel completely wrong, so ignore your sensory guidance and play. It can take a while to work it out.

Preparation (Fig. 12.21A)

- *Sit facing a wall, engaging legs and lower body (1).*
- *Place the flats of your hands on the wall, with the thumbs vertically up and the fingers splayed (2).*
- *Direct the tip of the elbows out, away from the top of sternum, to activate the deep back arm line (DBAL) (3).*
- *Pull the RBAP up and away from the sacrum, and the top of sternum forward and up from the RBAP – it will feel bowed. Do not let the shoulders rise with this, keep the elbows pulling away and down. Keep looking forward (4).*
- *Bend the elbows to lean you forward but stay back in the RBAP, as if they are resisting the forward movement (5) (Fig. 12.21A).*

Reverse whispered Ah (Fig. 12.21B)

- *Keep all the directions going: RBAP going back and up away from the top of the sternum, elbows forward and down (1).*
- *Take the RBAP back away from the hands (2).*
- *As the breath comes in, make a whispered sound, it can be quite loud, like a diver with an oxygen tank. The sound needs to be made very high and far forward in the mouth – it feels up in front of the face. You are stretching the muscular tube of the pharynx. (If the sound is made from back in the throat it will draw the pharynx down towards the larynx, and cause a sore throat) (3).*
- *Help the breath to go up by drawing the belly and pelvic floor up and back into the lower back and hold it there so that the lower body does not expand on the in-breath. Invite the costal arch not to move also (4).*

   Can you now do whispered Ah on both in- and out-breath, with no movement in the front of the shoulders or top of sternum?

# CHAPTER twelve

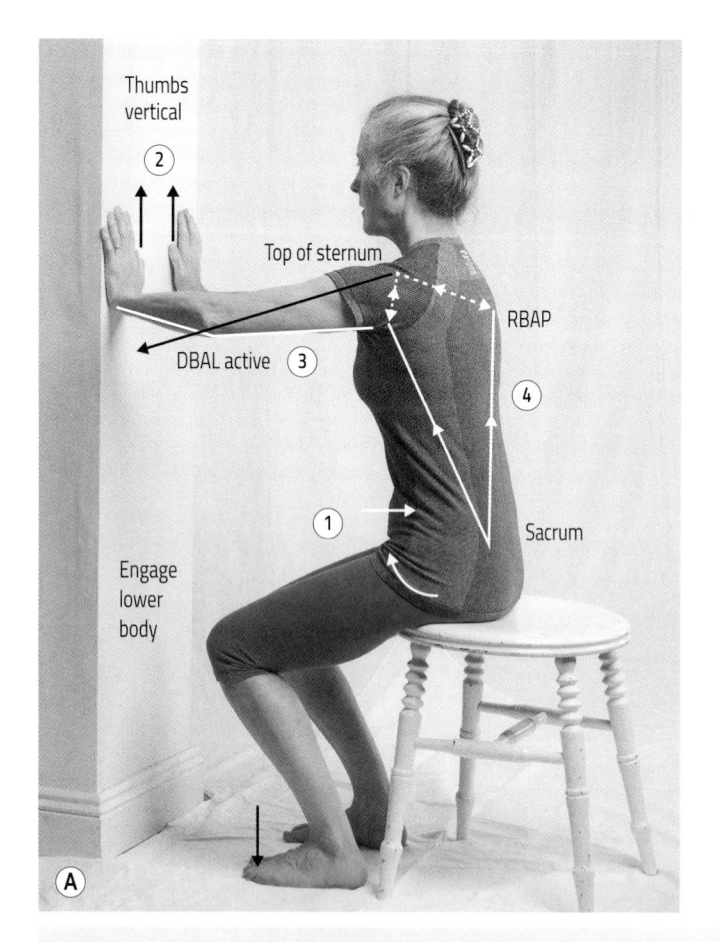

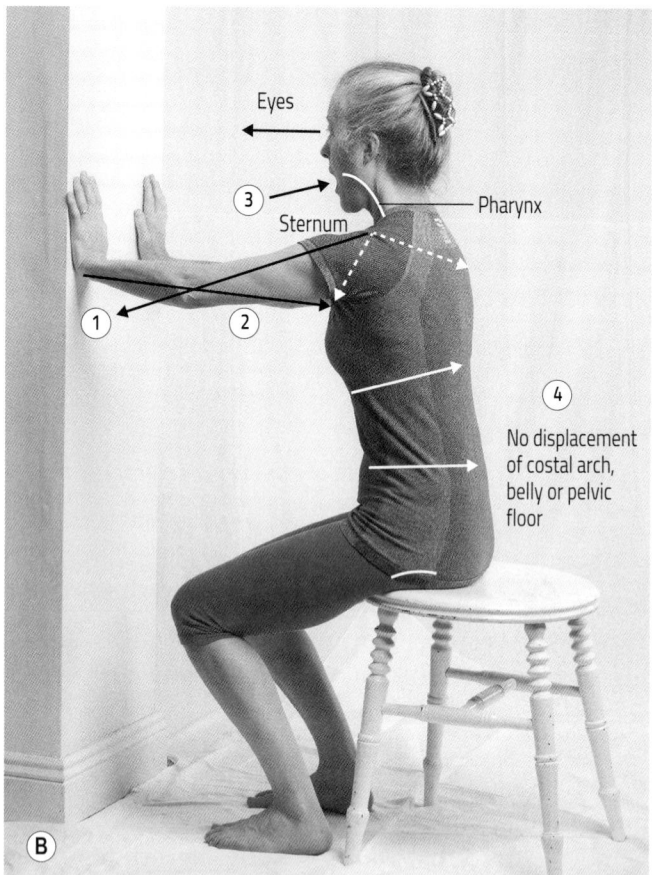

**Figure 12.21**
Reverse whispered Ah. **(A)** Preparation. **(B)** Directions

### Exploration 12.20  Cough up – combining the transversus thoracis with the lengthening of the pharynx

My first ever visit to an AT training course coincided with a bad cold and a cough. Just as Walter Carrington put hands on me, I began to cough – and to pull down strongly. His hands stretched my throat powerfully as he instructed "Cough up! Cough up!"

- *In exploration 12.9, we explored coughing without pulling down with the transverse thoracis. Now explore the CK sound of the word "cough," which uses this muscle. Put your hand gently on the front of your throat and see if you can allow the throat to lengthen forwards and up with this, without pulling your head back.*

## Lesson 6    Classic Alexander technique procedures for arms

These various explorations with arms provide the building blocks for Alexander's procedures (see my website for video tutorials of these).

*Hand on back of chair* (HOBOC) (Fig. 12.22) utilizes staying back at iliac spines, ribs, and RBAP, the pull to the elbow along with the oppositional pull to the wrist with ulnar deviation, the "beak" use of the fingers, then thumb leading the deep front arm line

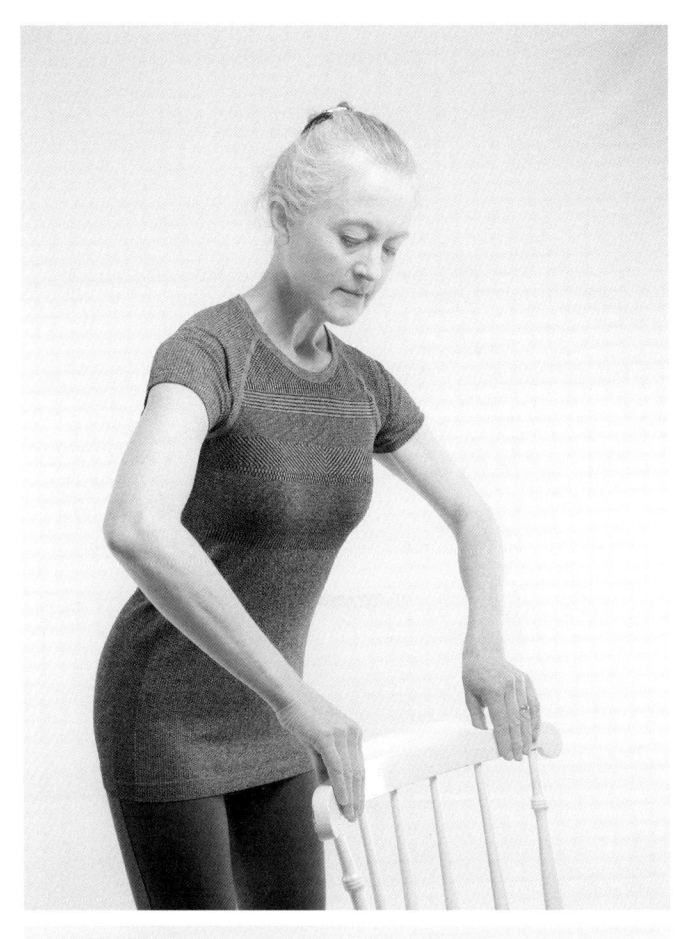

# Alexander's biomechanics for expansion of the upper body

**Figure 12.22**
Hands on back of chair

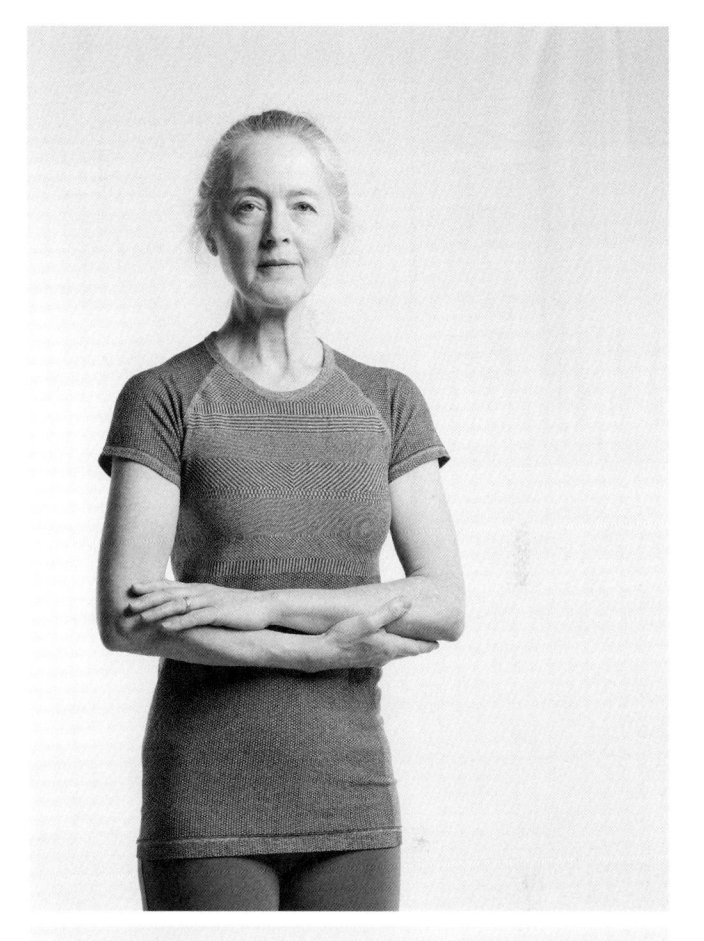

**Figure 12.23**
"Photoshoot" procedure

onto the chairback, all done from a true "monkey" (exploration 13.3). When all these directions are integrated together, it brings a dynamic strength through the body. I once asked Miss Goldie if she would do it with me as I did not understand it, and she replied I was nowhere ready for it. At the time I was puzzled. But when Jeando Masoero said the same some years ago, he was able to explain that there was not yet sufficient length and responsive tone in my arms. This could explain why many trainees find HOBOC so hard – it may be introduced too soon. All the Initial Alexander technique activations can be seen as *preparation* for it.

*The "photoshoot" procedure.* The position in which Alexander chose three times to be photographed is another procedure Masoero thinks Alexander used for himself but did not teach – a partial crossing of the arms, in which there is clear extension through arms and torso (Fig. 12.23 and Fig. 12.24). To maintain an open chest in this position, the fingers need to lead across the front of the body while the elbows and RBAP oppose them. If the ribs, top of sternum, and iliac spines stay on the unity line during this, and the sternum line is almost vertical, the line of the upper arm will also approach vertical.

*Sitting with the hands upturned on our thighs* is done by most teachers. The reason for this is obvious:

# CHAPTER twelve

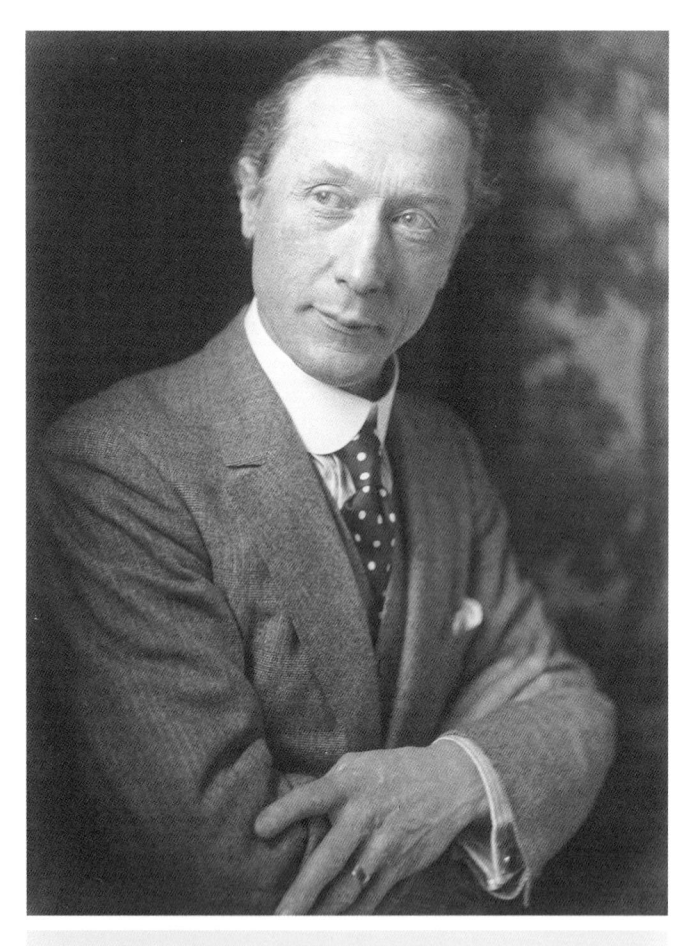

**Figure 12.24**
F. Matthias Alexander, c. 1910. Courtesy of © Mouritz 2020

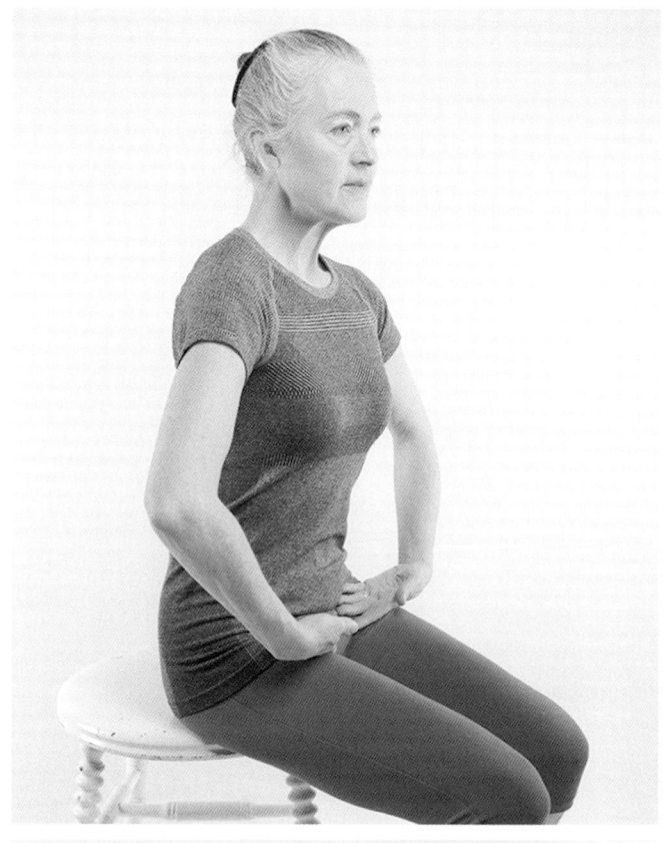

**Figure 12.25**
Sitting with upturned hands

with palms down the arms tend to pull on the back, while palms up support the back. But Goldie used it with me in a much stronger way – she wanted my back and arm to be fully expanded and working in such a way that the arm was self-supported and the wrist was not collapsed (Fig. 12.25). After some years she got my arms to cooperate by:

- ensuring my legs were aligned forward and fully conscious to provide real support for the torso
- continually tweaking each shoulder forward while widening the clavicle
- repeatedly poking my ribs and iliac spines back
- bringing my elbow much further forward than I thought reasonable
- angling my wrist so that the thumbs were almost in a straight line towards each other in ulnar deviation.
- My job in all this was simply not to collapse it immediately, which took a lot of focus.

I understood none of this till finding this understanding of our structure.

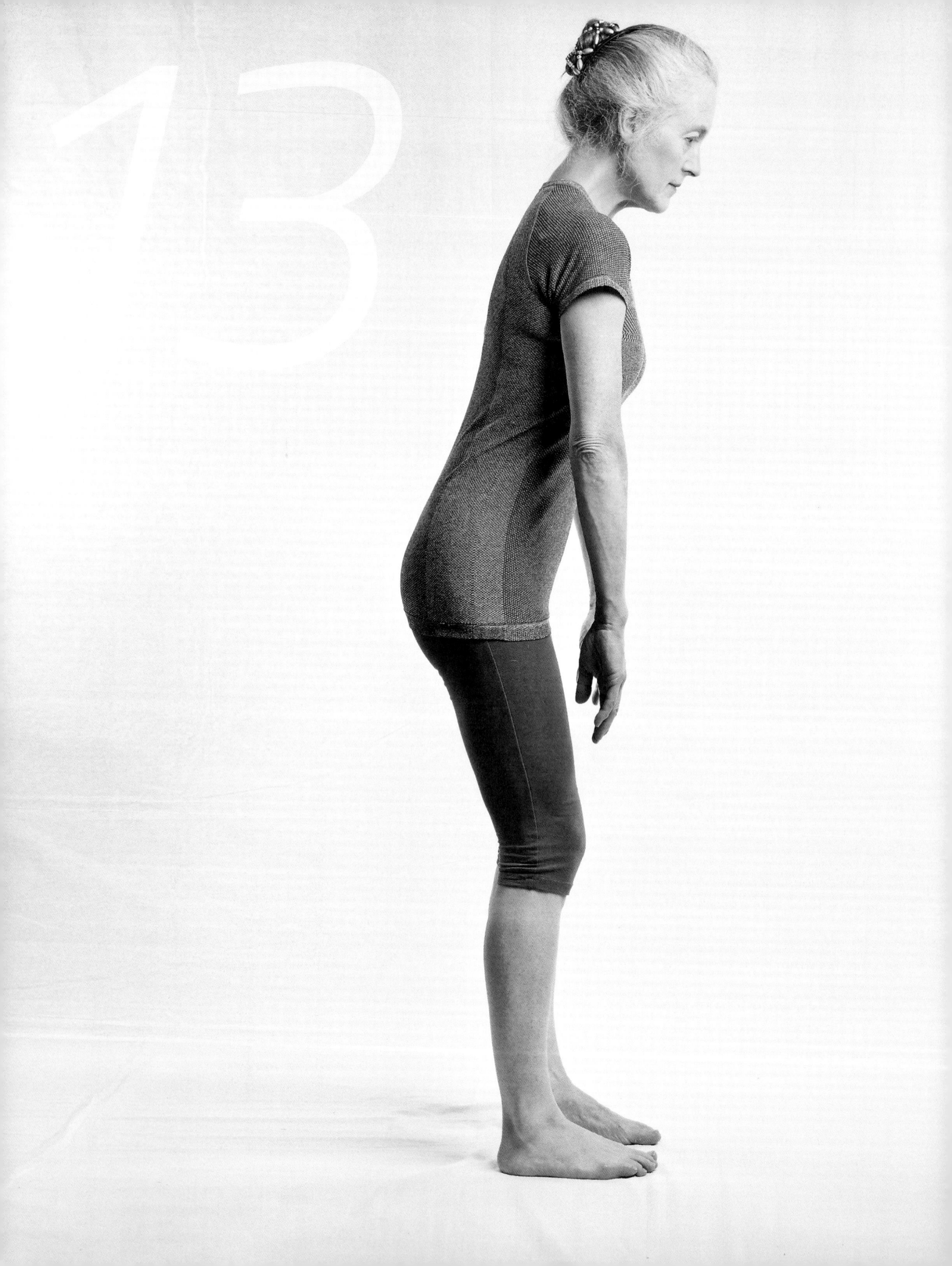

13

# Precise, springy alignment in sit to stand and "monkey" 13

Miss Goldie's work was incredibly precise and painstaking as she brought one's whole-body into play and kept it there, remorselessly prodding and instructing one to maintain the tone found, until she had created a whole new alignment and use that ran deep into one's being. It was a very different use than the one I had learned from most previous teachers or my training school. Through Masoero's analysis of Delsarte, biomechanics, and the Initial AT, I have gained understanding that finally enables me to teach the structural alignments she taught me.

This is a detailed exploration of how we need to maintain precise alignment and tone of limbs and torso for truly efficient, strong, and light movement.

## Lesson 1  Anatomy and engineering play

### Exploration 13.1  Stabilizing and controlling the tilt of the torso

I define three pivotal points on a pelvis: sitting bones, hip joints, and iliac spines (see Fig. 7.4), and they are roughly equidistant. To demonstrate this for yourself, push a stick up against your sitting bones, then keeping it horizontal, roll it round to the front of your leg – you will see that the level is surprisingly far down the thigh; measure the distance to your hip crease. Now measure how far your iliac spines are above your hip crease – is it roughly the same (Fig. 13.1)?

If you were to hold a stick loosely between finger and thumb, an inch (3 cm) from its base, it could swing freely between your fingers, but could easily fall. But if you were to put an elastic band on the base and another around the stick an inch up from your fingers, you could control and stabilize the angle of tilt (Fig. 13.2). The hamstrings, running from sitting bones to back of knees, and the transverse abdominals, working through the thoracolumbar fascia to engage psoas, quadratus lumborum and erector spinae, are there to stabilize and control the tilt of the torso from above and below the pivot of the hips, *as long as they stay responsively toned.*

- *Play with this now as you stand – relax your hamstrings and let the torso fall forward, notice the movement is hard to control (Fig. 7.18).*
- *Now tone the hamstrings and keep them engaged as you tilt. You now have control of the movement. (Fig. 13.3).*
- *Now let your iliac spines fall forward as you tilt. Notice that the lumbar spine will fall forward and arch, shortening the extensor line of the back of the body, and feeling heavy. The ribs will also fall forward (see Fig. 7.18).*
- *By keeping iliac spines and also ribs back as you tilt, the length of the back is maintained, and the torso feels lighter (Fig. 13.3).*

I observe that there are four ways to tilt forwards:

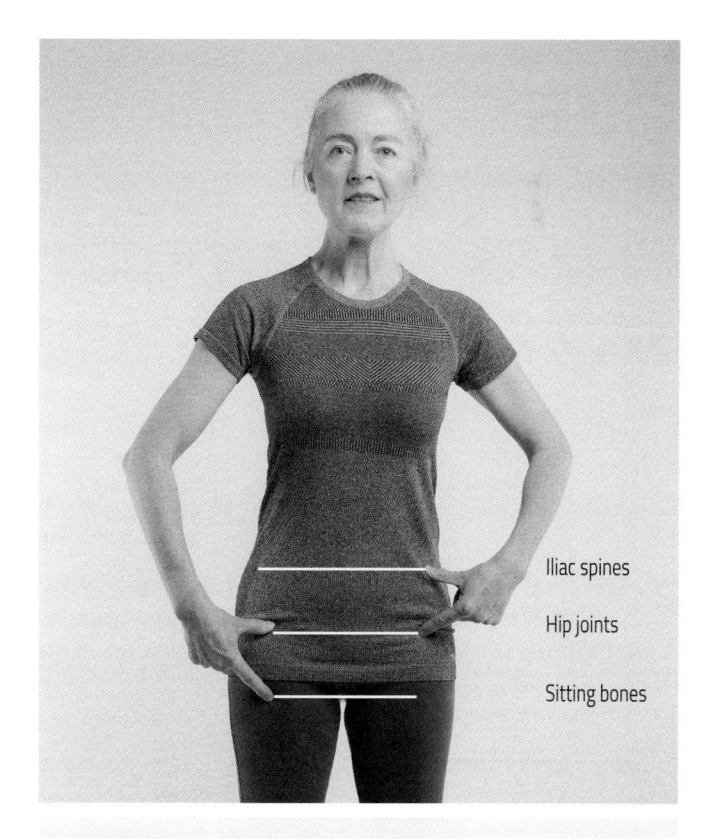

**Figure 13.1**
Spacing of iliac spines, hip joints, and sitting bones

# CHAPTER thirteen

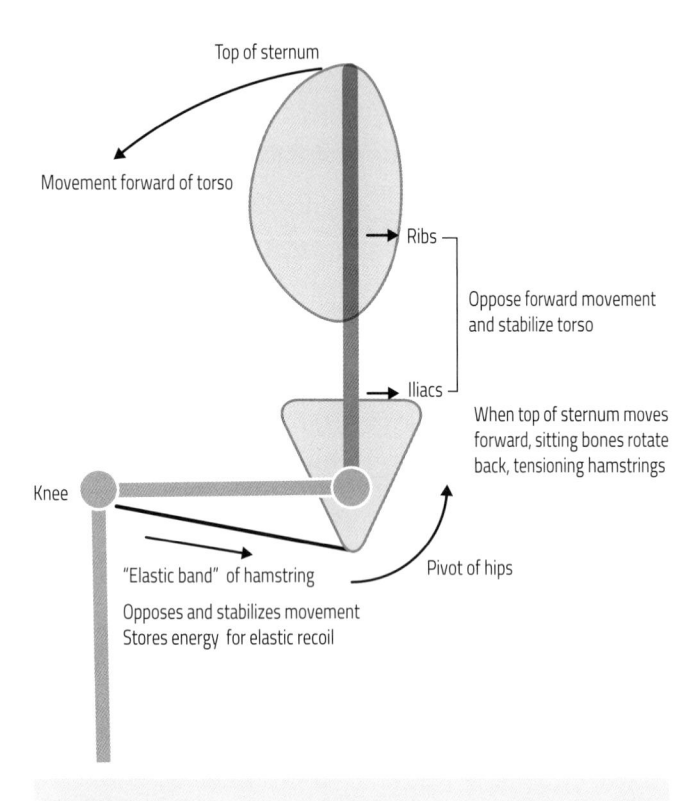

**Figure 13.2**
Balance of forces giving control, stability, and elastic resistance

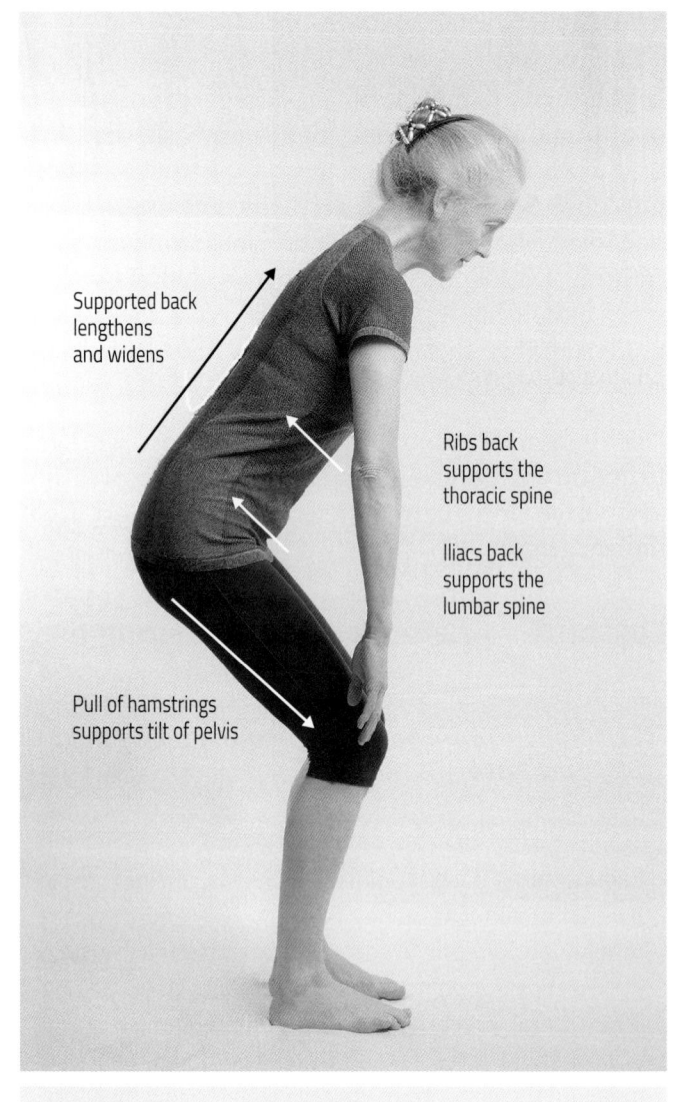

**Figure 13.3**
Tone at iliacs and in hamstrings gives control and support

1  Tilting from sitting bones tilts the pelvis and arches the back.

2  Tilting from the hip joints gives a straight back, but little link into the legs.

3  Tilting from the iliac spines engages the thoracolumbar fascial links front to back and down into the legs, bringing stability and control.

4  Tilting from the waist collapses the upper torso and does not utilize the hip joints fully.

- *Play around to see if you can find all four of these.*

Miss Goldie hated the word "release"; she saw that people often collapsed as they released tight areas. She wanted reorganization, which brings tight areas back into balance by re-engaging slack areas. Through her work I learned to keep the whole back and legs responsively engaged as I went into "monkey," taking the strain off the legs, which instead were springy and ready to lengthen up again at any moment. In part, this uses the elastic resistance in muscles and fascia, which resists being stretched then helps to power the return movement. (Though the elastic energy of a stretched muscle must be used quickly – within a second – or it dissipates as heat. If we hold a position for longer it will be gone, though elastic tone in connective tissue such as in fascial sheets or tendons can still be in play.)

# Precise, springy alignment in sit to stand and "monkey"

To engage all this fully, we need the hips to come back to the unity line to open up our full extensor capacity.

"The weight of the body, it should be noted, rests chiefly upon the rear foot, and the hips should be allowed to go back as far as possible without altering the balance effected by the position of the feet, and without deliberately throwing the body forwards. This movement starts at the ankle, and affects particularly the joints of the ankle and the hips" (Alexander 2011: 219).

### Exploration 13.2 Bringing the hips back by rocking back on the heels

Most people stand with hips pushed forward beyond their instep. This next exploration allows us to bring the hips further back, often out of our comfort zone, and open the lumbar curve. It builds on active hip flexing (exploration 10.7) and using the wall (exploration 12.1), and is a preparation for "monkey." You could check with your measuring sticks, before and after, whether your iliac spines are vertically over your instep, and the angle of your sacrum line (exploration 7.1).

Preparation

- Stand with your back to a wall, a few inches from it so that should you fall back it will catch you. Stand with heels hip-width apart, outside feet parallel.
- Put your hands on your thighs, fingers pointing downward.
- Find your breath into the lower body, and the psoas coming back and up on the out-breath.

Explore these directions, then program and move over a count of 1-2-3.

Initial AT instructions

*I send my heels down and send an up-force up the back of the legs to the sacrum and T8.*

*I pull my sitting bones towards the back of my knees, and iliac spines back.*

*I pull the tips of the elbows down and away from the RBAP and forwards.*

*I pull the top of sternum forward and up from RBAP.*

Keep your torso vertical. This strongly pulls the upper body forward.

Now we are going to pull the iliac spines back strongly, so that the hips come back in space, lifting the toes so that we rock back on the heels. To stop ourselves falling back, we oppose this by pulling the pubococcygeals strongly forward. This brings the pelvis to neutral and opens the lumbar spine. Bending forward to help yourself balance is cheating! Keep sending the top of sternum forwards and up.

- *Keeping the above directions going, add:*

  *I pull the pubococcygeals strongly forward.*

  *I pull the iliac spines strongly back in space, and the ribs back and up.*

- *Move as you count 1-2-3, to let your toes lift off (Fig. 13.4).*

Once you have the balance, you can play with walking on your heels, forwards and backwards, maintaining these pulls to open the lumbar arch. When you then walk forward normally again, you may notice that your knees do not need to bend as much. This is because the tight tensor fasciae latae have lengthened (Bowman 2017: 184). My "Lipizzaner horse" knees (see Chapter 6) were only a stage in the journey.

## Lesson 2 Tilting the torso forwards into "monkey"

"Monkey" is an important AT procedure. Properly called the *position of mechanical advantage*, it is the tilt of the torso forward on the hips, with the simultaneous bending of the knees. Ideally it is the start of all bending movements, such as squat or sitting. It is a movement we were evolved to do continually, but which most Westernized people have lost to some degree.

# CHAPTER thirteen

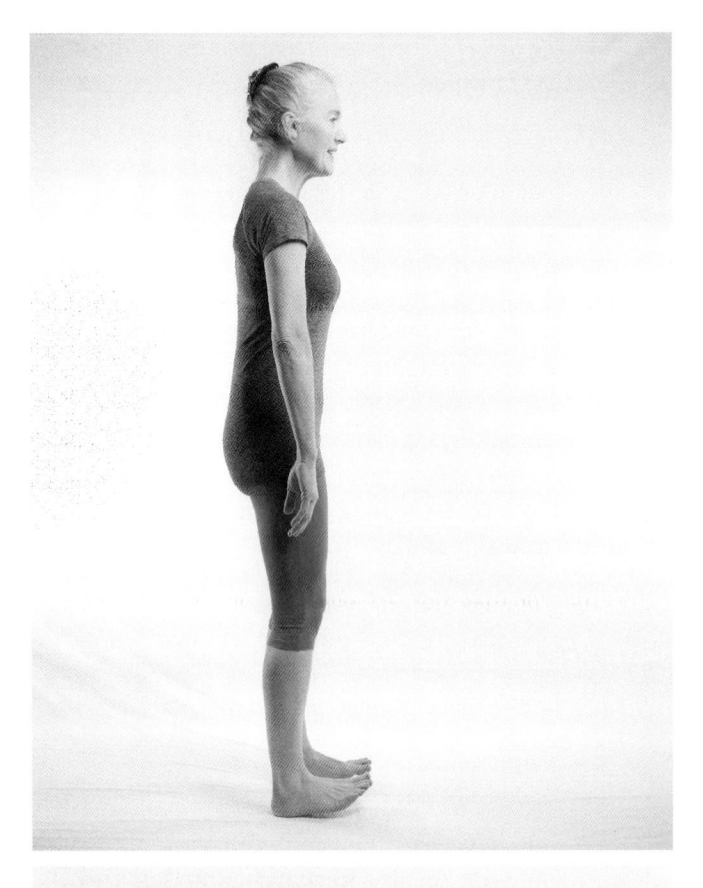

**Figure 13.4**
Balancing on heels to open the lumbar spine

Though "position of mechanical advantage" is nowadays the official term for this position, I prefer the term "monkey." Partly because originally there were many such positions (see Chapter 3, lesson 4, the flow of dynamic balance) and because it really is descriptive of the movement made and so is memorable for pupils.

Goldie always took me into "monkey" in a different way that I could not quite define. I only knew she poked me around the ribs and the iliac spines alternately to stop them moving forward. Now I understand why. When we tilt the torso forwards, and if we are not slumping into the movement, we usually rotate around the sitting bones, taking the thighs backwards, and sticking the backside out. This hollows and narrows the back. Rotating around the hip joints is better, but still hollows the back somewhat. Instead, we want to take the iliac spines back, which fully lengthens and widens the back, and bring the hips back in space. This also takes the ribs back, tilting the ribcage on the lumbar spine, which further uncurls the back. It requires that we do not let the knees bend forward or the ankles bend at all. Instead it is the thighs that draw back, upwards off the knees, which can feel completely unfamiliar.

This is an exercise in aligning the parts of our torsos with gravity. Think of anglepoise lamps that you can bend into different Z shapes (Fig. 13.5). I love playing with them: when you keep the arms balanced above each other they bend and straighten so fluidly. But if you pull one arm too far forward or let another tilt too far back the whole thing overbalances. We are like sprung anglepoise lamps and for us, the top of sternum and the knees and insteps are the key points that must stay above one another to maintain an easy balance.

Another way of thinking of it is like drawing a bow. The bowman must keep the top and bottom of the bow still (the top of sternum and knees) while the string is drawn strongly back (at the iliac spines and ribs). This uses the front to back connectivity of the thoracolumbar fascia to lengthen and widen the back (see Figs 6.5 and 6.6).

For stability and tone, our "bowstring" of the back must always be stretched lengthways and widthways together.

- *Stretch any piece of elastic material – it will lengthen but narrow. Stretch it widthways and see it shorten. When you do both together (as in a well-pegged tent sheet), then you will build much greater elastic resistance and resilience.*

# Precise, springy alignment in sit to stand and "monkey"

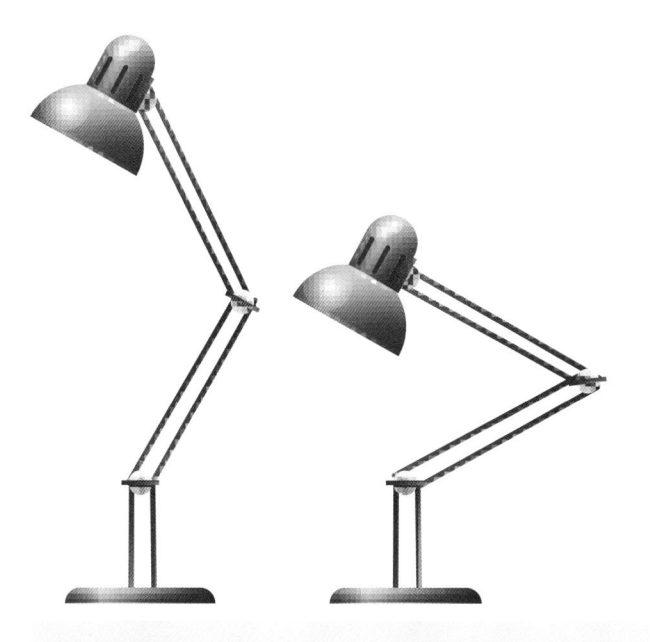

**Figure 13.5**
Anglepoise lamps fold in balance

How precise should a "monkey" be? Goldie's work was precise beyond most teachers. Masoero takes this into much more technically exacting realms to employ what he understands as the full potential of elastic resistance and the leverage of the torso, working alongside the adaptive organization of postural support through the muscles. There has been no research as yet on how much leverage and elastic resistance play a part in AT work, or whether potentially, with fully responsive musculature, one can sit and stand optimally at any angle. Personally I suspect not, as I observe this precision of alignment to be invaluable in bringing me springiness, poise, and strength. This is new ground, and I invite you to play with it and make your own decision.

You may or may not achieve this precise "monkey." However, any gain made here in torso stability and tone will give you a much stronger and lighter "monkey," and take pressure off your knees as you bend.

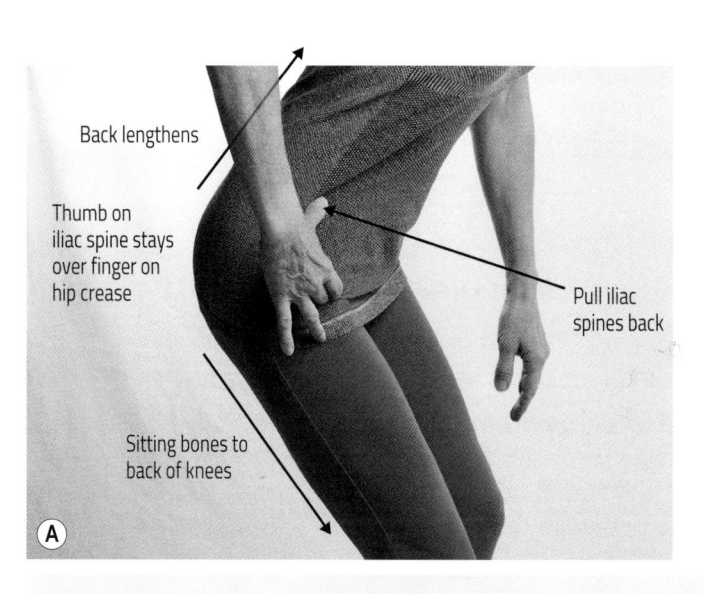

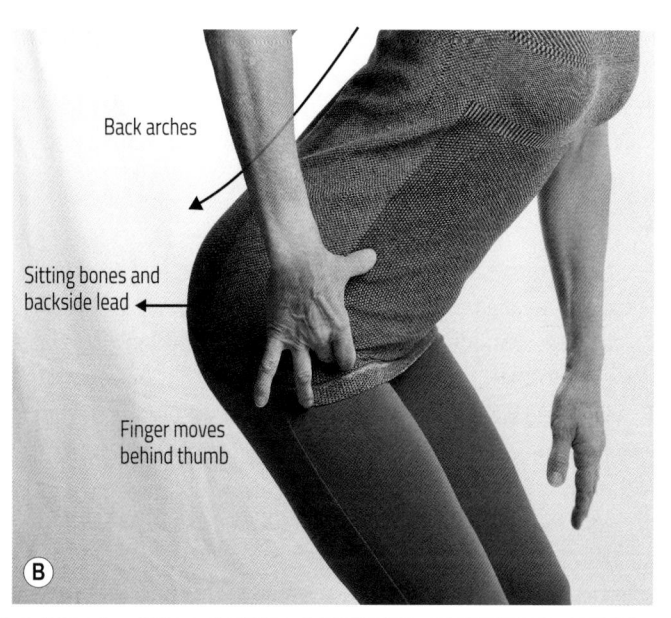

**Figure 13.6**
Finger check on how we tilt forward. (A) Tilt supported by pulling back at iliac spines. (B) Using thighs to tilt

# CHAPTER thirteen

### Exploration 13.3 Tilting into true "monkey"

To tilt to a true "monkey" we need to keep the top of sternum, knees, and insteps vertically aligned on the unity line, and take the iliac spines back behind that line. *Everything keeps going up.*

- *Check you are drawing back from the iliac spines by using the finger check (see Fig. 13.6, previous page).*
- *Start by finding your natural breathing throughout the torso. This gives internal support throughout, and ensures the torso is already lengthening and widening.*
- *Your eyeline needs to drop ('roll your raindrop' slightly), but not the head – the crown stays going up.*
- *Initially, keep the backs of your knees against a chair throughout: it will stop you from releasing the knees or ankles, which would collapse the extensor system and take you down. One less thing to think about!*
- *Give yourself a preparatory 1-2-3 for the legs and feet, lower body and upper body, separately or together as you are able.*

Preparing the brain programs: inhibition and direction

We need both *inhibitory thoughts,* which stop our usual habits, and *directions*, which are the instructions to bring about an adjustment.

Once you are familiar with the procedure, do this from spatial awareness and embodied intelligence, aware of "emails" connecting to points down your body.

Inhibitory thoughts (see Fig. 13.7):

*I do not pull the knees forwards or back (1).*

*I do not let the top of sternum move forwards or backwards (2).*

*I keep the arms by the sides, elbows outward, upper back widening, palms facing back (3).*

Directions to bring about a change (Fig. 13.8):

*I pull the iliac spines back, away from the knees, away from the top of sternum, back in space (Fig. 13.7).*

The bend will do itself. It is a subtle internal movement, and may feel strange.

- *Keep breathing throughout, deepening and widening into the pelvic bowl, and widening back and up through the torso, with support from psoas and quadratus lumborum (QLs) – the muscles that form the back wall of the abdominal cavity (see Fig. 6.3).*
- *To help the ribs come back, think of T8 lifting up from the heels; and ribs at the back of the armpit (RBAP) coming back, wide and up from the sacrum.*
- *Direct your eyes to look at your toes, move your eyes down but not your head (Fig. 13.8).*
- *As this subtle internal pull tilts your torso forwards, let the arms hang vertically from the shoulders.*
- *Keep the top of the sternum pulling up, away from RBAP, to keep the shoulders horizontal. (If you shorten down the front, your shoulders will probably droop forwards.)*
- *Keep the front of the chest widening into the front of the armpit.*
- *Still keep breathing. Your lower leg has stayed vertical.*

**Extend your fingers and stop the moment they point 2 inches (5 cm) in front of the instep.**

This is the alignment we are after.

> **Video link for exploration 13.3**

### Another anatomical surprise

- *The hips, knees, and ankles are not released into "monkey"; instead the torso inclines back, up and off the legs.*

This ensures full extension is always maintained, and keeps the spring in the system. It is crucial for coming into squat with the legs aligned, the root of human movement.

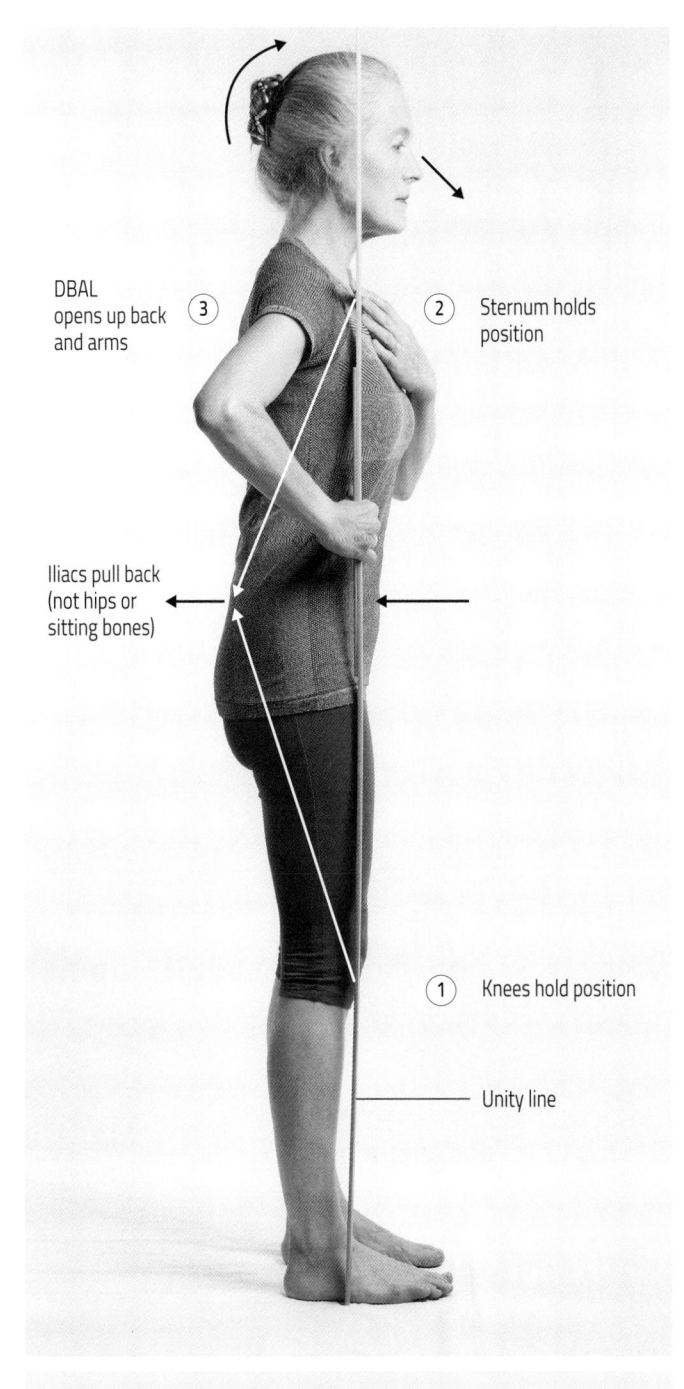

# Precise, springy alignment in sit to stand and "monkey"

**Figure 13.7**
Preparations for "monkey"

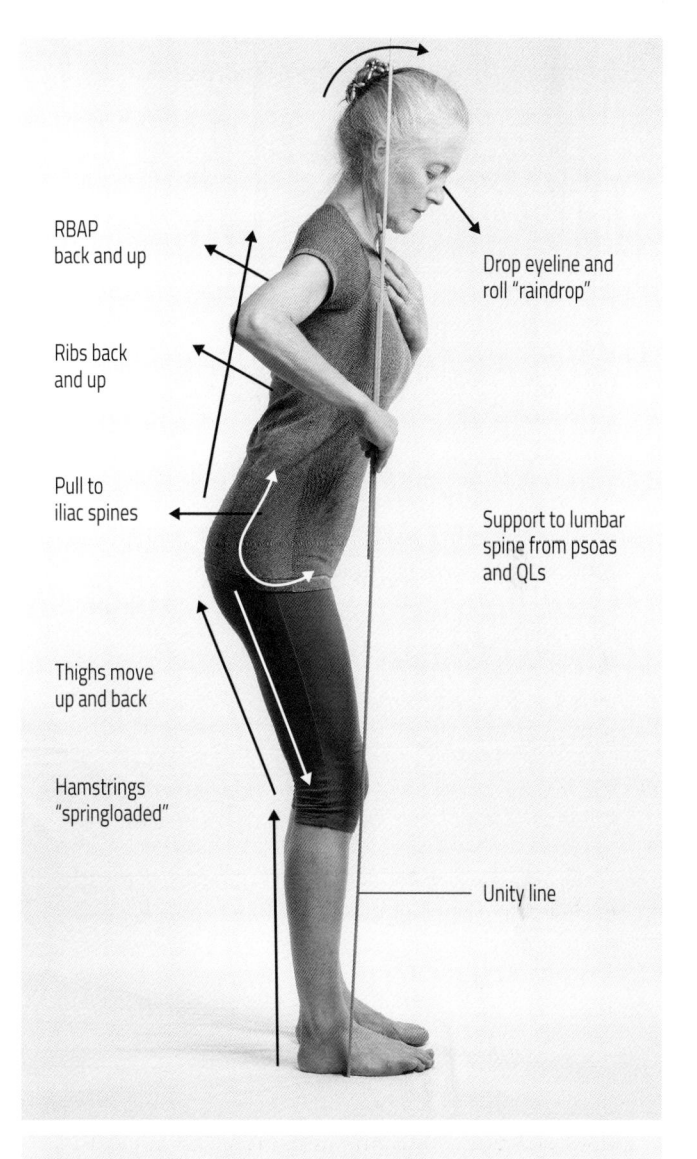

Labels (Figure 13.7):
- DBAL opens up back and arms ③
- Sternum holds position ②
- Iliacs pull back (not hips or sitting bones)
- Knees hold position ①
- Unity line

**Figure 13.8**
Drawing back and up into "monkey" away from the unity line, using iliac spines

Labels (Figure 13.8):
- RBAP back and up
- Drop eyeline and roll "raindrop"
- Ribs back and up
- Pull to iliac spines
- Support to lumbar spine from psoas and QLs
- Thighs move up and back
- Hamstrings "springloaded"
- Unity line

**AT info:** Alexander's directions to his readers were not precise. Masoero pointed out (Galway workshop, November 2017) that Alexander instructs to "order simultaneously the hips to move backwards and the knees to bend, the knee and hip-joints acting as hinges" (Alexander 2011: 223). He did not say: "the knee, hip-joints and ANKLES" (which he does shortly after when instructing how to stand), but this is how it has been interpreted.

267

# CHAPTER thirteen

### Exploration 13.4 Sitting from "monkey"

When a "monkey"' position is optimally aligned for gravity, the top of the sternum is directly over the instep and knees. This maintains the balance between the front and back of the body, so all the muscles can maintain their length. To keep this balance as we sit (or squat) we need to keep this aligned relationship of the parts of the torso as we bend the knees, like the angle-poise lamp in the illustration.

- *Find your "monkey" as above, with your fingers pointing to 2 inches (5 cm) in front of the instep.*
- *While keeping all the directions going, bend your knees. The top of sternum stays over the instep throughout.*
- *Keep the fingers pointing to 2 inches (5 cm) in front of the instep as you bend, until your backside reaches the chair (Fig. 13.9).*
- *STOP! Stay on the angle you now find yourself in. Do not release the tone in your body.*
- *Come back by thinking iliac spines back, to rock the torso back in one piece. Do not let the upper body fall or arch back.*
- *Continue to maintain the tone as you sit. There is no switching off!*

When Miss Goldie first said to me "There is no switching off!" I was shocked. Couldn't one just let go sometimes and "relax"? But I soon realized she was right: why throw away your hard-won tone? Once, when I was waiting outside Miss Goldie's door, I heard her instructing the pupil within. There were familiar sentences that meant she was taking the pupil into the chair, then I heard her expostulate: "Now look at you! You are like a sack of potatoes! No! That would be an insult to the potatoes, for potatoes have life, and in this moment, you have no life!" Evidently the pupil had "let go" on sitting. I could picture her prodding and supporting and reconnecting the hapless pupil, and heard her comments gradually become more positive again. When the pupil finally emerged, I was glad to see she was smiling, evidently as used as I was to Miss Goldie's tirades.

## Lesson 3 Balanced sitting – actively upright without bracing

Balanced sitting is an active state, in which everything is working. There is dynamic balance between the quads and other leg muscles lengthening down, and rectus abdominis and psoas lengthening up, that allows the erector spinae into play; the pelvis drops

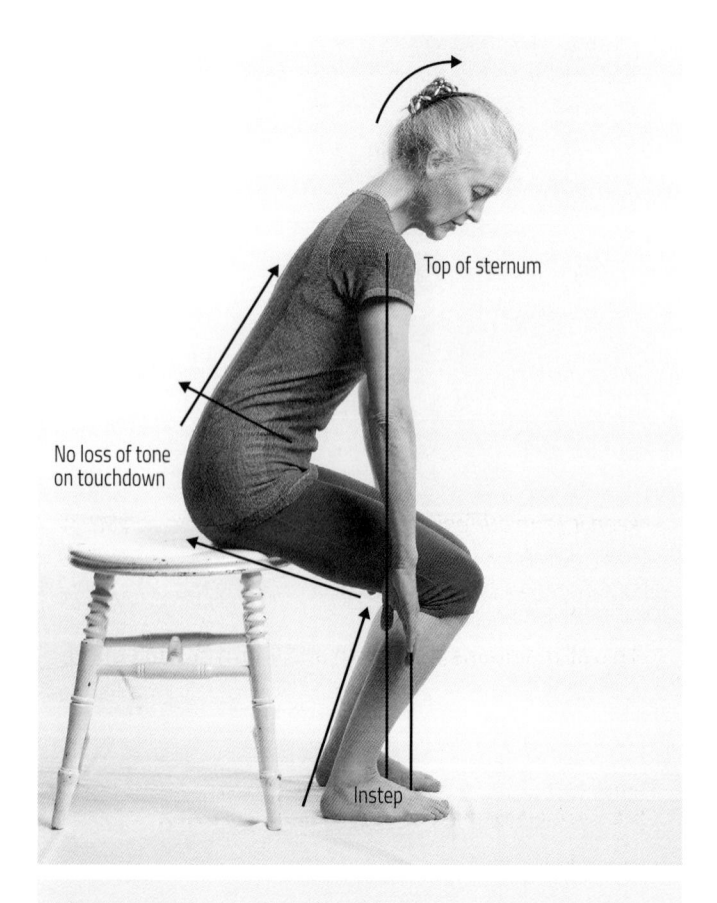

**Figure 13.9**
Sitting from "monkey," with a zed bend around the unity line

# Precise, springy alignment in sit to stand and "monkey"

fully into vertical, and the lumbar spine uncurls. This allows the deep front line to come into play right up to the inside neck, releasing tension from jaw, infra-hyoids, and clavicles. When the torso is fully supported in this way, the shoulders can engage forwards and outwards into their balanced position and the arms rotate forwards.

### Exploration 13.5  Active sitting

- *Keep your legs and feet engaged:*

  *big toe balls and inside heel on the floor*

  *pulling the inside ankle bone back and up (screwing the ankle)*

  *while pulling the iliac spines back and up from the outside of the knee.*

If needed, give another 1-2-3 to refresh their life and tone. Add in more directions to your integrative thinking.

- *The ribs at the back of the armpit (RBAP) come back, wide and up from the sacrum, helped by iliac spines and ribs pulling back. The upper back widens from the forward and outward pull of the elbows.*

- *The top of the sternum keeps its length away from the sitting bones, forwards from RBAP.*

- *Keep breathing, allowing the springy in-breath to expand your whole torso especially in the back of the body and keep it from stiffening with all these pulls. Watch you do not collapse on the out-breath but maintain your tone in the ribs. Keep spatial awareness externally and internally.*

This all maintains the length and width not just of the back, but of the whole system. Everything is working.

### Exploration 13.6  Testing the difference between sitting upright without bracing your back and slumping

If you do not brace, and the ribs are pulling back and up strongly, it can feel as if the back is in a curve, even hunched. But this is faulty sensory perception – unless your ribs really have slumped down toward your iliac spines.

- *Do a finger test of this, with a finger on your iliac spine and your thumb on your lowest rib. Feel the distance between them.*

- *Now slump a little, rounding your back, and notice that distance decreases.*

- *Take your top of sternum up away from the sitting bones and send your hip laterals down to sit yourself upright again.*

- *Now take your ribs strongly up and back, with ribs at the back of the armpit coming back, wide, and up. Notice the sensation of the back being curved, but the distance between your thumb and finger stays the same or even increases.*

The muscle we are working eccentrically (i.e. lengthening as it contracts) is the quadratus lumborum (see Fig. 6.3). (This runs from the top of the iliac crest to the lowest rib – the floating rib – and to the sides of the lumbar vertebrae.) You are lengthening the back of the ribcage up off the pelvic girdle.

## Lesson 4  Why the knees need to stay back as we tilt forwards to stand

Goldie would work to tilt me forwards in the chair and back to upright, getting my torso working, without any thought of standing. It was always hard work. There were several principles at work, but the main ones were that I did not sag the torso into the hip joints, nor let the upper body narrow or move forward and down, so that at the moment of standing, the full length, and so the full springy responsiveness of the whole back line of my body, was still in play and ready to spring into action. "I'm just going to whisk you out of the chair," she would say. And so she would – in such a way that my back would come back and up so strongly that it felt like it alone was taking me up, and all my legs were doing was lengthening underneath.

We have looked at standing from sitting in explorations 10.4 and 10.11. Here we will look at the

# CHAPTER thirteen

mechanics in more detail. To come out of the chair, we need to start in toned sitting, then to tilt forward without losing the extensor tone in back and legs. Then at take-off, there needs to be no forward movement of the iliac spines, ribs, knees, or top of sternum. Instead, the hamstrings (and their extensor chains), along with the deep front line, need to be actively engaged, which will control the lift off the chair. Masoero suggests we need to hold tone to utilize stored elastic energy to help to power the movement.

### What goes wrong is often that we "relax"

Normally when one inclines forward, one sags a little into the hips. This then allows a curve in the back which loses the continuity of the extensor line of the back of the body, and we need to push against gravity to stand. Or, as we go to stand, the upper body and ribs "relax" slightly, letting them drop forward and down. Or the knees slip slightly forward. Then we lose length and with it, springy responsiveness of the extensor line, so we push or jump instead.

To avoid all this, the knees must not slide forward as we tilt forward. Since this seems counterintuitive, let's discover the engineering basis of this.

### Exploration 13.7 To demonstrate that knees should not move forward as we stand

- Rest your forearm along a table. Hold a stick upright on the table, pivoting between finger and thumb an inch (3 cm) from its base. Since its bottom end cannot move back as the top end tilts towards your elbow, the fulcrum between your fingers must move forward instead, moving your lower arm and elbow (representing the thigh and knee) forwards. To detect this, lie a book on the table against your elbow. As the stick tilts, the elbow will push the book away.
- Observe there is no stability to the movement because there is no counterbalance, the stick is top heavy and will topple over.

- *If, when sitting, we tilt the torso forward by rotating around the sitting bones, the hip joints will move forward in space. The knees also move slightly forward. (Check by putting another chair an inch from your knees. Does the distance decrease?) Then the torso becomes heavy and could fall forward off the chair unless we push up in some way.*

This is why we need to keep the back back, and not let the knees go forward.

- *Instead, if we pull back at the iliac spines and keep the hamstrings engaged when we tilt forward, then the hip joints will hold their position in space as the pelvis rotates around them, so that the sitting bones move slightly back.*

As this happens, the whole weight of the torso going forward puts a backward pull on the knees (see Fig. 13.2).

The pull "spring-loads" the hamstrings with potential energy, like a stretched elastic band that when released straightaway into action will help to unfold us to upright.

Video link for exploration 13.7

### Exploration 13.8 To test whether you sag as you tilt forward

- Use finger and thumb on hip crease and iliac spine respectively as we did when going into "monkey." If the torso sags, the thumb will come ahead of the finger (Fig. 13.6).
- Test that you have not compensated by collapsing the upper torso onto the lower torso: use the second finger check, and watch that thumb on lower ribs and forefinger on iliac spine do not move closer together as you tilt.

# Precise, springy alignment in sit to stand and "monkey"

### Exploration 13.9  Not pulling the chin down

As we tilt, we can focus so much on the iliac spines and hips that we draw the chin down. But the answer is not to focus on the head leading, as this results in a weak movement. We need everything working together. The head and neck are above the torso.

Instead, work to engage the top of the torso:

- *Keep your length in the front by thinking to pull the top of the sternum up away from the sitting bones and heels.*
- *Widen the RBAP away from sacrum, breathe into front and back of the chest, engaging the deep arm lines through to tips of the elbows, and pull the top of sternum forwards and up from the RBAP (see explorations 12.13, 12.14 and 12.16).*

The more the legs and torso free, stabilize, and engage, the more the neck can free and lift up, and the head then can play its part to lengthen the movement upwards. (More on engaging the head leading in Chapter 14).

### Exploration 13.10  To tilt forwards in the chair and stand

Sit with your knees an inch (2.5 cm) from another chair.

- *Find your active, toned sitting (exploration 13.5), breathing throughout.*
- *Maintain the tone in legs and feet, which stops collapse in ankles or knees.*
- *Maintain the chest widening, front and back, with toned pendular arms (Chapter 12, lesson 4).*

  *I pull T8 up away from the heels (1).*

  *and top of sternum up away from the sitting bones (2).*

  *I pull the iliac spines back and the ribs back and up (3).*

  *I pull the RBAP away from the sacrum, and the tips of the elbows away from RBAP (4).*

  *Be aware of the psoas deep in the belly coming back and up (5).*

  **Push the heels forwards towards the toes (6).**

- *Give a count of 1-2-3 as you angle forwards over the feet without collapsing into the hip joints – it may feel as if you are coming up and over the hips instead.*
- *Your knees should not move forward at all.*

The arms hang vertically, and so will follow the torso's inclination at a slight lag (Fig. 13.10).

Lifting off the chair

STOP and give another 1-2-3 of the directions above to lift-off.

- *The RBAP are pulling up away from the heels, lengthening the superficial back line, while the pressure into the front of the foot lifts the superficial front line.*
- *The psoas, iliac spines, and ribs moving up and back stop the quads pushing, and engage the lifting of the lower body off the legs as in a pelvic lift.*

  *Let the sitting bones and knees move back slightly, to push the chair back.*

Trust the process, and you should lift off the chair.

## Lesson 5  Squatting and bouncing – testing our elastic resistance and mobility

If your alignment has changed with this work you may find it easier to squat with aligned feet and legs. This is more challenging than a wide-legged squat with splayed feet but will show your true mobility and adaptive, lengthening muscle tone. There is usually work to be done here.

# CHAPTER thirteen

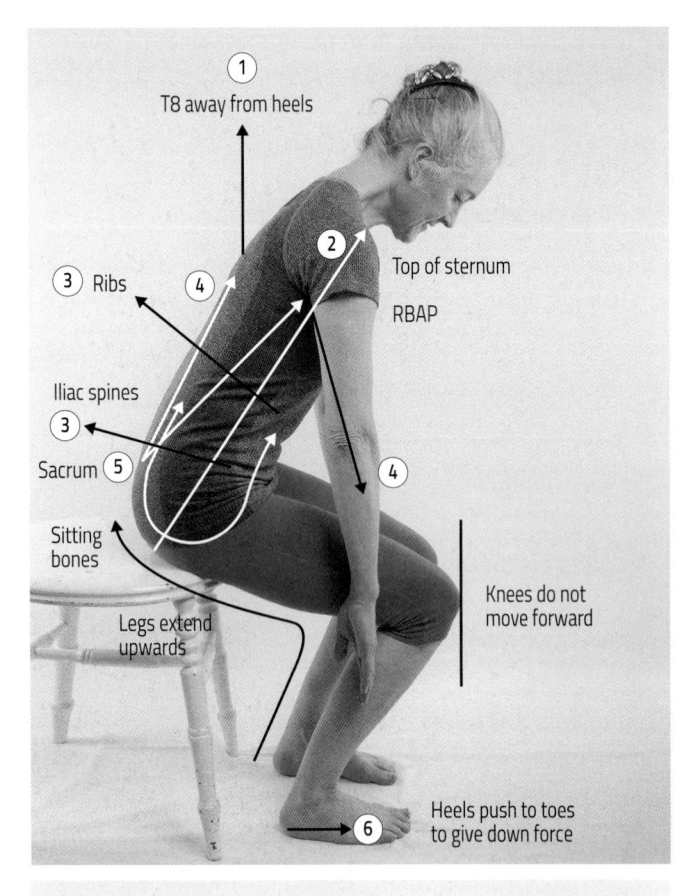

**Figure 13.10**
Tilting forward in a chair

Labels on figure:
1. T8 away from heels
2. Top of sternum / RBAP
3. Ribs
3. Iliac spines
4. (arrows)
5. Sacrum / Sitting bones
Legs extend upwards
Knees do not move forward
6. Heels push to toes to give down force

### Exploration 13.11  Squatting

Stand with legs hip-width apart and feet aligned. Breathe through the whole-body, engaging the psoas.

- *Engage the legs strongly by pulling the inner ankle bones back and up, and the iliac spines up and back from the outside of the knees. Pull the pubococcygeals forwards, and elbows outward.*

- *Pull the iliac spines and ribs back to come into a true "monkey" (exploration 13.3). Look down where you are going (Fig. 13.11A).*

- *Keep pulling iliac spines and ribs back, and also work your active hip folding: widening with the breath into the depth,* width, and back of the pelvic floor, working the psoas and deep belly muscles back and up to open the lumbar spine and flex the hip joints.

- *Keep thinking both the top of the sternum and the back of the armpits up away from the heels – don't let the upper body tilt forward beyond the feet (Fig. 13.11B).*

- *Keep lengthening the lower legs up off the ankles by continuing to bring the inner ankle bone up and back. The lower legs only come forward enough to balance. Nothing drops down as the body shape-shifts and lowers to the floor (Fig. 13.11C).*

However far you get, everything stays engaged and going up.

Only go as far as you can keep your alignment; if the feet or knees start to turn out, or the neck or back to arch, the inner torque chain is lost. Not only is extension then lost, but the misalignment causes co-contraction, reducing joint mobility. As muscles lengthen and alignment improves, co-contraction is reduced, joints open, and one day the full squat happens.

Take this into bouncing also (see Fig. 6.7).

- *As your lumbar spine opens, and the line sacrum to T8 lengthens, you will be able to "sit" more vertically back in the air, and maintain this as you bounce upward. To help this, engage all your directions and work particularly to bring iliac spines and ribs back, to help uncurl your lumbar spine.*

## Lesson 6  Constructive conscious guidance and control – using Initial AT for yourself

Our modern age is witnessing the excitement of discovering our feelings – our emotions, intuitions and instincts. They are now often seen as the voice of truth. After 2500 years of being told that only pure reason is to be followed while the body and its feelings are unreliable, we are discovering both neurologically and through somatics and psychotherapy that feelings are feedback in the flow of the body; they are

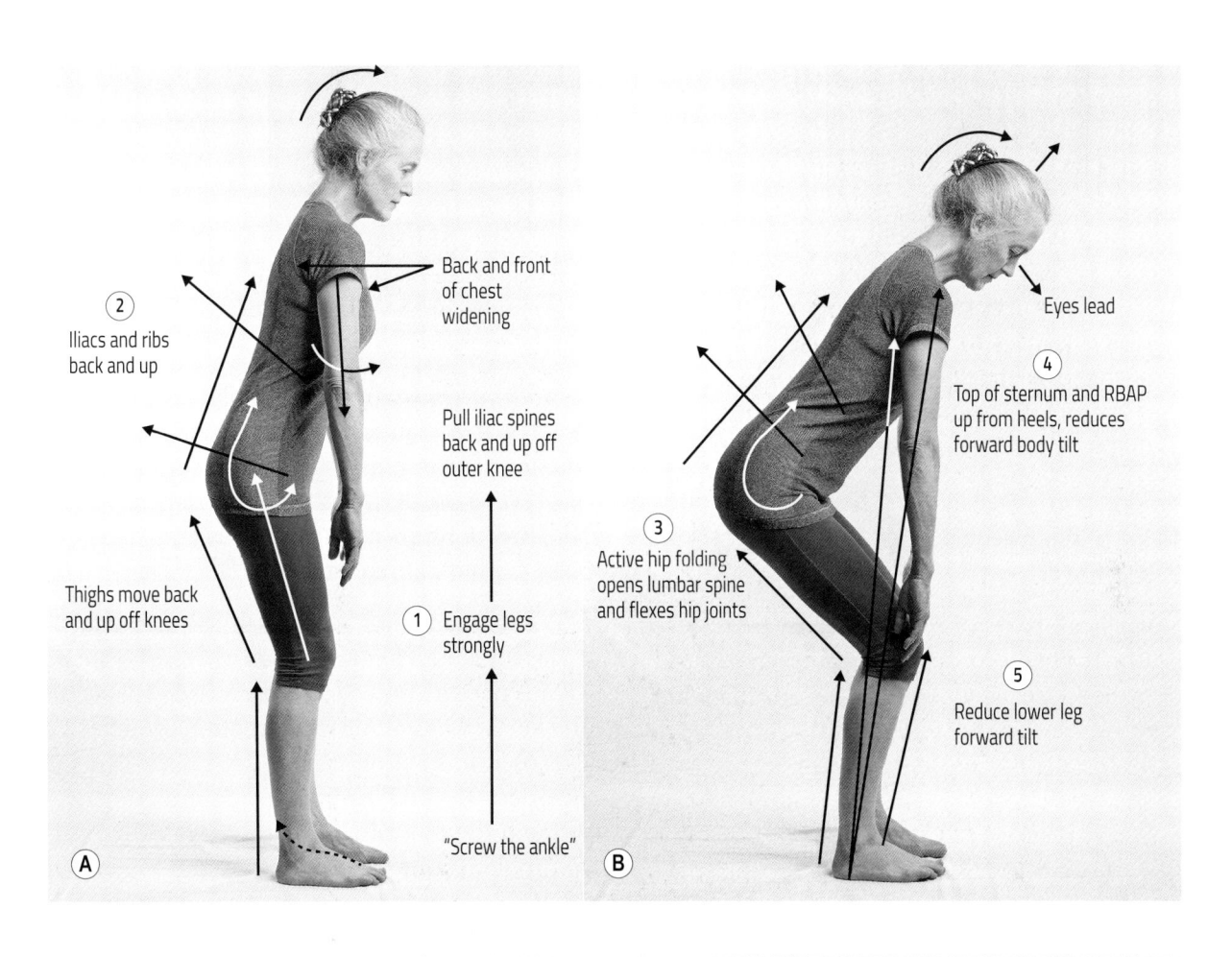

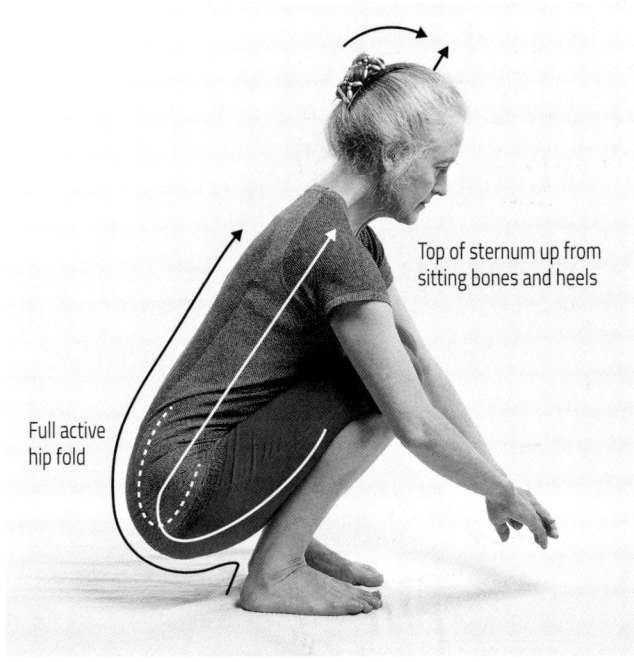

# Precise, springy alignment in sit to stand and "monkey"

**(A)**
- ② Iliacs and ribs back and up
- Back and front of chest widening
- Pull iliac spines back and up off outer knee
- Thighs move back and up off knees
- ① Engage legs strongly
- "Screw the ankle"

**(B)**
- Eyes lead
- ④ Top of sternum and RBAP up from heels, reduces forward body tilt
- ③ Active hip folding opens lumbar spine and flexes hip joints
- ⑤ Reduce lower leg forward tilt

**(C)**
- Top of sternum up from sitting bones and heels
- Full active hip fold

**Figures 13.11A–C**
Squatting sequence from "monkey" to full squat

# CHAPTER thirteen

crucial at every level of decision making for both conscious and unconscious processes.

I suspect it makes us less willing to use pure reasoning processes – they seem hard work and cold compared to warm feelings. But the word "feeling" is too broad. We are here specifically concerned with the unreliability of feeling feedback from the voluntary muscles that tries to tell us, mid-action, what to do. The problem is that our neurology is not wired to give us the detailed feedback from deep postural muscles that we need for balanced action (Ong 2017).

Alexander was very clear in his first two books about the discipline required for the conscious mind – observing and reasoning out solutions:

"The displaced parts of the body must be restored to their proper positions by re-education in a correct and controlled use of the muscular mechanisms" (2011: 226).

"He must learn to give the correct mental orders to the mechanisms involved, and *there must be a clear differentiation in his mind between the giving of the order and the performance of the act ordered and carried out through the medium of the muscles.* The whole principles of volition [direction] and inhibition are implicit in the recognition of this differentiation" (2011: 167).

"When the correct guiding orders have been practised and given by the mind … the muscles involved will come into play in different combinations under the control of conscious guidance, and a reasoned act will take the place of the series of habitual, unconsidered movements which have resulted in the deformation of the body" (2011: 168).

## Be "the architect of your own building"

To use Initial AT well for yourself:

- You need to have an "architectural" plan, knowledge of our optimal body geometry.
- Then to be able to observe where we deviate from this – the problem.
- We then need to reason what is needed to meet the plan. It helps to have a palate of possible directions to choose from and experiment with to bring about appropriate change.

Here is a starter "cookbook" of sample directions you might choose for different problems you observe, to begin to make your own discoveries.

Video yourself going through each exploration to identify where you need extra help. Don't try to watch it while it is happening, as you will be tempted to change it as it is happening, which is counter-productive. We are looking to write a program and test it. The directions are a brain-map to take you into previously unknown movement.

What do you see? Are the knees unstable? Is there still a lumbar arch and projecting ribs? Think through what is needed, and choose directions that could help. The key is to combine the directions you have chosen into one brain program, so that they can integrate together. Don't be tempted to add directions as you go through the movements. If the next video still shows up problems, stop, have a think, and refine your program. Then run it again and see what happens this time. It's a learning process which will take time and experiment.

A. *Anterior tilted pelvis*: pull iliac spines back, sitting bones to the back of the knees and pubococcygeals forward (exploration 7.17). Balance on heels (exploration 13.2).

B. *Arched lumbar spine, projecting ribs*: realign pelvis (A), plus pull ribs back; take T8 up from sacrum (exploration 12.2), using the wall (exploration 12.1).

C. *Bent arms that do not hang vertically*: pulls to the arms, and to RBAP (exploration 12.16; exploration 12.17).

D. *Bulging belly, abdominal problems*: (A) with natural breathing into the lower body (Chapter 6, lesson 2; Chapter 10, lesson 3).

E. *Collapsing torso when bending or tilting*: use finger checks (exploration 13.8).

# Precise, springy alignment in sit to stand and "monkey"

F. *Elbows falling backwards, projecting shoulder blades, upper body tilted back*: elbows pulled outward and forward (exploration 7.10); shoulder shrug (exploration 12.6); the ribs at the back of the armpits (RBAP) up and away from sacrum (exploration 12.13).

G. *Integration of torso when bending*: use a true "monkey" (exploration 13.3); active hip folding (exploration 10.7).

H. *Instability of hips*: use (L) and (A) plus widen into the sides of the hips or the sitting bones with the breath (exploration 8.13) and pelvic lifts (exploration 8.7).

I. *Lack of mobility of hips, e.g. to get over your legs when getting out of a chair*: engage the psoas and active hip folding (exploration 10.7) and pelvic lifts (exploration 8.7).

J. *Laterally tilted hips and shoulders, spinal curvature*: use (L) and (F) together; pelvic lifts (exploration 8.7).

K. *Narrowed or weak upper body*: (F) plus breathing across front and back of the upper body (exploration 12.14); bring RBAP away from front of shoulder, and vice versa (exploration 12.12).

L. *Unstable knees, unstable ankles or misaligned feet*: align and activate the pulls to the feet and legs (exploration 8.12).

M. *Upper body collapsed forward, forward neck*: sternum up away from sitting bones (exploration 7.6; exploration 12.4); ribs at back of armpits back away from tips of elbows (exploration 12.17); T8 away from heels (exploration 7.13 and exploration 12.2); pelvic lifts (exploration 8.7); reverse whispered Ah (exploration 12.18; exploration 12.19).

N. *Weak arms*: use (F) plus (M) along with general torso aligning and strengthening (A, H, I).

O. *Weak legs*: use (L) plus the thrust from friction with the floor (exploration 10.4).

# 14

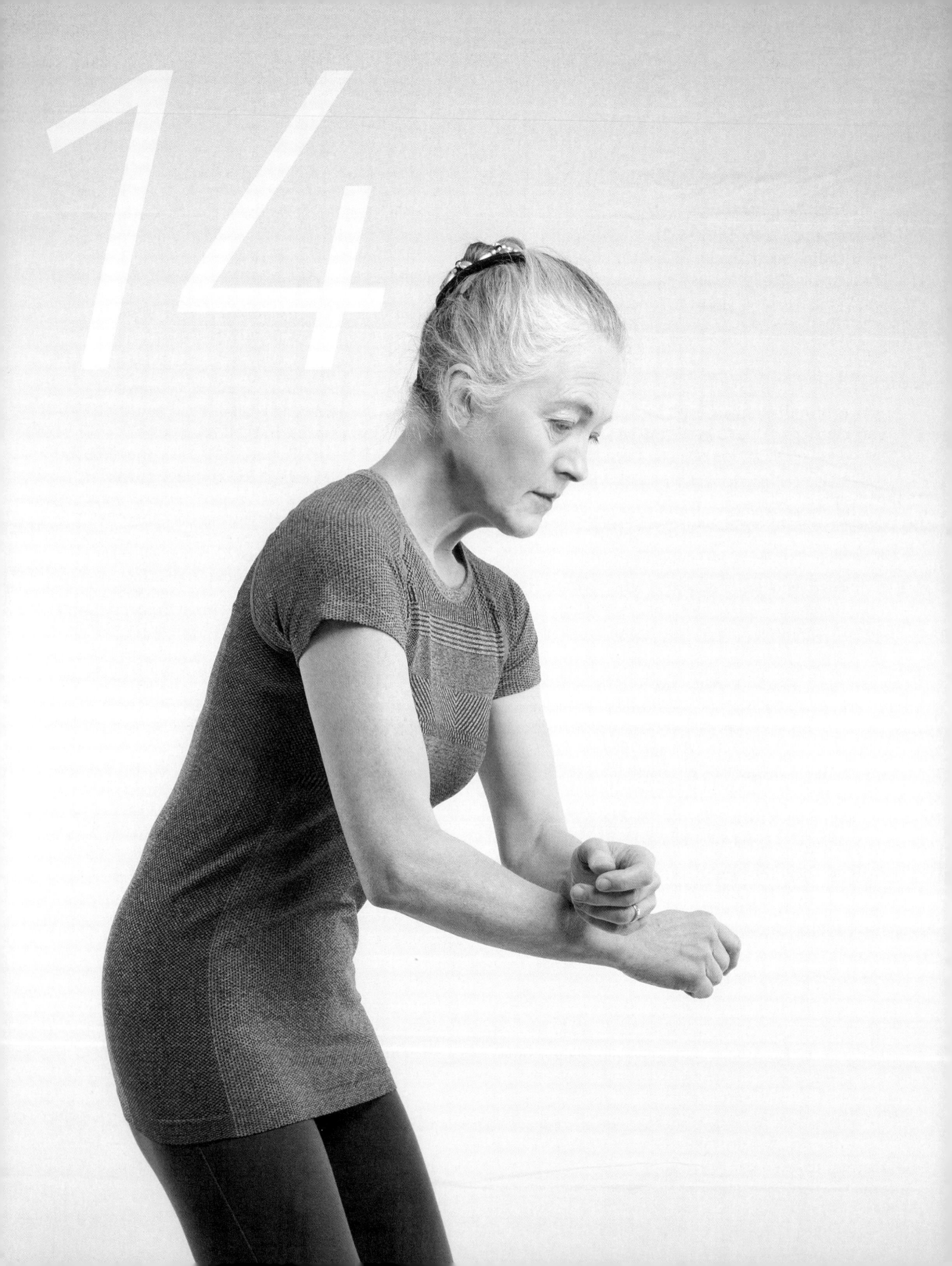

# Freeing the neck, and Alexander's primary directions    14

In 1988, at the Brighton International Alexander Congress where 500 AT teachers were gathered, a teacher visiting the ladies' cloakroom overheard the cleaners talking. "They're a strange crew we've got in this week, who are they?" "I dunno," came the answer, "But they've all got something wrong with their necks!" I suspect the cleaners were picking up on our over-involvement with our necks. Miss Goldie told me that Alexander, towards the end of his life, had said exasperatedly that he wished he had never instructed: "Free the neck." He added something like: "Their necks are all they think about. They forget that there is anything above their necks, and to come further up into their heads!" She told another teacher that in his later years Alexander never even said "neck free, head forward and up, etc." (Alex Farkas in email communication with author, February 18, 2020). She herself never used it. Instead she would say "*Not* the head back, *not* the body forwards, but the knees forwards."

In 1910, in his first book, Alexander wrote: "If there is any undue muscular pull in any part of the neck, it is almost certain to be due to the defective coordination in the use of the muscles of the spine, back and torso generally the correction of which means the eradication of the real cause of the trouble" (2011: 172).

He later makes what looks like a complete turnaround. In 1932, in *Use of the Self*, he writes: "After further experimentation I found at last that in order to maintain a lengthening of the stature it was necessary that my head should tend to go upwards, not downwards, when I put it forward; in short, that to lengthen *I must put my head forward and up. As is shewn by what follows, this proved to be the primary control of my use in all my activities*" (1985: 30).

In twenty-two years, the head/neck balance has gone from being the last to get involved to apparently being the leader. What do we make of this? It is interesting that both he and Delsarte, and also Mabel Ellsworth Todd who developed Ideokinesis for dancers, all started their investigations after voice training and subsequent problems. They were only too aware of the delicacy of this area.

## Lesson 1   Why we need to free the neck

I vividly remember driving away from my very first Alexander lesson thinking, Wow! My neck! It's so free!

The standard directions of the modern Alexander technique are:

*"Let the neck be free,*

*to let the head go forward and up,*

*to let the back lengthen and widen,*

*to let the knees go forward and away."*

This is the theory of primary control, that the balance of the head on the neck leads the whole-body into extension, as quoted above.

> "Free the neck" is a very imprecise instruction. In modern AT understanding, it refers only to freeing the atlanto-occipital joint, the head/ neck joint, then the axis joint (exploration 3.8; exploration 3.9), from which other cervical vertebrae will follow.

A free head/neck joint is important, and there is a certain amount of scientific evidence for this. Firstly, from the suboccipital muscles – the tiny muscles that link the occiput and the very top vertebrae, that so delicately help to balance the huge weight of the head on the top of the spine. These have a far higher density of muscle spindles (the stretch receptors, see Chapter 3, lesson 1) than anywhere else in the body. Why? These muscles are ideally placed to act as sensors of head movement, and it is known that their sensory input converges with vestibular, oculomotor, and visual inputs at various brain levels (Kulkarni et al. 2001). These inputs would presumably be feeding into the complex control of posture (see Chapter 8, lesson 2).

Secondly, Loram et al. (2017) showed that after some basic training, violinists (the subject group) could notice their neck tension and selectively inhibit

# CHAPTER fourteen

it; the result was a cascade of more efficient overall movement such as less pressure on the chinrest and reduced leg activity. Skin sweat reduction also suggested that people were calmer.

So freeing the neck really is important for integrated movement. But is it the whole story? Do we only need to repeat "let the neck be free" for everything to sort itself? Do we even want to think this at all?

### The neck is a complex zone

Ted Dimon writes: "This region [the throat and the underside of the jaw] is far and away the most complex part of the human musculature and includes dozens of muscles" (2011: 79). I want to put the muscle layers of the neck into an overview of what we have covered here, and how we can best work with its complexity and linkages, while staying out of interfering with it.

Consider the layers of the neck. At the back are the *trapezius*, under which are the *levator scapulae* (see Fig. 9.2), then the *erector spinae* (see Fig. 3.5), and below them the many deep tiny muscles between vertebrae. These include the deepest attachments of the head to the neck, the tiny but crucial suboccipital muscles (see Fig. 3.4). On the sides of the neck are the *sternocleidomastoids* (SCMs), then *splenius capitis and cervicis* (part of the erector spinae) (see Fig. 8.4), and below them the *scalenes*. I'll discuss the complex muscles at the front below.

### The head and neck are the top "stations" in all the muscle trains (except the front arm lines)

The head is often tightened back on the neck because of deep tensions in the erector spinae (see Fig. 3.18). These muscles – part of the superficial back line (SBL) and the spiral line (SpL) – shorten the whole spine, arching the neck and lumbar spine, so that the trapezius must take over to support the head.

I wonder how much hard-earned cash is spent yearly on massage and physio for tight traps. These are expensive muscles! The researchers in the neck tension study on violinists mentioned above (Loram et al. 2017) suggested that because the neck is the root of kinematic chains of head, trunk, and arms, less co-contraction at the neck would require less co-contraction further down the chain. Many people could benefit from learning voluntary control of their neck and spine muscles, and in doing so, improve the poise and adaptive tone of their whole framework.

### The neck is affected by fear

The startle reflex is our first response to danger (Fig. 14.1). It causes contraction and narrowing in the front of the body, down the superficial front line (see Fig. 3.22), caving the chest and protecting the vulnerable organs, in a return to primary curve. But the head is not pulled down with this. Because the sternocleidomastoids (SCMs) originate *behind* the pivot of the atlanto-occipital joint (the top of the neck), the shortening of the SCMs pulls the neck forward and the face up, to better observe the source of danger. Unfortunately for many, this becomes their permanent posture (Fig. 14.2). In this the trapezius, and beneath it the levator scapulae (in the deep back arm line; Fig. 9.2), become chronically short, lifting the shoulders up towards the head rather than hanging down from it, and tangling the shoulder girdle with the balance of the head.

The SCMs are also part of the lateral line (see Fig. 8.4). It can be interesting, when one thinks of lengthening the head up, if instead of thinking to let the *back* of the head go forward and up, to think of the mastoid bones – at the *side* of the head – going up and back to lengthen the SCMs. This will result in a lengthening of both the front and back superficial lines.

### Exploration 14.1 Lengthening the neck with the superficial front line and the lateral line

- *Stand and go into a startled slump, observing the double bend in the neck from the shortening of the SCM and shoulders hunching to support the forward neck. This pulls the superficial front line down.*

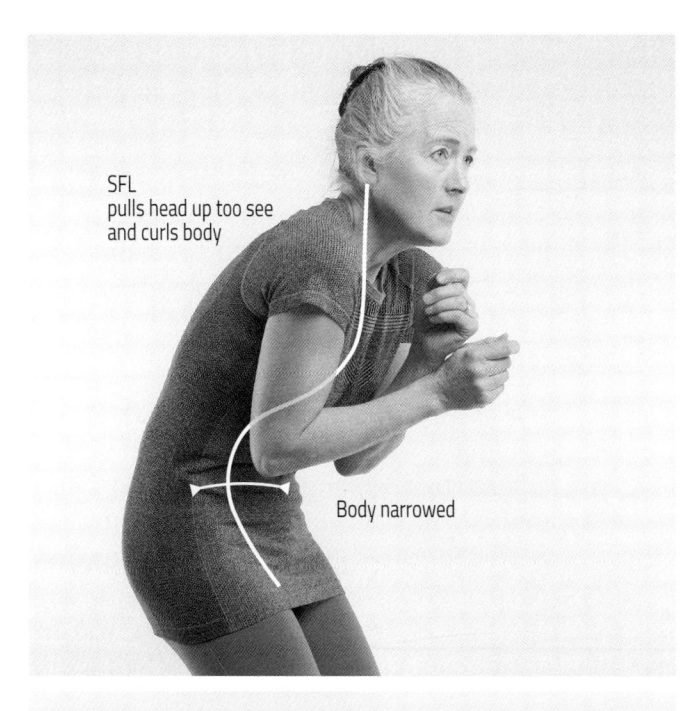

# Freeing the neck, and Alexander's primary directions

**Figure 14.1**
Startle pattern

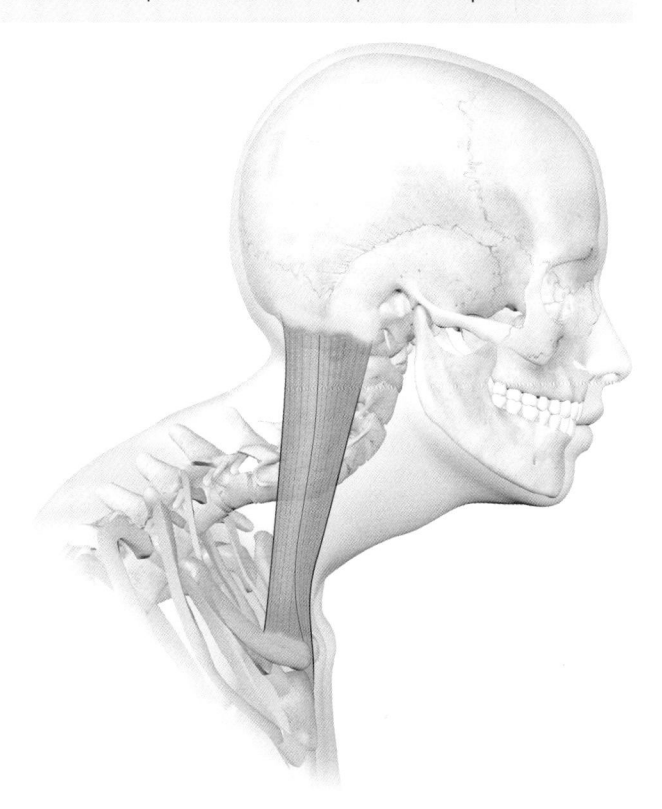

**Figure 14.2**
In the startle response, the contracting SCM pulls the neck forward at the base, while it pulls it back into hyperextension at the top. This can become a permanent posture

- Observe that, as the body narrows, we tighten into the inside legs, maybe with knees coming together, and come out of the lateral line (Fig. 14.1).

Coming up by engaging the superficial front line (SFL)

- *Put your fingers on your mastoid bones under your ears and take them up. Notice the neck lengthening up, and the front of the body is taken upwards as the clavicles and top of the sternum are then lifted by the SCMs. This lengthens the rectus abdominis upward, pulling the pelvis more vertically aligned. You have lengthened the superficial front line (Fig. 14.3).*

Coming up by engaging the lateral line (LL) (Fig. 8.4)

- *Find your pelvic lifts (exploration 8.7). Notice that when the hip lateral group (gluteus maximus, medius, and minimus, tensor fasciae latae, and IT band) pull down the outside of one leg, the criss-cross patterns of internal and external obliques and intercostals, with deeper quadratus lumborum, lengthen the side of the body up. Above them, the cross of SCMs and splenius capitis lengthen the neck and head up.*

This movement is also brought into play naturally when the head rolls forward on the atlanto-occipital joint, lengthening the superficial back line (SBL), and pulling the SCMs back and up to lengthen (tight underlying muscles permitting).

- *Play with this by "rolling your raindrop" (exploration 3.8).*

### Imbalances in the outer muscles cause tightening in all the underlying muscles at the front and sides of the neck

The muscles in front of the neck spine are:

- The *hyoid group* at the front. These include the complex muscle groups of the larynx and floor of the mouth. They run between the styloid process on the base of the skull, the hyoid bone, the larynx and the clavicles and sternum.

# CHAPTER fourteen

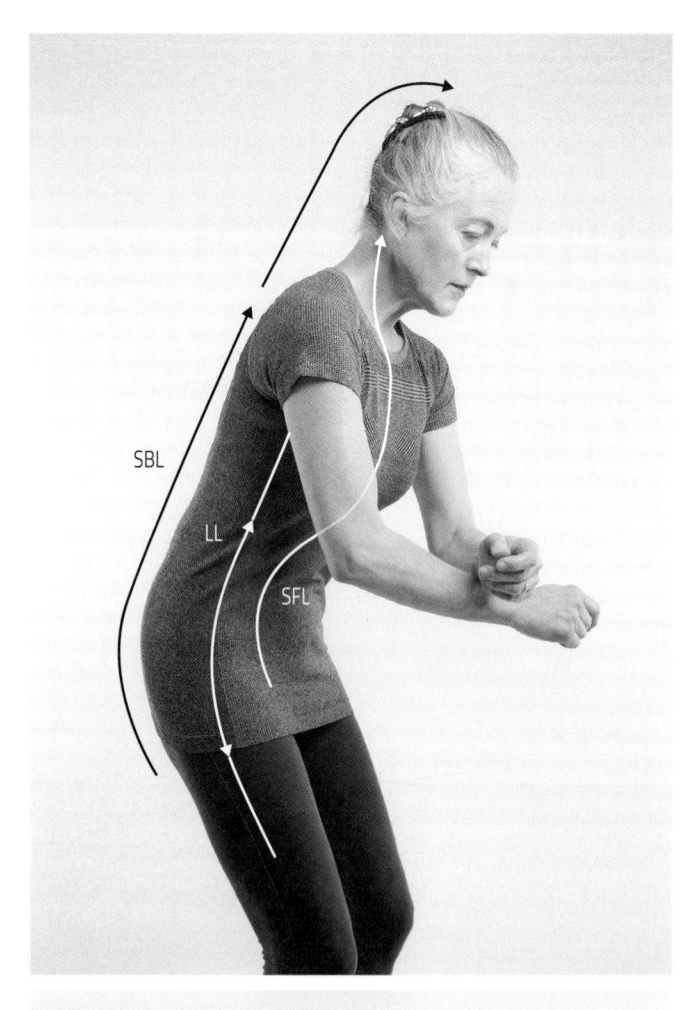

**Figure 14.3**
Lengthening through SFL, LL and SBL (see text for abbreviations)

- Under the hyoids are the *pharyngeal constrictors* of the throat – the swallowing muscles.

- Under these are the only muscles that actively balance or oppose the pulling back of the head: *longus colli and capitis* along the front of the spine, and the tiny *rectus capitis anterior*.

- The *scalenes*. These run between the side of the neck and the upper ribs. They are guy wires for supporting the ribcage from the upper spine, and not breathing muscles as is often thought. (If the scalenes are involved in heaving your upper chest up and down, say while running, then you have lost contact with the diaphragm and whole-body natural breathing.)

All these muscles are part of the deep front line (Fig. 10.9). This is why a major way of working with all these delicate muscles is through breathing and vocalizing with the whispered Ah (exploration 17.4). So to free the neck, we need to be present through the deep lines, and in all the outer lines also!

If we think of leading a movement with the head, we will often pull on these delicate mechanisms. One can suggest that leading with the head needs to be an indirect process, initiated instead by the vision (or other senses), as evolution surely intended. Sensory information is then collated in the brainstem with proprioceptive feedback, especially from suboccipital muscles, cueing the body to follow the head's intentions, with which the brainstem presumably then organizes the appropriate muscle patterns. Meanwhile, by not disturbing head/neck balance, the kinetic chains are also undisturbed and stay free for responsive action.

We need to stay out of the way of this – big-time! Ted Dimon voices an idea that I have now heard from many teachers: "Experienced teachers ... when working with a student, will leave the neck alone and trust that as the system comes into balance the neck will be able to let go on its own. Our job as teachers is to find out what is interfering with these conditions and in so doing to help reestablish system-wide balance, not to try to directly elicit neck reflexes" (2015: 47).

### Exploration 14.2   Alignment of the head/neck relationship

Following Masoero's work on Initial AT, I am contending that the head lengthens up off the neck not just from T1, but from T8 (Chapter 7, lesson 5). The aligned neck is much further forwards than usually thought, "ramped" forward, so that the base of the ear is over the top of the sternum. Further forward becomes a forward-held head. We have explored this by bringing the top of the

# Freeing the neck, and Alexander's primary directions

sternum forward (exploration 12.4). Now let's explore this from the neck itself.

This exploration is only valid if the line sacrum to T8 is straight (or nearly so). If the person is slumping in the upper back, then the ear may be over the top of sternum but this will be forward-held head. Check with a stick that the upper back below T8 is still on the stick. If not, or if you have a pronounced lumbar curve, and you still have work to do on aligning and expanding your torso.

- *Stand aligned, and play around with your head/neck relationship, raising and lowering the eyeline while using this finger test: put your thumbs in the hollows under your ears – the pivot – and your index fingers under the base of your nose, with the other fingers together, making a level plane. Play with the balance of the head around the pivot of the thumbs, between ears and nose, until you find the balance point where they are level.*

- *Bring your neck back so your thumbs are behind the top of the sternum, the base of the nose is still level. Your neck will now be quite vertical – your head is going up, but not forward and up. You may notice you are looking out of the tops of your eyes, from under your lids.*

- *Pull your thumbs forward again, keeping your fingers level. Find where your thumbs are over your top of sternum. This is the balanced position, where the head moves forward and up off the neck.*

- *Now take them further forward, so they are in front of the top of the sternum. This is forward neck.*

**Video link for exploration 14.2**

**AT info:** This is partly why AT teachers have the front hand under the chin when working on pupils, it is leading the throat forward to balance the up of the back of the neck from the back hand. Alexander instructed in whispered Ah – to take the jaw forward to free the throat. We are also working with this in reverse whispered Ah (exploration 12.19).

## Lesson 2  Finding length and adaptive tone in the neck extensors

We have been working over several chapters with the Initial Alexander technique model to sort the torso first and the head will sort itself out. By optimizing support from the feet and legs, the torso is supported; by lengthening, widening, and lifting the parts of the torso, the legs can lengthen, and the shoulder girdle and arms can open and relax, finding full strength and mobility. The opening of the shoulders and untangling of the upper ribs lengthens out the restricting trapezius and deeper muscles below, allowing space for the neck to spring up unimpeded from T8, so that the head can move forward and up.

For all this, we have applied lengthening and activating pulls to almost all the muscles of the body – except those of the neck. The following exploration allows us to lengthen and integrate the tight muscles of the neck directly, and integrate them with the upper thoracic spine. Once you have found the physical movements and pulls involved, can you let the head be led by the vision. Or, since one starts with the head down, by intent to see, letting the spatial awareness and embodied intelligence organize the movements dynamically.

### Exploration 14.3    Head leading in child's pose

**Preparation – active folding of the hips (exploration 10.7)**

- *Fold yourself into child's pose, with your forehead on the floor, your arms comfortably in front of you. Notice that in this position, the head naturally falls forward from T8 between the shoulder blades and the shoulders naturally widen forward of the back (Fig. 14.4A).*

1   *Engage the psoas group on the out-breath, drawing up and back along the spine. This will draw the thighs towards the chest, actively folding the hips from within.*

2   *On the in-breath, maintain the active hip folding as you widen the back into the pelvic floor and hips, and*

# CHAPTER fourteen

also into shoulder blades, backs of armpits, and down the deep back arm lines (DBAL) into elbows and little fingers (Fig. 14.4B).

**Finding your vestibular directions (Chapter 8, lesson 2) in child's pose**

- Find the "laser beams" of up/down, side/side and forward/back. However in child's pose, "up" points horizontally through the crown of the head, while "front/back" is from the nose vertically downward, and through the back of the head upward to the ceiling.

**Tractioning the spine from the head to reawaken adaptive tone in the upper vertebrae**

When we take the head forward in child's pose, usually the hips would take over the forward movement very quickly. The neck and back are then passively carried forward. If we stop the hips from moving, the head and neck then leads the movement and the spine is tractioned.

1   While keeping your hips actively folded from within and unmoving,

2   let the head follow the two vestibular directions of forward and up, so that it lengthens your neck away from the body.

- You are looking to lengthen forward until your neck is on a line with the back, with the head neither pulling back, nor dropping down. When the neck reaches full extension, return the forehead to the floor (Fig. 14.4C).

3   Do the same, but this time let the head traction the neck, vertebra by vertebra successively from C1 (top) to C7 (the base), and from there into the upper thoracic vertebrae. Use the active inner hip folding strongly to resist the body following. Again return your forehead to the floor. This is not about yanking your spine. You are making a conscious connection with each vertebra, while keeping expanded awareness of the whole-body, which itself will allow the traction to happen.

- Keep repeating this, each time finding traction into another vertebra and without letting the hips move forward at all, from thoracic, to lumbar, to sacral, until you can traction right down the spine (Fig. 14.4C).

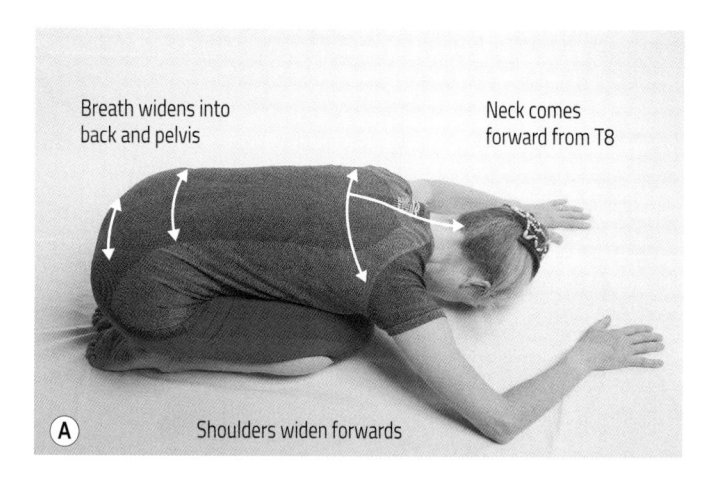

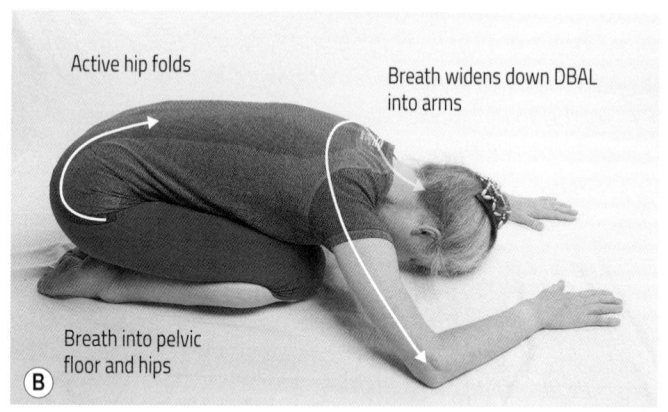

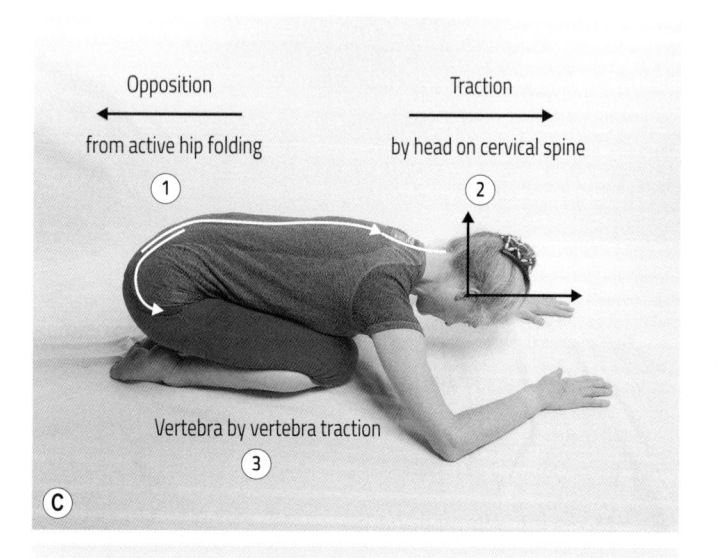

**Figure 14.4**
Child's pose. (A) Finding the position. (B) Engaging muscle tone with the breath. (C) Using opposition from active hip folding to traction neck and spine

# Freeing the neck, and Alexander's primary directions

*Exploration 14.4    Lengthening into all fours and plank*

### 1    Into all fours

When people go from child's pose into all fours, mostly they will push up with their hands and knees. Instead, with the head leading the spine with spatial awareness and embodied intelligence, the limbs will flow dynamically into new appropriate positions.

- *From child's pose, let the head lead the body forward, still resisting the movement in the hips somewhat, but now letting the head win. (Do not let the hips take over.)*
- *As the spine follows the head, the elbows and knees will unfold easily under you into all fours (Fig. 14.5A).*
- *Return to child's pose by actively folding the hips, while the head and neck now offer resistance by continuing to traction forward (Fig. 14.5B). Keep the breathing quietly going throughout. Repeat a few times.*

When we are on all fours, we tend to overuse the front (inner) arm lines (the flexors) for support. So also think of activating the back (outer) arm lines (the extensors). By expanding all the arm lines, we keep space for the head and neck spine to lengthen.

- *Think of the deep back arm line (DBAL) opening the shoulder blades through into the little fingers, while the deep front arm lines (DFAL) open across the chest into the thumbs. Like two nested hoops, one traces the inside line of arms and chest, the outer one traces the outside of arms and upper back (Fig. 14.6).*
- *You may also be aware of the top of the sternum leading the superficial front line (SFL) forward and up, which also helps support the arm lines.*

### 2    Move into plank position

- *From all fours, tuck the toes under, pull back in your iliac spines and ribs, and continue to take the psoas group back and up. Your pelvis will lift up, and as it does so, extend first one leg then the other back to take you into plank. Don't let your backside stick up in the air; the legs, hips, and back are all level (like a plank), the superficial back line (SBL) engaged throughout. Keep working your iliac spines and ribs back, working your arm lines (like nested hoops) out and down, engaging your legs, and you may well surprise yourself (Fig. 14.6).*

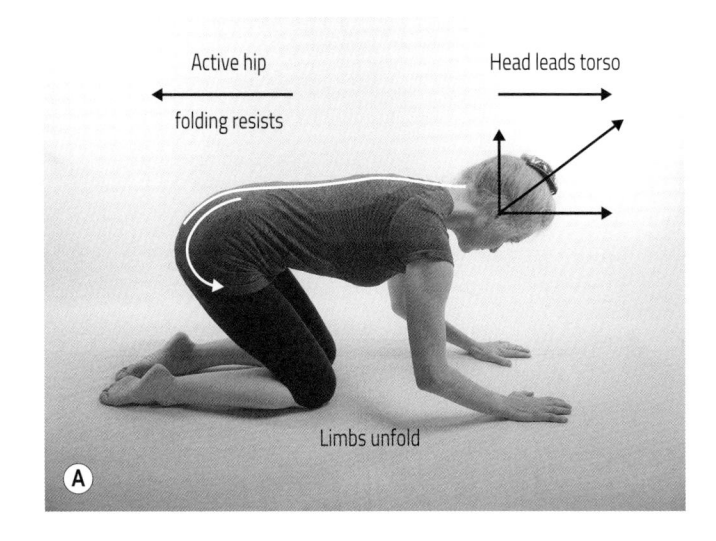

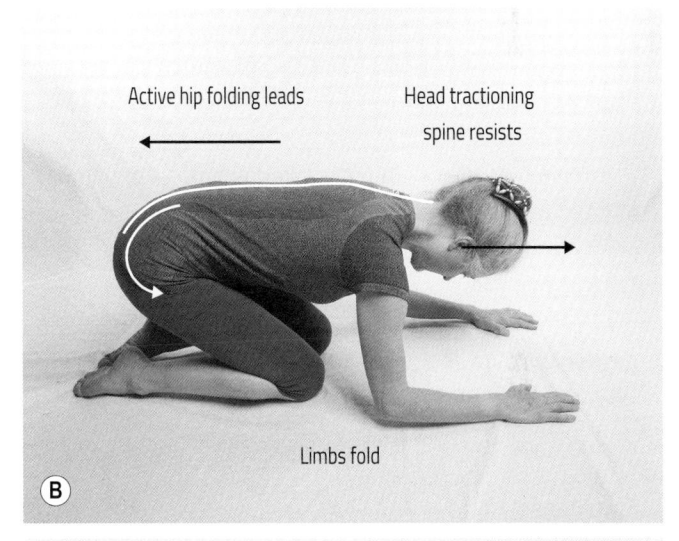

**Figure 14.5**
Morphing from child's pose to all-fours and back again. **(A)** Moving up, head forward and up draws torso. **(B)** Moving down, active hip folding draws torso

In plank, all the muscle trains need to work in balance together; you are using inner and outer torque chains, the vPNS and SNS engaged together with high vagal

# CHAPTER fourteen

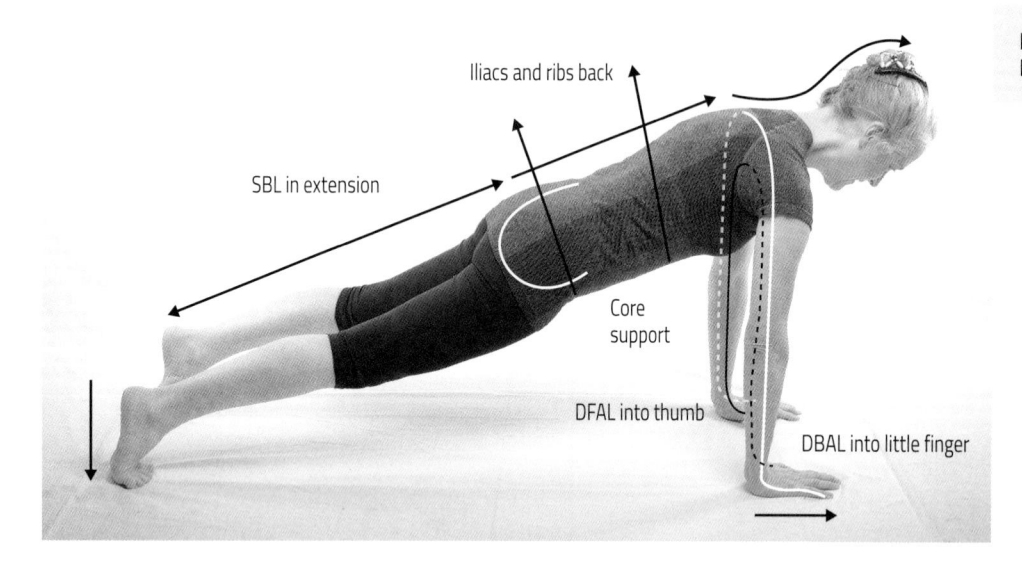

**Figure 14.6**
Plank position

*Labels on figure:* Iliacs and ribs back; SBL in extension; Core support; DFAL into thumb; DBAL into little finger

tone, so you can employ considerable muscular action from a place of quiet.

Can we now stand and move keeping this opposition of head and hips, and so let the whole-body move as a piece?

### Exploration 14.5 Returning to standing and walking with head leading and engaged hips

**Standing again**

- Draw yourself back into child's pose with active hip folding. You are still lengthening in opposition between head and hips and also widening throughout on every breath.
- Keeping this opposing balance of head tractioning forward and actively folding hips, let the head lead the spine to kneel up.
- Keep this opposition going as you bring one leg forward – does this bring stability to the movement? Tuck the back toes under and take yourself to standing.

**Walking**

- What happens now if you walk with head leading, but still have the alive opposition of the hips?

## Lesson 3 Primary control and directions revisited

### Exploration 14.6 Integrative directions

Should the primary control directions be thought one at a time, or all together? Alexander's answer was: "all together, one after another" – that they needed to be thought and acted upon concurrently (1985: 64). Let's explore this:

- Work through these directions, letting each action happen as you think it. Doing it this way, you may notice yourself feeling out or checking each part of the action.

  "let the neck be free,

  to let the head go forward and up,

  to let the back lengthen and widen back and up,

  to let the knees go forward and away."

- How did it go? Maybe you had a lovely sense of each part lengthening and floating away from the part below. Was the overall movement strong? Or was it like seaweed in the water, fluid but rather weak and ungrounded?

# Freeing the neck, and Alexander's primary directions

- *Now program these from mind in the brain, clearly thinking and understanding each in turn, while inhibiting any response. Then give yourself a 1-2-3 and action them all together in movement.*

What are you aware of this time? Is there more of a sense of the whole-body moving as one?

This was always my sense of how Miss Goldie moved me.

We have to STOP to formulate the integrative directions, allowing a moment of quiet (raising vagal tone), so that compression and extension forces are employed together in an integrating way. Marjory Barlow confirms this interpretation: "Keeping still and ordering is fine – you're laying down the pathway – but change is made through movement" (Barlow 2011: 119).

## Is there a primary control?

From reading Alexander's *Use of the Self* (1985), the primary control is often envisaged as some sort of master reflex, turning on innate patterns that take care of everything else. Certainly, a good lesson seems to give this experience; teachers talk of getting primary control working, from which everything then works. But is this what is really happening?

In Chapter 1, I observed that several different methods I encountered had their own models of primary control, all of which worked to give that unifying experience, and I asked how could they all be right? As we saw in Chapter 4, lesson 5, control is through neural networks. Modern neuroscience thinking is that there is no primary control system in charge, though there are self-organizing systems. This potentially means we can lead movement from many points: eyes or touch, pelvic floor, dan tien, even fingers – as any dancer or Tai Chi adept knows. I suspect that the nervous system can organize around the part leading, as long as the rest of the body follows in a dynamic flow, maintaining integration.

Tim Cacciatore (personal communication, February 7, 2020) told me of unpublished observations using the Twister (see Chapter 3, lesson 5). "Slowly rotating the hips causes changes in neck tone, and this seems to be a fairly robust and repeatable effect. If primary control is considered to be the influences on tone from the neck down, this would be similar but going in the opposite direction."

It would seem plausible that AT is switching on or biasing innate low-level patterns, some of which may be organizing deeper muscles of the spine to give spinal synergy. But such organization would likely be made up of a lot of different little patterns that join up, from multiple directions.

One of Marjorie Barstow's students described his second encounter with her work: "She spent about 30 seconds with me … The degree of coordination I experienced made me realize what superb athletes must feel like and where the impulse to move comes from: everywhere" (Ottiwell 2016: 2). (Barstow was on Alexander's first training course.)

## Summary of tools to "free the neck"

After *Use of the Self* was published, the Alexander world prioritized freeing the neck. But it is a trap to think of the head/neck balance in isolation. There are many roots to finding the freedom of the neck, and they all link to the whole spine and whole-body balance. Here are eleven different ways of freeing the neck.

A. Using innate brain pathways that engender whole-body balance and movement

- *The line.* The balance of the head on the neck follows the eyes. This utilizes visuo-motor pathways via the superior colliculus (exploration 4.2).
- *The vestibular system directions* (exploration 8.3). The vestibular organs are just above the atlanto-occipital joint. By thinking these lines outwards, we encourage expansion. Usually we think into the neck which causes us to contract around it.

# CHAPTER fourteen

- *Connect through the neck, not into it, with "liquid light"* (exploration 4.8). There are many neural relay stations level with the top of the neck – the hypothalamus, thalamus, and cerebellum. It is a pivotal point for alignment, and is also a fascial diaphragm. It is difficult to connect *with* our necks, and easier to connect *through* them. Don't get hooked up in the neck. If you do, think "let the neck be free," think it from spatial awareness.

- *Bringing the mind to the brain* – especially to the top of the brain – brings us out of over-involvement with the neck and allows it to free (exploration 4.7).

B. Mechanical means of freeing the neck

With these, Alexander's directions work in reverse: when the head goes forward and up, the neck will free.

- *The "raindrop"*. To find the balance of head on neck. The balance of the weight of the head will take it forward (exploration 3.8). This uses the superficial back line.

- *Thinking up through the crown* brings the head in stacking balance (exploration 3.11).

- *Head leading – lengthens the whole spine vertebra by vertebra, integrating the neck*. Use child's pose to all fours (exploration 14.3) to discover how the head leads the spine.

C. When you untangle the torso, the head will go forward and up, and the neck will free

- *By bringing the line sacrum to T8 vertical, and bringing the top of sternum forward from T8* (explorations 12.2 to 12.4). Only when the head is lengthening up from T8 does the ribcage hang down properly. Then the neck can be free.

- *Open the shoulders* (exploration 9.7). When the shoulder blades and clavicles open up by stretching the arm lines it allows space for the neck to sweep up out of the body and the head will balance on top.

D. Using natural breathing to open the deep front line and free the neck

- *Whispered Ah* (exploration 17.4). Voice is another connector of head and body through the neck. The sound links down the front of the spine to the coccyx, as we look out.

- Notice *when the in-breath gets caught in the throat* (exploration 6.8). Instead, bring it in through the sinuses and down the front of the spine (along the anterior longitudinal ligament) to the back of the lungs. You come into the deep front line.

### The full biomechanics behind Alexander's primary directions

Goldie told Fiona Robb that Alexander was always looking for simpler words (1999: 30) – and presumably simpler descriptions also. But was that wise? His discoveries opened a world of exploration that is complex, multifaceted, and still evolving. While the adept can see the simplicity behind this, the beginner must wrestle with the complexity first. If they are only given the simple answer, they will never get to this point of understanding for themselves. By coming to quiet, we help this along with right hemisphere/whole-body intelligence which can comprehend complexity.

The basic instructions of "let the neck be free to let the head go forward and up", etc., were written when Alexander had already been developing his technique for forty or so years. They can be seen as a goal by which the adept can organize the body. But for the novice, they are far too simplistic. There is much to be sorted before the back can work in one piece, or the knees move easily forward and away. And anyway, what do they actually refer to?

*Let the neck be free*: is specifically to open the atlanto-occipital and then axis joints. The other cervical vertebrae will then follow.

# Freeing the neck, and Alexander's primary directions

*To let the head go forward and up*: letting all the muscles lengthen at the back of the neck down to T8, rather than pulling back.

*To let the back lengthen*: the erector spinae of SBL need to lengthen down the full length of the spine to the coccyx. To allow this, the spinal curves need to open, becoming vertical (or nearer to vertical) between sacrum and T8, through realigning the parts of the torso: the pelvis, the lumbar region, ribcage, and upper torso.

*… and widen.* Every level of the torso widens: the pelvic floor, deep hip rotators, transverse and oblique belly muscles, all the ribcage, with the intercostals and the serratus posterior muscles, the latissimus dorsi, rhomboids, and trapezius. The serratus anterior muscles widen the shoulder blades.

Widening is dependent on lengthening, and vice versa. The floating ribs cannot widen unless the lumbar spine lengthens; the widening of the shoulder blades allows the thoracic and neck spines to lengthen.

*The back lengthens and widens back and up.* The psoas, quadratus lumborum, and erector spinae lengthen back and up along the lumbar spine, helped by iliac spines coming back and widening; the costal arch ribs and ribs at the back of the armpit come back and up to widen and lift the upper back.

*To let the knees go forward*: the thighs need to lengthen forward out of the hip joints, into which they are pulled when hip stability is poor. This opens the psoas and quads, and other muscles of the thighs can then lengthen. This then allows the lower legs also to lengthen and the heels and balls of the big toes to ground.

*… and away.* The counter-rotation of the thighs, brought about through the balance of the hip laterals, bringing stability from the lateral line.

You can also do the whole procedure the other way up, or start in the middle, with the base of the torso. When the feet and legs engage with the inner and outer, front, back, and spiral lines, truly supporting the body, they will send the torso up and wide, the head will lengthen forward and up and the neck will then free. Or, by engaging the core muscles of the torso, the legs and arms lengthen into action, and the head is free to lead with the senses.

# Part 3
## Living in a Flow of Dynamic Balance

15

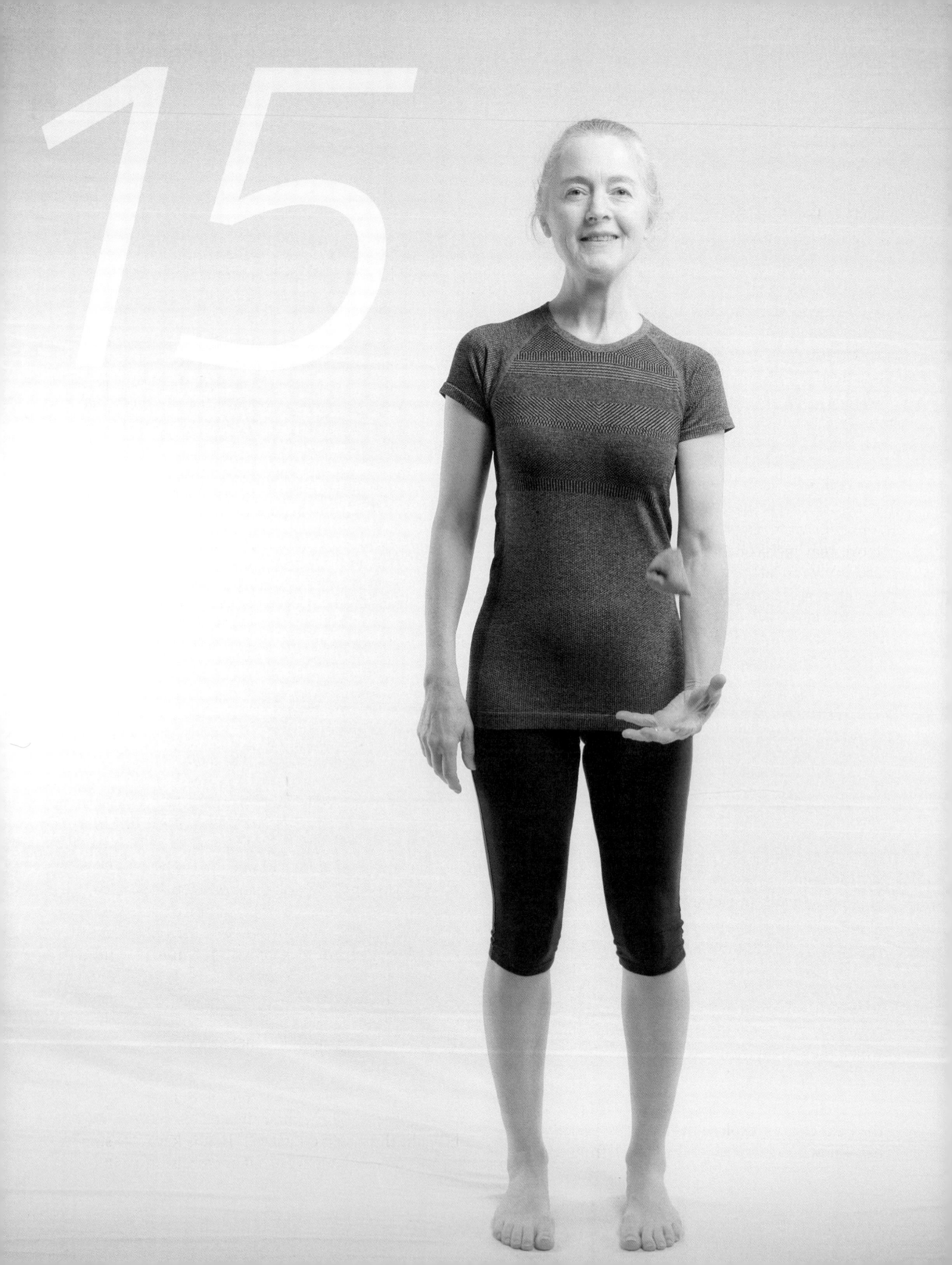

# Catching a ball – inhibition in action 15

## Introduction – discovering the core of Miss Goldie's work

When we first moved to Ireland, I watched our cat assessing whether he could jump from a 2 meter (6 ft 6) high stone structure in the garden to the rough cliff about 1.5 m (5 ft) behind it. He sat motionless, looking at the cliff, for at least five minutes, his eyes, I guessed, taking in all the information and relaying it to his brain and nervous system, which turned the information into a "program." Then he "gave consent" and the action – a beautiful leap – happened. He landed flawlessly on the rough, steep surface, then climbed up it to the field above. His brain and body intelligence had sorted the task out. I doubt he was consciously thinking: "If I get my front right paw just above that piece of moss, because it looks slippery, and my back left paw on that piece of slate, which should hold my weight …" Instead, his intelligence systems sorted all that, then organized the four limbs appropriately with different balances on the different rock, shale or plant surfaces.

Cats do that naturally, so can we?

Some months later I was on a beach watching a group of school kids jumping a shallow stream. An unfamiliar leap was needed, as it had been for the cat. There were the nervous kids, who stood on the stream edge, trying to work out where to put their feet. They dithered anxiously before they jumped and nearly all got their feet wet. Then there were the cocky ones who just ran and leapt without looking properly. They too mostly went in the water. But some were genuinely physically confident. As they ran towards the stream, I could sense them being aware of their movements, their eyes taking in all the information, and they cleared the stream neatly. Like the cat, they had allowed their intelligence systems to receive all the necessary information, then sort the task for them, which they could then execute flawlessly.

Although every chapter spring-boards, directly or indirectly, from my work with Miss Goldie, this and the next chapter explore the work for which she was best known – that of coming to quiet, from which one can move into the unknown and something new can come about. In Chapter 4, lesson 2, we distinguished between inhibition as an executive, cognitive *process*, and inhibition as a *state* we can inhabit, of quiet, tonic functioning, which enables the system to self-organize and modulate responsively. In this, I speculate that we side-step the learned habits of the left hemisphere, done out of conscious voluntary processes. This allows the right hemisphere to lead, allowing subconscious processes fuller access to our full sensory awareness and innate motor pathways, to transform movement and coordination, relationship and being. This is the work I have presented over the years in my "Goldie's Understanding" workshops, focused around mind in the brain, seeing out to the world in spatial awareness rather than being over-involved with the body, full embodiment, and coming to a true stop.

The true stop is a state of no preparation, which opens up a full range of possibilities. From this a fresh choice can be made, when we can step into the unknown and discover a whole new way of moving, whether for a new task like jumping an unfamiliar stream, or in a task we have done many times before. In the next chapter we will put these together and explore the science of movement using all twelve fundamentals.

It is all down to how we react. Life is full of stimuli, and we react to each one. The milk spills over, three urgent emails all come in together, a friend needs help … Mostly we respond in an imbalanced way because we feel an urgency of some sort, consciously or unconsciously. Perhaps to get it right, or prove ourselves, or to get it done and move on. These underlying drivers of our behavior are so habitual they mostly continue, perhaps unnoticed, even when we feel calm and there need be no urgency. We react poorly because our nervous systems are continually charged by these subconscious driving emotional urges.

To change the way we react, we need to calm the nervous system, we need to "come to quiet," as Goldie would tell me again and again. "Come to quiet and the right thing will do itself." "That is key – to 'stop' and be quiet. But not to opt out or collapse or go into a

# CHAPTER fifteen

trance or go to sleep. No – to 'stop', so that everything is alive. The brain is waiting and listening out for the new direction …" (Robb 1999: 39) This is truly a conscious process.

From this quiet place there is true choice of action. "The readiness is all" – a Shakespeare quote Alexander often used. Frank Pierce Jones, the first teacher trained by Alexander in the USA and great friend of Goldie, expressed this beautifully: "The Alexander technique opens a window onto the little-known area between stimulus and response and gives you the self-knowledge you need in order to change the pattern of your response – or, if you choose, not to make it at all" (Jones 2016: 4).

### Inhibition in action

"Mainstream" Alexander technique, the way most of us first learned the technique, usually has direction as the primary driver, often used in a piecemeal way. You free your neck, send your back up and your shoulders wide, you send your heels down, remember to breathe, etc.

Miss Goldie worked to organize the whole-body in one self-integrating hit. We have been exploring the physical aspect of this with Initial Alexander technique, sending a stream of directions to the brain, and inhibiting our response until we allow it all to happen together. She considered that most people were using directions from feeling, over-involving in the body. We have been using mind in the brain and spatial awareness to avoid this.

But here we are exploring a simpler way of discovering new use, which is to inhibit any urge to action, and to wait, and then to let movement happen. This uses tonic inhibition as the driver. We used this in finding our natural breathing: if we stop at the bottom of the out-breath and wait, the next in-breath will do itself. Then the self-organizing mechanisms of the whole-body intelligence come into play to recruit the appropriate muscles: the diaphragm drives the action and other muscles of the torso dynamically balance the body around it.

When we apply this process to voluntary action, it turns the "mainstream" AT process on its head. "If you're quiet, and really 'stop' – as none of us ever do – then you are doing nothing. In particular, you're not-doing the wrong thing, so that the right thing does itself. So the head-neck-back is secondary – it comes out of the 'stopping'" (Robb 1999: 53). Goldie's lessons worked slowly over months and years, to bring one to the quiet place where one could bring this about for oneself. Here we will play a powerful game that brings this about remarkably quickly.

### We need to break the stimulus–response chain

A stimulus produces a response. Take a ball and pretend to throw it to someone, but do not actually throw it. Chances are, he (or she) will pull up both their hands to catch, with quite a fast, exaggerated movement. When they realize they have been tricked, they will laugh, or get cross or puzzled with you. Do it again, and this time watch what else happens in their body. You might see the hands respond less this time, as they clue in to what you are doing, but that a chain of other things is still happening: their head tightens back on the neck, eyes widen, the shoulders might lift, they stop breathing for a moment, the legs and feet may stiffen. In other words, we are seeing a whole-body response (one could call it a surprised, defensive response).

In this moment of whole-body change, the thought to keep the neck free is too little, too late, as everything has changed so fast in one go. To continually put it all back through executive inhibition and directions to each individual part of the body, or even just to release the neck and let the primary control take care of the rest, is clearly not the answer. Doing that is shutting the stable door after the horse has bolted. We are trying to keep our necks free in everyday life, and yet life is full of stimuli that pull us continually out of shape. The answer is not to respond in the first place. But how?

Scientists tell us that the response to a stimulus is almost immediate. Within a fraction of a second

# Catching a ball – inhibition in action

of perceiving a stimulus, the brain starts to fire out instructions to alter every muscle in the body to the "set" required in that situation. Every learned movement has pre-formed default settings – our automated patterns for writing, answering a phone, catching a ball, etc. Even thinking about these activities begins to engage them.

If we are truly to keep our bodies and spatial awareness expanded in any situation, we have to break the stimulus-response chain, and be able to do this reliably and fast. This requires us to discover a deeper place of quiet, which can then deepen our work on ourselves and with others.

## Catching a ball in seven stages

### Exploration 15.1  Throwing a ball from hand to hand

This is a fantastic tool to access calm and coordination when needed. I suggest using this before each day's teaching or therapy work, or musicians to use it before practicing, as it brings the hand into an alive relationship with the body.

Video link for exploration 15.1

**Stage 1:** observation

- Throw the ball from hand to hand as you would normally, and observe yourself, on video or in a mirror. Are your hands held in front of you, does this take tension?
- Does a shoulder lift as you throw? Does the throwing hand jerk the movement?
- Does the catching hand come up to catch?
- Does it stay up afterwards?
- Does the catching hand easily close around the ball, or does it snatch, or is it sluggish so the ball drops out of the hand?
- Do you pull your neck back/stop breathing/tense in the legs, etc.?

**Stage 2:** come to quiet, breaking the stimulus response chain

- Let the hand holding the ball rest by your side, with the palm rotated normally backwards. Think through the task from mind in the brain: I know where my hand with the ball is, and where the other hand is. I track the intended trajectory from one hand, past my nose, to the other hand.
- We do not need to prepare the hand to throw. When you are quiet, give consent, and let the hand throw the ball in an arc to the other one. Let your spatial awareness and whole-body intelligence sort the throw – what joints to use, how much force is needed.
- This is too complex for us to work out, so stay out of the way and let it happen spontaneously. Your brain may take several goes before it sorts the problem you have set it.
- See the ball as it goes past. (If you don't, then throw higher, or lower.) Do not catch but allow the ball to drop the floor.
- If the ball hits you, allow that to be okay.
- Keep coming fully to quiet between throws.
- Let the hand return to hanging fully by the side, the ball just resting in the hand, the palm facing back. It is useful to use a mirror to check that you have fully returned to quiet between throws. Most people resist!
- Give the hands equal turns. Do not be afraid that your non-dominant hand cannot do it! It sometimes has less "baggage" and so can sort the task more easily.

**Stage 3:** making decisions

- You may have throws that are perfectly landing by your other foot. But if some of your throws go wild you have an opportunity to practice decisions: "could I catch that easily or not?" Simple decisions, yes or no. There is no "maybe." (If your decision turns out to be wrong, you have had a learning experience.)

## CHAPTER fifteen

**Stage 4:** allowing the catch to happen

- *The first decision was: Can I catch it? The second is: Will I catch it?*
- *Give your hand permission to catch, but still to let most balls fall. Keep coming to quiet between each throw, do not attempt to catch till the urge to do so is gone.*
- *Only give permission to catch throws that land right next to the hand. You are watching for a catch that "does itself." You may even feel surprised to find the ball in your hand!*
- *Allow that your brain may take many attempts to "sort out" this task. Trust that if you keep coming to quiet, coming back to first principles, then your whole-body intelligence can organize this task with incredible efficiency.*
- *After each catch attempt, say no to catching the next ball, and return to quiet. Do not build a new habit, but keep coming back to the quiet unknown (Fig. 15.1).*

**Stage 5:** does the catching hand come up to meet the ball?

- *The catching hand does not need to reach up. The hand will turn as the ball arrives, and the ball will fall into it. It can take a lot of trust to allow this (Fig. 5.1).*
- *Play with "gluing" your elbow to your side so the hand can turn but not lift.*

**Stage 6:** the next ball

- *Once mastered, give yourself more challenging throws, e.g., out to the side or slightly behind you. Trust your intelligence systems to work out where to place the hand to catch; all you need do is stay out of the way.*
- *Remember to stop fully, to come to quiet, between each go, and come back to first principles. From time to time let the ball drop.*

> Goldie instructed me always to work from first principles, i.e., the instructions needed by the brain to bring about a new use. This is the same as the Zen phrase "beginner's mind." Here, the instructions would be come back to quiet, know the trajectory, give consent to throw without preparation.

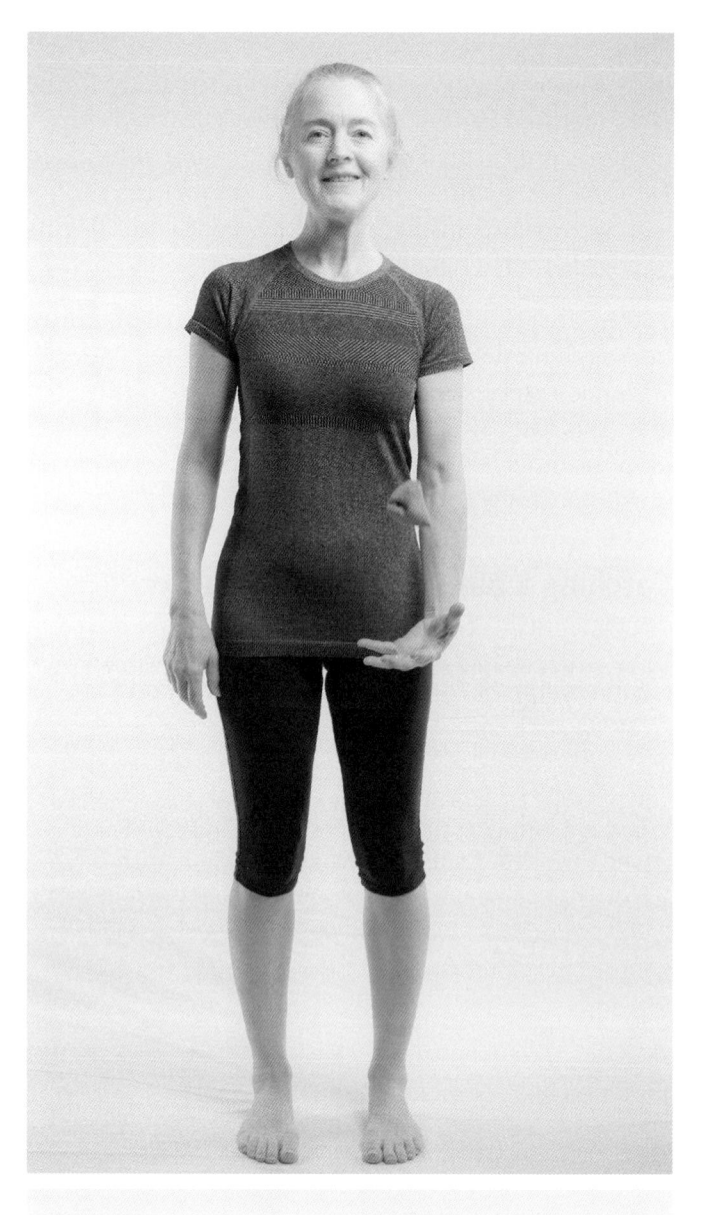

**Figure 15.1**
Trusting the quiet catch

Problems catching:

- *If your hand is unable to catch, then use exploration 15.3 below for yourself. Do both hands.*

**Breath-holding patterns when throwing and catching**

- *Throw the ball from hand to hand and notice your breath – does it stop as you throw?*

# Catching a ball – inhibition in action

- *If so, do you stop at the end of the in-breath, or out-breath? Or somewhere in-between?*
- *Do you always throw on the same point of the breath?*
- *Having observed this, find your natural breathing. Then choose an unfamiliar part of the breath to throw, such as halfway through the in- or out-breath, and choose to keep breathing! This may feel very strange!*
- *Play around with throwing on different parts of the breath cycle until it no longer matters where you throw or catch, your breath carries on regardless.*
- *You can then observe whether you breath-hold on other tasks – opening a door, turning a tap, even climbing stairs, etc. – and work to break the patterns.*

### Exploration 15.2    Ball catching with a pupil or partner – modeling our responses to life

Find a family member, friend or long-standing pupil for this. Children love this game. If you do not have a partner available right now, then read through this anyway for the commentary. If you can, arrange to play it with someone soon though, as the process can be clearer when we are not both thrower and catcher.

Use soft balls or beanbags. Rolled socks also work! If you have quite a few balls, you will get more of a flow and with less picking up.

For maximum effect, don't let your partner read this first, so you take them by surprise!

**Stage 1:** observing the catcher's reaction

- *Stand opposite your partner, 2–3 m (6–10 feet) away. You will be thrower and your partner will be catcher. Come to quiet yourself.*
- *Tell them you will throw the ball for them to catch, but only pretend strongly to do so – you are providing a stimulus.*
- *Observe and discuss the reactions to this stimulus throughout their body. Keep giving pretend throws until you have identified all their reactions.*

Ball catching has been a big deal for most of us, and that makes it a very strong stimulus. In school games, a duff catch was often shameful, and these memories run deep. But this game is not just about catching a ball. Life is full of stimuli, of "balls" that should be caught: a spilt drink that must be quickly wiped, a phone ringing, traffic lights changing to green. When we are too busy we may comment that we are trying to keep a lot of balls in the air, and our lives often can feel like a juggling act of work, chores, kids, etc.

**Stage 2:** come to quiet, breaking the stimulus–response chain

- *Explain to them now that you are not going to throw, it is purely a visual stimulus. Continue to pretend to throw – gently now – until all response, not just the visible response, has stopped.*
- *Be inventive to help them stop responding. Help to break the visual stimulus by turning back to back as you continue your pretend throw – their reaction will stop – then turn back slowly to face each other again, inviting your partner to maintain the non-reaction.*
- *Invite them to think of the space between you as large, and to stay grounded and breathing. Ask them to go between over-focusing on the pretend throw, and seeing it as part of the bigger picture, with depth perception and peripheral vision.*

When we come to quiet, we shift gear. It can feel very different. Things begin to relax. What seemed so urgent no longer looks so necessary. The shift from reactive to quiet is the shift from sympathetic to parasympathetic, from flight/fight survival mode, to peaceful calm.

**Stage 3:** not catching the ball

- *Tell them you will throw but they are not to catch, they are just to witness the balls going past and dropping. Do this until they drop any urgency to respond and are comfortable to let the balls go.*

We need to know that when life throws balls at us, we can safely let them drop. It is not all down to us. I do not have to prove myself. Someone else can catch them just now.

# CHAPTER fifteen

**Stage 4:** letting yourself be hit by the ball

- *Ask them if they are willing to be hit by the ball (NB: use soft balls and take care!) Keep quiet yourself throughout, or your unquiet will stimulate your partner. The first throws will often cause reaction, so invite them to keep grounded and breathing and to keep seeing the space between you.*

- *If they find this one difficult (some people don't admit this so use your intuition), ask them to watch the ball's trajectory right to the point of impact on them. This usually allows it to become a neutral experience. Continue till they can allow this without making any response.*

**Stage 5:** making decisions – can I catch it?

- *Now throw unpredictably, some going right to them and some falling short or wide, etc.*

- *Ask them to say out loud whether they would be able to catch each throw easily or not, as they continue to let the ball fall. To simply say yes or no, with no complicated thinking, no maybes. (If their decision turns out to be wrong, they have had a learning experience.) This practices pure decision-making, simple yes or no. It decouples "can I" from "will I."*

- *The decision cannot to be taken till the ball has left your hand – which can feel too quick, so invite them to see the space between you which will expand their experience of time. Keep quiet yourself, give them space!*

The deeper your embodiment, the more you will be in whole-body intelligence, with fully expanded spatial awareness. For the right hemisphere, time is an endlessly unfolding moment.

**Stage 6:** allowing the catch to happen – will I catch it?

- *The first decision was: Can I catch it? The second is: Will I catch it?*

- *Give your partner permission to catch but instruct them still to let most balls fall. Ask them not to attempt a catch until they have no urgency to do so. The very act of giving permission will probably reawaken the urgency.*

- *Keep coming to quiet between each throw, inviting spatial awareness and embodiment, and watch that they do likewise. There is no preparation needed on either side. Everybody can catch if they come to sufficient quiet for spatial awareness and whole-body intelligence to organize the body for them. Take your time and watch for the moment when a catch "does itself," there is no effort of any sort involved. Allow that your partner's brain may take many attempts to "sort out" this task for itself.*

Quiet is not asleep. Quiet is completely conscious, completely present. Then when a simple decision is made to catch, the hand and arm respond so economically. In that moment we are not mentally aware of our movement; it seems to happen of its own volition. We can feel surprised that the ball is now in the hand. Compared to the initial, over-stimulated and protective movement in response to the first pretend throw, this movement could not be more different. It is so beautiful it can make one laugh.

You may have walked past a shelf at some time, knocked something off, and caught it before you were even conscious that you had knocked it off. You almost wonder how it came to be in your hand.

**Stage 7:** the next ball

- *After saying "yes" to catch, whether it is successful or not, always say "no" to the next ball to return to quiet. This is needed because once nerves are firing, they have feedback loops that re-stimulate the initial neurons to keep firing. After catching one ball, you will want to catch the next and the next, regardless of how it is done. Every throw and catch is different, and needs the same quiet attention and awareness. Be aware that the brain will attempt to shift us into "I know how to do this now, just get on with it" mode, which makes assumptions and is less awake. Instead, stay awake, quiet, in an encounter with the unknown.*

Problems catching

If the catcher's hand looks floppy/asleep and just misses every ball, or touches but does not grasp well, then use exploration 15.3 below.

**Stage 8:** throwing accurate, quiet, non-stimulating throws

# Catching a ball – inhibition in action

- *Make no preparation but stand with spatial awareness and embodied consciousness, and look at where the catcher's hand is. Keep breathing. While maintaining this quiet presence, give consent and allow the throw to happen. This gives quiet non-stimulating throws. (This is now very different from the deliberately over-stimulating show of throwing in stage 1.) After a catch, invite the catcher to do the same process to return the ball.*

Swap roles and have a go yourself!

For full tuition videos for this valuable game, see the inside front cover. These include bonus videos on how to proceed to two and then three balls for those who want a further challenge!

## Fully responsive action for optimal coordination

We have just discovered that when we come to quiet, we can respond to what is happening in the moment without expectation, and the result is ease of movement and precise coordination. How does this occur? I call this "fully responsive action" – that we are responding anew in the moment. However, current science is more interested in how we use predictive mechanisms.

For instance, when subjects must hit a moving screen image, they used the speed information from the previous attempt to plan the next move (de Lussanet et al. 2001). I think anyone who has played goalie and been wrong-footed knows this one – the brain extrapolates from what just happened to predict what happens next. The researchers concluded that we do this because there is limited time to process the sensory information and plan the interception. Instead of waiting until all the information is in and integrating it for a perfect outcome – which could take longer than the time available – the brain selects which information to prioritize and runs with that, accepting a margin of error in the interest of getting the job done (Brenner and Smeets 2001).

> There are puzzles in the optical system. Incoming visual information from the retina travels along the optic pathway to the primary visual cortex. The information is then deconstructed to extract information: such as edge-detection to understand spatial organization, distinguishing of depth and foreground, direction and speed of objects, motion of objects relative to the background, self-motion, and simple shape recognition. This is then processed in many different centers. It is as yet a total mystery how the cortex then puts it all back together.

So what is so different about what we just did? I suggest that in the state of quiet tonic inhibition we are using different brain and visual pathways that allow more integrated processing to happen and give very different outcomes. To me, this is what top sports people are doing, and it would be worthy of research.

### Coordination for catching a ball and the two visual streams theory

We think of the purpose of vision as giving us a unified, detailed perception of the external world. As a result, precise focus is the only function tested by the standard eye tests, and most vision research has been perception-based with no thought of the behavior it might serve. But vision evolved to locate us in our environment, to avoid obstacles or predators, and to catch prey. Frogs have no cortex – all sensory data is processed in the base of their brains. Their primitive vision sees only moving dots, which triggers their targeted tongue reflex (Milner and Goodale 1995: 5). Every mouthful must be a surprise! Our ability consciously to see and name a detailed, colorful world evolved relatively recently.

Vision is of no use unless it relates us to where we are in space, and *in relationship* to objects around us with eye–head–body orientation. Just as there are two competing needs of brain function requiring two separate hemispheres, it turns out there are two distinct

# CHAPTER fifteen

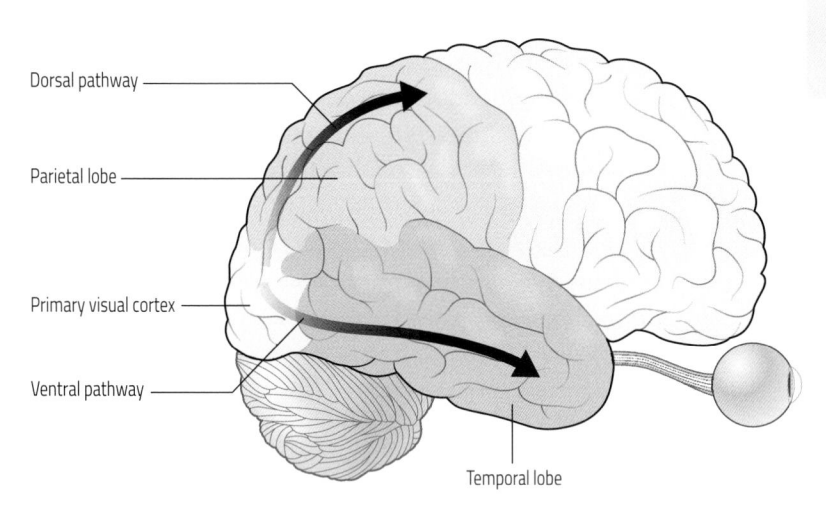

**Figure 15.2**
The two visual streams, for perception (ventral) and movement (dorsal)

requirements for vision, which likewise require two distinct visual systems (Goodale and Milner 2006) (Fig. 15.2). One requirement is for accurate vision to identify objects, known as the perception or "what" stream. We are conscious of what we see. The other is vision for movement, or action – the "where" and "how" stream, and amazingly, this operates at unconscious levels. In the ball game, by coming to quiet, I speculate that we are facilitating the dorsal pathway to operate optimally.

The ventral "perception" visual stream connects to the temporal lobes (through which we access long-term memories) for recognition of complex shapes, objects, and faces. Like the left hemisphere, this stream is self-referencing, working from memory and known facts, in past and future. It allows us to form or interpret images, enabling us to watch a film as the frames of reference are entirely within the screen – the mountains, houses, and people on-screen relate to each other but bear no relationship to your physical reality; and you cannot make an action that links to it. It enables us to envisage a plan of action "offline." And like the left hemisphere, this visual stream has no direct link to the body, to movement and coordination.

The dorsal "action" stream connects to the parietal lobes, where our spatial maps of the body are held, and where skilled movement is organized. This stream is head-centered (called egocentric referencing): it calculates the coordinates of objects relative to the viewer's own eyes. To move, one must always know "here" and "there" and the distance between; action must be in relationship of self to object. So this stream works with real metrics of space and time in the present, as it guides the programming and unfolding of our actions moment by moment. However, the action stream, like much of the experiential right hemisphere, operates subconsciously. So when you knock something off a shelf and have caught it before your consciousness has processed that you have knocked it off, it is this "instinctive" dorsal subconscious process that perfectly coordinates a link between a moving object and the hand to grasp it. If we think too hard about coordinating an action – its where and how – we cannot do it. We have to let it happen (Table 15.1).

The standard literature does not deal with meditative/mindful states. When we look at a flower, and come present to it without naming it, seeing it as it is, I think we are in right hemisphere-led experiential consciousness, in which the flower is known yet unknown. All aspects of the visual experience are present: full color, texture, three-dimensional, in relationship to ourselves; any touch would be appropriately gentle yet accurate. Which visual stream is operating now?

# Catching a ball – inhibition in action

My guess is that we are now using both together in a fully integrated way. In contrast, I wonder if our two visual streams are operating more separately when we are bumbling along on autopilot with our thoughts elsewhere. As when you realize while driving that you haven't been present for the last ten miles. How did we do it? It seems the dorsal stream and our automated movement habits can operate nicely without us as we drift in our thoughts – until the unexpected happens and we come back to the present.

The pathways interplay to give us whole vision. For instance: you see an apple on the table. Your ventral stream identifies the apple, remembers they are good to eat. Meanwhile, the dorsal stream has updated the visual map of the scene in the parietal lobes, linked it to knowledge of where you are in space and the current configuration of your body and hand, and links directly to the movement centers for accurate reach, rotation of the wrist, and pre-configured hand posture to grasp successfully. It is a weird thought that when we touch something, we are not seeing it with the same part of the brain as we use to touch it.

One experiment that demonstrates this is the hollow mask illusion, in which we see a convex face, despite the reality being concave. This is because the ventral stream which recognizes objects knows from past experience that faces are convex and reconfigures the image we see. *This is "top-down" processing – it uses past experience to compute reality.* But if you ask the viewer to flick a bug off the nose of the mask, their hand will go unerringly – though unconsciously – to the bug, as the dorsal stream organizes the hand unconsciously and correctly to reach the real distance inside the mask to flick the bug (Kroliczak et al. 2006). *The dorsal stream is not taken in by the illusion, because it works "bottom-up" – i.e., it takes the actual incoming sensory information of depth and contour and uses it in real time.*

Current research is focusing on how these work together. For instance, the ventral stream allows us to look away as we reach for a cup and yet continue the action – we are using the visual memory to continue. The dorsal stream has no visual memory. So, for the dorsal stream to improve performance through experience requires the memory of the ventral stream. "Most of our visually guided actions are as skilled as they are precisely because of their being well-honed by practice. It seems likely that as our initially slow and painstaking efforts become more automatic, the contribution of the ventral stream retreats and is replaced by more streamlined circuitry involving the dorsal stream, related frontal cortical areas, and subcortical structures in the brainstem and cerebellum (Goodale and Milner 2006). But I wonder if we are over-involving the ventral stream in this. By coming to quiet with spatiotemporal awareness, we are allowing the self-organizing systems to sort the learning

| Table 15.1 The two visual streams | |
|---|---|
| Dorsal "action" stream | Ventral "perception" stream |
| Unconscious vision for movement | Conscious perception of objects |
| Connects to parietal lobes | Connects to temporal lobes |
| Fast processing | Slow processing |
| On-line processing – sees in real time | Off-line processing, works from memory |
| Real metrics – distance is always measured between eyes and objects | Scene-based reference frames (such as on TV!), unconnected to metrics of observer |
| Sees in 3D | Sees in 2D |
| Sees in present | Sees in future and past, links to memory |
| Takes information from the whole retina | Takes information from the central retina only (the fovea, that detects detail) |

# CHAPTER fifteen

for us with much greater efficiency, and stepping out of using "our initially slow and painstaking efforts." More on this in Chapter 16, lesson 3.

I hope you had a new experience with the ball games, of letting an action simply happen. If so, when you caught the ball, did you surprise yourself? I often see people laugh with wonder that they have a ball in their hand. When action just happens, we often do not process it consciously till afterward.

## Discussion points

### A true stop versus a pause

Perhaps you remember playing music on a cassette tape recorder. When we pressed the pause button, the music stopped. But only one thing could happen when we released the pause button: the same music started again from the same place. However, if we pressed the stop button, there were many more possibilities. We could press play again, rewind or fast forward, take that tape out and put in another, or go off to do something completely different. From a true stop, in quiet tonic inhibition, the possibilities are completely open. We can catch or not, even look at the ball thrower or not, and to respond to the ball wherever it is thrown because we have not prejudged the situation.

The deeper we are embodied, more present to the right hemisphere with its sense of spatial awareness and temporal flow, the more our experience of time and space expands. Then the "stop" becomes a moment of standing back, observing from a neutral space.

### When catches do not happen – there is no such thing as failure

If the catches are not successful it does not matter. What matters is the way we set the process in motion. Initially when we do not catch, we will probably laugh, grimace, or apologize. Invite your partner to do none of these and stay neutral yourself. This can be quite hard to do, for both parties. Catches are not right or wrong, they are all simply part of the brain learning process, as new connections are made.

We are programmed so early for success and failure.

> It was Christmas evening. Our daughter Amelia was four months old, lying on the floor and continually attempting to roll over. The whole family was sat around her, only half-watching her attempts.
>
> Halfway through the evening she succeeded, and everybody woke up to her and clapped, exclaiming: "Well done! Now have another go! See if you can roll back again." All eyes were on her, her every move was commented on. "Oh, never mind, try again." "Well done, you've rolled back again!" I was appalled. This small baby was doing something for herself for the first time ever, and there were six adults all teaching her success and failure.
>
> But on Amelia's baby face there was no sign of "success" or "failure." If an attempt did not work, she simply had another go. If it did work, she moved onto the next stage. It was not until nine months old that I saw her first "failure" grimace, when I saw her pull herself up on the bars of her cot, not succeed and fall down again. No wonder firstborns, particularly the firstborn of the next generation as she is, tend to be high achievers, very anxious about success and failure. Everyone knows that child number two will crawl, will walk, will feed himself, and it is not the big deal that it seems for the first child.

### When someone cannot catch – keeping the hands and eyes alive

#### Exploration 15.3   Limp and uncoordinated hands

Sometimes, after going through all the steps above, the catcher's hand just does not coordinate. It seems limp, does not move with any conviction. Or goes to the wrong place or does not close around the ball so the ball

# Catching a ball – inhibition in action

bounces out. Hands go sleepy or "switched off" like this when there is little or no embodied linkage between brain and hand. Use this with your catching partner, or even with yourself.

- *Touch the crown of their head lightly with your left hand, ask them to be aware of where their crown is, and that their mind is in the brain.*
- *With your right hand trace a line down the head to the neck base, asking them to be aware of the connection and the distance between the two hands, by saying something like "and your neck base is all the way down here."*
- *Leave your right hand where it is, and with your left hand trace out to the tip of their shoulder. Again, ask them to be aware of the connection and the distance between the two hands, by saying "and your shoulder is all the way out to the side here."*
- *Continue down in the same way, physically tracing and verbally naming, down to the elbow, down to the wrist, the knuckles, the fingertips.*
- *Now ask them whether their two hands feel different. They will probably find the traced one feels more present, more alive. So do the other one too.*
- *Now try the catches again, in the same non-doing way, always keeping calm and quiet yourself.*

## Do we need to watch the ball?

Jugglers do not watch the ball – there are too many balls to watch, and they are engaging with their audience. We do not need to see our hands to catch, *but we do need to keep seeing*. If the eyes glaze then we will stop catching. While some people need to watch the ball's trajectory for a while, ideally, we move beyond this stage. Once connections to catch are made, we only need a peripheral glimpse of the ball's trajectory for the hand to find the ball.

## The intelligence networks take time to sort the task out

Sometimes a person cannot make the new connections on the first session. If so, do it again the next day, or on a subsequent occasion; it will probably work then.

Goldie would say: "You are sending the messages from your brain, but they are not getting through yet."

## "Quiet" and "limp" are not the same thing

There is a real confusion for many people between a state of quiet and a limp state. Real quiet – tonic inhibition – is coordinated and ready to go. Think of a cat lying in the sunshine, completely relaxed, eyes closed, just being. But if a dog comes near, the cat is immediately up and taking appropriate action. Compare a dog lying in the sun, waiting for somebody to throw the ball, waiting for something to happen. Being or waiting, both cat and dog are fully alive in the process.

Now compare a person sitting on their sofa waiting impatiently for a pizza delivery. At the slightest noise he is on his feet, halfway to the door, then realizing it was a false alarm. Eventually he gives up, lies back in a doze. When the doorbell finally rings, he is taken off-guard. Many comedy sketches have used this to great effect. Most humans live between overstimulated and this dozy switched-off place. Miss Goldie would say: "There is no switching off!" The modern word is "mindful."

## Find the challenge just beyond your current level of competence

For those for whom this presents no unfamiliar challenge, please move to more advanced games. I suggest you play with applying the same principles to juggling with more balls, alone or with a partner (see the inside front cover). For myself, the current challenge is juggling four balls: when I come quiet and alive throughout, suddenly I can bring about this seemingly impossible task!

### Exploration 15.4  Watching your response to household/daily tasks

- *Notice your reactivity around daily tasks. If you, say, take a load of washing from the bedroom to the washing machine, do you get there in one? Or do you have to stop to pick up a stray sock on the stairs, or get caught into clearing the kitchen, etc.?*

I have heard people say that by the end of the morning everything else is done but the washing still is not in the washing machine! This builds huge frustration in our systems.

- *Having noticed your patterns, see if you can make some clearer choices. Tell the sock and the kitchen they will need to wait their turn. Or else make a deliberate choice to stop and action them, before carrying on with the washing.*

When you only action a task for which your whole being is on-board, it removes a huge stress-burden from the nervous system.

### What have we achieved?

- *By breaking the stimulus–response chain, we are no longer reacting to a stimulus.*
- *We are quiet but fully alive, with the full possibilities of choice to act or not.*
- *When we then give consent to act, the whole-body intelligence can sort out the task in a new way.* This then brings in a hand–eye coordination that is beyond anything we can achieve by trying. "If you 'stop', then it can have a chance to sort itself out" (Miss Goldie, in Robb 1999: 118).
- *We are moving into the unknown, allowing an unfamiliar way of doing an action to come about.*

This is the process of making discoveries. "Each time it is a discovery – you're not trying to 'do' anything or reproduce an experience you've had. You don't know what it is for your knees to go forward – you're discovering it anew each time" (Miss Goldie in Robb 1999: 145).

*To reframe these steps in scientific terms*: I speculate that we have inhibited our current maladapted automated habits, to come to the state of tonic inhibition, in which we have responsive muscle tone, but no feed forward anticipatory movements.

We are then in a right hemisphere-led experiential state, spatially aware, and in the temporal flow, where we can allow new information to generate new pathways of self-organizing action, in which cortex and hindbrain are in networking balance.

We have re-established the dominance of the parasympathetic, the self-engagement system, and come out of stress responses.

This new way is responsive to the present, rather than predictive and based on past experience.

The action is not organized around the head-neck-back but around our intention.

"Come to quiet" was Miss Goldie's refrain, the key principle underlying everything. After I had come to an understanding of all this, Miss Goldie unexpectedly told me that learning the technique was like progressing through the alphabet: A to B to C ... Then she declared I had now reached letter A!

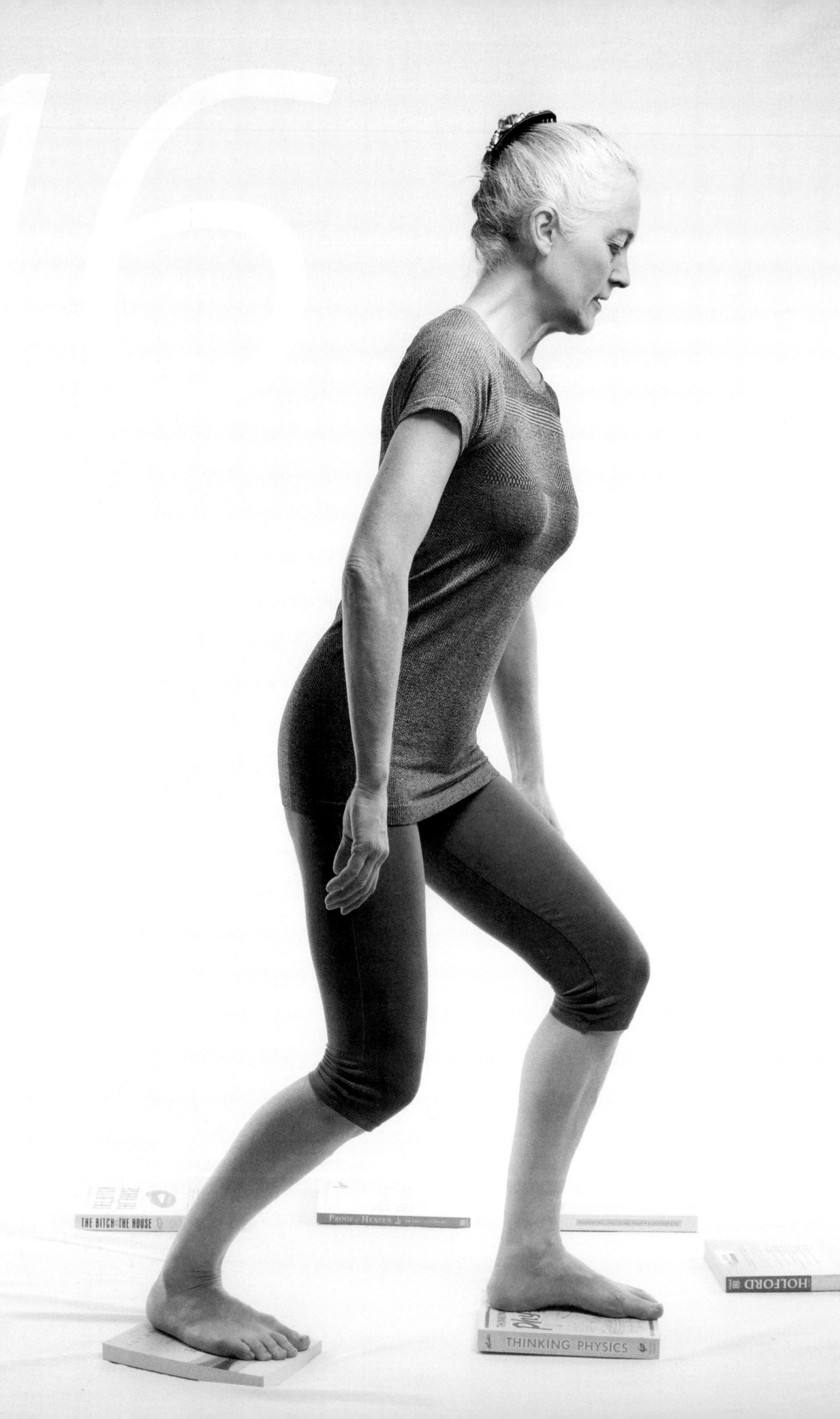

16

# New models of coordination and learning  16

In Chapter 15, we explored how bring about unconscious optimal coordination in catching a ball, and how we can bring conscious awareness to the process without interfering in it. Now we will explore this for three major aspects of coordination: locomotion, the daily task of our legs; reaching, grasping, and other daily tasks of our arms; and learning and coordinating complex tasks such as for instruments or dance moves.

## Lesson 1    Coordinating locomotion by using the whole-body intelligence network

I first started asking how we make unconscious coordinating decisions in 1990 when walking Rufus, our hairy, big-footed bearded collie. Beardies have hair falling over their eyes; we felt Rufus often navigated by smell. The park had no poo bins, so for the first 100 m (110 yards) or so I would be dodging dollops of excrement every few steps. Walking behind him, I'd be fearfully anticipating his big hairy feet splodging into one. Then, I realized that he never stepped in any dog mess, ever. That's what humans do. Neither was he dodging round them, but just plodded along in a steady rhythm.

How did he do it? I pictured that his eyes and nose detected the location of each dollop, passing the information to his brain, like a radar passes information to a ship's computer about rocks in a bay. Then just as the computer calculates the simplest line to take and coordinates the steering accordingly, so the dog's brain must create an internal map of his environment, calculate the simplest course for all four feet, and organize the muscles accordingly. This process has to be continually responsive, very different from the old model of preformed reflex responses.

> **Where do stretch receptors fit?**
>
> Stretch receptors were once thought to be the sole organizers of movement through generating reflexes. Now they are understood to be just one of many sensory inputs in the equation of movement outcomes (Prochazka and Ellaway 2012). New models of movement are being developed to understand how central pattern generators (CPGs) interface with reflexes and kinematics. Prochazka and Yakovenko (2007) coined the term "neuromechanical tuning" to describe the matching of the CPGs to the kinematics of the movement. The spinal cord self-generates the rhythm, leaving the rest of the nervous system free to send in sensory input – including those of stretch receptors – to help time the duration of swing and stance phases as we navigate around obstacles or over uneven surfaces.

### Solving the movement challenge

The brain does not send instructions to the body like water down a pipe. The spinal cord has interneurons interconnecting both within and between spinal segments, bringing inputs together from many places. These give the spinal cord its own integrity and organization. Brain and spinal cord microcircuits work together cooperatively to solve the movement challenge of the moment (Turvey et al. 1982).

Many components work together to solve the movement challenge.

### CPGs, brainstem maps, and predictive mechanisms for fast responses

The nervous system creates accurate internal representations (maps) against which it can understand subsequent information. We know that central pattern generators (CPGs) generate innate rhythmic patterns in the spinal cord and brainstem for breathing, walking, and bouncing (Chapter 6). But to be useful, they need to be appropriate to the activity of the moment. Proprioceptive information streams constantly to the brainstem from stretch receptors and mechanoreceptors in the muscles, joints, and fascia, along with information from ligaments and skin, especially soles of the feet or other contact points.

# CHAPTER sixteen

From the proprioceptive information, the brainstem creates maps of the spatial orientation of the limbs relative to the body. These allow the organization of local body and limb movements in a directed and coordinated way. These maps are updated moment by moment, so that information about limb position is instantly available at the moment of a stimulus: CPGs are always ready to operate – they are predictive as reflexes are not. (In the reflex model: after a stimulus, feedback information would need to be processed before action could be taken (Rosenbaum et al. 2007). This would create a time delay, unacceptable to the best tennis or baseball players!)

While plans to move are made in the frontal lobes, innate movement is sorted from lower down. Movement is switched on and off by motor programs in the brainstem. When we are resting, these motor programs are kept under powerful tonic (on-going) inhibition, so that CPGs are inactive. When we move, the basal ganglia (below the cortex) are involved in choosing which programs are then activated. If basal ganglia functioning is lost, people lose automatic movement – as in Parkinson's disease (Grillner et al. 2008).

*This local autonomy that generates and organizes locomotion hugely simplifies the task of the higher cortical centers in directing activity. The higher brain does not have to micromanage our movements!*

---

Rugby player Jonny Wilkinson was taught by scientists to take a multi-map approach when taking a try, in the rugby world cup in 2003. The scientists worked out a formula for him,

KP=CSP-(EnC(s+w+r+yn) + PsS(cr+sc+mt+xn) + PhS(ctw).

It recognizes four crucial factors: Wilkinson's technique, or closed skill performance (CSP), environmental conditions (EnC), psychological state (PsS) and physiological status (PhS), which all determine his kicking performance (KP). His EnC has to contend with pitch slope (s), wind (w), rain (r) and other factors (yn); the psychological conditions need to include the mood of the crowd (cr), the current score (sc), how much remaining match time (mt), and other factors (xn), while the physiological factors include fatigue as a factor of time (c and t) and workload (w). It is impossible to put a figure on each of these factors, yet that is what Wilkinson's brain did subconsciously. The *Times* report (Henderson 2003) called it his Sci-Q, the natural ability of his brain to perform hundreds of thousands of mathematical and engineering equations without actively thinking about them.

On the field, one watched Jonny lining up a kick for a conversion of a try, as other players would, but then spending maybe a minute looking intently, from the posts to the ball, to the crowd, to the wind, etc., as he "inputted" each factor of the data to his brain, in a sensory, not mental, way. Then the crowd watched amazed as kick after kick sailed over the bar and won England the title.

---

### Prediction and perception – the integration of internal maps and external facts

In an unfamiliar environment we "get our bearings" before we take a single step. Incoming sensory information is collated in "place cells" in the hippocampus, making and continually updating our own internal GPS system. If the ground surface is unfamiliar, even our first steps will be cautious as information is gathered.

Locomotion is not just about the generation of movement. It is about orienting the body and navigating it through the world, interactively with the surroundings. *Without a sensory relationship to the environment there cannot be integrated movement.* In this, feedback and feed forward mechanisms work together. The nervous system has evolved to provide contextual plans, made from goal-oriented, mostly short-lived predictions, verified by moment to moment sensory input (Llinas 2002: 18).

# New models of coordination and learning

The more we pay attention and maintain awareness of all our senses, the better will we gather information for our brain maps. Vision and perception are not the same. **Perception** is when we bring to awareness the differences between what we expect to be happening and what actually is happening. We do this by comparing the internally generated sensorimotor images with the real time sensory information (Llinas 2002: 4).

For instance, I can plan to walk the length of a pebbled beach. While conscious plans are made in the frontal lobes, my immediate neurological goal is to take steps in a certain direction. My predictive CPGs organize the mechanism of walking, for which the internal maps of my limb positions and orientation are continually updated. Alongside these, my brainstem map is also registering the increased strain in the muscles of my legs and feet from the rough terrain, the challenge to stability in the joints, and are factoring this into the stride length and type of step generated. My sight is collecting information about the terrain and adding specific information that generates conscious or unconscious decisions about where the safest placement of each foot might be.

If I am paying attention – visually and to body awareness – then my CPGs will have good information to work with and will generate appropriate movements. My higher cortex is concerned only with the choice and organization of behavior, such as when to begin, which overall direction to choose, and that walking would be safer than running. Knowing Alexander technique, I can also add conscious awareness to inhibit any micromanaging of movement. Then I can navigate the beach more enjoyably without twisting my ankle.

Now we can refine how Rufus avoids the dog poo. Moment by moment, sensory information from his nose and eyes generates and updates internal maps of his environment. This is fed to "place cells" in the hippocampus, which are both remembering what the park was like yesterday and plotting his position relative to the landmarks around him right now, i.e., the poo dollops of today (Moser and Moser 2016). This allows an appropriate path to be found, moment by moment. Meanwhile sensory information streams continually from his muscles and joints, skin, soles of feet, and ligaments, informing his brainstem where his limbs are, along with ground surface information. The CPGs generating his walking patterns are modified by all this other information, recruiting slightly different spinal circuitry to create subtle shifts in muscle patterns, such as a slightly longer stride, a slight diagonal, etc., so that Rufus's hairy feet land smoothly and evenly along the path without stepping in anything smelly.

## Sense of self and the organization of movement are inextricably linked

Most people think about movement in a cortico-centric way: assuming that they need to direct the movement of their hands and feet more or less consciously. But dogs and horses cannot see their feet as they place them. So do we need to see ours? Research shows clearly that too much conscious control makes coordination worse, not better (Wulf 2007: 11). Over-thinking seems to interfere with the high level of precision and organization at the deeper brain and spinal cord levels. Just as importantly, to let these deeper brain levels do their organizational work makes higher-level cortical control much simpler and faster.

The information that gathers in the brainstem is sufficiently complete to make a whole-body map that can organize and synchronize whole-body movement. The superior colliculus, a part of the brainstem, is our primary whole-body awareness center, which then has links to the motor centers of the cortex (Damasio 2010: 70). It has direct connections to the retina and primary visual cortex, with a topographical map of the retina. Layered under that are topographical auditory maps and somatic maps – with input from hypothalamus (interoceptive and homeostatic information) and spinal cord (proprioceptive information). The vestibular information also assembles here. This superimposition of maps allows more complete multisensory integration than that of any other area of the brain.

# CHAPTER sixteen

In particular, it acts as the center for visual orienting movements. When we turn the head towards something that has "caught our eye," this action is organized by the superior colliculus and can also result in locomotion (Grillner 2008). I assume that this is part of the mechanism by which the head and vision leads the body into movement – when we let it.

Feed forward pathways stabilize us before a movement is initiated, but it seems that we often use unnecessary anticipatory movements. When participants were asked to carry a tray across a room (a goal-oriented task) it was observed that they pushed their necks forward when preparing to walk, and this increased with potential task difficulty. The participants who showed the most forward necks also scored lowest on tests of inhibition (Baer et al. 2019). Loram et al. (2017) noted that when violinists inhibited neck tension, it reduced unnecessary anticipatory movements along with other unnecessary muscle activity.

### Exploration 16.1    Navigating across and around obstacles without looking down

- *Scatter ten or more objects across your floor – cushions, books, etc.*

- *Stand and look across the room to something (e.g. an ornament) level with your eyeline, then walk across to pick it up. Do you have to look down to navigate all the scattered objects?*

- *Return to your starting point, stand and come to quiet, with spatial awareness and natural breathing; allow your expanded awareness between your whole self and the room. Notice your physical body expanding upwards and downwards, fully into your back and front, and sideways. You and the world are three-dimensional. (Play around to find the keys you need today to find this quiet, receptive and physically expanding state.)*

- *Let your eyes arc downwards, nodding your head slightly, then up again. Notice that when you see forward with a balanced head, the whole floor is in your peripheral vision.*

- *Now, while maintaining spatial awareness, focus the object level with your eyeline. Let yourself walk towards it as if you are drawn across the space to it. Do not look down to navigate the scattered items, simply let the object draw you, and allow your connection between peripheral vision and brainstem to look after the rest.*

- *Notice what happens. Can you navigate like Rufus, allowing your sensory radar and on-board computer to work out your stride length and placement?*

## Lesson 2    Coordination of reaching and grasping in everyday actions

One might reasonably expect our nervous systems to be wired both to give us optimum movement patterns and to make us desire this. But for Westernized people at least, neither seems true. Most people are content when movement works adequately enough to get them through, even when there is some discomfort. Scientists are finding that the nervous system seems set up to provide a good-enough result only, rather than an optimal one; they call it "satisficing." Alexander defined "end-gaining" as being so over-focused on achieving a task that one pays little or no attention to the "means whereby" the task is carried out. Science is now giving us clues why end-gaining is so prevalent, and so hard to overcome.

That the nervous system is set up to work from predictions is easily seen in catching and reaching movements.

### Exploration 16.2    Demonstrating prediction

- *Try suddenly throwing a ball to someone a few times, always aiming to their right; then throw to their left and they will probably reach in the direction of the previous throw.*

- *To demonstrate that movements are planned in advance: pick up a few different wide and narrow objects and watch your hand form the appropriate shape before each. Then try the same but with eyes closed and feel your hand maximize the opening shapes to be certain.*

# New models of coordination and learning

Reaching and grasping movements are learned and stored – each new kitchen gadget or trouser button requires a rethink; we are continually adding to our store. Evidence shows that when we encounter a new task, we don't develop a new optimal movement from scratch, but that "we satisfice – we draw on our memory of stored movement plans, mentally simulate a few to find a good one, tweak it a bit, and call it adequate. The amount of fine tuning probably depends on how pressed we are for time, how important we think the action is, and how refined our internal simulation ability is. Movements made directly from memory with very little fine tuning could be said to be habitual" (Cohen 2019).

Rosenbaum et al. (2007) showed that we make use of stored postures from previous experiences, and plan the movement required beforehand by using the initial and goal postures, in which the movement itself is little regarded. For instance, if I am to put a cup in an unfamiliar dishwasher, my brain uses the information of how I stand by the counter-top holding the cup, and an idea of the end-shape I will make to put it in the dishwasher. It does not consider the movement between. The new movement required is generated by a two-stage process of finding the best-fit stored posture (maybe from previous encounters with dishwashers) and tweaking it to fit. If the final posture is not adequate, the brain will prioritize completing the task over posture comfort – resulting in an awkward movement. This is all consistent with Alexander's concept of end-gaining: the words "end" and "purpose" are often used synonymously.

The more often we do a movement, the easier it becomes for the brain to use a previously stored posture, and a habit forms that can be done unconsciously. There is now no advantage in generating a new posture when the old one does the job. We have lost the exploratory engagement within the task, and shifted to achievement orientation in which we are already thinking ahead.

Science may be interested in how the average Western individual goes about their largely unmindful day, "satisficing" to get by. They are demonstrating the depth of our endgaining patterning. But in AT, I suggest we are interested in optimizing movement patterns. We know that movement with AT is qualitatively different, as we found with the ball game – smooth, precisely coordinated, easy, light, etc. But there is more than this. By coming fully present, we can become less predictive in our movements and more responsive to what is actually happening in real time. The science of this is not known, but I will speculate that several elements are involved.

### A new model of coordination in catching a ball

Now we can speculate how, in so short a time, we can awaken our ability to catch a ball with amazing precision and ease of coordination.

1. By using directions to find our whole-body organization, we bring ourselves grounded and balanced, which allows us to return to a calm, spatially aware, embodied state. Our whole-body intelligence networks are then available.

2. By coming to quiet, we quieten our reactivity – our impulse to use habitual responses to a stimulus. We come to a place of no preparation – "an open plane of possibilities" (Siegel 2010: 10).

3. When the frontal lobes are quiet (inhibited), the back of the brain can come more fully alive. The right hemisphere will now be prioritized over the left hemisphere, bringing us present.

4. Coming present brings fuller perception, internally and externally. Embodiment wakes up the sensory feedback, giving more proprioceptive information of our limb positions to the spinal cord and brainstem body-maps. By paying attention to the whole visual/sensory field, we provide more exteroceptive information for place maps, brainstem, motor cortex, and other coordinating systems. These together make our moment by moment sensorimotor maps far more accurate.

# CHAPTER sixteen

5. Spatial awareness prioritizes the right hemisphere. This accesses sustained attention and temporal flow so we are more aware of movement, not just position.

6. This all brings in the dorsal visual stream, which operates in real time, and links to the movement centers. With the frontal lobes turned down, we come out of trying to do the movement consciously. Instead we let the self-organizing systems of whole-body intelligence come back into play that will generate movements for us.

7. By attending to the continuity of real time and space, we are integrating all the sensory information as it happens, experiencing it moment by moment. In this responsive process, space looks bigger and time seems to slow down. When we only work from the start and end-points we must generate an end-point before it happens; this predictive process will limit our responsiveness.

8. With presence, we perceive when reality is different from our prediction, as when the throw comes from an unexpected direction, and can allow an appropriate response. Our consciousness is not micromanaging our response, it is simply making the decision to catch or not catch.

9. We usually repeat an experience by adapting what we have done before. Here, we want to start from "beginner's mind" each time, coming afresh to the experience of the moment, so we can discover our end-point of catching. We are using all of the above every time so that the whole-body intelligence solves the movement puzzle responsively.

> Tthe famous physicist Niels Bohr tested the typical Western movie show-down scene, where the good guy and the bad guy face off on the main street. In the movies, the bad guy always goes for his gun first, but the good guy still beats him to the draw. Bohr tested this in his lab by giving his assistants water pistols and observed that it worked every time – the person who drew first was consistently the slower one. The good guy – his senses responding to the situation – allows his whole nervous system to self-organize his limbs to operate and coordinate, which is faster than the bad guy's consciously controlled action (Barba 1995, cited in Shepherd 2010: 176).

Ball catching is a stimulus–response game. Life is full of external stimuli: mobiles ringing, emails pinging, children shouting for attention. But I suspect more of our activities happen from internally generated stimuli (called ideomotor responses), such as thoughts that I should help the kids, send an email, ring someone. Or a mixture of the two, such as seeing a used coffee cup and feeling an urge to tidy it. I think Miss Goldie considered that not to be enslaved to these habitual responses, and to choose our subsequent action, was the real goal of the AT work.

The games that follow were evolved through working first with Miss Goldie, and then with Erika Whittaker. Erika emphasized seeing our goal of movement, keeping full vitality like a child, discovering the responsiveness of the body to the task of the moment.

### Living in a flow of dynamic balance in daily life

#### Exploration 16.3    To walk to and pick up a chosen object

- *Stand across a room from a variety of objects and come to quiet, with spatial awareness and embodied consciousness (as in exploration 16.1).*

  Your nervous system is now open to any possibility, preparing for nothing.

- *Mentally choose an object in your visual field that you intend to walk towards. (Don't choose something you really desire: untidy papers you want to rearrange, etc.)*

- *Have you made a subtle preparation for movement? Is there still three-dimensional space between you and the object, or not?*

# New models of coordination and learning

Notice whether you have made an intent that you might perform a task, or a decision that you will, that is already being put into effect. If so, your nervous system now has no choice, it is locked onto the object.

- *If you are now committed, however subtly, to this object, then let go again. Break the visual link by looking away, and come back to quiet three-dimensional awareness.*

How easy is that for you? Does your mind resist changing, once a decision has apparently been taken?

- **Play "no" games** *with the objects. Say "I'll pick up that one ..." then, if you detect response in your system, say "No, I won't" and let go again. Do this with object after object, until the nervous system gives up preparing, and you can choose an object without disturbing your quiet system.*
- **Or use spatial awareness:** *invite your eyes to track across objects and the spaces between them. See the space between you and the objects from your whole-body, until there is no pull or loss of self. Can you now choose one of the objects, without disturbing your quiet nervous system? Keep tracking until the intent to pick up the object no longer matters.*

The first is a more left hemisphere, cognitive approach, in which saying yes or no feels like switching on and off. It uses executive inhibition. The second is a more right hemisphere/embodied approach, where one mentally steps back, and urgency simply diminishes. It finds inhibition as a tonic state.

This is slow patient work and some people find it easier than others. If your nervous system is very reactive it may take a while before you can do this.

- *Once you can stay quiet as you make a choice, then play "no" games (as above) while walking towards it. Think: "I'll walk towards it, I'll walk backwards, no, sideways, no ..." Notice any subtle (or less subtle) responses. If needed, look away to break the visual link.*
- *Seeing from your whole-body expanded field of awareness will help.*
- *Continue until you stop responding completely to your own suggestions.*

Once you have got to this place of quiet:

- *Give consent to walk towards it.*

  As you are walking ask: can I stop?
- *Stop in your tracks and observe whether you have once again locked onto the object.*
- *If you have, then look away and come to quiet again.*

Keep playing with all this until you can reach the object without attachment to it. Then you will still have full spatial awareness of yourself and your surroundings.

We are looking in detail at just how quickly our nervous system kicks into a reactive state. This can initially be very frustrating for those with a very reactive nervous system. *Don't give up!* Trust the process. Like any learning process it may feel like nothing is changing for a long time. You may feel a failure (adults hate this) and want to abandon the whole attempt. You are not failing, you are learning something new. Once it begins to change, and it will, you will be able to trust the process better.

What did you observe?

- *Did end-gaining for the object creep in as you moved closer, or could you stop and make a new decision at any moment?*
- *Was this walk a careful act (trying to be "Alexandered") or a natural, purposeful walk?*
- *Did the integrated movement come in by itself? Was it freer? Lighter? Did you discover something about moving?*

Goldie again and again emphasized that we do not have to "do" directions, we simply have get out of the way and the body will grow, lengthen, and lighten.

**Video link for exploration 16.3**

### Become familiar with coming to quiet

It may take time and careful, patient observation to find this level of quiet in something as simple as walking towards an object. We are learning to step from a state of more left hemisphere/head dominance to

# CHAPTER sixteen

more right hemisphere/whole-body presence; from over- (or under-) focusing to spatial awareness; from pre-formed ideas to experiencing; from predictive satisficing to responsive action. Once your nervous system understands that it is safe to make these shifts, you can find it more easily and can play with it in your daily life.

### Exploration 16.4  Pick up a chosen object

- *Stand near the object, seeing it with spatial awareness. Bring in its detail without losing this.*
- *Notice if you have stood close enough. So often, we choose a distance from which we will strain to reach, distorting our alignment and snatching the object.*
- *Play "no" games with which object you are choosing, break the visual link as needed, until you come to quiet.*
- *Once all desire to pick up the object has evaporated, and it no longer matters, give consent and pick it up.*
- *Keep connecting to the object visually, while keeping spatial awareness throughout the whole task, including any recovery moment such as standing upright again. This stops us flicking back in to check on ourselves.*

What did you notice?

- *Did you organize your hand or did it move simply, by itself?*
- *If a bend was required, did you organize it, or did a "monkey" bend happen by itself?*
- *Did you notice the sensitivity of your fingers as you picked up the object?* Often there is heightened sensitivity when touching from this quiet yet alive place.

**Video link for exploration 16.4**

### Exploration 16.5  Allowing the fundamental bending movements of "monkey" or squat

Play in this way with picking things up at different heights.

- Off a table *at your level, where you only need to extend the hand and arm.*
- Off a lower surface *requiring a "monkey" or lunge movement. Can you let these organize themselves by sustaining focus on the object?*
- Off the ground, *requiring a deeper bend or squat. Let the movement organize itself, then stop and renew your parameters before you stand again: you may discover how to let your legs extend by themselves.*

Alexander writes (1985: 45) that he used these methods ("no" games as I call them) to make the breakthrough in speaking without contraction. He gave himself the choice to speak, or lift an arm, or do nothing. Only when he perceived he was no longer preparing did he give consent to let the movement happen. Then he was able to "stay out of his own way" and could allow unknown movement patterns to discover a new way of speaking.

### What new habits do we build?

The aim is not to build a new "how to move" habit that we can perform on autopilot. Instead we are looking to build up new habits of consciousness:

- Coming present.
- Letting the movement be organized in relationship to an activity.
- Letting the whole-body move as an integrated whole, rather than only using the part involved.

Movement that is responsive to the activity has to be done from consciousness every time.

### Exploration 16.6  Coming conscious in all of life – explore a daily task

Over time, aim to cover all the small actions of which life is made: opening a door, putting on a shoe or sock, turning on a tap, so that over time we are conscious in most of our lives.

# New models of coordination and learning

1   *First stop and come to quiet. See from your expanded field of awareness.*

2   *Play "no" games around doing that task or different tasks instead.*

3   *And/or come quiet, present, and spatially aware in your whole being.*

4   *When your urgency to do the task has gone, and it no longer matters, let yourself go ahead.*

You will probably need to break up the task into little stages, being alive to how fast end-gaining (prior assumptions) sets back in for each. For example, in putting on a sock, we need to bend forward (let the bend organize itself); pick up the sock (conscious of the quality of touch); allow the foot and hands to work together, alive in each moment to the degree or angle of action or force required (the hands and foot can have a quality of separateness from the rest of the body, which is uninvolved); and finally put the foot down and straighten up. Initially only to work on the first one or two parts of these actions may be enough.

Can we at any point put the sock down and go to another task, or look out of the window? Ensure you see each stage as you do it. Keep playing "no" games. Trust that you will get your sock on eventually!

Erika Whittaker would say: "If at any point, in anything you are doing, you cannot put it down and go to look out of the window, then you are doing too much!" I now keep my "grabbing" left hemisphere under control by working with a ten-minute timer – especially when on a computer or gardening. The requirement is only to walk across to my phone, reset the timer and return to the task in hand. It provides a few seconds of movement and the reminder to look out again at my surroundings, which resets me to whole-body intelligence, from which I can return with more consciousness to the task.

## Fitting exploration into busy lives

We cannot come into total consciousness in all of our lives in one go; we would go mad. Miss Goldie suggested to me that I take one task each week, and for that week, every time I come to that task, e.g. opening the bedroom door, that I stop, and fully go through the process above. She called it "giving yourself a lesson." After a week, I will have built up new habits of consciousness during the discovery process of door opening. Rather than learning a new move that I repeat, the process can surprise me with its newness each time I open this door. This brings us fully alive.

Try this for yourself. After a week, you may notice that the sight of the door handle reminds you to be conscious. So being conscious throughout the task will then become much easier, and we can begin becoming conscious in a second task, and so on. The key is to be fully present in this daily self-lesson, as we so often only do in a real lesson; in life we often have one eye on what we will do next, and so don't fully engage with the process. This is the real work.

It took me about two years to get round all the little tasks of life; some of them took many stages. The difference in my nervous system – of calm and resilience – was well worth the effort.

## What do we mean by "predictive" and "responsive"?

It seems to me that the word "predictive" is being used in two ways, according to the level of motor maps involved. CPGs (along with other spinal microcircuits) have the basic building blocks of movement ready to deploy – and so are predictive, unlike reflex models of action, which required sensory input to activate them. But CPGs are modulated moment by moment by incoming sensory information which makes them responsive to the current circumstances. Then there are higher order maps of our stored habitual moves, which allow us to perform tasks predictively (automated actions) and be much less present as we do so, and so less responsive to the moment.

Compare these two passages from Sandra Blakeslee (Blakeslee and Blakeslee 2008):

"Another interesting thing about these higher-order maps is that they represent all your movements before you carry them out. Your actions, and your

# CHAPTER sixteen

ability to imagine them, are driven by internal models in the mid- and high-level echelons of your body mandala, rather than directly by what is happening in the world outside your body. These models are locked and loaded and ready to deploy by the time you become consciously aware that they are, in fact, what you intend … You need to predict what is happening in the world to cope with its complexity" (2008: 61). Blakeslee is interested in the predictions made by a sportsman's nervous system to anticipate ahead of the event where the ball will be, by reading the body movements of the opponent. She says that without this there would be no time to respond appropriately.

I am interested in the way that when one comes truly present, and chooses *not* to allow these predictive responses, the time opens up allowing one time to make decisions. The Brazilian soccer player Pele, approaching the goal, would watch the goalkeeper's response to his body movements, make a small stop, and kick the other way. If he has time to do this, why not the other guy?

Turvey and Fonseca (2009) would seem to agree. They point out that when an outfielder catches a fly ball, getting to the right place at the right time cannot be solved by prediction, but only by adapting action to information. Likewise, when you balance a stick on your fingertip. In these, I suggest we are using the first order of prediction within the nervous system, but not the higher order maps. However, the experienced outfielder's whole-body intelligence has had practice at solving the movement puzzle of catching flyballs, giving him many neurological connection possibilities to draw on.

Blakeslee's second passage (2008: 115) discusses the old and new models of sensory and motor input. The old model was that we receive sensory information, and then we choose to act, and they are two separate units. Science now sees that ordinary perception almost always involves multiple senses, and that perception and action are functionally one unit.

"It turns out the sensory maps of your parietal lobe are also de facto motor centers, with massive direct interlinkage to the frontal motor system. They don't simply pass information to the motor system, they participate directly in action. They actively transform vision, sound, touch, balance, and other sensory information into motor intentions and actual movements. And by the same token, the maps of the motor system play a fundamental role in interpreting the sensations from your body. Your parietal lobe is not purely sensory, and your frontal lobe is not purely motor." This gives a better model from which to understand responsive action.

When operating well, the whole system is far from predictive. Instead, it is perceptive and responsive, because the predictive map is compared against the latest information, moment by moment, and the response is changed accordingly. It seems to me that, for instance, great musicians are present with every note, however fast, as great sportspeople are present with every movement, and could at any moment make a subtle change of direction. With responsive presence, there is no sense of rush.

### Exploration 16.7   Lifting a heavy object such as a chair

- *Stand back and look at the chair from your expanded field of awareness.*
- *Play "no" games until the urge to lift the chair is gone, then walk close enough to be right on top of it.*
- *Let your vision lead the body into an appropriate "monkey" with the arms hanging, and strong, straight back connected to your buttocks and thighs. Don't reach out for the chair, just take yourself low enough.*
- *Stop when the hands encounter the edge of the chair seat. Let the hands* gently *fold around it.*
- *Keep your spatial awareness as you give consent to let yourself pick the chair up.*
- *Notice what happens. Was it heavier or lighter than you expected? Did you notice your back or legs engage in a different way?*

# New models of coordination and learning

We are coming from **predictive action**, where the brain predetermines the muscles/force, etc., used, into **responsive action**, where the brain facilitates the body to respond appropriately to the task moment by moment, in often unexpected ways, and we discover anew how to move.

We might have assumed the chair was heavy, and so tensed our arm muscles in advance above the level needed. Alternatively, we might have assumed it was light, and the insufficient preparation could then cause us to stagger with the unexpected weight. In both these, the arms take charge of the action – a partial pattern. By acting responsively, the muscles can engage only as much as is needed. This allows the whole-body to perform the movement, and results in a completely different and integrated action. Cacciatore et al. (2020) call this **force matching,** and comment that AT seems to improve one's ability to match forces, especially in a postural context.

### Our nervous systems are information networks, and not top-down hierarchies of control

The new thinking is that our nervous systems are information networks. So how is sensory information processed? The brain has often been envisaged as a machine with localized areas doing specific bits. We learn that visual information is processed in the visual cortex, hearing in the auditory cortex, etc., all in the head-brain. New thinking is that the brain operates in looping networks, and that information from different senses is always linked together. For instance, each area of the body has its own map of personal space, created through spatial multisensory processing (Cardinali et al. 2009). One can speculate that it is whole-body systems that coordinate with the environment not just the brain. The whole-body attunes to the world and then responds to it as a whole. Many writers have expressed this idea poetically; we can now begin to understand it scientifically.

Miller and Clark (2018) ask how the predictive processing model of the cortex fits with the emotions and subcortical contributions. They suggest that to achieve fully embodied action, the many circuits that connect cortical and subcortical structures are allowing feedback and feed forward with the body, of both proprioceptive and also emotional/homeostatic information (allowing for motivational drives). This gives us a unified sense of what's out there and why it matters.

### The role of Alexander technique and the fundamentals of integrated movement

The following is a summary of my own speculative model of how the technique works as presented throughout this book, based on my own and others' observation and experience, and drawing on some established ideas. This model goes way beyond established science, but could provide a basis for further research.

- When we bring about our optimal geometry, aligned with gravity and in whole-body coordination, our muscles are in lengthening antagonistic relationships, and our proprioception will function optimally. This links up our kinetic muscle chains, so that we have the full range of movement possibilities.

- When we come to quiet presence – tonic inhibition – we are perceptive both internally and externally, giving our brain maps full information. Our whole-body intelligence is in play – the right hemisphere with spatial awareness and temporal flow, our grounded intuitive senses, our hindbrain's organization of innate movement, our skin and limbs alive with their own perceptual fields. We are open to the unexpected, in an open field of possibilities.

- We can inhibit automated cortico-centric habits, so that our innate movement patterns re-emerge, giving smooth, easy movement from dynamic modulation of postural tone. We can stay calmer for longer in response to the stimuli of life. All this brings about an ease and coordination of

# CHAPTER sixteen

movement that most people do not even dream of having.

What of this is known from a scientific standpoint? Cacciatore et al. have developed a neurophysiological model for AT (2020), based on currently available quantifiable data (though they tell me the body schema aspect needs more verification). Postural tone and body schema are the core of their model, on which executive processes of attention, inhibition and motor plans act through feed forward processes, while force matching adaptive tone processes act in feedback loops, to produce smooth, integrated movement.

### Poorly coordinated movement becomes micromanaged rather than emergent

In contrast, when the body is out of alignment, there are co-contracted joints and compromised muscle patterns. I suggest that these compromise the whole-body flows of information or movement. There will then be less sensory feedback from the body, and a reduced sense of embodiment. This stresses the system to a greater or lesser degree. As we lose access to whole-body self-organizing movement patterns, we must use voluntary control to move, using partial patterns. Movement becomes micromanaged at the cortical level, using feeling feedback from our muscles.

Decisions become based on what I think will happen, or what I think needs to happen, rather than on what I observe. This could include trying to catch balls that have not been thrown yet, or reaching to catch on the predicted trajectory though they are flying in an unexpected direction; or trying still to catch when you have been instructed to leave it.

The patterns produced then will be less attuned to the environment, and more attuned to what I believe I need to or can do. Because this is now the status quo, we believe this is all we are capable of. Learning now becomes a laborious process in which we attempt to coordinate our limbs or actions through conscious instruction.

## Lesson 3   New models of learning a complex task

A friend of mine, Emer, recently went skiing for the first time with her sister, an experienced skier. Emer has been a fellow adventurer exploring Philip Shepherd's work of *The Embodied Present Process*.

Emer was a worrier who lived in her head chatter, which was telling her she was foolish to attempt skiing at age fifty-three, she'd break a leg … The first day she learned to take her ski boots on and off, and how to slow down. On day two they set off down a beginners' piste. Emer's head was full of negatives, spoiling any enjoyment, blocking her learning so that making the simplest changes took great focus. Then she realized she was headed down a slope towards some trees … and a drop. The head, panicking, redoubled its chatter. But suddenly, her embodiment learning kicked in. Her body took over and knew exactly what to do to avoid an accident: she sat back without thinking, and stopped before going over the edge.

Now everything changed for her. She realized her body knew how to ski! She now found the teacher's instructions got in the way, she just knew to bend one knee slightly to turn, etc. In the evenings she skied with her sister on more difficult terrain, and could be both in herself and her environment, enjoying the beauty around her, while taking in the detail of the snow quality, and knowing how to respond to it on her skis.

My husband's response to this tale was that she must be a natural. But had she let her chattering head stay in charge she would have had the same long hard learning curve as most people. I am suggesting that everyone has the potential to be a natural if they can sidestep the traps that stop us learning.

> The brain, once thought to be fixed beyond age ten, is now known to be plastic and changeable. New learning occurs most effectively when we pay close attention – when we open the mind fully to present experience. This

# New models of coordination and learning

> activates the nucleus basalis – that part of the brain that is very active in young children but switches off at adolescence. With full, undivided attention – being fully present – then change happens in the brain maps and it holds – we remember the learning. When tasks are performed automatically, brain maps do change but the changes do not last (Doidge 2007: 53, 62).

### *Acquiring a new skill – cortical-led learning is hard*

Our current model of learning a new action is cortical based, and seen as hard work, taking much repetition. It is seen as happening in three stages (Wulf 2007: 3); the brain areas involved are from Blakeslee and Blakeslee (2008: 58).

1 *The cognitive, or verbal stage.* Learners are given instruction on what to do. This uses the higher motor regions, such as the supplementary motor area, important for engaging in any complex and unfamiliar motor task. I remember, when learning a tennis serve, being told to step sideways with the right leg, keeping the knee bent, extend the arm and sweep it forward as the racket encounters the ball. It takes a lot of conscious cognitive activity – mental effort and attention – to control the body in this way; it is a slow laborious process, in which people often verbalize the instructions to attempt to focus what is required. The result is halting, inconsistent and slow, with abrupt movements, as new movement patterns are built.

2 *Associative stage.* As the basic movements are acquired, the process of smoothing them begins through more subtle movement adjustments. The result is more consistency and smoothness, and some movements start to become automatic. Less cognitive control is required. This process is deeper in the brain, in the premotor cortex.

3 *"Motor" or autonomous stage.* Smooth, accurate and seemingly effortless movements are now reliably made with little or no cognitive activity or attention needed; instead they happen automatically, they "do themselves." The movements have mingled intimately with the motor primitives in the fundamental motor maps in the brainstem.

Research shows that in these processes, the cortical brain maps of the body areas involved change visibly. For instance, with novice piano players, an experiment showed that the size of the finger maps were significantly bigger after a week of daily practice. The following week, half the group were asked to stop practicing, and their finger maps returned to pre-practice size within a week. The other group kept practicing daily for four more weeks. Surprisingly, their finger maps also got smaller, even as their performance improved. "While you are still a novice, your finger maps grow in an exuberance of neural wiring, seeking and strengthening any connection patterns that maximize your performance. If you then stop practicing, your finger maps stop adapting and slump back to their original size. But if you stick with practice over time, you reach a new phase of long-term structural change in your maps. Many of the novel neural connections you made early on aren't needed any more. A consolidation occurs: the skill becomes better integrated into your maps' basic circuitry, and the whole process becomes more efficient and automatic" (Blakeslee and Blakeslee 2008: 57–9). True expertise, the virtuoso level, where the complex motor skill has been practiced day in, day out, for years on end, show motor maps that are again increased in size. Professional pianists will have enlarged hand and finger maps "crammed full of finely honed neural wiring that gives them exquisite (and hard earned) control of timing, force, and targeting of all ten fingers."

> Each night, the brain does an operation called synaptic pruning, removing any neural connections that are not currently being used, or which have been superseded. This is "use it or lose it" in action – those who stop practicing a skill, particularly early on, lose it as the brain wipes it out again. It also means that as skills become more efficient, the maps get smaller as neural connections are refined (Walker 2017: 109).

# CHAPTER sixteen

*Embodied learning – learning to be a "natural"*

But is this the only way of learning something? Or is there an easier way, as my friend Emer found? Can we learn complex skills simply by getting out of our own way?

One way of coming out of over-thinking is to envisage the action directly, which activates the motor maps almost as completely as physical performance, with every needed brain area working except the final motor stimulation the muscles. Simply visualizing it like a spectator doesn't work, there needs to be the embodied sense of physical participation (Blakeslee and Blakeslee 2008: 60). Formula One drivers now practice on virtual circuits to learn the corners and rhythms of a circuit before they drive it for real, while musicians often practice by hearing the music in their heads and envisioning their movements. I suspect we use this in ball games when we first envisage a throw's trajectory.

Skiing does not count as a complex use; it is a derivation of locomotion patterns. Complex uses include the hands of a pianist, or the feet of ballet dancers. How can we ease the learning process here?

Matthew Noone is a professional sarod player (an Indian instrument similar to a twelve-stringed sitar). In 2015 he lost the tip of his left middle finger in an accident. He came for lessons six months later, when the fingertip had healed, but he feared he would never play again. He told me: "All the hours of practice I have done over years, building up movement patterns in the fingers of my left hand are now invalid, as my hand is a different shape. I cannot do that all over again." We started with general Alexander work. On his third lesson he told me he had agreed to do a small informal concert, but had worried that it would not be good enough. We worked with non-reaction to stimuli using ball games, and he experienced how he could allow his arm simply to respond, meeting different and unexpected catches. Then I asked him to take his instrument, and from the same place of no preparation, to allow responsive movement of the left hand to touch the instrument's neck, or the strings, or his own head. I then asked him to come to a simple chord in the same responsive way. To his wonder, his hand formed the chord perfectly where it was needed on the strings, allowing for the new length of the shortened finger. He found it also brought much greater sensitivity in his fingertips.

Matthew is a meditator and understood this process straight away, incorporating it straight into his playing. He realized he had found a method to rediscover new ways of playing, fresh in every moment. The concert was only three weeks later; friends who heard it told him his playing was better than it had ever been. His phone soon rang with bookings for well-paid gigs.

I met him after another concert a year later. I was curious whether, with time, had pre-set patterns returned? "No," he said, "pre-set patterns don't work any more." But, I asked him, in the year since we had worked, have new pre-set patterns formed? Emphatically no, he was working never to let pre-set patterns form again. "The way I practice now has changed. When I first pick up the instrument, I use the process you told me of not catching the ball, so I don't play for a moment, so that when I do play it happens fresh in the moment. I'm working not ever to go into the pre-set patterns again. I don't now do a whole routine of scales and exercises, instead I just work with saying no."

He wants to ensure that, every time he plays or performs, he is on an adventure into the unknown, to let the music inform him.

Gaby Wulf is a scientist who discovered this same process after attempting to learn to windsurf. First, she memorized the instructions from a magazine article. But after a few unsuccessful hours on the water, attempting to control her body consciously to achieve the correct movements, she decided to focus instead on the turning of the board. The change of attentional focus produced a dramatic change, and she was soon jibing more fluently, consistently, and faster too. Since then, she has researched attentional focus and learning (2007: 35). The results are so far consistent for any sport or learning.

# New models of coordination and learning

Focusing on the body makes matters worse, not better. This was demonstrated at the simplest level in a group who were asked simply to stand still, observe their natural body sway and attempt to control it. The result was more sway, not less (Wulf 2007: 26). In novice skiers on a ski simulator (2007: 8, 37) no instruction proved better than verbal instructions directing people how to use their bodies to perform the task correctly. But another group, instructed to focus on the movement of the platform, did better, and this learning was retained after a period of time, showing it was real learning.

Wulf discovered that an internal focus – on trying to control the body – makes learning harder, while an external focus – on the effect of the movement – makes learning easier and more automatic. External focus can be on an object: the ball you are kicking, rather than the foot that is doing the kicking; on the racquet, golf club, surfboard, or skis. It can be further out from the body – on the rim of the basketball net, the height of a jump, or the end of a corner a driver is navigating. There are many possibilities that also will depend on an individual's skill level. It was also seen to be more helpful when tutors' instructions and feedback to learners were directing the learner's attention externally rather than onto themselves, for example instructing someone to notice what happened to the surfboard, rather than what their feet did.

This fits with Emer and Matthew's experiences: Emer discovered how to ski when she experienced the effect of her body movement on the skis, while Matthew focused on letting his hand come to the A chord position on the guitar, rather than making an A chord shape with his hand and bringing it to the guitar. It also fits with our explorations: in the ball game of Chapter 15, we focused the trajectory of the ball, never the hands themselves, while in walking and picking up objects (in explorations 16.3 and 16.4 above), the focus is on the goal of movement.

Wulf concluded that internal focus inadvertently interrupted automatic control processes that bring about effective and efficient movement. With external focus, unconscious, fast and reflexive movements can take over and "the desired outcome is achieved almost as a byproduct" (2007: 113). She observed that external focus also allowed high frequency small corrections rather than the slower, abrupt corrections of internal focusing. It also made movements more accurate, with a reduction in muscular activity, showing more fine-tuned movements. An internal focus seemed to hamper fine movement control.

To me, this finding stems from relationship. By using external focus with spatial awareness, relationship of self with the external environment is a given. With internal focus, we tend to micromanage, losing any spatial awareness or sense of relationship. This is why Delsarte instructed his pupils to give the directions to their reflections in a mirror. Loram et al. (2017) did something similar when asking violinists to reduce their neck tension by giving an external presentation (on a monitor) of intrinsic feedback (neck tension), so avoiding the problem of internal focusing. But in Alexander work, we do often give instructions to the body – so what is different? I suggest that when we use internal focus with spatial awareness – maybe from mind in the brain – then we can use internal focus productively.

Wulf saw that with external (or relational) focus, the body is free to explore different muscular options, maybe working from pre-existing forms as starting points. It can then find its own way to successful moves, whereas with internal focus, this learning from intrinsic feedback is not encouraged. I saw this clearly years ago when I ran a four-week juggling workshop, with four adults and four children. The adults all started with preconceived ideas of juggling being difficult, tried to control their hands, made tense faces when they dropped balls and at the end of the four sessions had only reached two balls. The children played, explored, threw wild balls and let their unconscious processes sort the task, and by the fourth week were all juggling three balls happily.

Loram et al. (2017) see learning in terms of feedback loops. They point out that muscle action and movement operate within a feedback loop that includes the nervous system, muscles, tendons, and

# CHAPTER sixteen

biomechanical interaction with the environment. When they are closed, there is no new input to change the patterning. The musician has multiple automated movement patterns compatible with performing the task, but these have varying costs such as fatigue, extra loading, or more sympathetic arousal (stress), which can reinforce the development of problems over time. Neck tension was part of these automated sensorimotor loops; when they inhibited this, it required that all the automated solutions were inhibited. This would open the loops, allowing new sensory and motor information to feed into different – and I presume experiential – brain pathways to allow new learning.

Continued feedback by watching the monitors for neck tension ensured that the less effortful new solutions were chosen. They commented that while problems with maladapted automated pathways only show over time, "sensorimotor learning works by immediate reward."

They noted that musicians' highly trained pathways are usually inaccessible to modification. But with this sensorimotor learning, "the generation of new behavior was uncomplicated, relatively instantaneous and self-chosen."

I presume that using temporo-spatial perception and embodied intelligence also encourages the feedback loops to open, to receive the new sensory information. When the focus is external, we are in relationship to the task, and in relationship to ourselves. Our whole intelligence is then in play – it is as if the hands and feet see, the eyes feel, and one can confidently use unfamiliar parts of the body to join in the task – such as holding shopping against the curved car door with your belly and your parking ticket with your teeth while contorting to find the car keys. The body schema is fully awake, accurate and humming with activity!

In contrast, when misaligned, there will be faulty sensory perception, and the areas of the body not being used effectively cease to be fully embodied. Our connection to the body is diminished. Then lacking the direct link to it, we must control the body cortically. We are then more likely to drop the shopping while finding the keys!

When we learn to stay quiet and in embodied awareness, inhibiting any reaction to stimuli, and paying full attention to visual and kinesthetic input, the forebrain is toned down. Instead of thinking about what we are doing, we are experiencing it. Then the hindbrain can recruit all the muscles appropriate to the task, and nothing else, and with precision timing. This brings us into the flow of dynamic balance, being in the "zone." This is often described as an altered state of awareness, as if it is not they themselves who do the incredible feats of skill and coordination. "I didn't realize I'd caught the ball till I saw it in my hand!" "It wasn't me dancing, something else took over." This sounds like nonsense but is accurate because the sense of self and self-awareness is in the forebrain. The hindbrain has no connection to language, decision making or a sense of self, so we do not experience its actions as "me" (Vineyard 2007: 149).

## Our culture determines how we learn

So why do many of us now have so little access to natural movement? What was our experience of learning? Newly born horses, who seem to be all wobbly legs, stand within hours, but we are born at a much more immature stage. We rely on a secure community of adults around us as we learn to walk, talk, and develop manual dexterity. Our development is then very much linked to the culture that we land in. In our Western culture, parents are often impatient with the slowness of development and learning. Children are pushed to walk, potty-train, or read ahead of the nervous system's development. I once watched a mum and her baby on a beach, the baby's speed crawling was a delight to see. But the mum kept catching the child's fingers and attempting to make him walk. "He's lazy," she told me. "He won't try to walk!" I gently pointed out that when she lifted him his legs still stayed bent, they were not yet extending fully from the hips – and that when this happened he would walk by himself.

# New models of coordination and learning

Till then, enjoy his crawling phase! She got it – and I left her happily praising his crawling.

Potty training doesn't happen till the sensory nerves are fully grown to the bladder, somewhere between two and three years old. Reading mostly doesn't come fluidly till about seven years old, when the brain's neural connections are formed to distinguish basic letter sounds, such as A from O, or D from T. I watched my daughter's utter frustration and despair as her school tried to drill her in reading between four and six, when this process had not yet happened. The school was oblivious to this; they assured me she was doing about average. Later, we home-educated for two years, and I observed children who had not begun reading until seven or even ten years old, and then progressed with amazing speed.

How many of us went through this pushing to do something before we were ready? To be part of noisy classrooms, deal with overwhelming social situations, or to be good at maths before our intelligence had processed and understood it. What scars of feeling inadequate did that leave? No wonder we leap to get out of a chair rather than trusting to our own bodies to know how to unfold us, the phrase "not good enough" ringing unconsciously in our inner ears.

Alexander wrote of a man he knew (actually himself), who by employing the principles of conscious control, was able to mount and ride a bicycle downhill without mishap on the first attempt (Alexander 2011: 183). Missy Vineyard told me she astonished a boyfriend on her one and only visit to a golf driving range: "By thinking my overall inhibition and spatial direction, as well as clarifying in my mind the direction in which I wanted to hit the ball, my shots were remarkably consistent for a beginner in distance and direction" (email correspondence, January 18, 2020). The first time I tried archery I scored three bullseyes. My pre-Goldie record with darts was of not even being able to hit the board, and people would back away fast when I had darts in my hand! I taught a disabled woman who had been to a school that had emphasized physical skills like ball catching, but had never once succeeded. When we first tried, her hands even missed each other in the air. With inhibition and paying close attention, she caught the eighteenth ball I threw to her. I suggest that these kinds of events are not so much a learning process, but a connection process.

## Learning as a connection process

What might we see on a CAT scan? Could complex motor patterns originate in or closer to the primary motor cortex, rather than having to work their way laboriously into the higher motor cortex before moving downwards?

In the 1940s, Bernstein stated that when we learn, we are not creating and imprinting movement formulas in some motor center. Instead, motor skill is solving problems in the moment, encountering and surmounting every variable of it (Latash and Turvey 2016, essay 6). The ecological psychology group of scientists, who took their lead from Bernstein's ideas, theorize that organisms are *coordinating with* the environment – *process informing,* rather than *processing information about it* (Fultot et al. 2019). They cite a proliferation of recent work on the linkage of perception and action in bacteria, fungi, and slime molds: despite having no nervous systems, these primitive forms can perceive how to navigate their cluttered environments and what to do (or not do) with what they encounter.

The classic model of the nervous system is that a stimulus, such as seeing a flower, is received by a sense organ (the eyes) and activates nerves to fire. This is relayed to the brain, which then engages in hugely elaborate processing to extract information in bits and then reassemble it, in order to decide what is being perceived. From this, a model of current reality is created, from which a motor output response is generated. These mechanisms, which neuroscience has so painstakingly discovered, may be part of information flow, required to coordinate a complex, multi-jointed, organism. But they cannot be the primary processes of engagement. To make an analogy with language, one can say "I am hungry, let's go and forage" either simply

# CHAPTER sixteen

or complexly, depending on the language and culture. But the basic communication is made non-verbally, which is more evident in babies or pets.

Modern cell recording techniques are showing a multitude of ways in which neurons fire and connect, which are far removed from the binary on/off model that came out of viewing the brain as a computer (another mechanical image). Instead, the picture emerging "is one of a large variety of intermodulating processes taking place at a multitude of partially overlapping spatiotemporal scales" (Fultot et al. 2019). So the nervous system is already active, primed and ready to respond, at speed, by modulation to what is perceived.

This runs in parallel to the new ideas of the musculoskeletal system. Rather than being switched on by action and then off again, our muscles are always switched on in antagonistic lengthening relationships, toned and ready to morph or power into action, to connect with the task in hand.

Rather than processing and modeling what is happening, learning what to do in advance, our systems are primed to get in there and connect, and to learn from that connecting process.

As I understand it, the new model of Fultot et al. takes a perceptual route – that the organism "tunes into" environmental information and spatial layouts, modulating the active nervous system. We are drawn by the apple because we are hungry. We navigate through the environment with moment by moment perception/response (as we saw with Rufus and the poo piles). Our systems do not need to decode the information so much as coordinate with it. How primitive humans operate by these means is beautifully described in Robert Wolff's book *Original Wisdom* (2001). I suspect there is much we do not yet know about the harmonic processes of attunement and resonance (see Chapter 18).

These two theoretical approaches, classic neuroscience vs the ecological approach, sound like left vs right hemisphere approaches. McGilchrist's main point throughout his book (2012) is that if right hemisphere leads, left hemisphere is also in play, looking after the details of life, and can take its place contextually. But if left hemisphere leads, right hemisphere is dumbed down, which is a problem. We are learning to step from a state of left hemisphere/head dominance to more right hemisphere/whole-body presence; from internally generated ideas (information processing) to more external experiencing and connecting; from over-focusing on the task to including more spatial awareness; all of which will take us from predictive satisficing to responsive action. There are, as McGilchrist says, two ways of being in the world. When we make a shift from one to the other it can feel distinct, like a gear shift, or like stepping from a cold room to a warm one. We all can learn to shift a little in the experiential direction, and experience better coordination and easier learning patterns as a result.

17

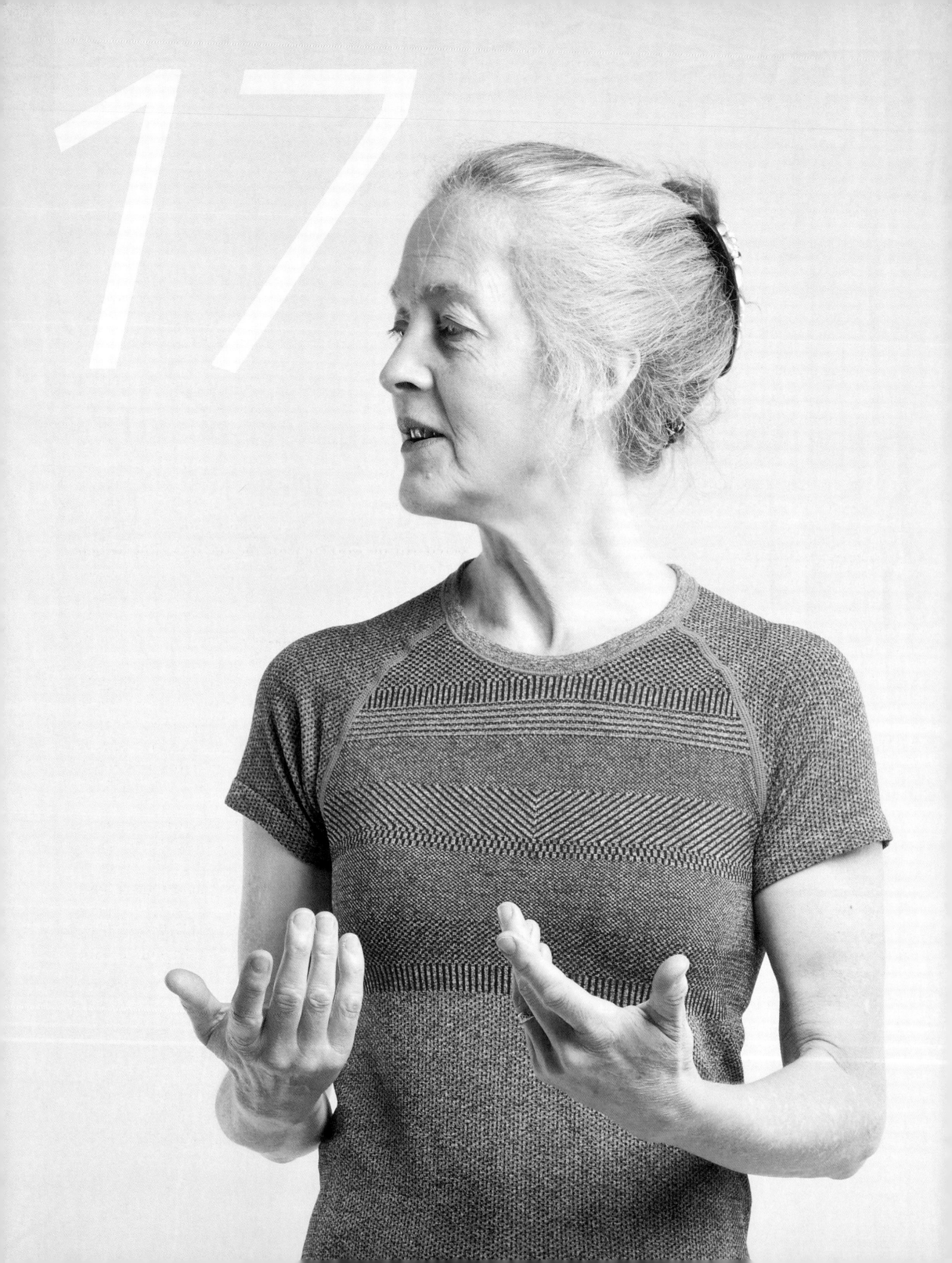

# Embodied speaking

## Introduction

Goldie had a voice that commanded attention. It could be soft and crooning, business-like, clear and emphatic, or hugely angry. It could go from pianissimo to fortissimo, very soft to *very* loud. She was, of course, a fine actress. We have no idea if this is something that came out of the Alexander work or whether it was something she was already developing when she met him. Her voice, as many people have commented, had the quality that whatever she said was for ever burned into your brain and your soul, never to be forgotten. I interviewed ten AT teachers that worked with her, and they all mentioned her voice.

"She had a way of speaking which felt as if she were dropping words into your ear. Her voice was sweet but had a bit of an edge to it. The very first instructions from her were: 'Now as Mr Alexander used to say, just let yourself be very quiet inside so that something different can happen'" (Alex Farkas).

"I was listening very actively, acquiescing with movements of the head. I suppose I wanted her to see how present I was to her teachings. She suddenly burst out: 'And stop doing this thing with your head.' The sound of her powerful voice acted like a slap in the face: I stopped. With quiet tears, I realized how hard I had been trying all my life to please, to show I was worth acknowledgment" (Louise Herard).

"More than anybody I can still hear her voice. The phrase which most burned itself into my brain was her saying almost in a whisper, an ethereal voice: 'not the head back, not the body forward, but the knees forward and away.' The emphasis always on the word 'not.' 'Not the head back, now not the head back; you come to quiet. Just come to quiet.' And I don't have anybody else's voice that I can hear from that length of time ago. Sometimes I find, when I use these phrases with pupils, that I'm saying it in her voice!" (Penny Spawforth).

I often wondered how she did this. Particularly as my own history of voice was very different. As a shy young teenager, I would sit among, or rather on the edge of, my school social circle, trying to think of something to say to join in. Eventually I would think of something, but when I came to speak, the words would come out as either a squeak or a growl. I would blush furiously, and notice that nobody had heard anyway. Even when I came out of this extreme, and found the confidence to speak, I was often aware still I could not rely on my voice to do what I wanted. Both volume and pitch could be rather erratic.

My first Alexander lessons sent my voice even lower: as my tight throat opened up, my voice got deeper and deeper until at one point it disappeared completely! Just as nobody ever suggested working on my breathing, so nobody ever taught me whispered Ah or worked with me on speaking, which could have been so helpful. In retrospect, I wonder why not, since Alexander had started as a breathing and voice coach. It seems here is another area where the roots of the technique were abandoned by many. Alexander worked with his first trainees on two Shakespearean productions, and all those first-generation teachers had beautiful, powerful voices that commanded respect. Natural speaking, is now being rediscovered, but in the intervening years it was often viewed as too easy to interfere with and so better left alone.

Because of my issues around voice it was something I wanted to remedy. I wanted to be able to speak in public without shaking to my boots, take a spoken part in a simple play or ritual, or sing a song. I have worked on this over the years with various Alexander teachers, natural singing teachers and more recently, with actor Philip Shepherd, all underpinned with Goldie's work to forge my own discoveries.

Speaking, almost more than any other activity, involves the whole of us. Not just our physical being, but including our expression of ourselves as we relate to our world. This influences how the world responds to us – our voice sends messages of safety or danger according to tone, pitch and modulation (Chapter 5). Finding our calm embodied voice is crucial for all

# CHAPTER seventeen

therapists, Alexander technique teachers, and indeed anyone who wants to be viewed as safe. Without embodiment, a voice that is gentle can be weak; a voice that is strong can be scary. Embodiment allows us both strength and gentleness together that inspires safety and trust.

## Lesson 1  Being present as you speak

### Exploration 17.1  Slowing down one's speech

This game comes from a choir instructor. Although it was intended for classical singing, it is an inhibition game that works beautifully for speech. Goldie never rushed her speech – it was always slow, measured, and deliberate. Many of us nowadays gabble, hurrying to get our words out; speaking faster seems a modern trend. When we rush speech, we often then clutter it with unnecessary phrases and repetitions, and even slight stammering.

- *Speak a sentence, lingering as long as you can on every vowel, saying no to landing on the consonants. For example, Mary had a Little Lamb might come out as: Maaaaa-reeeee haaaaaaaaad aaaaaaa liiiiii-tuuuuuuul laaaaaaaaaaaaamb ...*

- *Once you can do this, speak simple phrases to your pets or houseplants in this way: Jaaaaspeeeeeeer wooooooooould yooooooooooou liiiiiiike yooooooooour diiiiiiiiineeeeeeeer noooooooooooow? The dog won't mind as long as he gets his dinner! It's also fun game to play back and forth with others. Then explore bringing sentences back to a normal speed but keeping a watch for when you rush over the vowels for the consonants.*

With time you can then become conscious of slowing your vowels in normal speech. I notice that slowing the vowels in this way means that one can give emphasis to every word in every sentence, and unclutter one's speech. This brings a presence to speaking such as Goldie had. It also gives you time to think!

### Exploration 17.2  Envisaging what you say before you speak it

Peter Grunwald taught me that, when speaking, if we envisage what we want to communicate from the upper visual cortex, then speech is simpler, clearer, stronger, and more easily comprehended. When I was on Peter's Eyebody retreats (Wales, August 2016 and 2017) he often told me he found it hard to understand me because I would speak too fast. The excitement of the moment would take over and I would forget to stop and envisage what I wanted to say before saying it. When I eventually managed to inhibit myself from blurting out my thoughts, I could then let the thought of what I wanted to say grow in my upper visual cortex till I could speak it from this different place. Then even the words spoken would change, taking me by surprise, becoming simpler, more expressive, more real.

- *Before you say something, even quite a simple thing, stop and envisage what you are asking or describing before you speak, and notice what then happens.*

### Exploration 17.3  Explore not smiling and laughing as you speak

With all these speaking explorations, it helps not to smile or laugh, even if what we are doing seems somewhat hilarious, or embarrassing. For most adults, smiling and laughing is accompanied by a strong pulling back into the jaw that tightens the top of the neck, and shuts down any connection with the body. These are usually not real smiles such as a baby or small child gives, radiant with joy, but are social smiles, designed to appease and please. This is also why most smiles and laughs look or sound somewhat strained, even false, especially to the camera. Not to smile can allow us to connect to the body and its real feelings, which may be quite different from our apparently smiley face – and possibly uncomfortable. Later when we can keep our connection to true body feelings, we can let real, spontaneous smiling and laughing happen, connecting from our depths, and discover them happening in a different way.

# Embodied speaking

- As you are speaking, notice laughing or smiling and invite yourself to let it drop. You may have to be quite firm with yourself, and it may feel very wrong or rude not to smile. Do you smile or laugh a lot as you engage with people? If so, notice that not everyone smiles all the time, and they are ok too! Later, if something truly funny or touching happens, notice the different quality to any smile or laugh that then spontaneously comes.

## Lesson 2    Embodying the voice

### Exploration 17.4    Taking the whispered Ah down the body

Voices that come only from the head are often squeaky or harsh. A full resonant voice connects to the depths of the body. But as we connect down for this, we also need to connect out to the world and those listening to us. To play with this:

- *Stand or sit, and see out. Track your vision along an imaginary or real line, out to the distance and back again. Find your whole-body natural breathing: the in-breath connects us down to the base of the body, and the out-breath connects us back up and out to the world.*
- *Use this whole-body out-breath to blow an imaginary leaf across the room, using an ffff sound. Track its imaginary path with your eyes. If you can, let the in-breath "come in" through the feet and pelvic floor. You will notice this brings support for the breath from the legs and will lengthen the out-breath.*

Now as we sound a whispered Ah, we will take the awareness of the out-breath in two directions at once. The sound and breath connects simultaneously down the front of the spine, and out to the world. For this, we need mind in the brain and spatial awareness (Fig. 17.1).

- *Start with a very soft Ah sound, just a whisper, no vocalizing.*
- *Keep looking forwards, and allow your jaw to drop, the lower back teeth dropping away from the upper back teeth. Let the sound connect you down the front of the neck spine into your throat. (Notice that if you allow the mind to follow the jaw and sound down, then you will shorten down the front.)*
- *Thinking to lift the soft palate and thinking something amusing so you smile a little (both part of Alexander's rather complicated instructions for whispered Ah) will help, but only if you can get your head round these. If you can't, never mind them for now!*
- *Think of seeing from the back of the head, if you can.*
- *When you can let the sound connect down to your throat, then take it further, down the front of the spine to your heart. Keep letting it drop down the front of the spine to your solar plexus, to your belly, and finally to your pelvis. It may take you a few sessions to get this far, or you might do it in one. The aim is to connect the sound with the whole length of the front of the spine, as you continue to look forwards. You are fully in and fully out together.*
- *On the in-breath, do not let the breath gasp or the chest lift, but let the diaphragm and ribs work gently.*

There is no preparation needed to make a sound, no "taking a big breath." You need no more air to make the sounds than you do to breathe normally.

- *When the sound and breath start together, it is often harsh. Play with letting a little out-breath happen before beginning the sound, letting the sound emerge from the breath.*
- *If the note runs out quickly, you will probably draw immediately away from the point you have got to. Choose not to do this, but to rest there, continuing to breathe out, maintaining awareness at that point and inviting the "block" to melt. You may find that the voice returns, and you can carry on down a little further, before you need to breathe in again.*

**Video link for exploration 17.4**

Once you have this non-vocalized, then play around with vocalizing the Ah sound, keeping it gentle. Use

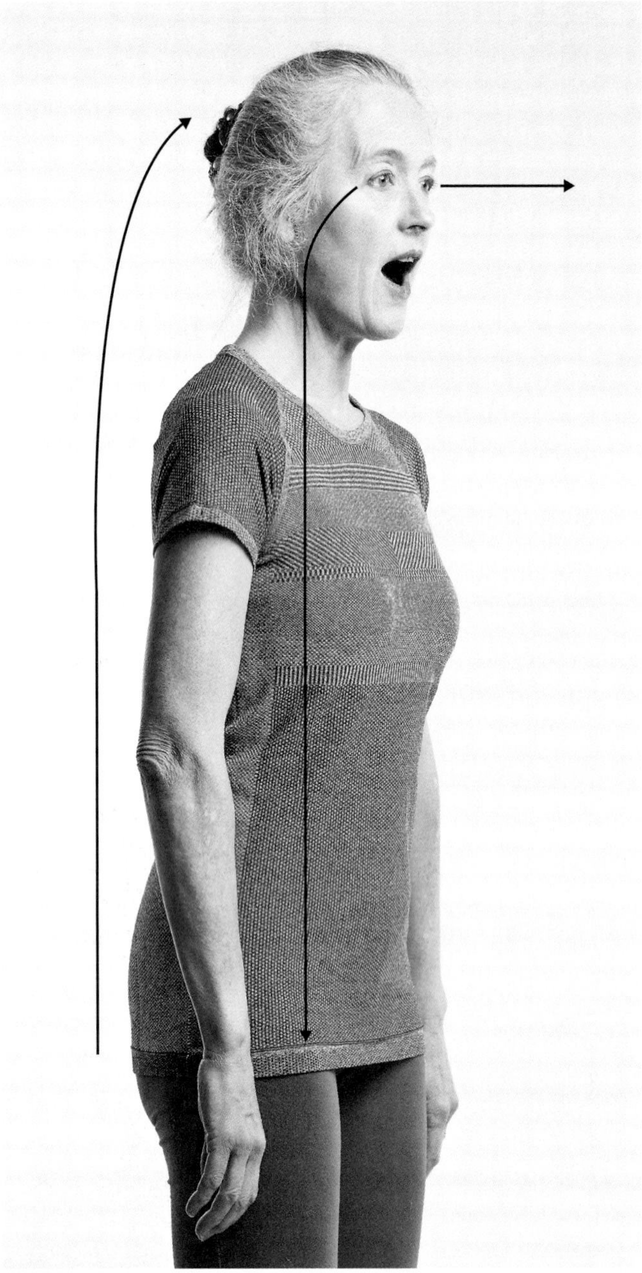

# CHAPTER seventeen

### Exploration 17.5. Letting words ride on the breath

This is my version of one of Philip Shepherd's games from his Radical Wholeness workshop (www. EmbodiedPresent.com).

- Speak three words on one breath leaving a space between: floor – window – ceiling. Notice whether you prepared your breath before speaking, maybe drawing breath up into the chest or pausing it. As you spoke, did you stop the breath between the words, or alternatively run them into each other?

Now breathe in with no preparation to speak:

- Allow a long out-breath, pause and allow a responsive in-breath.

- The moment the breath turns to go out, allow a little breath to go out then make a Ffffffff – as if blowing a leaf across the room. There is no preparation.

- Repeat this, then when your leaf is half-way across the room let it become the word "floor": ffffffffflooooooor-rrrrr. The out-breath begins and the word rides on the breath.

- Explore it with other words – window – ceiling. Can you draw these words out? "Wwww-iiii-nnnnnn-dooooow-ww. Sssceeeeeeeeeeeei-linnnnnnnng." Play with sea shell, theme, frisbee.

- Now say three of these words on one breath with pauses between them, in which the breath is not held but keeps going out. It can help to use an "fff" between words to keep the breath going out.

Notice how gentle your voice now is.

**Video link for exploration 17.5**

**Figure 17.1**
Expanded awareness with Whispered Ah

spoken and sung sounds, with the pitch maintained, dropping or even rising as you link down with your awareness.

# Embodied speaking

### Exploration 17.6    Embodying and speaking experiences of food

Once we have this vocal connection to the body, we can connect thought to it. These games, of how to take our felt experience down the body and speak from there, are all from Philip Shepherd's Radical Wholeness workshop (www.EmbodiedPresent.com).

- *Think of what you had for breakfast. You will probably think the thought in your head. Speak the name of it out loud – perhaps porridge, or cappuccino, or orange juice – being aware of the quality of the sound you make. Is it rich with experience and sensation, or is it just a word?*

- *Now take the thought of what you ate down the body to the belly and pelvic floor. The food itself has already traveled this path, and your body has experienced it. Did you enjoy this food? Did your body enjoy it? Connect again with the experience of eating that food. What were its qualities? What did you enjoy?*

- *While continuing to look out, maintain contact with this experience of the food in the belly. You are holding the experience as if it were still happening, not just the memory of it. As you continue to experience this, speak the name of the food out loud as you look out to the world. What is the quality of the sound you make this time, is it richer than before? In the sound, can you hear the hot creaminess of the porridge, the frothiness of the cappuccino, the slight tang of the orange juice, whatever you are re-experiencing?*

Again it may take you a while to connect with this.

### Exploration 17.7    Embodying your experience of a beautiful object

Now take the thought of an object down the body. I suggest a rose, tree, or cloud, or maybe a Ferrari if you connect better to mechanical things!

- *Hold the thought of the object in your head. Be aware of the experience that arises there, and say the word that connects you to that experience. Perhaps "red," "oak," "soft," "expensive."*

- *Now let the felt experience of the object travel down with an Ah sound to your throat. Rest there and let your throat experience this wonderful object. Feel the throat's experience, and let a word form that expresses it, then speak it from the throat. Can you let the throat speak that one word? Or do you bounce back into your head? Often my pupils initially say something like, "the word I'm finding is 'beautiful' (or whatever)." They are expressing the head-thought about the word, and not the word itself. It can take a while to speak only one word, that comes from the body and expresses its feeling.*

- *Take the thought down to heart, solar plexus, belly, and pelvic floor. You may find that some zones are harder to connect with, while others are easier.*

### Exploration 17.8    Speaking a poem from the perineum

Now you can take a poem, or words of a song, and speak it from the perineum.

- *Hold the felt sense of each line, or initially even each word, connecting with your experience, and attempt to speak it from there, out to the world.*

When you manage this, you may notice a richness in your experience of the poem. Since most of us have been brought up not to feel this deeply, it can take real courage to go there; we can feel quite vulnerable.

- *It can be even more powerful to come into a deep lunge, arms outstretched sideways, while you speak the poem. Your legs may shake from the strain of this, but this can help you connect right into your legs and feet, so that the speaking comes from your feet, through your legs, through your perineum, through your being and out to the world.*

I remember Bob Britton saying (Dublin workshop, 2013) that if an actor was not connected to the muscles

# CHAPTER seventeen

of the lower legs – particularly the tibialis anterior, he would never be heard on-stage. This doubtless is why Alexander was told to take hold of the stage with his feet as he recited, an instruction he misunderstood, and the ensuing harm to his voice started him off on this great exploration! (Alexander 1985: 33).

### Exploration 17.9   Connect and speak to everyday objects from your whole being

We need to connect this experiential speaking with life in the present. We will start with an object, as it is often easier to connect to objects than people.

- Look at an object (maybe your mobile phone or hairbrush) with spatial awareness. Take an Ah down the body as you continue to look, connecting to the depths of your being. Seeing from the back of your head, be aware of the fullness of space between you and the object.

  Say the phrases out loud and see what you notice:

  I see the phone and the phone sees me.

  My throat sees the phone and the phone sees my throat.

  My chest sees the phone and the phone sees my chest.

  My solar plexus sees the phone and the phone sees my solar plexus.

  My belly sees the phone and the phone sees my belly.

  My pelvic floor sees the phone and the phone sees my pelvic floor.

- Seeing and experiencing the phone from your pelvic floor, speak its name from there. "Phone." Do you have the sense that the phone can hear you? This may seem mad, but we are in relationship to everything in our world, and everything in our world is in relationship to us. (This makes much more sense at the quantum level than a Newtonian one.)

- Speak the object's name again, but this time let your hand unfold to make contact with it. What is the experience of the phone? We are allowing our whole selves to come alive to the world, and the world comes alive to us. It can be easier initially to do this in a garden – in a living environment.

It occurs to me that we have built ourselves a strange world, where we live surrounded by dead things. Even if we choose natural materials – wooden floors rather than vinyl ones, cotton trousers rather than polyester – they are still dead. Mobile phones and computers are even further from natural rocks and plants. To let ourselves perceive mutual relationship with our possessions is to allow our world to be alive as it was for our ancestors in the rainforest.

This path to embodied speaking has taken me several years. It has connected me to poetry as never before, as I allow myself to experience and express the words from the fullness of my being. I often speak a poem while I prepare food, and it connects me fully to myself and to what I am doing. (It's also a great excuse to memorize my favorite poems!)

### Exploration 17.10   Finding the power in speaking

So far, we have worked to come down the body to find the voice, which has probably resulted in low, quiet, slow speaking, far removed from how we might speak to buy a loaf. Now we need to find the voice coming the other way, as the opera singer prepares for her performance in the basement of the opera house, and then climbs the stairs, comes out on to the stage and her voice flows out to the audience. Here are four games to explore this.

- Play with taking an Uh sound down the body. Then bounce as you vocalize, noticing the power coming up as the feet touch down.

- Play with doing a whispered Ah, then a poem, as you do pelvic lifts on the out-breath (exploration 8.6).

- Continue throughout to see from the back of the head and out to the world.

- For a truly dynamic, forceful expression of our core being, also powerfully connecting us to the world, play with combining the "fffff" that connects us out to the world,

# Embodied speaking

*the "Uh" that goes so forcefully down to the gut and back up from the feet, and the "CK" sound that lengthens the pharynx forward and up (exploration 12.20). No wonder the resulting word is so expressive, defiant, and energizing. Add in pelvic lifts, stamping, kicks and punches (little finger knuckle leads) to mobilize more power. (For those of delicate temperament, I suggest the word "Yuck.")*

- *Contrast this with the similar yet opposite qualities of "love" with its embodied resonances.*

### Exploration 17.11    Expressing ourselves fully in daily life

We want to be able to express ourselves in the moment from our whole being.

- *Be aware of what you are thinking in this moment. Can you speak it from the fullness of your being? Can you let its intent resonate? Can you let the emotion behind it communicate? To start with you may only manage a word or two. Explore waiting a moment even, to see if your body wants to use different words or phrases than your head's instant formulation. Bodies, I notice, often speak more simply! Try talking in this way to your dog or your houseplants, then slowly see if you can bring it to expressing yourself to people. To speak your real feelings from the core of your being is an incredibly powerful thing to do!*

### *Irene Tasker on the importance of speech work*

Tasker (1978: 2) was one of the first AT teachers and ran the Little School.

"I don't think too much importance can be placed on the application of the work to speaking. I do not mean specific speech training or elocution, as such, but the connecting of the conscious directions especially the preventative ones with the ordinary give-and-take conversation of everyday life. I think it should be part of the training of Alexander teachers. It is true that we teach with our hands to convey sensory experiences, but it is speech which conveys the ideas of which the sensory experiences are the counterpart ... I have a personal interest in this aspect of the work, as one of my worst symptoms of misuse has been a shockingly rapid speech. I have had to keep working at it, and during my period of helping F. M. [Alexander] both in America and at Ashley Place, he would send me little notes, reminding me to 'watch it'. I can never be grateful enough for those reminders! The putting on of the Shakespeare plays during the Training Course gave me a welcome opportunity for experiencing this particular application of the Technique. F. M. invited me to join the students' class when I could be spared from the schoolroom, and I valued greatly the sessions when he combined working on us with giving us the Shakespeare lines to speak. I shall never forget one experience I had of this. I was standing; and after he had worked on me a minute or two he placed a hand on the top of my head and then told me to speak the lines, still maintaining my directions. I realized for the first time the meaning of 'thinking in activity.' The activity of speaking was part of the whole use of myself, and the experience of my voice expressing the meaning of the words without any decision on my part 'to speak well' or to 'put expression into it' is one of my most valued recollections."

Tasker continued by saying that she felt that the children of the Little School benefited hugely from work on speaking (in which incidentally she first ensured that they understood the meaning of what they were saying – there is nothing so dreary as hearing children recite by rote, in which they are so disconnected both from their beings, and from the sense of what they are saying). She adds: "Indeed I would go so far as to say that it contributed more than anything to their improvement *as a whole*."

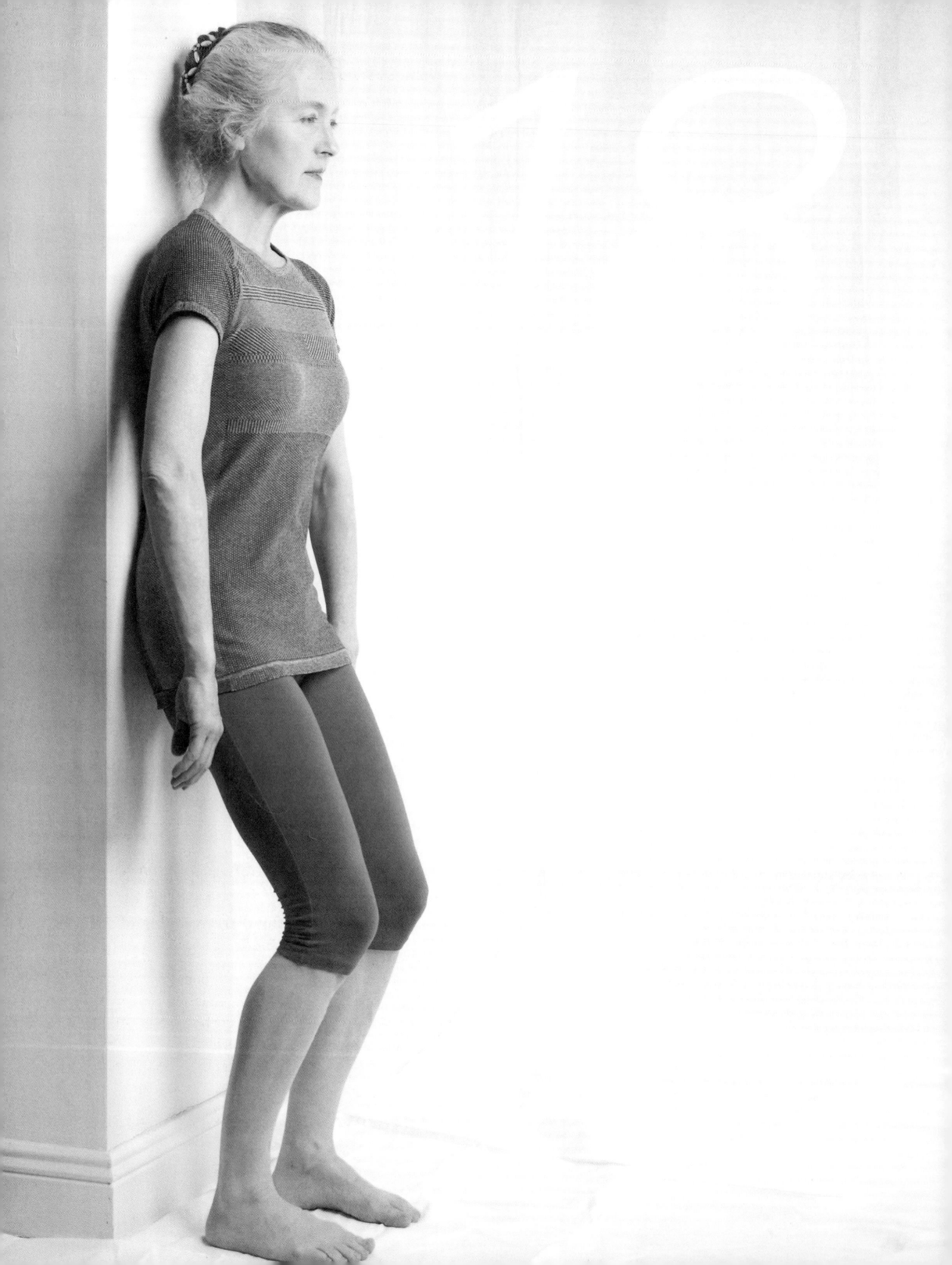

# Relating and attuning to people for putting hands on others    18

## Introduction – we are not machines but self-integrating systems

> "Alexander ... takes you in his very powerful, sensitive and discerning hands and ... begins reshaping you ... Then he stands off from you a minute, takes a long deep critical gaze at you ... studies the poise and stresses of your body, X-rays down through you with a look – through you and all your inner workings from the top of your head to the soles of your feet. Then he lays hands on you and works ... slowly and subtly once more, all the while giving orders to you softly not to help him ... with your preconceived ideas ... Then when you have removed all obstructions and preconceptions in your own mind – and will stop preventing him from doing it, he places your body in an entirely new position and subjects you to a physical experience in sitting, standing, and walking, you have never dreamt you could have before ... until you walk out of the studio feeling like somebody else." Description of lessons with Alexander in 1919 (Lee 1920, cited in Staring 2005: 165)

It would be easy to assume that touching another person with the aim of freeing tight muscles or improving body linkages is a mechanical process, like tuning a car – tightening some joints and loosening others to find a better mechanical balance. One can certainly touch and be touched in such a way – I am remembering certain osteopathic and massage sessions – and they were effective but not pleasant. Or early memories of my mother tugging at my coat fastenings when she was in a hurry to get us out. But we are not mechanical beings, and in Alexander work and all good therapy, there is vastly more going on than this.

Alexander's discovery circa 1914 was that he could use his hands to bring about profound postural changes in his pupil without verbal communication. He did this by intentional thinking to bring about the change required in his own body, while making connection through his hands. This is the process that most AT training courses seek to impart: such as that in order to make a change in my pupil's back, I have to bring about a change in my own back. Miss Goldie taught me that before putting hands on, I had to get my own use going, and then all I need to do is connect to the pupil and that information would go across. I subsequently found that this can even begin before hands are placed. In this chapter you'll learn to bring this about for yourself. This skill is increasingly relevant as the AT profession branches into online teaching, enabling deep work to happen over the Internet.

But how does this information transfer happen? Until recently this has been inexplicable and hard to learn, requiring a lot of trial and error. I notice it often takes students years or decades even to trust the process until repeated experience renders it more reliable. This process is rarely spoken about to the public, perhaps because it sounds too esoteric, something which the AT has always scrupulously avoided. It is not my purpose here to describe the detailed hands-on instruction given in training schools. Instead, we need to understand what is going on, and then explore the key elements by which we access this. Then we can discover hands-on work as A. R. and the very first teachers learned it. (F. M. Alexander's brother, Arthur Redden, maintained that he only needed six lessons (Jones 2016: 18) during which F. M. never put hands on him (Barlow 2011: 46)).

> **We are not machines – we are self-organizing systems**
>
> I have at times used a machine or computer image to explain how we work. This is because the left hemisphere, which needs explanations, can best understand the logical, sequential world of machines which we have created. While physiology has made great strides in understanding the living body by applying engineering principles to it, modern medicine is limited by solely taking this approach. Living bodies have many mechanical properties that are the opposite of non-organic non-living materials. These include the following:
>
> - Machines are eroded and destabilized by friction, shearing forces, tension, or pressure; living tissue strengthens in response to these forces.

# CHAPTER eighteen

> - Machines have no self-repairing facility; broken parts must be replaced. Living organisms are self-organizing systems that can self-repair, and if allowed, will always work towards integration.
>
> - The parts of a machine are not in relationship to each other: if the windscreen wipers break on a car, it does not affect the gears. In living organisms, all parts are in relationship, and their functioning is affected by the functioning of every other part.
>
> - While machines are self-contained systems, living systems are simultaneously self-organizing and organized in *relationship* to the environment.

## How is non-verbal information transmitted?

Several avenues of explanation have been developed over the last twenty years or so.

### Fascia, mechanotransduction, and the linking of brain maps

As we saw in Chapter 4, lesson 5, the fascia provides a communication network of mechanotransduction. "As a hands-on therapist, what you touch is not merely the skin – you contact a continuous interconnected webwork that extends throughout the body" (Oschman 2000).

How might consciousness and thinking interact with our physical structures? When a skilled therapist or AT teacher puts hands on, they can "tune in" to what is happening in another part of the body. Maybe while holding the neck or head, they become aware that the knees are locked, or that there is pain in the back. They may experience this in their pupil's body or in their own. Then by thinking an appropriate response to this, maybe by giving instruction (inhibitory and/or directive) to their own bodies, they can bring about a change in the pupil or client. How might this thought communicate and create change?

In Chapter 4 (lesson 6), and Chapter 16 also, we met our constantly updating brain maps, containing topographical information about the body. These can be extended beyond our body's physical limits. For instance, when we hold a fork, our sensorimotor maps extend to include the fork tip as accurately as to our fingertips, and we then feel the food through the fork (Blakeslee and Blakeslee 2008: 141). This is how we know where the bumpers are when parking the car, and how great drivers can drive "through the seat of their pants." When we link into another human in this way, and they link into us, the brain maps of each extend to include the other's maps also. This sets up a flow of information. For instance, when horse and rider or a pair of ice skaters are in tune together, each knows instinctively what the other is doing or planning. Blakeslee calls this blending personal space (Blakeslee and Blakeslee 2008: 135). Natural horsemanship employs this: the rider has only to look right – or even think it – for the horse to turn.

Is this information flow only through the neural networks? New work shows that the glial cells (which are part of the fascia), which make up 50% of brain tissue, are not simply providing mechanical and nutritional support, but interact in many ways with the neural tissue. The relationship between fascia and nerve tissue is a whole new field of current research (Oschman 2012). This linkage between the nervous system and fascia supports the speculation that consciousness travels in the fascia, and could link our consciousness to every cell.

### Attunement, resonance, and mirror neurons

But this connection between two people does not even need touch. When I returned to work following a long illness, having had a year in profound quiet, I somehow knew what was going on in my pupils from across the room, and only had to become conscious of their distress for it to change. This profound state was soon lost when I returned more to living in the outer world, but the essence of it has remained. This attunement to the state of another person, and the resonance that it creates between people, is being

# Relating and attuning to people for putting hands on others

studied by psychotherapists and neurobiologists as the field of interpersonal neurobiology. It is a key part of any deep relationship, and especially a good therapeutic relationship. Dan Siegel (2010: xx) identifies three primary steps to bring it about.

The first step is to *come present:* the process we explored in Chapter 15, where the nervous system comes to quiet, open to any possibility. When present we can flow easily between activity and quiet, so that we are always open to the unknown: it is a state of receptivity. To come present we have to feel safe, with the ventral parasympathetic in charge of the nervous system.

From there we can *attune to another person*, in which we take their current state into our own inner world to experience and understand it. Attunement happens from a place of presence, openness and with no judgement. If we are already fitting what we observe to some theoretical model, planning a course of action or worrying about outcomes, we are no longer present, receiving and attuning. Many of the games in this book are about attuning – whether to your own breath or body, visually to the world around you, or when scooping an object into the hand (exploration 9.12). Any time we are aware of coming into relationship, we are attuning.

The neurobiology of attunement with people has been hypothesized as follows (Iacoboni 2008, cited in Siegel 2010: 39). When we are present and receptive to another person, we are detecting myriad subliminal cues about their state of being from facial expression, intonation, timing and intensity of responses, gestures, body language and more. These are all thought to be detected by mirror neurons – the 20% of our motor neurons whose role is not to initiate action, but to create simulations in our own being of the other person's state. The information is carried via the brainstem and limbic areas into our bellies, our guts, heart and organs, our muscles and tissues, where it produces tensions, pains, emotions, changes in rhythms or speeds, to model the other person. This interoceptive information is then relayed back up to our posterior insula, and so to the anterior insula. As each part of the nervous system is included in this process it enables another quality of understanding, a fuller experience of the other person; then we can become conscious of the way we feel and can modify our response. This brings us to empathy with the other person. This only works when we come from a place of safety and can be informed by our interoception.

Then we have *come into resonance* with them and information flows between. In an experienced therapist, this right hemisphere embodied process can happen alongside left hemisphere rational observations and deductions, each feeding the other. When ideas or links are made by the left hemisphere, the intuitive processes check whether they fit with the pupil's state right now. When the rational path is uncertain, the intuitive systems can feel their way forward.

> While mainstream biological science doggedly continues to insist that consciousness is a product of the brain, many quantum physicists now understand consciousness to be an intrinsic part of the universe, pervading everything, and key to many processes. I feel sure that thought and consciousness will one day be understood as quantum processes. At this level of reality, there is no time and space. Many therapists and healers can attune and resonate with clients while they are not physically present. When I first learned this with reiki healing, my science head took a long time to believe and trust it. But, however much mainstream science distrusts it, this is a common experience – such as when you know who is phoning you before answering, or have a gut feeling that something is wrong with a loved one.

For the pupil or client, being experienced in attunement, without judgment, enables them to feel truly seen by the therapist. Then they can begin to trust, and through this feel safe to turn and face what is happening for them, to witness it, without reacting to fears. They can begin to understand their thought

# CHAPTER eighteen

and feeling processes, to name them, and find different responses to move forward. They can begin to move down the ANS ladder (Chapter 5) to a place of safety and a much stronger sense of self, from which they can build much more resilience.

Often, people have observed that Alexander work helps them be a nicer person. It is, in a sense, psychotherapy for the body. As we return to calm, we can allow ourselves to perceive our interoceptive processes, bringing self-engagement, and then can find our social engagement. Embodied speaking is a key part of this (Chapter 17).

Though this quality of resonant connection has been described for emotional processes, the quality of resonant physical connection that we strive for in AT work is identical. This makes sense since there can be no emotion without a physical response, and vice versa. All physical therapists need this understanding. Our clients are often frightened or angry as they encounter their pain or problem, or may bring past or present traumatic life events with them which is unconsciously affecting their behavior. I think that by not reacting to their emotions or physical tensions by tightening ourselves, but instead letting the feelings wash over us, experiencing and empathizing with them, we then model trust and safety for them as physical lengthening. In this we are re-parenting them, helping them find secure attachment (Chapter 5) during which they may be needy of us for a while. But this will pass as they find trust and safety in themselves and can again parent themselves, maintaining their own expanded use.

## Five key elements to bring about resonance with a pupil

The physical procedures we have worked with all act to lengthen, widen, and expand the body into responsive tone. But, as I hope you are discovering, this only works optimally if we are using the sensory and consciousness fundamentals as well as the physical ones: being calm to make embodied conscious choices, and linking with our expanded field of awareness – being both within ourselves and with our surroundings.

The process is the same with pupils. However well we learn to maintain our own lengthening and widening while touching, if we have reactivity to the pupil in any way, agendas to help them, or anxiety about our work, then we will either crowd them or pull back from them. We need to recognize such patterns and let them go so that, as I and others experienced with Miss Goldie, we can be anywhere in the room and yet fully present to our pupils; close in beside them and yet never crowd them. To do this, we need to embody several key elements that enable the state of resonance from which the work will flow. These bring all twelve fundamentals into play for ourselves and the pupil as we work. Explore them initially with a friend, colleague, or experienced pupil and see what you notice.

### Element 1   Starting a session – let them land in the room and attune to you

1   Let your pupil land

The moment of greeting a pupil is often a flurry of emotions. I show them into my workroom and often leave them for a minute to arrive in the space without having to focus on me. (It also gives me a moment to rebalance if needed.) The first requirement of our whole-body intelligence in a new environment is to map the surroundings. A small child – if allowed – will run around an unfamiliar room, checking out the corners, the furniture and objects, before beginning to notice and then interact with people. Where possible, it is good to give your client this time.

2   Let the pupil attune to you

Most AT lessons (and many other physical therapies) move immediately to touching the pupil, being in their personal space. While pupils agree to this contractually, I feel they are often being polite while subtly shutting down. We can unintentionally force our techniques on our clients. I prefer to sit a little way away for a few minutes and talk about their week and

# Relating and attuning to people for putting hands on others

issues, partly to get the chat out of the way and partly to allow them to attune to me, and me to them. Are they distressed? Do I sense they need the comfort of hands on, or need to find themselves? Are they calm and ready to engage with thinking and directing? If they are agitated I may do a lesson where I let them talk, but bring them to awareness of their physical responses to what is happening, guiding them gently into letting the breath deepen, the voice to soften or strengthen, the body to open, ground and lengthen up. I may guide them with hands on where the comfort of touch is required, or guide them verbally and through modeling to find it for themselves, which can empower them. Always I am engaging with any instruction myself, whether my hands are on or off.

3   Keeping the pupil's mind out of interfering – give them a job

"In lessons, FM attached enormous importance to the eyes; he was watching all the time to see if the pupil was going into a trance or a dream. He'd say to people, 'You're not looking out; you're not seeing something'" (Carrington and Carey 2004: 11).

### Exploration 18.1   Guiding your pupil's vision

- *Assuming the pupil is sufficiently calm, ask them to sit or stand but do not immediately put hands on. Instead verbally guide them – and yourself – to look at what is in front of them. To let their eyes track around without jumping or glazing, noticing textures, unexpected colors, etc., as in explorations 4.1 and 4.2. The language given there is precise – use it for your pupil until you find your own phrases.*

This now is their job. It helps to bring them – and you – to the present, to a place of calm focus, and keeps their minds from interfering in your work. It keeps them in spatial relationship to the surroundings, and so also to themselves and to you.

### Element 2   Finding spatial relationship to the pupil

One can do splendid parodies of a "bad" Alexander lesson, in which the teacher comes close in by the side of the pupil, then shuffles their feet into a grounded position. They focus on themselves for a few minutes, freeing their necks and finding primary control and a decent "monkey," until they notice the pupil again, lifting limp hands up carefully until flopping them onto the front and back of the person's chest. Then nothing happens again for a few minutes while they return to themselves and their directions in the hope of generating a response in the pupil, who is often feeling uninvolved and vaguely bored by the proceedings.

This is not what we want! In this parody, the teacher is alternating between their inner world and outwardly focusing on the pupil. There is no resonant connection between them to give intuitive guidance of what is needed. Without this, all work must be done through procedures, which may or may not be what the pupil requires. It is boring and repetitive. That point where one thinks – I've freed their neck, lengthened their arms, loosened the hips, what do I do next?

The paradox is that to make a resonant connection, one must give the pupil space. With the right spatial relationship, we can move in and out of a pupil's space while continuing to be present to them, yet always giving them freedom to expand.

### Exploration 18.2   The four spaces around the body

The idea that bodies were surrounded by an energy field was always rubbished by science, and our need for space – "elbow room" – was considered metaphorical. Blakeslee (Blakeslee and Blakeslee 2008: ch. 7) discusses our brain maps of the space around the body – named as our peripersonal space. This is a 3 ft (1 m) wide zone all around us – about an arm's length. Then scientists found a second mapped area another arm's length beyond that, which they named extrapersonal space. The brain detects clearly when objects or people come within these zones.

# CHAPTER eighteen

She also cites the cultural anthropologist Edward Hall, who identifies that in USA and Northern Europe we have four zones. Intimate space up to 18 in (50 cm) for touching; personal space, 18 in to 3 ft (0.5–1 m), for conversation with a close friend; social space 3 ft to 6 ft (1–2 m) such as when talking to a group of friends; and impersonal space outside this, for public lectures. These spaces can be bigger or smaller in different cultures or individuals.

- *Stand side on to your partner, about 10 ft (3 m) away, out of their space.*
- *Walk forward slowly, being aware of crossing firstly into their social space, then personal and finally intimate space. Then notice as you step backwards out of each in turn.*
- *Ask for feedback from your partner, can they feel it too? I have rarely found anyone who cannot feel these zones clearly.*

### Exploration 18.3    Background and foreground

When Americans were shown a picture of a tiger in a jungle, their eyes fixated on the tiger – they only saw the central feature, the foreground. When East Asians were shown the same picture, their eyes took in the jungle – the background – first, and only then fixated intermittently on the foreground (Blakeslee and Blakeslee 2008: 127). Seeing only the central image is more left hemisphere-led, while seeing the whole scene, the context and relationships in which the object moves, is more right hemisphere-led.

- *Concentrate fully on an object, switch off your peripheral vision. How does it feel?*
- *Now see the rest of the scene, using your peripheral vision only, but don't focus on the object. How does this feel? This is meditative seeing, calm but diffuse.*
- *Maintaining this background awareness, bring back the focus of the object. Notice whether you are now in spatial relationship to the object.*

### Exploration 18.4    Playing with this with a partner

"Habit can lead you to think you know someone – and that the background to her presence … is irrelevant. If … you allow your awareness to dilate such that the background gently shifts into the foreground of your attention, you will sensitize yourself to her presence in your life right now, in all its specificity" (Shepherd 2017: 191).

- *Stand side on to your partner, so they can feel the quality of your presence but not see directly what you are doing. Begin outside their space.*
- *Focus your eyes on them totally, losing your peripheral vision – the background, and walk in towards them till you are close. How do you and they feel? Most people really don't like this. Step back again.*
- *Now let your eyes have the background only, defocusing your partner, again walk in. Although this is initially more comfortable, people may feel you are ghost-like, invisible, which is also unsettling.*
- *Now while maintaining this background awareness, bring your focus back on them. Most people are very comfortable with this; they feel you there, in relationship but not crowding them.*

How we are seen by another person can determine how safe we feel. Over-focused seeing feels like a spotlight, with the potential for criticism (unless you love performing). With under-focused seeing, we can feel we do not matter (though people with low self-esteem can be more comfortable being invisible). When background and foreground are seen together it brings presence, allowing attunement and resonance. This way of seeing brings us into right relationship so the person feels seen and held. (People with attachment issues or trauma can have skewed responses to these, which can normalize with time as they find a stronger sense of self. See Chapter 5.)

# Relating and attuning to people for putting hands on others

### Exploration 18.5  Seeing from the whole-body for full embodiment

The root of the word "consciousness" is from the Latin *con-sciere* – to be mutually aware. In quantum physics, the Copenhagen interpretation is that observation brings something into being, and this is two way – it also brings us into being. I do not know of any objective biological research on this, but we can explore it subjectively.

- *Begin outside your pupil's space, and invite them to choose an object in front of them, say a vase while also maintaining background vision.*
- *Ask them to say: "I see the vase and the vase sees me."*
- *Ask them whether they are comfortable with this statement. Most people will be, though I have worked with several who were not. If this is so, leave it until their systems strengthen. If they are comfortable, then carry on, asking for feedback at each stage. Areas that are uncomfortable can indicate unresolved emotions/lack of embodiment, for example, overweight people often do not want their belly seen. This can resolve with a few repetitions of the sentence.*
- *Then do the same for each area of the body, inviting it to see and be seen by the vase. This may make no logical sense, but most people can sense it.*
- *"My chest sees the vase and the vase sees my chest." Then "my solar plexus sees …" my belly, hips, knees, feet, back, hands, heart – any part that feels appropriate.*
- *While talking them through this, you can check out your own embodiment vis-à-vis the pupil: "I see the pupil and the pupil sees me." Etc.*
- *Only when you can be comfortable with every part of you seeing the pupil are you fully present to them. When you are fully present in this non-judgmental way, you will be attuning to the pupil and receiving a stream of information to your right hemisphere and whole-body.*

I feel this exploration wakes up embodiment, brings the pupil fully present, and brings our whole being into relationship with the room and the pupil. I speculate that in this, the incoming visual information is mapped onto the spatial map of each body area.

### Element 3  Stepping out of our agendas around helping the pupil

Many therapists, particularly inexperienced ones, are keenly aware of the agendas in any session. One can feel a pressure to sort the client's pain and give value for money, to please or entertain them, not to offend them, etc. These may be your issues, while some clients steam with agendas that one can get drawn into. Stepping out of this requires maintaining our spatial relationships so we are not "pulled in." This gets harder the closer in we get to them physically, so we will explore this in stages. Goldie was insistent that I learn to "stay back" from pupils emotionally and energetically, and for a while, when putting hands on, I donned an imaginary space suit complete with gloves. It changed everything – my teaching life became much easier for me and more effective for the pupil.

When we truly get out of a pupil's way, and teach them to get out of ours, then we teach them to stand on their own two feet, without co-dependency games.

### Exploration 18.6  Creating space between self and pupil

> Video link for exploration 18.6

These explorations involve walking away from your partner, and then walking in and out again, without anything obvious happening. To explore this yourself with a pupil, stay behind them so they cannot see what you do, and keep talking them through vision games so they know something is happening. If they question what you are up to, ask how they feel: calmer? Relaxing? Expanding? When you give them space, they can physically open. The lesson is in progress.

- *Stand back from your pupil or partner and notice where you pull towards them.*

# CHAPTER eighteen

- *Walk away till you are right out of their personal space. Keep the sense of space between yourself and the pupil – if necessary, look away from the pupil to break the visual "pull," or turn completely away. Think: I can do nothing for the door/window, etc. in front of me. Or think of the pupil as being just like a vase of flowers, needing nothing from you. Have you now fully let go of emotional pulls towards them?*

- *Turn back to face them, keeping that detachment, and giving yourself permission to do nothing.*

- *See the background, then include them as foreground. See them from your whole-body. Your whole-body gives them space and sees, especially solar plexus, hips, feet. See what is actually there – with the eyes of an artist – light, form, texture, etc.*

- *Both we and they are letting go of all agendas for the lesson, expectations, etc. It can be useful to voice this.*

Fly pasts

- *Take a step towards the pupil – does anything change, in you or them?*

- *Do a "fly past," where you walk in through their spaces and out the other side. Can you do this with no response from either of you? Check in with your pupil, ask them what they notice. You could explain that we are waking up their self-observation of how we anticipate human interaction and touch.*

- *Now let your hand brush against a chair-back or wall as you pass it; be aware of the finger sensation. The hand just brushes, without making a tightening response. Walk past your pupil, likewise, brushing the back of their chair.*

- *Do the same but stop (without stopping) and leave the hand on the wall or chair-back, again without a tightening response. Then repeat on the pupil: your hand is doing nothing but is alive and sensing. Don't settle as you come to stand by the pupil.*

## Element 4    Putting hands – "put them where they are needed"

Alexander worked by first standing back and looking at the pupil, rather than by feeling into them with his hands. Erika Whittaker felt that in his last years, all Alexander's students were attempting to copy how he used his hands. He commented, "All they want to do, is to use their hands. But I am looking for the one who doesn't!" Whittaker described that instead, he worked with all his senses and his whole being. "I always think that he listened with his eyes and saw with his ears" (Taylor and Tarnowski 2000: 134). Erika gave workshops in which she taught us to stand back and look, and then respond.

### Exploration 18.7    Letting unconscious (intuitive) visual pathways inform you of what is needed

We are all processing vast swathes of information through unconscious brain pathways. When we come truly present to our pupils (or anyone else), information will be streaming from them about their physical and emotional state, which we take right into ourselves, process in the insula and then maybe bring it back to conscious awareness. We just know – say – that they are pulling down in their chest and that is where my hands are needed. These are quiet internal voices or impulses that initially we may think are imagined, but that we need to learn to trust.

- *Stand outside your pupil's space, probably side on, and just look at them, seeing background and foreground. Track round them, take in what you are seeing. Let your eyes and whole being absorb what you are seeing, and let go any agendas or protocols that you think you should work to. Just look, and absorb them into your being.*

- *What do they need in this moment? It could be a need to free a part of the body, move it, or simply be with it to help the tissues come alive.*

- *Before you move, while continuing to see them with background and foreground simultaneously, think that process in yourself first, so that the change or element is alive in you as you approach them.*

- *Then move to them, still seeing the background also, stop without stopping, and allow that to happen.*

# Relating and attuning to people for putting hands on others

### Exploration 18.8  Bringing the hands onto the pupil

In his article 'The teaching of Frank Pierce Jones, a personal memoir' (1982), Tommy Thompson describes a moment in his training.

"Frank explained that neither F. M. nor A. R. 'showed' him how to 'use' his hands. A. R., in fact, remarked that since Frank was fully capable of using himself, he was certainly capable of using his hands. '*But where do I put them?*' quizzed Frank. '*Put them where they're needed*' replied A. R."

I was taught on my training that to put hands on the pupil I was to come into "monkey," then let my wrists and elbows lead my limp hands onto the pupil. This is to confuse non-doing with not-doing; limp hands are switched off, and information from the back then cannot get through. Non-doing, embodied hands are enlivened without being reactive, and will communicate the whole-body. In rolling out of semi-supine (exploration 4.18), when picking something up (explorations 9.11–9.17), and in household tasks (exploration 16.6) our quiet, alive hands lead, in spatial relationship to our attention and intention, and we allow the whole-body to follow, morphing into movement. The process of putting hands on the pupil is no different.

- *While standing near the pupil and hands by your sides, do not go into a pre-prepared "monkey" position. Instead, bring mind to the brain, and find a spatial awareness of the full length of the arms. Then one can send the fingertips away, and the whole arm will stream after it.*
- *If the fingertips lead onto the pupil, to where the eyes see they are needed, then the body will morph into whatever position of mechanical advantage is needed to balance.*

Video link for exploration 18.8

### Exploration 18.9  Touching without being over-involved with the pupil

- *When we put hands, it is natural to think forward into the hands and into the pupil and so lose ourselves.*
- *With hands on the pupil, think of the touch balancing you. This keeps you in spatial relationship to them, and keeps you present to your whole self. Then information flows between you. (Thanks to AT teacher Bob Britton for this one; AMSAT conference, New York 2019).*
- *Keep seeing foreground and background. Foreground is no longer the whole pupil, but detail of clothing texture/ individual hairs or texture of skin. I notice that when these come into sharp focus, I come into resonance and information flows.*

### Exploration 18.10  Not responding to tensions

Once hands are on, we may try to move the pupil, but find nothing moves without a push. Often, joints are co-contracted, or there are restrictions in the fascia or muscles. Any of these will impede the kinetic chains or fascial continuities, so nothing flows. It is tempting to rub or manipulate such problem areas. But the real problem is not in the muscles and fascia themselves, but in the brain-patterning of the neuromuscular regulation.

A little piece of evidence for this is that under general anesthetic, restrictions of mobility lessen or disappear (Schleip 2012). The key is not to respond to the pupil's tensions or pain, which would pull you down into the problem, but instead to stay with your spatial awareness of yourself and your surroundings. This invites overall integration so that their whole-body and your whole-body are held in consciousness together. It invites their embodied intelligence to become conscious of the imbalance, from which it can begin to address it.

- *Now you have your hands on the pupil, balancing you. You are letting touch information inform you. You may be sensing tensions in the pupil's and/or your own body,*

# CHAPTER eighteen

which may make you want to move or make some other response.

- Instead, choose not to respond, but invite the areas concerned to do less, while you keep overall expansion patterns open in yourself. What happens?

- Stay there and let the process have time to work without any agenda of doing anything. Be aware when the process is complete, take your hands off again and step back.

## Element 5    Using directions and moving the pupil without interfering in the process

Have you ever given someone's car a jump-start? The jump-leads plug from one car battery to another, and the second battery kickstarts the first. In hands-on work, one might think the hands are doing the work. Instead, one's communicating hands are the jump leads, and one's whole-body aliveness is the car battery jump-starting the other car. It is the ongoing integration of the teacher's body that informs and generates integration in the pupil's body.

### Exploration 18.11    Preparation for moving a pupil – connecting up your muscle trains and spirals

- First find the movements required. Revisit weight transfer (exploration 11.8). The medial (inside) back of each knee leads away over the ball of the big toe to open all the leg spirals. Lead also with attentive, calm eyes to engage the head leading the body. These together keep both core muscles and extensor systems engaged, so that the torso works as a whole.

- Now revisit the arm oppositions of exploration 9.9. With the arms held up in front of you as if enclosing a ball of space, lead left with the tip of the left elbow, then right with the right one. Be aware of the deep back arm line opening and linking into the latissimus dorsi and other muscles, expanding and moving the whole back.

- Bring the wrists into this, rotating from the inside wrist (the very base of the thumb), so that this linked opening of the wrist also leads the movement. Anyone familiar with Tai Chi will know these spiraling movements well, and that they can take you anywhere.

- Play around with them for a while, going lower or higher, forwards or back, etc., keeping back in iliac spines, ribs, and back of armpits.

**Video link for exploration 18.11**

### Exploration 18.12    Directing movement of the pupil through your own body

Now we will find the same with hands on your seated pupil, first with hands on the chest, then around the neck. Once the principles are understood, you can work out other moves for yourself.

With the hands on front and back of the chest:

- Lead first to the left with eyes and head, left knee and big toe, elbow and wrist, and then to the right. Does your pupil come too, swinging in the hips?

- Does thinking back in your iliac spines, ribs and back of armpits help their hips open to move more freely? Invite them to send these thoughts too as they keep looking forward with spatial awareness.

- In this position, the wrists cannot make much rotation, but the intention will activate the connection.

With hands around the top of the neck:

- In this, the back hand wraps around the base of the occiput, linking physically and mentally to the superficial back line, the extensor line that takes us up.

- The front thumb and forefinger are just inside the jawbone, leading both the superficial front line of the body (which ends at the mastoid processes behind the ears) but also the deep front line through the floor of the mouth and throat. But the key is to focus a link here to the front of the spine itself (to the anterior longitudinal ligament – see Chapter 10, lesson 3, and exploration 6.6). (I understand that both Tai Chi and yoga teach that the deepest energy line in the body is an upward flow, and runs up the front of the spine.)

# Relating and attuning to people for putting hands on others

- *The other fingers of this hand can stretch down onto the sternum and ribs, sending messages to the torso to stay back when the head moves forward and up. This is multi-task thinking, which requires spatial awareness.*
- *Think of the two hands making a connection together through the pupil.*
- *When we intend to swing the pupil forwards in the chair, it is the front wrist that rotates to lead, while in opposition to this the hand maintains good physical contact with the pupil, and a felt sense of contact with the other hand (presumably through blended body maps and/or mechanotransduction). To lead the pupil back in the chair, lead from the back elbow and knee.*

Always you are keeping all your directions going, maintaining tone throughout, and softly inviting the pupil to do likewise; there is no need to pull. If we or they come into over-involvement with the body, this is when spatial awareness is lost, and the mind goes frantically running round the body firing out directions to try to keep it all together. When we maintain spatial awareness by seeing background and foreground, with embodied intelligence receiving our full body awareness, then these multiple directions happen naturally together for you and the pupil.

With the anatomy play and integration work of Part 2, we discover the lines of pull and opposition, bringing all the muscles into play. Then finding these directions from embodied intelligence will be easier, as the connections will be fully alive. I always explore the pulls involved with pupils before asking them to think directions, so that mind and body fully understand what is asked, and the connections are there.

We are looking for the pupil to swing easily in the hips, from responsive tone in the kinetic chains rather than from slack allowance in particular joints. Then you may find that if you take your front knee and wrist forward, the pupil will come with you and out of the chair. Keep inviting them not to interfere – to stay back in iliacs, ribs, back of armpits, and forwards and up from sacrum to T8, sitting bones to top of sternum, and T8 to crown, and they will follow up, out of the chair. We are working to get the pupil to stay with quiet tonic inhibition, to trust that the whole-body intelligence will self-organize us to extend upwards in dynamic flow. Once this basic move is achieved, it can be refined over many lessons, as the new anatomy described in Part 2 is taught and assimilated into their movement. You are teaching them to morph into movement – to use force matching and dynamic modulation of postural tone.

With time and experience, these dancing movements can become much more subtle. Footage of Alexander working does not show these outward Tai Chi-like moves, but I think they were happening internally. The more subtly the lateral aspects of the movements happen, the more the whole-body up-current is engaged as everything spirals together away from the ground and the pupil must come too. Then real core strength is built, strength in every level of our being, as those first teachers had.

## What inhibitory processes are we using?

When there is reactivity, from trying to follow preconceived ideas or habits (these probably link to the left hemisphere), then we need to "stop" physically and let these interfering thoughts go. Using reactive inhibition makes for a stop/go process.

But the right hemisphere-led processes of this chapter sidestep this, by bringing us to quiet, alive presence. Then we are in a flow state, and flowing the pupil along with us, in a symphony of interconnections. From discussion with Tim Cacciatore (see Chapter 4, lesson 2) I see this as a *state* of quiet tonic inhibition. If we or the pupil lose connection to this, by pulling down, making assumptions, trying to achieve a known goal, etc., then we need to pause the process. This allows the space to become aware of what has happened, and decide what new course to take: bring mind back to the brain, re-establish spatial awareness or new directions, etc. In this we may be using proactive or selective inhibition. In Miss Goldie's later lessons, her murmuring reminders were continually keeping me present yet uninvolved so that over perhaps twenty minutes of sustained work

# CHAPTER eighteen

there was no break in this flow state, and something completely different could be built.

## Summary for hands-on work with a pupil or client

For other therapists, some of this won't apply – the client may have eyes closed. But the key elements for yourself of keeping spatial relationship while attuning to your client, listening to intuitions alongside following protocols, and working on yourself alongside working on them, can bring more flow, connection and power to your work, while easing backs and wrists.

1. Coming to quiet, fully alive and present, is primary for all that follows.
2. Speak always from a fully embodied, resonant, modulated voice.
3. Give your pupil a job to stay present, probably vision work, and think it alongside them.
4. Rather than zoning in on the pupil, keep an expanded field of awareness as you work. Include all of your own body and the pupil's, the space behind you, the space behind the pupil, the rest of the room, etc.
5. Get your own springy, dynamic expansion going, using Initial AT procedures, ball games, vestibular directions, natural breathing or other methods.
6. See the pupil like a vase of flowers. See the detail of clothing, etc. without zoning in/peering. This brings space and connection together between self and pupil and enlivens everything.
7. Rather than having a pre-formed idea of procedures, step outside the pupil's personal space, observe them and attune to what is needed from your whole-body knowing. Work with right hemisphere intuition and left hemisphere knowledge together.
8. Step in beside the pupil, stopping without stopping, then allow fingertips to lead to bring the hands on in an alive way, balancing you, informed by your back and your springy legs.
9. Allow your arms and body to follow your fingers, morphing responsively into an appropriate position of mechanical advantage. Rediscover a working "monkey" or lunge, etc., each time they are needed. Let your legs be fully alive and responsive in this process, bending, stepping, or smoothly transferring weight as appropriate. The whole-body will be organized around the pupil, and will be continually reorganized as movement is made. This is a dynamic process; there are no pre-set movements.
10. Don't spend time "releasing" hands/shoulders, etc. Instead connect up your own body, and enliven your arms/hands/fingers by connecting them up to your back. You are like a battery with jump leads, your hands need a good connection to the aliveness of your back and springy legs.
11. Stay out of your usual habits, or creating new habits! Keep every moment real. Keep seeing.
12. When you sense an opening to move the pupil, go with it by directing or envisaging yourself to move, and let something happen. Let there be life in it!
13. Move your own body by envisaging the flow of movement upward from the ground through to the crown, and sending backs of knees, elbows, and wrists away so that the muscle trains all engage, and the pupil will come too.
14. When the life goes from what is happening, take your hands off: step back and start again.

*Each moment is an exploration into the unknown. Always be an explorer, as you discover the rewards of fully integrated movement for your yourself, and for your pupils or clients.*

# References

Alexander, F.M., 1985. *Use of the self.* (First publ. 1932, Methuen). London: Gollancz.

Alexander, F.M., 1987. *Constructive conscious control of the individual.* (First publ. 1923, Methuen). London: Gollancz.

Alexander, F.M., 2000. *Aphorisms.* London: Mouritz.

Alexander, F.M., 2011. *Man's supreme inheritance.* 7th ed. (First publ. 1910). London: Mouritz.

Alexander, F.M., 2015. *Articles and Lectures.* London: Mouritz.

Arshad, Q. and Seemungal, B.M., 2016. Age-related vestibular loss: Current understanding and future research directions. *Frontiers in Neurology*, 7: p. 231.

Baer, J., Vasavada, A. and Cohen, R., 2019. Neck posture is influenced by anticipation of stepping. *Human Movement Science*, 64: 108–22.

Balk, M., 2006. *The art of running. Raising your performance with the Alexander technique.* London: Collins and Brown.

Barlow, M., 2002. *An examined life.* Berkeley, CA: Mornum Time Press.

Barlow, M., 2011. *Alexander technique: the ground rules.* London: Hite.

Barton, R. and Venditti, C., 2017. Rapid evolution of the cerebellum in humans and other great apes. *Current Biology*, 27(8), pp. 1249–50.

Berger, J.M. et al., 2019. Mediation of the acute stress response by the skeleton. *Cell Metabolism.* 30(5), pp. 890–902.e8.

Berkowitz, A., 2016. *Governing behavior.* Cambridge, MA: Harvard University Press.

Bernstein, N.A., 1967. *The co-ordination and regulation of movements.* Oxford: Pergamon Press.

Blakeslee, S. and Blakeslee, M., 2008. *The body has a mind of its own.* New York: Random House.

Bojanek, E.K., Wang, Z., White, S.P. and Mosconi, M.W., 2020. Postural control processes during standing and step initiation in autism spectrum disorder. *Journal of Neurodevelopmental Disorders*, 12 (1).

Bordoni, B., Varacallo, M.A., Morabito, B. and Simonelli, M., 2019. Biotensegrity or Fascintegrity? *Cureus*, 11(6): e4819.

Bosco, G. and Poppele, R.E., 2001. Proprioception from a spinocerebellar perspective. *Physiological Reviews*, 81(2), pp. 539–68.

Bowman, K., 2017. *Move your DNA. Restore your health through natural movement.* USA: Propriometrics Press.

Brenner, E. and Smeets, J.B.J., 2001. We are better off without perfect perception. *Behavioural and Brain Sciences*, 24(2), pp. 215–16.

Buchanan, P.A. and Ulrich, B.D., 2001. The Feldenkrais Method: A dynamic approach to changing motor behavior. *Research Quarterly for Exercise and Sport*, 72(4), pp 315–23.

Cacciatore, T.W. et al., 2011. Increased dynamic regulation of postural tone through Alexander technique training. *Human movement science*, 30(1), pp. 74–89.

Cacciatore, T.W., Mian, O.S., Peters, A. and Day, B.L., 2014. Neuromechanical interference of posture on movement: evidence from Alexander technique teachers rising from a chair. *Journal of Neurophysiology* 112 pp. 719–29.

Cacciatore, T.W., Johnson P.M., and Cohen, R., 2020. Potential mechanisms of the Alexander technique. Toward a comprehensive neurophysiological model. *Kinesiology Review.* Available at: <https://doi.org/10.1123/kr.2020-0026> [Accessed 3 September 2020]

Cardinali, L., Brozzoli, C. and Farne, A., 2009. Peripersonal space and body schema: Two labels for the same concept? *Brain Topography*, 21, pp. 252–60.

Carrington, W. and Carey, S., 2004. *Explaining the Alexander technique.* London: Mouritz.

Cohen, R., 2019. "Science catches up": An overview of research on the Alexander technique. *General AT.* [online] 2 Sept. Available at: <https://www.alexandertechniquescience.com/general/overview/science-catches-up/> [Accessed 17 January 2020]

Corballis, M.C. and Haberling, I.S., 2017. The many sides of hemispheric asymmetry: a selective review and outlook. *Journal of the International Neurophysiological Society*, 23, pp. 710–18.

Craig, A.D., 2003. Interoception: the sense of the physiological condition of the body. *Current Opinion in Neurobiology*, 13(4), pp. 500–5.

Damasio, A., 2006. *Descartes error.* London: Vintage.

Damasio, A., 2010. *Self comes to mind.* New York: Pantheon books.

Damasio, A., 2017. *The strange order of things. Life, feeling, and the making of cultures.* New York: Knopf Doubleday.

Dana, D., 2018. *The polyvagal theory in therapy.* New York: Norton.

Dart, R.A., 1950. Voluntary musculature in the human body: The double-spiral arrangement. In: Dart, R.A., 1996. *Skill and poise. Articles on skill, poise and the Alexander technique.* London: STAT books. (First publ. *British Journal of Physical Medicine*, 14(12), pp. 265–8, Dec. 1950).

Delsarte, F., 1854. DC, box 1, folder 24/items 2–6, document 6, p. 9. In: Waille, F., 2009. *Corps, arts et spiritualité chez François Delsarte.* PhD. l'Université Jean Moulin-Lyon 3, France. (Language, French). Available at <https://scd-resnum.univ-lyon3.fr/out/theses/2009_out_waille_f.pdf> [Accessed 3 September 2020]

de Lussanet, M.H.E., Smeets, J.B.J., and Brenner, E., 2001. The effect of expectations on hitting moving targets: influence of the preceding target's speed. *Experimental Brain Research*, 137, pp. 246–8.

Dimon T., 2001. *Anatomy of the moving body A basic course in bones, muscles, and joints.* Berkeley, CA: North Atlantic Books.

Dimon, T., 2011. *The body in motion. Its evolution and design.* Berkeley, CA: North Atlantic Books.

Dimon, T., 2015. *Neurodynamics.* Berkeley, CA: North Atlantic Books.

Doidge, Norman., 2007. *The brain that changes itself.* New York: Viking Press.

Easten, P., 2004. *Lessons with Miss Goldie.* [Photocopied booklet]. Available at <http://alexandertechniqueinfo.org/shop-alexander-technique.html> [Accessed 18 January, 2020]

Easten, P., 2020. *A new history of the Alexander technique.* [blog]. Available at: <https://www.alexandertechniqueinfo.org/blog/> [Accessed 21 August 2020]

Eilbert, J.L., 2014. The vertebrate strategy for brain evolution. *Procedia Computer Science*, 41, pp. 233–42.

Evans, J.A., 2001. *Frederick Matthias Alexander. A family history.* Chichester, UK: Phillimore.

Ferber, R., Noehren, B., Hamill, J. and Davis, I., 2010. Competitive female runners with a history of iliotibial band syndrome demonstrate atypical hip and knee kinematics. *Journal of Orthopaedic & Sports Physical Therapy*, 40(2), pp. 52–8.

# References

Field, D., 2009. *The other brain*. New York: Simon and Schuster.

Fultot, M.P, Frazier, P.A., Turvey, M.T. and Carello, C., 2019. What are nervous systems for? *Ecological Psychology*, 31(3), pp. 218–34.

Gauthier, B., 2011. *Critical edition of manuscripts by François Delsarte and examination of their epistemological relevance in the formation of a modern scenic body*. [PhD. Montreal University of Quebec, Montreal. (Language, French)] Available at <http://www.archipel.uqam.ca/id/eprint/7835> [Accessed 21 January 2020].

Gazzaniga, M., 1998. The split-brain revisited. *Scientific American*. [online] Available at: <https://www.scientificamerican.com/article/the-split-brain-revisited/> [Accessed 20 January 2020]

Gershon, M., 2003. *The second brain*. New York: HarperCollins.

Goodale, M.A. and Milner, A.D., 2006. One brain, two visual systems. *The Psychologist*. 19, pp. 660–3. Available at: <https://thepsychologist.bps.org.uk/volume-19/edition-11/one-brain-two-visual-systems> [Accessed 16 January 2020]

Gopnik, A., 2016. Feel me. What the new science of touch says about ourselves. *New Yorker*, 16 May 2016.

Gracovetsky, S., 1988. *The spinal engine*. New York: Springer-Verlag.

Grillner, S., 1996. Neural networks for vertebrate locomotion. *Scientific American*. 274(1), pp. 64–9.

Grillner et al., 2008. Neural bases of goal-directed locomotion in vertebrates – an overview. *Brain Research Reviews*, 57(1), pp. 2–12.

Grunwald, P., 2010. *Eyebody. The art of integrating eye, brain and body*. 2nd ed. Auckland, NZ: Condevis publishing.

Guertin, P., 2012 Central pattern generator for locomotion: Anatomical, physiological, and pathophysiological considerations. *Frontiers in Neurology*, 3, p. 183.

Guimberteau, J.C., 2014. Strolling under the skin. [Video online] Available at: <https://www.youtube.com/watch?v=eW0lvOVKDxE> [Accessed 13 January 2020]

Gurfinkel, V.S., Cacciatore, T.W., Cordo, P.J. and Horak, F.B., 2011. Method to measure tone of axial and proximal muscle. *Journal of Visualized Experiments* (58), p. 3677.

Henderson, M., 2003. KP=CSP-(EnC(s+w+r+yn) +PsP(cr+sc+mt+xn)+PhS(ctw)… but will Jonny's magic formula work? *UK Saturday Times*, 15 Nov. p.1c

Herbert, N., 1994. *Elemental mind*. New York: Penguin.

Horak, F.B., 2006. Postural orientation and equilibrium: What do we need to know about neural control of balance to prevent falls? *Age Ageing*, 35(Suppl.2), pp. 7–11.

Hunter, J., 2013. The first training course in 1931, a different perspective. *Upward Thought*. [blog] 13 August. Available at: <https://upward-thought.com/category/history-and-development/> [Accessed 14 January 2020].

Johnson, P., 2019a. Debunking biotensegrity. [video online] Available at: <https://www.alexandertechniquescience.com/biomechanics/debunking-body-tensegrity/> [Accessed 11 January 2020].

Johnson, P., 2019b. The science of inhibition and end-gaining. *General AT*. [online] 9 Dec. Available at: <https://www.alexandertechniquescience.com/general/science-of-inhibition-end-gaining/> [Accessed 2 February 2020]

Jones, F.P., 2016 *Freedom to change. The development and science of the Alexander technique*. 3rd ed. London: Mouritz.

Kroliczak, G., Heard, P., Goodale, M.A. and Gregory, R.L., 2006. Dissociation of perception and action unmasked by the hollow-face illusion. *Brain Research*, 1080 (1), pp. 9–16.

Kulkarni, V., Chandy, M.J. and Babu, K.S., 2001. Quantitative study of muscle spindles in suboccipital muscles of human foetuses. *Neurology India*; 49, pp. 355.

Latash, M.L. and Turvey, M.T. eds., 2016. *Dexterity and its development, with 'on dexterity and its development', by Nicholai A. Bernstein*. Oxford, UK: Routledge.

Lee, I-M, Shiroma, E.J and Katzmarzyk, P.T., 2012. Effect of physical inactivity on major non-communicable diseases worldwide: an analysis of burden of disease and life expectancy. *The Lancet*, 380 (9838), pp. 219–20.

Lindstedt, S.L., LaStayo, P.C. and Reich, T.E., 2001. When active muscles lengthen: Properties and consequences of eccentric contractions. *News in Physiological Sciences*, 16, pp. 256–61.

Llinás, R., 2002. Prediction is the ultimate function of the brain. In: Llinás, R. 2002. *I of the vortex: from neurons to self*. Massachusetts: MIT Press. Ch. 2.

Longo, U.G. et al., 2013. Prevalence of accessory ossicles and sesamoid bones in hallux valgus. *Journal of the American Podiatric Medical Association*, 103(3), pp. 208–12.

Loram, I. et al., 2017. Proactive selective inhibition targeted at the neck muscles: This proximal constraint facilitates learning and regulates global control. *IEEE Transactions on Neural Systems and Rehabilitation Engineering*, 25, pp. 357–69.

Lou, D.W., 2014. Sedentary behaviours and youth: Current trends and the impact on health. *Active Living Research*, *Research Review*. [online]. Available on: <https://activelivingresearch.org/sedentaryreview> [Accessed 14 January 2020]

McAndrew, D., Gorelick, M., and Brown, J.M.M. (2006). Muscles within muscles. A mechanomyographic analysis of muscle segment properties within human gluteus maximus. *Journal of Musculoskeletal Research,* 10(1), pp. 23–35.

McDougall, C., 2009. *Born to run*. London: Profile Books.

McLeod, R., 1994. *Up from down under. The Australian origins of Frederick Matthias Alexander and the Alexander technique*. London: Mouritz.

McGilchrist, I., 2012. *The master and his emissary. The divided brain and the making of the Western world*. New Haven, CT: Yale University Press.

McNeill, D., 2012. *How language began. Gesture and speech in human evolution*. Cambridge, UK: Cambridge University Press.

McAndrew, D., Gorelick, M. and Brown, J. M. M. (2006). Muscles within muscles. A mechanomyographic analysis of muscle segment properties within human gluteus maximus. *Journal of Musculoskeletal Research*, Vol. 10, No. 1: 23–35.

Medline Plus. (2020). Guide to good posture [Online] <https://medlineplus.gov/guidetogoodposture.html> [accessed 20 August 20]

Mian, O.S. et al., 2006. Metabolic cost, mechanical work, and efficiency during walking in young and older men. *Acta Physiologica*, 186, pp. 127–39.

Miller, M. and Clark, A., 2018. Happily entangled: prediction, emotion, and the embodied mind. *Synthese*, 195(6), pp. 2559–75.

Milner, A.D. and Goodale, M.A., 1995. *The visual brain in action. (Oxford Psychology Series 27)*. Oxford: Oxford University Press.

# References

Moser, M.-B. and Moser E.I., 2016. Where am I? Where am I going? Scientists are discovering how the brain navigates. *Scientific American*, 314(1), pp. 26–33.

Murray, A.D., 2015. *Alexander's way*. Urbana, IL: ATCU.

Myers, T., 2014. *Anatomy trains. Myofascial meridians for manual and movement therapists.* 3rd ed. Edinburgh: Elsevier.

National Collaborating Centre for Primary Care (UK). (2009). Low back pain: Early management of persistent non-specific low back pain [Internet]. London: Royal College of General Practitioners (UK). (NICE Clinical Guidelines, No. 88.) Available from: <https://www.ncbi.nlm.nih.gov/books/NBK11702/> [Accessed 14 January 2020]

Nettl-Fiol, R. and Vanier, L., 2011. Primary and secondary curves. Looking at movement through a new lens. Excerpt from Chapter 4, in *AmSATNews*, Spring 2011, 85: pp. 28–31. *Dance and the Alexander technique: exploring the missing link.* Illinois: University of Illinois Press.

Ong, C.P., 2017. Spinal engine and waist power from Taijiquan viewpoint. *Journal of Integrative Medicine and Therapy*, 4, pp. 1–12.

Orlovsky, G.N., Deliagina, T.G. and Grillner, S., 1999. *Neuronal control of locomotion*. Oxford: Oxford University Press.

Oschman, J., 2000. *Energy medicine: The scientific basis*. Edinburgh: Churchill Livingstone, 2000: 46–8.

Oschman, J., 2012. Fascia as a body-wide communication system. In: Schleip, R., Findley, T.W., Chaitow, L. and Huijing, P., eds., 2012. *Fascia, the tensional network of the human body.* Edinburgh: Elsevier. pp. 103–10.

Ottiwell, F., 2016. Let us now praise Marjorie Barstow. In: Conable, B., ed. *Marjorie Barstow: her teaching and training: a 90th birthday offering.* 3rd ed. Mouritz, London.

Pert, C.B., 1998. *Molecules of emotion. Why you feel the way you feel.* London: Simon and Schuster.

Pineau, J., 2018. Understanding torque with Julien Pineau of StrongFit. [video online] [Accessed 10 January 2020]. Available at: <https://www.youtube.com/watch?v=j9KfETcuQTc>

Porges, S.W., 2011. *The polyvagal theory. Neurophysiological foundations of emotions, attachment, communication, self-regulation.* New York: Norton.

Porges, S.W., 2017. *The pocket guide to the polyvagal theory: the transformative power of feeling safe.* New York: Norton.

Porte, A., 1992. *Francois Delsarte. Une anthologie.* Paris: Editions IPMC.

Preece, S.J., Cacciatore, T.W. and Jones, R.K., 2017. Reductions in co-contraction during a sit-to-stand movement in people with knee osteoarthritis following neuromuscular re-education. *Osteoarthritis and Cartilage.* 25, S121.

Prochazka, A. and Ellaway, P., 2012. Sensory systems in the control of movement. *Comprehensive Physiology*, 2, pp. 2615–27.

Prochazka, A. and Yakovenko, S., 2007. The neuromechanical tuning hypothesis. In: Cisek, P., Drew, T. and Kalaska, J., eds., 2007. *Progress in brain research, Vol. 165.* Amsterdam: Elsevier BV. Ch. 16.

Reed, E.S. and Brill, B., 1996. The primacy of action in development. In: Latash, M.L. and Turvey, M.T., eds., 2016. *Dexterity and its development, with 'on dexterity and its development', by Nicholai A. Bernstein.* Oxford, UK: Routledge. pp. 435–9.

Robb, F., 1999. *Not to 'do'*. London: Camon Press.

Robinson, B., 1907. The abdominal and pelvic brain. [online] Available at: <https://archive.org/details/abdominalandpel00robigoog/page/n7> [Accessed 15 January 2020]

Rosenbaum, D, Cohen, R. Jax, S. Weiss, J. and Van der Wel, R., 2007. The problem of serial order in behaviour: Lashley's legacy. *Human Movement Science*, 26, pp. 525–54.

Scarr, G., 2018. *Biotensegrity, the structural basis of life.* Pencaitland: Handspring.

Stern, J.T. (1972). Anatomical and functional specializations of the human gluteus maximus. *American journal of physical anthropology.* First published: May 1972 Volume36, Issue3: 315-339. Issue Online:28 April 2005. https://doi.org/10.1002/ajpa.1330360303 [Accessed 9 December 2020]

Scheirling, R., 2017. Fascia as a proprioceptive organ and its relationship to chronic pain. Destroy chronic pain. [blog]. Available at: <https://www.doctorschierling.com/blog/fascia-as-a-proprioceptive-organ-and-its-relationship-to-chronic-pain> [Accessed 20 January 2020]

Schleip, R., 2012. Fascia as an organ of communication. In: Schleip, R., Findley, T.W., Chaitow, L. and Huijing, P., eds., 2012. *Fascia, the tensional network of the human body.* Edinburgh: Elsevier. Ch. 2.1.

Schore, A., 2003. The seventh annual John Bowlby Memorial lecture. Minds in the making: attachment, the self-organizing brain, and developmentally-oriented psychoanalytic psychotherapy. In: J. Corrigall and H. Wilkinson, eds., 2003. *Revolutionary connections. Psychotherapy and neuroscience.* London: Karnac.

Schultz, L. and Feitis, R., 1996. *The endless web. Fascial anatomy and physical reality.* Berkeley, CA: North Atlantic Books.

Sharkey, J., 2016. Ep. 55. A new paradigm of anatomy with John Sharkey. *Liberated Body podcast, by Brooke Thomas*. [podcast]. Available at: <https//:www.liberatedbody.com> [Accessed 10 January 2020].

Shepherd, P., 2010. *New self, new world.* Berkeley, CA: North Atlantic Books.

Shepherd, P., 2017. *Radical wholeness.* Berkeley, CA: North Atlantic Books.

Siegel, D., 2010. *The mindful therapist.* New York: Norton Books.

Sporns, O., 2010. *Networks of the brain.* Cambridge, MA: MIT Press.

Staring, J., 2005. *Frederick Matthias Alexander 1869-1955. The origins and history of the Alexander technique.* Nijmegen: Integraal.

Stebbins, G., 1885. *Delsarte system of expression.* New York: Edgard S. Werner.

Stern, J.T. (1972). Anatomical and functional specializations of the human gluteus maximus. *American Journal of Physical Anthropology,* 36 (3), pp. 315–39. [online: 28 April 2005] Available from: <https://doi.org/10.1002/ajpa.1330360303> [Accessed 9 December 2020]

Tasker, I., 1978. *Connecting links.* London: The Sheldrake Press.

Taylor, C. and Tarnowski, C., 2000. *Taking time: Six interviews with first generation teachers of the Alexander technique on Alexander technique training.* Denmark: Novis Publications.

# References

Thompson, T., 1982. *The teaching of Frank Pierce Jones, a personal memoir*. [online] Available at: <https://www.easeofbeing.com/the-teaching-of-frank-pierce-jones> [Accessed 17 January 2020]

Turvey, M.T., Fitch, H.L., and Tuller, B., 1982. The Bernstein perspective, I: The problems of degrees of freedom and context-conditioned variability. In: Kelso, J.A.S., ed., 1982. *Understanding human motor control*. Hillsdale, New Jersey: Lawrence Erlbaum Associates.

Turvey, M.T. and Fonseca, S., 2009. Nature of motor control: Perspectives and issues. In: Sternad, D. (eds.) *Progress in motor control. Advances in experimental medicine and biology, vol. 629*. Boston, MA: Springer.

Vasavada, A.N. et al., 2015. Gravitational demand on the neck musculature during tablet computer use. *Ergonomics*, 58(6), pp. 990–1004.

Vineyard, M., 2007. *How you stand, how you move, how you live*. Massachusetts: Da Capo Press.

Walker, M., 2017. *Why we sleep*. London: Penguin.

Westfeldt, L., 1985. *F. Matthias Alexander: the man and his work*. (Text copyright 1964). Long Beach, CA: Centerline Press.

Williams, C., 2018. 'The brain's secret powerhouse that makes us who we are. *New Scientist*, 4 July, 2018.

Williamson, M., 2015. Speaking with the tongues of men and of angels. In: Rennie, C. Shoop, T. and Thapen, K., eds., 2015. *Connected perspectives*. London: Hite, pp. 136–63.

Wolf, J., 2014. *Art of breathing*. [video download] Available at: <http://www.jessicawolfartofbreathing.com/rib-animation/>

Wolff, R., 2001. *Original wisdom. Stories of an ancient way of knowing*. Rochester, Vermont: Inner Traditions.

Wulf, G., 2007. *Attention and motor skill learning*. Champaign, IL: Human Kinetics.

Zügel, M., Maganaris, C.N., Wilke, J., et al., 2018. Fascial tissue research in sports medicine: from molecules to tissue adaptation, injury and diagnostics: consensus statement. *British Journal of Sports Medicine* 52, p. 1497.

# Index

## A

*The Abdominal and Pelvic Brain* (Robinson), 82
abdominal cavity, 116f
abductor muscles, 166f, 170
Achilles tendon, 50f–51, 120, 155
action muscles, 37–38
active hip folding, 203, 209f–210, 272, 273f, 275, 281–284
adaptive tone, 111, 271, 281–282, 316, and see responsive tone
adductor muscles, 63, 164, 168, 169f, 171, 206–207f, 207f, 214, 221f, 223f, 229–230
Alexander, Frederick Matthias (F.M.), 19, 61, 64, 78, 90, 127, 131f, 145f, 153f, 238, 255, 257, 258f, 277, 325, 331, 340
    *Constructive Conscious Control* (CCC), 128–129
    directions, 47, 92, 187, 267, 274, 281, 284, 286–287
    development of AT, 7–9, 75–76, 125–129, 141, 286, 333
    fundamental concepts, 16, 19, 21, 25, 28, 60, 70, 72, 75, 103, 141, 240, 308
    *Man's Supreme Inheritance* (MSI), 128–129
    procedures, 60, 126, 212, 256–258
    quotes and book refs., 9, 60, 75, 92, 126, 128, 129, 141, 145, 146, 180, 198, 205, 212, 249, 255, 263, 267, 274, 277, 284, 292, 312, 321, 330
    *The Use of the Self* (UoS), 129, 141, 277, 285
Alexander, A.R., 128, 212, 333, 341
Alexander technique, 7–9, 79, 96, 128, 197, 307, 326, 336, 337
    modern/mainstream AT, 9, 60, 89–90, 129, 212, 237, 277, 292
    re-evaluation of, 5, 284–287, 315
    teaching tips, 64–66
anatomical surprises, 145, 152, 266
*Anatomy of the Moving Body* (Dimon), 66, 180
*Anatomy Trains*® (Myers), 50, 66, 132
animal body movements, 21–22, 225, 305, 307
ankles, 43f, 150f, 164f, 170–174, 173f, 177, 219–221, 220f, 224, 263–267, 275
antagonistic action, 105–106, 128
antagonistic balance of lengthening forces, 53
anterior superior iliac spines, see iliac spines
"anti-gravity" (force), 48, 88, 211
"anti-gravity" line, 88–89
armpit, back of, 179, 181, 185, 187, and see ribs at back of armpit
arms, 193, 237–239, 247–248, 251–254f
    alignment, 132–135f, 139, 239f, 252–253f, 274
    classic AT procedures for, 256, 257f, 258f
    lines, 181, 182f, 189f, 282f, 283, 284f
    pendular, 212–213f, 253, 271
    walking/running, 217, 218f, 225–227, 230–231f, 234
arousal states, 95–101
*Art of Breathing* (Wolf), 66, 105, 111
atlanto-occipital joint, 43–46, 44f, 45f, 121f, 153, 277, 285, 286
attachment, 20, 99, 336, 338
attention, 4, 15–18, 22, 27–28, 69–70, 72, 81, 84, 85
    feeds brain-maps, 29, 307–309
    left hemisphere/fragmentary, 15–17
    organizes body response, 87–89, 316–319, 321
    sustained, 70, 73, 181, 310, 338, 341
attuning, 28, 65, 315–316, 322, 334–336, 338
autonomic nervous system (ANS), 20, 69, 82, 95
    dorsal/ventral branches (dPNS), see PNS
"autopilot" mode, 29, 73, 81, 299, 312
awareness, see spatial awareness, expanded/unified field of awareness
awareness of body, see proprioception, interoception
awareness vs feeling, 76–77
axis joint, 45–47, 46f, 69, 133, 277, 286
Arshad, Q. and Seemungel, B.M., 161

## B

back muscles, three layers to, 37, 38f, 39f, 40f
back (stays) back, 213, 222f, 230f, 250, 270
Baer, J., Vasavada, A. and Cohen, R., 308
balance, 159–161, and see flow of dynamic balance; head/neck balance
    control mechanisms of, 61–62, 161–162
balance organs, 15, 159, 161–162, and see vestibular system
balancing with touch, 161–162, 341
Balk, Malcolm, 217, 226
Bojanek, E.K. et al., 161
ball of big toe, 164, 168–169f, 171f, 172, 173f, 222f, 287
Barlow, Marjory, 9, 25, 90, 129, 153, 212, 285, 333
Barstow, Marjorie, 72, 285
Barton, R. and Venditti, C., 22
Bates's natural vision technique, 8, 105
beginner's mind, 6, 33, 73, 294, 310
belly brain, 19, 74, 83f, 103
belly muscles, four layers of, 205, 206f
Berger, J.M. et al., 97
Berkowitz, A., 104
Bernstein, Nikolai, 20–21, 54–55, 131, 321
Best, Robert, 153, 240
Bible creation story (Genesis 1), 19–20
biomechanics, 20, 48, 52, 58, 131, 238, 261, 286
biotensegrity model/theory, 20, 52–54, 53f, and see tensegrity
biotensegrity, Living, 54
bipedalism, 22, 63, 104
Blakeslee, S. and Blakeslee, M., 20, 22, 66, 74, 79, 86, 160–161, 188, 313–314, 317–318, 334, 337–338
body as gravity-stacked structure, 48–49f
body geometry, 55, 126, 132–135f, 131f, 133f, 138f, 154, 176f, 238, 239f, 240, 243f, 244, 250, 253f, 274
*Body in Motion* (Dimon), 66, 180
body maps, 78, and see brain maps
body schema, 79, 86, 160–161, 316, 320
Bordoni, B. et al., 54
Borneo, 3–4, 6, 8, 41, 88, 136
*Born to Run* (McDougall), 156, 217
Bosco, G. and Poppele, R.E., 61–62
boss in the office, 75, 78, 111
bottom-up (experiential) processing, 14, 16–19, 20, 21, 111, 299
bouncing, 41, 103, 120, 121f, 122, 145, 150, 154–157, 272
Bowman, Katy, 12, 15, 66, 131, 136, 153, 154, 166, 170, 177, 203, 205, 217, 238, 263
brachiation, 22, 104
brain/body intelligence network, 24, 82, 83f, 92, 141, and see whole-body intelligence
brain/body links, 125, 126, 136, 179, 301
brain/cortex, control of movement, 5, 13, 19, 54–55, 61–62, 103, 110–111, 122, 277, 297–299, 305–310, 319–322 and see control, theories of movement
brain/nervous system, evolution of, 22, 80–81, 103–104
    communication network, see networks
brain, and see forebrain/hindbrain; hemispheres; mind in the brain
    inhibition, 70–73
    maps/body maps, 26–27, 74, 78, 86, 160–161, 298–299, 305–307, 309, 313–315, 317–318, 334, 336, 337, and see brainstem body maps
    messages getting through, 76–77, 93, 301
    plasticity, 5, 20, 73, 316–317
    programming/programs, 93, 126, 127, 141–145, 266, 274, 291
brains, head/cranial, heart and belly, 19, 74, 82–84, 83f, 100, 103
brainstem body-maps, 26, 305–309, 317
brainstem/spinal cord and movement control, 20, 28, 61–62, 70, 86, 88, 110–111, 280, 305, and see control of movement theories
breathing, 15, 99–100, 109f, 104–112, 143, 251f, 280
    action of diaphragm, fixed and floating ribs, 108–112, 109f
    and speaking, 327–328
    and swimming/walking/running, 110, 119, 221
    from the back, 138f, 146, 251f
    from pelvic floor, 114–117, 116f
    imbalanced/false breathing patterns, 105, 106–107, 138t, 294–295
    into top of lungs, 247, 254–256
    natural, 8, 80, 104–106, 108–112, 114, 117, 119, 143, 221, 254, 292, 295, 344
    natural support for, 107, 115–116
    postural support from, 106, 108, 114–115, 249
    relation with nervous system, 99–100, 107–108
    stopping or straining, 107, 294–295
    to widen front of chest, 248–249, 251f
Brenner, E. and Smeets, J.B.J., 297
Britton, Robert, 162, 329–330, 341
Brown, Graham, 103–104
Buchanan, P.A. and Ulrich, B.D., 28

## C

Cacciatore, Tim, 20, 62, 71, 100, 113–114, 160, 197, 285, 315–316, 343
calf muscles, 47f, 50f, 51, 120, 200, 221
calm nervous system, 22, 23f, 24, 26, 95, 104, 132
Cardinali, L. et al., 315
Carrington, Walter, 131, 145, 153, 256, 337
catching a ball, 292–297, 294f, 300–301, 305, 308, 309–310, 316, 318, 321
Cathcart, James, 126
cat's body movements, 21–22, 291
central pattern generators (CPGs), 5, 20, 28, 61, 103, 110, 122, 305–307, 313
cerebellum, 19, 61, 62, 83f, 104, 286, 299
cervical (neck) spine, 133f, 238
chair, getting in and out of, 33, 197, 201–203f, 213, 269–270, 343
child's pose, 115, 175, 281–283, 282f, 286
Chinese/East Asian worldview, 52, 338
choices, 5, 21, 25, 70, 74, 75, 128, 302, 307
    and true stop/"no" games, 291–292, 311–312
    clear (brain), 22, 24, 27, 70–71, 82, 84

# Index

embodied conscious, 23f, 336
unconscious, 81
chronic fatigue syndrome (CFS), 7, 8
clavicles, 132, 180–181, 183, 244–249, 245f, 246f, 247f, 254, 258, 269, 279, 286
co-contraction, 38, 41, 60, 71, 121–122, 148, 218, 272, 278, and arthritis, 218
Cohen, Rajal, 71, 113, 309
come to quiet, 69, 95, 111, 286, 291, 293–297, 302, 308, 310–313, 315, 325, 335, 344
communication network, see networks
compensatory movement patterns, 41, 52, 60, 110, 165, 168, 217, 229
compressive forces of gravity, 49f, 51–52
concentric contractions, 106, 112, 113f, 155
connection process, learning as, 30, 300, 321–322
conscious (guidance and) control, 55, 126, 141, 238, 272, 274, 321
consciousness, 14, 18, 21, 23f, 26–27, 73, 77, 79–82, 84, 89, 96, 161, 298, 310, 334–336, 341, and see embodied consciousness
and directions, 128
and tone/balance, 89, 120, 155, 161, 181
building new habits of, 312–313
cloud, 80, 79, 91
definitions, 27, 339
fundamentals, 23f, 24, 26–27, 336
primary, 19, 20
taking deeper into body, 82, 115, 206–207
consciousness in fascial network, 80, 334
constructive conscious control, 25, 126, 127, 157
*Constructive Conscious Control* (CCC), 128–129
contraction, three types of muscle, 112, 113f, and see concentric; eccentric; isometric
patterns of, 35, 36f, 37f
phasic and tonic muscle, 113–114
control, theories of movement, see balance, control mechanisms of; brain/cortex; brainstem/spinal cord; central pattern generators, posture
coordination, 28–29, 61, 103, 113, 145, 152, 161, 223, 293, 297–298, 302, 305–309,
optimal, 55, 297, 305
new model of in catching ball, 309–310
Corballis, M.C. and Haberling, I.S., 18
core muscles, 61, 100, 106, 112, 115, 117, 159, 164, 171, 198, 201–202, 205–208, 225, 287, 342
cortex, parietal and body-maps, 78, 86, 317
cortical control/patterns vs hindbrain pathways, 72, 110–111, 113, 233, 299, 302, 316, 320
costal arch ribs, 108–109f,132f–133f, 240f, 255–256f, 287
counter-rotating the thighs, 172–4, 177, 200f, 201f, 287
Craig, A.D., 74
craniosacral therapy, 8, 62, 82
critical voice, 33, 134
crown of head, 47, 120, 286, 343–344
curve patterns, 58, 60, 101, 130, 132, 135, 136–7, 154, 214 and see primary curve; secondary curve

## D

Damasio, Antonio, 20, 74, 103, 307
Dana, Deb, 20, 99
Dart, Raymond, 50, 52, 56
Darwin, Charles, 19, 20
decisions, 71, 74, 81–82, 84, 88, 129, 293–294, 296, 305, 307, 310–311, 314, 316, 320, 331

deep back arm line (DBAL), 138, 181, 182f, 185–189f, 186f, 244, 251, 282f–284f
deep cervical flexors, 40, 208, and see longus colli and capitis
deep front line (DFL), 61, 63, 198, 205–208, 207f, 221f, 227f, 228f, 230f, 269–270, 286
deep hip rotators, 171, 173f, 175, 208, 287
default patterns/settings, 34, 73, 141, 293
Delsarte, Camille, 126
Delsarte, François, 9, 63, 75, 125–128, 130, 135, 141, 143, 156, 170, 261, 277, 319
Delsarteism, 125
deltoids, 38, 40f, 55, 63, 118, 182f, 186, 190
de Lussanet, M.H.E., 297
depth perception, 85, 87, 106, 119, 142–143
Descartes, René, 13, 19–20, 81
descriptive anatomy, 48–49
descriptive muscle theory, 57
Dewey, John, 128
diaphragm, 63, 95, 105, 108, 109f, 111, 114, 115, 116f, 204, 207–208, 221, 292
digestive system/digestion, 5, 95–98, 103
Dimon, T., 66, 175, 180, 280
directions, 8, 46–47, 72, 131, 277, 284–287, 292, 311, 319, 331, 337, 342–344
"all together, one after another", 9, 141, 284
and Initial AT, 126, 128, 135–136, 141–142, 146, 266, 274–275
defining, 25, 92–93,
integrated, 141–145, 152, 156, 284–285
Doidge, Norman, 20, 73, 317
doing or non-doing, 197, 198, 237, 341
dorsal/ventral PNS, see parasympathetic nervous system (PNS)
double spiral of muscle, 56–57
dynamic modulation of postural tone, 24, 28, 30, 61–62, 72, 88, 106, 113, 315, 343

## E

eccentric contractions, 61, 114, 155–156, 112, 113f
Eilbert, J.L., 104
elastic recoil/elasticity, 61, 109, 121, 154
elastic resistance, 61, 121, 125, 154–156, 262, 264–265, 270–271
elbow, 132, 133f, 137–139, 183, 186, 247, 252–253, 257–258, 275, 341–344
as lever on back muscles, 137, 138f, 139f
oppositions with, 192f, 194f, 245f
pull to the, 127, 184f, 187–188f, 256f
"string", 184f–185, 188f
embodied consciousness, 27, 81–82, 93, 155, 201, 336
embodied intelligence, 23f–24, 80, 198, 206, 320, 341, 343
embodied speaking, 6, 325, 329–331, 336, 344
embodiment, 23f–25, 27, 69, 78–82, 87, 100, 296, 309, 316, 326, 339
definition, 79
emergent movement, 28, 145, 150, 152, 316
emotional awareness, 73–75
emotions, processing, 81–82, 101, 335–336, 339–340
empathy/empathizing, 20, 335–336
"end-gaining", 25, 160, 308–309, 313
erector spinae, 12, 13f, 14f, 38f, 39f, 47f, 50f, 51, 57f, 62, 63, 116, 117, 119f, 153, 203–204f, 210, 261, 268, 278, 287
Evans, J.A., 127

evolutionary hypotheses and perspectives, 19–20, 95–96, 103–104, 156, 225
expanded/unified field of awareness, 77, 127, 143–144, 156, 336, 344
experiential learning, see learning processes
experiential processing, 14, 18, 30
external perception/exteroception, 15, 23f, 24, 26, 74
extensor system, 62, 232, 266, 342
EyeBody Method®, 8, 85, 160, 326
eyes and balance, 160–162
and emotions, 81, 97, 98, 100, 292
eyelids, lowering the, 160
seeing, 76, 78–79, 85–86, 114, 298–301
tracking, 15, 44–46, 69–70, 88–93, 100
use of, and F.M. (Alexander), 337
eyes/perception lead head/movement, 8, 44, 45f, 69–70, 88–89, 157, 221, 285, 291, 305, 307–308, 342

## F

FACTISPAL acronym, 127, 198
Farkas, Alex, 277, 325
fascia, 21, 34, 48, 50–51, 54, 62, 80–82, 117, 155, 334, 341, and see thoracolumbar fascia
fascial continuity/network, 23f, 24, 26, 54, 82, 334
fascintegrity, 26, 54, 58
faulty sensory perception, 16–17, 33–34, 41–42, 70, 81, 89, 107, 126, 140, 152, 242, 244, 320
feedback (pathways), 61, 161, 296, 306, 309, 315–316, 319–320
feed forward (pathways), 161, 302, 306, 308, 315–316
feet,
anatomy of, 155, 162–163f, 170, 227–228
lifting the arch, 174
placement of, 168, 170–174, 172f, 173f, 175–177, 263, 271–272, 275, 307
stability of, 153, 162–164, 170, 227
walking, 217–224, 227–230, 232–233, 307
feet and legs while sitting, 199–202, 200f
Ferber, R. et al., 174
fibularis longus, 57f, 166f, 173f, 174, 200
Field, Douglas, 80
fight/flight system, 95–96, 97, 99, 105, 107, 295
finger checks and tests, 211, 269–270, 281
fingers/fingertips leading, 91, 246, 257, 266, 268, 285, 341, 344
fingers, oppositions with, 187–189, 188f, 191–193, 192f, 252, 257, 283–284
first principles, working from, 73, 294
first training course, 8, 9, 78, 153f, 238, 240, 285, 331
Fischer, Jean, 129
flexibility vs mobility, 198
flexor and extensor chains, 51
flexor system of arms, 186–188f, 283
floating ribs, 105, 108–109, 111, 133f, 204, 255, 287
flow of dynamic balance, 58, 60, 88, 154, 289, 310, 320
flow state, 97–99
focus,
attentional/external/internal, 318–320
clear focus of intent/attentiveness, 23f, 24, 27, 88
narrow, 15–16
over/under focus, 100, 308, 312, 322, 338
force of contraction, sensing, 33, 61
force-load, 51, 52
force matching, 315–316, 343

# Index

forebrain/hindbrain, 30, 72, 110, 113, 302, 315, 320
forward-held head, 35, 153, 280–281
forward neck and head, 38, 45f, 308
freeing the neck, see neck, freeing the
free movement, 3–5
free will, free won't, 74
freeze state, 96, 97t, 99, 105
frisbee throw, 57, 226f, 227f
front of the shoulder (FSh), see shoulder, front of
Fuller, R. Buckminster, 52
fully responsive action, 297
Fultot, M.P. et al., 321–322
functional anatomy, 21, 50, 163, 179–180, 198
functional line, 63, 193f
fundamental bend, 87–89, 312

## G

Gauthier, B., 125
Gazzaniga, M., 17
Gershon, Michael, 82
gesture, 20, 141, 156–157, 194–195f, 335
gluteal muscles, 12, 14f, 38, 148, 229
gluteus maximus, 13f, 40f, 63, 117, 118f, 149, 166f, 171, 193f, 217, 228
    upper/superior part, 168, 170, 214
gluteus medius, 166–170, 167f, 168f, 169f
going up on toes, 126, 164, 172, 174, 228f
Goldie, Margaret, 7, 9, 25, 69, 82, 105–106, 128–130, 135, 153, 179, 198, 237, 257, 285, 286, 192, 325–326, 333, 336, 339, 343
    approach to structural work, 118–119, 125–127, 131, 152, 180, 199, 212, 258, 261–262, 264–265, 268, 269, 292
    key teaching ideas, 27–29, 49, 71–73, 75–78, 92–93, 199, 277, 292, 294, 302, 310, 311, 313
    quotes, 64, 73, 75, 95, 118, 268, 277, 291–292, 301, 302, 313, 325
    tablework, 90, 118, 153, 208
    teaching on "stopping", 6, 28, 292
Goldie's procedures, 159, 162, 165, 212
Goodale and Milner, 20, 298–299
Gopnik, A., 84
"grab and go" culture, 179, 189
Gracovetsky, S., 225
gravity, and see compressive forces of gravity; "anti-gravity",
    alignment of body with, 41, 51–52, 88, 130–136, 154, 159, 161, 201, 264, 268
    fighting, 35, 38, 41, 62
    force, 49, 51, 88, 172, 243
Grillner, Sten, 20, 104, 110, 122, 306
grounding, 69, 86, 96, 99–101, 118, 153, 254, 284, 287, 309, 315, 337
ground reaction force, 51, 218f
Grunwald, Peter, 8, 66, 85, 100, 160, 326
Guertin, P., 62
Guimberteau, Dr. Jean Claude, 80
Gurfinkel et al., 62

## H

habits, changing our, 15–16, 18, 70, 73, 312
habits, unlearning/inhibiting, 19, 28, 302
hamstrings, 14f, 47f, 50f, 63, 148–152, 155, 171, 217, 222f, 228–229, 261–262, 267f, 270

releasing and toning, 150f, 151f
hands, and see fingers and palms
    catching, 292–297, 294f, 300–301, and see catching a ball
    functional anatomy, 183, 190–191
    on pupil, 54, 126, 128, 333–334, 337, 339–344
    on the back of a chair, 126, 129, 256–257f
    upturned on thighs, 257–258f
    use of, 28, 33–35, 179, 188–195, 189f, 190f, 191f, 192f, 194f, 195f, 237, 252, 308, 312–313
head,
    centre of gravity of, 43, 44f
    forward and up, 44f, 128, 145, 153, 238, 240, 242, 277–278, 281, 283f–284, 286–287, 343
    rebalancing of, 43–45
    stability of, 226
head-neck-back relationship, 103, 129, 225, 292
head/neck balance, 43-47, 46f, 51, 129, 153, 277–278, 280–281, 285–286
healing methods, establishing processes, 64–65
heart brain, 74–75, 82–84, 83f
heel strike, 217f, 218f
hemisphere of brain, right, 23f, 98
hemispheres of brain, 27, 29–30, 33, 35, 77, 83f, 99, 291, 298, 309–311, 322, 335, 338, 343–344
    and inhibition, 71
    McGilchrist's theory of, 16–19
    space/time processing, 17, 70, 296, 310
Henderson, M., 306
Herard, Louise, 325
Herbert, N., 84
hip joint, 42, 43, 92–93f, 165–167, 171, 175, 212, 218–219, 261f–262, 264, 267, 269–270, 287
hip laterals, 166f–170, 214, 219f, 222f, 223, 229f, 287
hip lifts, see pelvic lifts
hip stabilizers, 159, 165–168, 177, 197, 232
homeostasis, 55, 82, 95, 98, 307, 315
Horak, F.B., 161
human evolution, 22–23, 103–104
hump, the, 153, 238
Hunter, John, 105

## I

"I can do less", 71–72, 101, 107
ideomotor theory/responses, 128, 310
iliac spines (anterior superior), 133f, 157, 243, 261, 274
    and counter-rotating thighs, 173f
    and transverse abdominals, 146–147f, 175
    and unity line, 130, 132f, 134f,
    and walking, 155, 214, 222, 231–232
    inclining back/forward on chair, 210–214, 270–272f
    opening lumbar spine, 111–112, 151f–152, 240f, 254, 261f–262f, 264–267f, 265f, 272–273f, 287
iliac spines, posterior, 147f, 214
iliacus, 115, 116f, 171, 203, 204f
iliotibial tract (IT band), 56f, 57f, 166f–168, 170, 173f, 174, 214
inhibition, 24, 25, 27–28, 30, 70–71, 92, 100, 103, 125, 132, 141, 266, 274, 308, 316, 321, 326, 343
    and brain hemispheres, 71
    as process or state, 71, 291, 343
    executive/reactive, 30, 71, 291–292, 311, 343
    giving negative directions to activity, 72
    to change patterns of use, 70–73, 334

tonic, 30, 100, 105, 292, 297, 300–302, 306, 311, 315, 343
inhibitory process, deeper, 30, 71, 143
Initial Alexander technique (Initial AT), 93, 125–157, 179, 198, 237, 238, 243, 257, 261, 272, 274–275, 280–281, 292, 344
innate brain/motor pathways, 285, 291
instep, 132, 134f, 170–174, 171f, 173f, 200f, 202, 228f, 234, 263–264, 266–268f
    in walking, 217f, 220f, 229f
integrated movement, 23f, 24, 29–30, 156, 225, 278, 306, 315–316, 344
integrated change, making, 93, 141–144, 149, 152
intercostal muscles, 105, 108, 166f, 287
internal awareness/perception, 17, 18, 20, 24, 26, 96
interoception/interoceptive awareness, 15, 23f, 25–26, 73–75, 96, 98, 100, 335
interpretation vs experience, 18
intuition/intuitive processes, 15, 24, 30t, 65, 74, 82, 97f–98, 100, 315, 335, 337, 340, 344
IT band, see iliotibial tract
isometric contractions, 112, 113f

## J

James, William, 128
jaw, freeing of, 46–47, 107, 208, 269, 281
Johnson, Patrick, 54, 71, 100, 113
joint receptors, 33, 42
Jones, F.P., 66, 292, 333, 341
Jull et al., 40

## K

Kallen, Horace, 128
kinematics, 55, 243, 305
kinetic/kinematic muscle chains, 21, 23f, 50, 55, 58, 60, 88, 278, 280, 315, 341, 343
kinetics vs kinematics, 243
knees,
    alignment of, 172–174, 177, 199–203, 275
    away/in, 36f, 173f, 174, 200f, 203, 211, 277, 287
    forwards, 93, 118, 121f, 147f, 219, 223f, 241f, 277, 287
    freeing of, 42, 177
    in stabilizing torso tilt, 261–273f, 262f, 267f, 272f
    in walking, 118–119, 220f, 232, 233f, 263
    to initiate movement, 60, 221, 342–344
Kulkarni, V. et al., 277
Kuperman, Yehudah, 93

## L

ladder of the ANS, 96–101, 97f, 336
ladybird, 88–89, and see visual arc
Langley, John, 82
language, development of, 20, 22
Latash, M.L. and Turvey, M.T., 321
lateral line (LL), 63, 166f, 174, 203f, 214, 230f, 278–279, 287
latissimus dorsi, 38, 40f, 58, 63, 117, 118f, 119f, 180, 182f, 184, 190, 193, 204, 227f–228, 287, and see "lifter muscles"
Lawrence, Esther, 128

351

# Index

learning (processes), 4–5, 13–15, 18, 21, 29, 30, 55, 64, 113, 274, 296, 299–300, 311, 313, 316, 318, 321
    as process of connection, 30, 300, 321–322
    models of, 316–322
Lee, I.-M. et al., 12
leg spirals, rebalancing, 168, 170–174, 173f, 177, 199–200, 226, 229f, 230f, 342
    and pain/soreness, 177
lengthening antagonistic relationships, 24, 26, 29–30, 155, 179, 315
lengthening the back top to bottom, 151f–152
levator scapulae, 249, 278
Levin, Stephen, 53
Libet, Benjamin, 74
"lifter muscles", 180
lifting a heavy object, 314–315
limbic brain/system, 83f, 96, 98, 335
Linden, David, 84
Lindstedt, S.L. et al., 120, 155
"liquid light", 78–79, 81, 88, 114, 286
Llinas, R., 306–307
load, 38, 41, 51–54, 60, 63, 135, 154, 179, 203, 205, 270
locomotion, 5, 62, 63, 103–104, 122, 225–226, 305–308, 318
Longo, U.G. et al., 162
longus colli and capitis, 207f, 208, 280, and see deep cervical flexors
Loram, I. et al., 277, 278, 308, 319
Lou, Deborah, 12
lower body, balancing, 146–151, 148f
lumbar arch, 12, 38, 134–135, 210, 239, 263, 274
lumbar curve, 111–112, 135, 136, 140, 150f, 151–152, 218, 239f, 281
lumbar spine, 133f, 153, 225
    compromised, 35, 135, 147f, 175, 203, 213, 261, 274
    support for, 115, 152, 203–204f, 209f, 213, 222, 240, 262f–264f, 267f, 269, 273f, 287

## M

MacDonald, Patrick, 9, 153
machine (analogies), 13–14, 16, 20, 30, 237, 315, 333–334
MacKaye, Steele, 125–126
Magnus, 129
*Man's Supreme Inheritance* (MSI), 128–129
maps, see brain maps/body maps; brainstem body-maps
Masoero, Jeando, 9, 93, 125–126, 130–131, 136, 141, 150, 156, 170, 198, 237, 238, 255, 257, 261, 265, 267, 270, 280
    *The Master and his Emissary* (McGilchrist), 16
McAndrew, D. et al., 214
McDougall, C., 156, 217
McLeod, R., 127
McNeill, David, 20
"means whereby", 25, 92, 128, 212, 238, 308
mechanical advantage, 128, and see position of mechanical advantage
mechanotransduction, 54, 58, 80, 117, 136, 334, 343
Medline Plus, 130
mental illness, 100
Merrick, Kitty, 9
Messi, Lionel, 145
Mian, O.S. et al., 122
Miller, M. and Clark, A., 20, 84, 315

Milner, A.D. and Goodale, M.A., 297
mind, definition, 27, 75
mind in the brain, 23f, 24, 26–27, 75–79, 85–87, 90–92, 286, 291–292, 319
    vs mind in the body, 76–79
mirror neurons, 20, 334–335
mirrors, use of, 125, 126, 133, 141, 164, 165, 319
mobility (of joints), 41, 198, 218, 271–272, 275, 341
modern/mainstream AT, see Alexander technique, modern
modulating an action, 71, 322
molecules of emotion, 81, 101
"monkey", 60, 126, 257, 262–268, 267f, 272–273f, 275, 312, 337, 341, 344
morphing (into movement), 23f, 28, 30, 58, 88, 233, 322, 341, 343–344
Moser, M.-B. and Moser E.I., 307
movement, and see responsive movement, adaptive movement, integrated movement, solving the movement problem
    animal (various), 21–22, 103–104, 225, 305
    control/organization of, 61–62, 103–104, 110, 285, 298, 305–310, 316, and see brain/cortex, control of movement, and brainstem/spinal cord, movement control
movement patterns, 6, 11, 15, 19, 22, 34, 56, 60, 61, 69, 73, 86, 121, 238, 308–309, 312, 315–318, 320, also see compensatory movement patterns
    breathing, 108, 111
    innate, 8, 28, 103, 122, 306, 315
moving into the unknown, see unknown
multi-joint muscles, 50–51
Murray, A.D., 127–128, 153, 240, 255
muscle, see concentric, eccentric, isometric contractions; action, phasic, postural muscle
    as shock absorbers, 156
    health and physiology, 12, 136
    spirals, 50, 52, 168, 342
    tone, 29, 38, 41, 61, 89, 100, 159, 180–181, and see tone; releasing (muscle tension)
muscle/myofascial trains, 50–51, 60, 80, 238
Myers, Thomas, 49–51, 54, 66, 80, 132, 163, 166, 181, 193, 204, 205, 238

## N

natural breathing, see breathing, natural
natural running, 233–234, and see running
neck, and see forward neck and head
    neck extensors, 281
    freeing the, 153, 246, 249, 271, 277–278, 280, 285–286, 292
    muscles, 38, 208, 246f, 278–281
Nettl-Fiol, R. and Vanier, L., 57, 101
networks, brain/nervous system, 18, 20–21, 82, 83f, 84, 99, 285, 315, 334
neuroception, 96, 100
neuroscience, 19–21, 28, 61–62, 76, 79, 285, 321–322
neutral balance, 137, 140
NICE guidelines, 11
Nicholls, Carolyn, 46
noble posture, 130, 138f, 154, 170, 176, and see posture, "correct"; plumbline posture
"no" games, 311–313
non-doing vs doing/not-doing, 25, 197, 198, 237, 341
nose feather, 69–70, 85, 88, 91
no switching off, 49, 268, 301, and see switching off

## O

obdurator externus/internus, 171
oblique muscles, external and internal, 56f, 116f, 119f, 166f, 168, 205, 206f, 227, 287
obliques, external, 240, 254
Ong, C.P., 226, 274
opening the palm of the hand, see palm
optimal alignment, 131–132
optimal coordination of movements, 55, 297, 305
organ health, 128, 129, 175, 205
organ massage, 106, 108, 128, 205
orientation, 21, 71, 161–162, 297, 306–307
*Original Wisdom* (Wolff), 322
Orlovsky, G.N. et al., 103
Oschman, J., 80, 334
Ottiwell, F., 285
over-straightened spine, 150, 152
Owen, Edward, 129

## P

pain, 11, 15, 34–35, 40, 74, 80, 91, 154, 177, 205, 218, 334–336, 339, 341
pain control, 87, 91
pain receptors, 80
palms facing backward, 131, 134, 139f, 144, 145, 230–231f, 293
palms, opening, 142f–143
parasympathetic nervous system (PNS), 8, 26, 82, 95t, 179, 295, 302
    and breath, 105, 107, 159
    dorsal (primitive) branch (dPNS), 95t, 97f, 96–101
    ventral (modern) branch (vPNS), 95t, 97f, 96–101, 283–284, 335
Parkinson's disease, 306
Parmenides, 13, 15
patterns of contraction, 35, 36f, 37f
pectoralis major, 57, 58, 182f, 184, 186, 193
pectoralis minor, 182f, 184–186, 251
pelvic arch and femoral triangle, 164, 174f, 175, 223
pelvic floor, 12, 14f, 114–116f, 119, 149, 207f, 287
    and breath, 106, 108, 111–112, 175
    in core musculature, 63, 104, 164, 171, 205
pelvic girdle, 51, 111–112, 114, 146–147, 166, 180
pelvic lifts, 167–170, 169f, 214, 229
pelvic rotation (lateral), 225–226, 229–230f
pelvic tilt or rotation (anterior/posterior), 12–14, 13f, 135, 136, 146–152, 147f, 150f, 171, 199, 204, 211, 262, 274
Penfield's homunculi, 86, 224
perception, 21, 24, 26, 29, 69, 84, 86, 88, 89, 160, 161, 297–299, 306–307, 309, 314, 321–322, and see depth perception, faulty sensory perception, spatial perception
personal space, 87, 315, 334, 336–340, 344
peripheral awareness, 77, 79, 86, 115
peripheral vision, 45, 85–86, 338
Pert, Candace, 66, 81–82, 101
Peters, Everard, 166–167
phasic muscles, 30, 37, 110, 112, 113–114
"photoshoot" procedure, 257, 257f, 258f
physical fundamentals, 23f, 26
physical problems, 11, 35
Pilates, 79, 93, 117
Pineau, Julien, 57–58, 59f, 96, 100

# Index

plank position, 283, 284f
plumb line posture, 130, 154, 239f, and see posture, "correct"; noble posture
polyvagal theory, 20, 95
Porges, Stephen, 20, 66, 95, 96, 98
Porte, A., 141
position of mechanical advantage, 60, 154, 212, 264, 341, 344, and see "monkey"
postural alignment model, new, 5, 29, 125–157
postural muscles, 37–38, 130, 274
posture, 20
    control mechanisms, 21, 61–62, 161, 277, 309, 316, and see control
    "correct"/ideal Western, 130, 131f, 239f, and see noble posture; plumb line posture
    feelings and, 81
    "good" posture vs slump, 130, 131f, 138t
    impacts of poor, 40, 53
    secondary curves and external torque patterns, 58, 130
preconceived ideas, 72, 92, 128, 319, 333, 343
predictive (mechanisms), 21, 188, 297, 305–310, 313–315, 322
predictive vs responsive, 20, 28–29, 309–310, 312–315, 322
Preece, S.J. et al., 218
present (coming/being), 6, 16–18, 22, 26–29, 34, 73, 79, 84, 100, 101, 106, 160, 197, 296, 298–300, 302, 309, 312–314, 316–317, 326, 335–341, 343–344
primary control, 8, 21, 103, 129, 225, 277, 284–285, 292, 337
primary curve, 56–58, 101, 131f, 136–137, 138t, 140, 278, and see curve patterns
    undoing, 137, 214
Prochazka, A. et al., 61, 104, 305
programming the brain, 93, 126, 127, 141–145, 266, 274, 291
proprioception, 15, 21, 23f, 24–26, 33–34, 79–80, 87, 103, 160–161, 179, 315
    and faulty sensory perception, 33
proprioceptive sensors, 34, 80
proprioceptive information, 110, 280, 305, 309
psoas, 116f, 119f, 171, 204f, 275, 287
    and leg spirals, 214
    imbalance from sitting, 12, 13f, 14f, 204, 217
    in core/deep front line, 63, 104, 115–117f, 203–204f, 207f, 206–209f, 213f, 219, 221f, 222f, 230, 241f, 267f–269
psychophysical unity, 76
pubococcygeal muscle, 116f, 117, 149, 151, 168, 201f, 209f, 222f, 253f
pull to the elbow, see elbow, pull to the
pulls, why we apply precise, 126–127, 135–136, 140–141, 154

## Q

quadratus lumborum muscles, 116f, 115–117, 119f, 203–204, 207f, 261, 266, 269, 287
quadriceps (quads), 13f, 14f, 52f, 116, 117f, 148, 150, 193f, 204, 209f, 210–212, 217, 219, 221, 229, 268, 287
quantum physics, 21, 30t, 330, 335, 339

## R

Radical Wholeness, 8, 19, 115, 198, 328, 329
"raindrop", 43–47, 44f, 46f, 65, 70–71, 119–120, 267f, 286
"ramping the head", 153, 238, 239f, 248f, 280
reasoning, 14, 20, 74, 141–142, 272–274
receptivity/receptive, 26, 64, 80, 87, 335
rectangle of the torso/back, 165f, 180, 218
rectus abdominis (abdominals), 52f, 116f, 119f, 148f, 169, 175, 204–207, 205f, 206f, 209, 211, 254, 268, 279
Reed, E.S. and Brill, B., 55
reflexes, 5, 13, 61, 103, 110, 161, 285, 297, 305–306, 313
reflex model (Sherrington) vs CPGs, 110, 305–306, 313
reflex, knee jerk/startle, 61, 278
Reiki, 335
relationship (between body parts), 26, 30t, 38, 50–51, 53, 55, 60, 72, 76, 112, 205, 208, 212, 243, 268, 293, and see lengthening antagonistic relationships; head-neck-back relationship
relationship (self to pupil/objects/environment), 11, 17, 20, 22, 25, 28–30t, 76, 78–79, 155, 179, 188–190, 297–298, 306, 312, 319–320, 330, 334–335, 338–339
relaxation, 60–61, 72, 101, 112
releasing (muscle tension), 72, 90, 149, 150f, 152, 344
repetitive movements, 11, 15, 187
resilience, 96, 98, 99, 112, 153, 264, 313
resonance, 322, 334–336, 338, 341
responsive movements/action/process, 5, 22, 114, 249, 309–310, 312, 314–315, 318, 322
responsive (muscle) tone, 41, 61, 100, 198, 302, 336, 343, and see adaptive tone
reverse curve, 12, 130, 238, 242
rhomboids, 38, 40f, 57f, 118, 181, 182f, 244, 287
ribcage, tilting the, 152, 264, 248f
ribs, and see costal arch
    anatomy, 62–63, 109f, 132–133f, 134f, 140f, 180, 238–239f, 242f–243f, 247f–248f, 251f, 287
    free breathing, 108–109f, 184, 185f, 186, 248–249
    support from, 240–241f, 262f–264, 266–267f, 269–272f, 273f, 284f,
    at the back of the armpit (RBAP), 132–133f, 250–254, 251f, 253f, 272f, 287
    untangling first rib and clavicles, 247f, 254
Rizzolatti, Giacomo, 20
Robb, Fiona, 286, 292, 302
Robinson, Byron, 82
Rosenbaum, D. et al., 110, 306, 309
rotation of the lower arm and hand, 189–190, 194
rotator cuff muscles, 181, 182f, 183, 185
running, 156, 217, 217f, 225–227, 233–234

## S

sacral plexus, 83f, 225–226
sacrum, 133f, 132–134, 146, 250, 253f, 254f, 256f, 272f
sacrum line, 134f, 146–147
sacrum to T8 line, 150, 210, 211f, 238–239, 242, 281, 286–287
safety state/feeling safe, 97f, 99, 183, 335–336
sartorius, 174
satisficing, 29, 308–309, 312, 322
scalenes, 63, 108, 207f, 249, 278, 280
scapula, see shoulder blades
Scarr, Graham, 53–55
Scheirling, R., 34
Schleip, Robert, 34, 80, 341
school, 11–13
Schore, Alan, 19, 20, 98–99
Schultz, L. and Feitis, R., 111
science model, old vs new, 30
screwing the ankle, 172, 173f, 177, 200f, 201f, 229, 273f
secondary curves, 56–58, 101, 130, 131f, 134, 136–138t, 140, 170, 179, 214, 226, 230f, 247
*The Second Brain* (Gershon), 82
self-awareness, 25, 95–96, 97f, 161, 320
self-engagement system, 96, 302, 336
self-organization of body, 28, 30, 61–62, 179, 233, 343
self-organizing structure, 24, 26, 111
self-organizing/integrating systems, 30, 285, 291–292, 299, 310, 333–334
self-regulation, 98–99
semi-supine, 89–93, 90f, 109, 115, 153, 209, 341
    rolling out of, 91f, 92f, 93f
senses, five, 15
sensorimotor information/maps/learning, 29, 161, 307, 309, 320, 334
sensory feedback, 60, 309, 316
sensory fundamentals, 23f, 24, 26, 336
serratus anterior muscle, 40f, 56f, 57f, 140f, 181, 250f, 287
serratus posterior muscles, 39f, 63, 208, 249, 287
sesamoid bones, 159, 162–164, 163f
Sharkey, John, 54
Shepherd, Philip, 8, 14, 15, 19, 66, 69, 74, 115, 157, 198, 310, 315–316, 325, 328–329, 338
Sherrington, Sir Charles, 103, 110, 129
shoes, five essential criteria, 224
shoulder, 36f–37f, 91, 112, 130–140, 145, 151, 169f, 181–186f, 184f, 190, 194f, 232, 234, 239f, 244–248, 246f, 253, 258, 269, 275, 278, 281, 286
    blades (scapula), 130–131, 134, 139f–140f, 153, 185–186, 239, 244–245f, 275, 281, 286–287
    front of (FoS), 132–135f, 133f, 183, 249–253, 250f, 251f
    girdle and arms, 54, 63, 179–180, 181–183, 238, 247, 278, 281
    joint, see rotator cuff muscles
    shrug, 244–246, 245f
Siegel, Daniel, 18, 20, 66, 77, 96, 309, 335
sitting,
    active/balanced, 14f, 199–201, 210f–212, 268–269
    harmful effects of, 11–14, 36–37
    inequality of muscle use, 12–14, 13f, 14f, 148, 166, 198, 204, 217
    with legs crossed, 41f
sitting bones, 115, 132, 133f, 149, 175, 199, 208, 210, 261f–262f, 264, 274–275
sit-to-stand (STS), 11, 35, 71, 88, 197, 201–203, 213, 269–271
skeleton, human, 35
Skinner, John, 129
slump/slumping, 12–14f, 47, 53, 58, 69, 114, 120, 130, 136–138, 140, 160, 180, 198, 204, 269, 278, 281
smiling, 326–327
social engagement (system), 96, 97f, 99, 100, 336
Solomon, Sara, 197–198
solving (a movement problem), 30, 41, 55, 305, 310, 314, 321
spatial attention and right hemisphere, 18
spatial awareness, 23f, 24, 27, 79, 83f, 84–91, 104, 161, 319
    for coordinated action, 119, 291–293, 296–297, 300, 310–315, 319, 322,
    for sounds and smells/pain control, 87
    in integrating directions, 141–144, 149, 152, 187, 233, 240
    of body/waking up brain maps, 85–86, 90–91
spatial multisensory processing, 315

# Index

spatial perception, 22, 25, 29, 100, 127, 141
spatial relationship, see relationship (self to pupil/objects/environment)
Spawforth, Penny, 325
spinal engine theory, 225–226
spinal microcircuits, 5, 61, 62, 103, 111, 305, 313
spiral arrangement of muscle, 23f, 24, 26, 55, 56f, 57f, 168, 170
spiral line (SpL), 56f, 57f, 63, 168, 170, 174, 181, 202–203, 190, 229f, 230f, 278
spiral patterns, 30t, 58, 140, 154, 161
spirals, 55, 226, 342, and see leg spirals
splenius capitis, 57f, 166f, 278–279
splenius cervicis, 57f, 278
Sporns, Olaf, 84
springiness, 11, 53, 60, 120–122, 125, 145, 154–156, 237, 265
squat, 3–4, 11, 126, 197–198, 263, 266, 271–273f, 312
stable/secure base, 41–42, 162–170
stability
 and co-contraction, 60, 122, 148
 and coordination, 30, 113, 223
 and hip laterals/lateral line, 166, 287
 and mobility, 29, 41, 50, 112, 198, 218, 225–226
 of head, feet, 226, 227,
 of self/being, 99–100, 159
 tone and control of tilt, 150, 262, 265
stance leg, 218, 219f, 220f, 228–229
standing, upright, 35
Staring, Jerome, 126–128, 333
startle reflex, 278–279f
sticks (assessing body geometry), 132f, 134f, 135f
Stebbins, Gertrude, 125, 141
*Stephen Fry's Victorian Secrets,* 129
Stern, J.T., 214
sternoclavicular joint, 132, 137, 183
sternocleidomastoids (SCMs), 40, 51, 52f, 63, 166f, 169, 278–279f
sternum, top of, 130, 132–136, 133f, 139f, 217, 234, 240, 242–249, 252–257, 262f–273f, 283, 286
sternum line, 242–245, 242f, 243f, 257
stiffness, 11, 40, 121–122, 140
stimulus-response chain, 292–293, 302, 310
stopping without stopping/losing tone, 120, 344
stimulus, not reacting to, 70, 292, 295, 302, 309
stretch receptors, 33–34, 42, 61–62, 80, 110, 277, 305
StrongFit system, 57, 59f, 100, 197
structural fundamentals, 23f, 24, 58
suboccipitals, 38f, 39f, 277, 278, 280
superficial and deep front arm lines, 181, 182f, 278, 283
superficial back line (SBL), 47f, 50f–51, 63, 88, 148, 203f, 230f, 278–280, 283f–284f, 286, 342
 lengthened or shortened, 47f, 48f
superficial front line (SFL), 51, 52f, 63, 203f, 204, 278, 279f, 280f, 283, 342
superior colliculus, 88, 285, 307–308
sustained attention, 17, 70, 73, 181, 310
swing leg, 217 –223, 219f, 220f, 228
switched on legs/feet, 198–200f, 233
switching off, 12, 14f, 49, 62, 73, 78, 89, 148, 155, 180–181, 223–224, 268, 301, 322, 341
sympathetic nervous system (SNS), 95t, 97f, 96–101, 283–284, 295
 and breath, 107

## T

T8 (8th thoracic vertebra), 121f, 130, 132–133f, 149–153, 210, 238–240, 242–245, 248–251f, 250f, 272f, 274–275, 280–281, 286–287
tablework, 90, 209
Tai Chi, 5, 8, 60, 79, 177, 226, 285, 342–343
Tasker, Irene, 25, 128, 331
Taylor, C. and Tarnowski, C., 340
tensegrity, 52–54, 53f, 65, and see biotensegrity
 problems with, 54
tension, releasing, see releasing (muscle tension); tone
tensor fasciae latae, 56f, 57f, 166, 166f, 171, 174, 263
*The Body in Motion* (Dimon), 180
*The Embodied Present Process* (Shepherd), 316
thinking, and see top-down processing/thinking
 changing our, 15, 18–19, 30, 49, 52, 70, 73, 84, 99
 conscious (embodied), 19, 27, 73, 93, 99, 101
 directions, 25, 46–47, 92–93, 141–144, 266
 evolution of, 22, 104
 from the body/visual cortex, 326, 329
 separating from doing, 141–142
 up heels to sacrum and T8, 51, 119, 146, 151, 156, 232
Thompson, Tommy, 341
thoracic spine, 133f, 153, 262, 281
thoracolumbar fascia, 117, 118f, 119f, 148f, 193f, 198, 261–262, 264
tibialis anterior, 52f, 56f, 57f, 168, 173f, 174, 193f, 200f, 229f, 330
tilting/inclining back on a chair, 90, 210–211f
tilting forward on a chair, 202f, 213f, 269–272f
tilting torso on hips/into monkey, 261, 262f, 263–267
toe push, 217, 221, 228
tone, and see adaptive tone, dynamic modulation of postural tone, muscle tone, responsive tone
 in core muscles, 203, 205, 207–209, 222
 increasing tone with precise pulls, 135, 140, 154–156
 in legs /hamstrings/pelvis, 119–120, 148–152, 175, 198, 261
 in natural breathing, 110–112, 114–115, 254
 in shoulders and arms/upper body/neck, 63, 180–181, 193, 237, 250, 253, 285
 in sitting / standing / "monkey", 197, 199, 264–265, 268–271
 maintaining, 29, 38, 60, 63, 72, 117, 159, 261–262
tonic inhibition/state, 30, 100, 105, 292, 297, 300–302, 311, 315, 343
top-down processing/thinking/learning, 5, 14–16, 18, 30, 33, 35, 111, 299 and see bottom-up processing
torques, 52, 57–58, 130, 132, 225, 243
 external and internal torque chains, 57–58, 59f, 61, 101, 132, 168,
 170, 172, 174, 229–230f, 232f, 272, 232, 283
torso,
 balanced, 210, 232, 239f, 342
 imbalance patterns, 13f, 35, 51, 136, 204, 212, 218, 239f, 277
 integrating with Initial AT, 126, 128–129, 261–275, 281
 support for, 42f, 168–170, 171, 180–181, 198–199, 253
 support from, 51, 179–180, 238, 244
touch, and see balancing with touch
 quality of, 29, 191, 237, 298, 312–313, 333–334, 336–338
 sense of, 26, 79–80, 87, 160, 299, 314, 341

tracking a visual line, 69–70, 120, 285, and see nose feather
transversus abdominis, 63, 116f, 119f, 146–148f, 175, 203–206f, 261, 287
transversus thoracis, 248f, 248–249
trapezius, 38, 40f, 63, 117, 118f, 180, 182f, 185–186, 190, 249, 278, 281, 287
trauma, 12, 20, 99, 101, 161, 336, 338
triceps, 40f, 118, 181, 182f, 238f
true stop, 291, 300
"tuck your bum under", 146
turning joint, 45–46
Turvey, Michael, 21, 54, 55, 305, 321
"Twister", 62, 285
twisting, 225, 226f, 227f

## U

ulnar deviation, 183, 187–189f, 252, 256, 258
unconscious/subconscious processes, 5, 18, 24, 27, 98, 100, 113, 274, 291, 298, 319, 340
unity line, 130–134f, 132f, 137, 144, 154, 257, 263, 266, 267f, 268f
unknown, (going into the/open to the), 6, 16, 18, 19, 28, 89, 291, 296, 302, 312, 318, 335, 344
upper body, balancing of, 136–141, 138f, 139f, 179, 237–258, 253f
 effect of primary and secondary curves on, 136–137, 138t
 programming integrated change, 144–145
 removal of unnecessary tension in, 140–141
*Use of the Self*, 129, 141, 277, 285

## V

vagal brake mechanism, 95, 98
vagal tone, 98, 100, 101, 283, 285
vagus nerve, 74, 82, 83f, 95, 98, 99
Vasavada, A.N. et al., 38
vertebral discs, compression of, 52, 154
vestibular directions, 161–162, 282, 285, 344
vestibular information, 161, 277, 307
vestibular organs (VSO)/system (VS), 15, 27, 159, 161–162, 285
Vineyard, Missy, 66, 72, 161, 320–321
visceral awareness, 20, see interoception
vision, 30, 69–70, 76–77, 79, 160, 280, 307
 and calm/presence, 99–100, 337, 339, 344
 peripheral/3D, 45, 84–86, 338
 purpose of, 5, 20, 280, 297–299
visual arc, 88, 89f, 90f, and see ladybird
visual cortex, 297–298f, 307
 seeing/envisaging from the, 19, 85, 326
visual streams, 18, 20, 27, 88, 297–299t, 298f, 310
voice, embodied, 100, 325, 337, 344, and see embodied speaking
voluntary action/processes, 28, 291–292

## W

Walker, M., 101, 317
walking, 110, 118–120, 155, 164f–167, 170, 193, 214, 217–234, 218f, 220f, 222f, 229f, 230f, 231f, 263, 307–308, 310–311
 sequence, 219, 220f

# Index

uphill/downhill, 170, 229, 232f, 233f
walking sticks, 8, 11, 159, 162, 201
wall game/work, 126, 153, 240–242, 241f, 263
Webb, Ethel, 128
weight distribution, 162–164f, 173f
weight transfer, 223f, 342, 344
Western culture/thinking, 52, 77, 82, 99, 101, 128, 156, 320
Westfeldt, Lulie, 9, 129
whispered Ah, 126, 129, 280–281, 286, 325, 327–328f, 330
whispered Ah, reverse, 254–256f, 275, 281
Whittaker, Erika, 9, 25, 129, 130, 310, 340

whole-body awareness, 78–79, 307
whole-body intelligence, 29, 79–80, 83f, 84, 87, 302, 305, 309–310, 314–315, 336 and see brain/body intelligence
whole-body movement, 3, 60, 285, 307, 312, 315
whole-body being/system/organization, 19, 28, 103, 148, 309, 315
Williams, C., 19
Williamson, Malcolm, 127
Wilson, Donald, 104
wobble boards, 160–161
Wolf, Jessica, 66, 105, 111
Wolff, Robert, 322

wrist, 132–133f, 138f–139f, 183, 194f, 341–344 and see ulnar deviation
Wulf, Gaby, 21, 307, 317–319

# Y

yoga, 8, 79, 93, 105, 131, 135, 177, 209, 342

# Z

zone, living in the, 4, 6, 320
Zügel, M. et al., 51